HUMAN FERTILITY CONTROL

Human Fertility Control

Theory and practice

D F HAWKINS DSc, PhD, MB, BS(Lond), MD(Mass), FRCOG, FACOG
*Reader in Obstetric Therapeutics, Institute of Obstetrics and Gynaecology,
University of London; Consultant Obstetrician and Gynaecologist,
Hammersmith Hospital, London*

M G ELDER MB, ChB, MD, FRCS, FRCOG
*Professor of Obstetrics and Gynaecology, Institute of Obstetrics
and Gynaecology and the Royal Postgraduate Medical School,
Hammersmith Hospital, London*

BUTTERWORTHS
LONDON – BOSTON
Sydney – Wellington – Durban – Toronto

United Kingdom	Butterworth & Co (Publishers) Ltd
London	88 Kingsway, WC2B 6AB
Australia	Butterworths Pty Ltd
Sydney	586 Pacific Highway, Chatswood, NSW 2067
	Also at Melbourne, Brisbane, Adelaide and Perth
Canada	Butterworth & Co (Canada) Ltd
Toronto	2265 Midland Avenue, Scarborough, Ontario, M1P 4S1
New Zealand	Butterworths of New Zealand Ltd
Wellington	T & W Young Building, 77–85 Customhouse Quay, 1, CPO Box 472
South Africa	Butterworth & Co (South Africa) (Pty) Ltd
Durban	152–154 Gale Street
USA	Butterworth (Publishers) Inc
Boston	10 Tower Office Park, Woburn, Massachusetts 01801

First published 1979

© Butterworth & Co (Publishers) Ltd, 1979

ISBN 0 407 00127 1

British Library Cataloguing in Publication Data

Hawkins, Denis Frank
   Human fertility control.
   1. Contraception
   I. Title II. Elder, M G
   613.9'4   RG136   79-40088

   ISBN 0-407-00127-1

Typeset by Scribe Design, Medway, Kent
Printed and bound by Camelot Press, Southampton, Hants.

Additional contributions by

Zara L Whitlock BTech, MPhil
Research Assistant, Institute of Obstetrics and Gynaecology, Hammersmith Hospital, London

Jack Parsons BA
Senior Lecturer in Population Studies, David Owen Centre for Population Growth Studies, University College, Cardiff

Preface

In the last decade, family practitioners have come to realise that their patients' family planning needs involve more than a prescription for 'the pill' or the occasional referral for consideration of a legal abortion. At the same time, specialist obstetricians and gynaecologists have taken an increasing interest in fertility control procedures and realised that family planning has come to be a major part of their practice. Once it is understood by these groups of practitioners that there is no 'best' contraceptive, only the most appropriate procedure for a given patient, much background knowledge is required to individualise effectively.

Most of the books on fertility control which have been published in recent years are either instruction manuals for the tyro or volumes dealing with either one or many specialised topics. We feel that the needs of the most potent groups currently involved in clinical fertility control practice, the family practitioners with a special interest and the obstetricians and gynaecologists, have been neglected. The present volume is intended as a textbook for both of these groups, which will enable them to tailor their counselling and practice to the needs of their patients as individuals. We have dealt with practical clinical procedures in some detail, and also discussed the basis of the methods at a depth which should be appropriate for the specialist. It is our intention to present both reasoned evaluations and firm opinions on controversial topics, so that these conclusions may assist medical and postgraduate students, and nurses and midwives concerned with family planning, as well as enable specialists in training to assess the evidence. This book is not a 'recent advances' volume, and we have tried to emphasize points of view which will survive in future years. One partial exception to this is that we have given a full account of the use of intra-amniotic hypertonic saline instillation for legal abortion, as it is still employed in some centres in the United States of America.

We have provided numerous references to the literature, both to deal with matters which need 'chapter and verse' for substantiation and to enable readers to pursue authoritative individual sources.

It was a pleasure to invite Mr Jack Parsons to write an epilogue for us. Doctors find it expedient to pay lip service to the sermons of population experts and economists, but they weary of being asked to implement programmes which have little respect for the intellectual ability of the doctor or the needs and rights of the individual patient. Clinical practice is based on a doctor's assessment of each situation as it presents and the welfare of the patient is paramount. Mr Parsons is one of the few in his field who have appreciated the need of those in the health professions to have some understanding of the demographic principles of fertility control at a level which is meaningful with respect to the individual. We are also grateful to one of his former pupils, Miss Zara Whitlock, for writing the chapter on motivation, which is based in part on the extensive behavioural studies she has conducted with the aid of patients at the Hammersmith Hospital family planning clinic.

We are greatly indebted to the late Professor J C McClure Browne for his encouragement both of our work in this field and of the production of this book. Mr J Duncan Murdoch had started the fitting of intra-uterine devices at Hammersmith Hospital in 1961 and in 1968 Professor Browne gave one of us the remit of developing this nucleus into a comprehensive clinic in which the training of doctors could take place and clinical trials could flourish in close relation to laboratory studies. Much of our knowledge of these aspects developed in relation to the Hammersmith Hospital clinic.

We are grateful to Miss Nancy Philcox for typing the manuscripts, the staff of the publishers, Butterworths, and, not least, to our wives for their tolerance over the last six years.

D F HAWKINS
M G ELDER

Contents

PART I HORMONAL CONTRACEPTION 1

1 Introduction 3
2 The clinical pharmacology of oestrogens and progestagens 7
3 Combined oral contraceptives 49
4 Other hormonal contraceptive procedures 91
5 The relative effectiveness and risks of hormonal contraception 127

PART II BARRIER METHODS 131

6 Condoms, diaphragms and caps 133
7 Spermicides 145
8 Coitus interruptus, periodic abstinence 151

PART III INTRA-UTERINE CONTRACEPTION 161

9 Intra-uterine devices 163
10 Procedures for intra-uterine contraception 201
11 Complications of intra-uterine contraception 213

PART IV LEGAL ABORTION 235

12 Abortion counselling 237
13 Techniques 263

PART V STERILISATION 317

14 Sterilisation counselling 319
15 Methods of operative sterilisation 343

PART VI FAMILY PLANNING COUNSELLING, CLINICAL TRIALS 371

16 Motivation and contraception 373
17 Special groups of patients 383
18 Contraception in patients with medical disorders 399
19 Clinical trials 409

x *Contents*

PART VII THE FUTURE   **427**

20   Developments in fertility control methods   429

EPILOGUE   **441**

21   Doctors and demography   443

       Index   471

Part I
Hormonal Contraception

1 Introduction

In 1937 Makepeace *et al.* discovered that progesterone inhibited ovulation in rabbits. Three years later Sturgis and Albright (1940) found that oestrogens used in the treatment of dysmenorrhoea also inhibited ovulation. In the early 1950s research was carried out to develop orally-active progestational steroids to be used to suppress ovulation. Norethynodrel was the first such compound to be synthesised in 1952, followed by norethisterone in 1954. Norethynodrel is the progestational component of the first oral contraceptive, Enavid (Enovid), which was shown to inhibit ovulation in the rabbit by Pincus *et al.* (1956) and in the human by Rock *et al.* (1958). The first clinical trials with Enavid were carried out on Puerto Rican women during 1956 and were followed by more extensive studies (Pincus *et al.*, 1958).

Enavid was marketed for the treatment of menstrual disorders in 1957 and as an oral contraceptive in 1960. The initial dose of norethynodrel was 10 mg, but with the introduction of more effective progestational agents and the realisation that an oestrogen component is the main factor in suppressing ovulation the hormone content of oral contraceptives has been considerably reduced. Most combined oral contraceptive pills now contain 0.5—2.0 mg of progestagen; some contain as little as 0.15 mg of norgestrel.

After Inman *et al.* (1970) suggested that the thrombo-embolic side-effects of the combined pill depended on the oestrogen dose, this was generally reduced from 200 to 100 to 50 µg of ethinyloestradiol or mestranol. Some oral contraceptives now contain as little as 20 µg of synthetic oestrogen.

The realisation that oestrogens were responsible for many of the major metabolic side-effects of the combined pill caused a return of interest in the study of products containing only progestational steroids. The first such preparation was chlormadinone acetate which became available during the mid 1960s. Tablets containing only norethisterone (norethindrone), ethynodiol diacetate, lynoestrenol, quingestanol acetate, norgestrel or clogestone have subsequently been tried or marketed with varying degrees of success. They are not widely prescribed but are useful for the woman who desires oral contraception and is advised against the use of the combined pill for medical reasons or is reluctant to accept any small risks that might be associated with synthetic oestrogens.

TYPES OF ORAL CONTRACEPTIVE

The Combined Pill

The combined pill contains an oestrogen and a progestagen. One tablet is taken daily for 21 days, though with a few preparations 20 or 22 days are advised. The tablets are stopped for seven days and consumption continued cyclically.

Oestrogens presently used in combined oral contraceptive tablets are ethinyl-oestradiol or its 3-methyl ether derivative, mestranol. The latter may be partly converted to ethinyloestradiol in the body. Most preparations now available contain 50 μg or 30 μg of one of these oestrogens.

The progestagens used belong to two groups, the 19-nortestosterone and the 17α-hydroxyprogesterone derivatives. The former group includes norethynodrel, norethisterone, lynoestrenol, ethynodiol diacetate and norgestrel. The latter group includes chlormadinone and megestrol. The doses of progestagens used vary from approximate equivalents of 0.5—4 mg of norethisterone. The absolute amount of each progestagen used is supposed to be related to its progestational potency.

A list of some of the combined pills available is given in *Table 3.1*, p. 50.

The Sequential Pill

Sequential pills were marketed for several years. All the 21 pills for a cycle contained an oestrogen, but usually only the last seven or eight contained progestagen. This sequence was an attempt to mimic the hormone pattern of the normal menstrual cycle. During the seven pill-free days some manufacturers included a placebo so that a pill was in fact taken every day. Poorly motivated patients found this confusing. A placebo tablet might be taken in error for an active pill at the mid cycle with the possibility of pregnancy resulting. The amounts of oestrogen and progestagen in the sequential preparations were similar to those in the combined pills. These preparations went out of favour despite the better menstrual cycle control provided. The failure rate was higher and it was also suggested that the sequential pills predisposed to the development of carcinoma of the endometrium.

Long-acting Oral Contraceptive Pills

These contain relatively large doses of a potent long-acting oestrogen and a progestagen. They were developed to provide a contraceptive which can be taken as a single oral dose once a month. This method best suits two classes of patients, highly motivated women with good memories who do not want the bother of taking a daily pill, and poorly motivated patients who can ingest the pill monthly supervised by a visiting nurse. The problems of the method are predictable — the metabolic and other side-effects of a high dose of oestrogen and the consequences on menstruation of initially high hormone levels falling throughout the month.

Low-dose Progestagen Pills

These preparations contain only a progestagen such as ethynodiol diacetate, 0.5 mg, norethisterone, 0.35 mg, or *dl*-norgestrel, 0.075 mg, and are taken daily with no break during menstruation. Their virtue lies in the very low dose of progestagen and the freedom from exogenous oestrogen therapy. The major problem they present — finding a drug whose dose is small enough not to cause menstrual irregularity and yet large enough to prevent pregnancy consistently — has not yet been entirely resolved.

The Postcoital Pill

The search for a pill which can be taken after intercourse and still prevent pregnancy has been pursued despite criticisms that such an agent essentially provides very early abortion on demand and contributes to promiscuity.

Effective regimens of oestrogen therapy have been developed to be initiated within 72 hours after a single episode of coitus. The object is to prevent pregnancy in rape victims and in women who subsequently regret their participation in unprotected intercourse.

Attempts have also been made to develop progestagen postcoital oral contraceptives for regular use — a pill to be taken after each episode of coitus. The concept is sound and involves using small doses of relatively harmless steroids at the most appropriate time. Some would also argue that motivation is strongest after intercourse. Unfortunately some of the early trials included women who undertook coitus several times a day. This resulted in an intake of progestagen sufficient to cause major disturbances of menstruation.

INJECTABLE HORMONES AND IMPLANTS

Depot steroid preparations have been developed to cater both for a small sophisticated group of women who do not wish to be bothered with personal involvement with contraceptive methods and for underdeveloped populations where it is necessary for professional personnel to participate actively in contraception programmes. These products contain relatively large doses of steroids and are injected or implanted at intervals of one, three or even six months.

Monthly injections of oestrogen—progesterone preparations have no advantage over monthly pills and carry the same risks. Injections of progestagens in doses which produce an effect lasting for several months have been used in selected groups of patients. Whether they carry any risk of an increased incidence of breast or other cancer has yet to be evaluated.

REFERENCES

INMAN, W.H.W., VESSEY, M.P., WESTERHOLM, B. and ENGELUND, A. (1970). Thrombo-embolic disease and the steroidal content of oral contraceptives, a report to the Committee on Safety of Medicines. *Br. med. J.*, **ii**, 203–209

MAKEPEACE, A.W., WEINSTEIN, G.L. and FRIEDMAN, M.H. (1937). The effect of progestin and progesterone on ovulation in the rabbit. *Am. J. Physiol.*, **119**, 512–516

PINCUS, G., CHANG, M.C., ZARROW, M.X., HAFEZ, E.S.E. and MERRILL, A. (1956). Studies of the biological activity of certain 19-norsteroids in female animals. *Endocrinology*, **59**, 695–707

PINCUS, G., ROCK, J. and GARCIA, C.R. (1958). Effects of certain 19-norsteroids upon reproductive processes. *Ann. N.Y. Acad. Sci.*, **71**, 677–690

ROCK, J., PINCUS, G. and GARCIA, C.R. (1956). Effects of certain 19-norsteroids on the normal human menstrual cycle. *Science, N.Y.*, **124**, 891–893

STURGIS, S.H. and ALBRIGHT, F. (1940). The mechanism of estrin therapy in the relief of dysmenorrhoea. *Endocrinology*, **26**, 68–72

2 The Clinical Pharmacology of Oestrogens and Progestagens

Oestrogens

Oestrogens are the principal functional hormones produced by the ovarian follicles. They are trophic hormones which play a part in growth and development of the non-pregnant woman, having a specific function in promoting the development of the female genitalia and secondary sexual characteristics. Cyclical increases in oestrogen production by the ovary are involved in the processes of ovulation and of the menstrual cycle. A massive addition to oestrogen production occurs in the feto-placental unit during pregnancy.

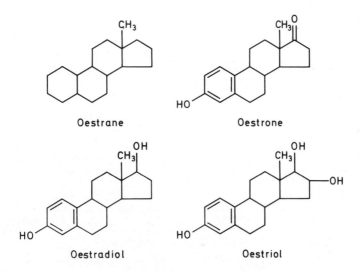

Figure 2.1 Formulae of the steroid nucleus, oestrane, and the three naturally occurring oestrogens

In the human female the three major oestrogens are oestrone, oestradiol and oestriol. Oestradiol is the most biologically active of the three, oestriol the least active. They are C-18 steroids, that is, derived from oestrane, which has 18 carbon atoms. The formulae of the steroid nucleus and the three naturally occurring oestrogens are shown in *Figure 2.1*.

7

8

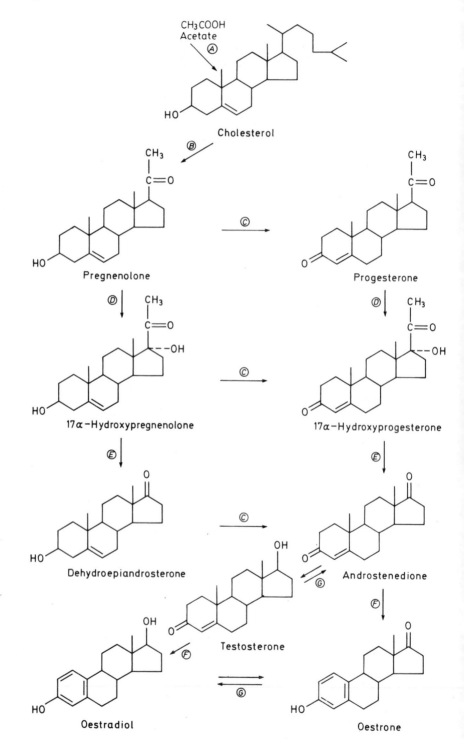

CH₃COOH
Acetate
(A)

Cholesterol

(B)

Pregnenolone

(C)

Progesterone

(D)

17α-Hydroxypregnenolone

(C)

17α-Hydroxyprogesterone

(D)

(E)

Dehydroepiandrosterone

(C)

Androstenedione

(E)

Testosterone

(G)

(F)

Oestradiol

(F)

Oestrone

(G)

Metabolism

Oestrogen is secreted by the theca interna cells of the Graafian follicle, and in addition it is synthesised in the adrenal cortex and produced peripherally. The principal metabolic pathways in the ovary are shown in *Figure 2.2.*

During pregnancy precursors produced by the placenta are sulphated in the fetus and then converted to oestrogens in the placenta. Large amounts of oestriol, oestrone and oestradiol then pass into the maternal circulation and are conjugated and excreted by the mother.

Physiological Role

Oestrogens have an anabolic action, favouring retention of nitrogen, calcium and phosphorus. They promote skeletal growth and epiphyseal closure. They act on the kidney to cause retention of water, sodium and chloride. In connective tissue, water content is increased and the mucopolysaccharides binding collagen are altered, rendering the tissue more supple. There is some evidence that oestrogens increase the blood volume and are involved in the consequent vasodilation by a direct action on the smooth muscle of vessel walls. Whether or not oestrogens have a generalised action on the process of ageing is not clear but they tend to prevent osteoporosis and, in the case of the natural oestrogens, atherosclerosis.

The tissues of the female reproductive tract have a much greater ability to incorporate and retain oestradiol than other tissues (Jensen and Jacobson, 1962) and this may account for its specific actions on the development of the genitalia. This binding capacity is due to a specific receptor protein for 17β-oestradiol within the genital tract epithelium. There are 4000–5000 such receptor molecules in each target cell. These receptors take up oestradiol from the blood as they have an affinity about 100 000 times greater than the binding carrier proteins in the blood. Oestradiol is then transferred from the cell cytoplasm to the nucleus where it is bound to a new receptor; progesterone may impair this transfer (Taylor, 1974).

Oestrone passing into the cell is rapidly converted to oestradiol before it can combine with the nuclear receptors and exert an influence. Oestriol probably competes for the oestradiol receptors but is less potent.

Under oestrogen influence the pelvic blood supply increases, the uterus grows and the vessels, glands and connective tissue of the endometrium proliferate. As the cervix grows its glands develop, secreting mucus. The development of ovarian primordial follicles is stimulated. Superficial vaginal squamous cells cornify under the influence of oestrogen. Oestrogen is also involved in the development of the breasts, controlling growth of the ducts, proliferation of lobules and development of the areolae.

Figure 2.2 Metabolic pathways for the ovarian biogenesis of oestrogens. A, formation of the sterol nucleus; B, cleavage of the cholesterol side chain with formation of C-21 steroid; C, isomerase reaction with changing of double bond from Δ^5 to Δ^4 position and dehydrogenation at the 3 position by 3β-ol-dehydrogenases; D, 17α-hydroxylation; E, cleavage of side chain, converting C-21 to C-19 steroids; F, aromatisation, introducing double bonds into ring A and converting C-19 to C-18 steroids; G, 17β-ol-dehydrogenase reactions, reversibly converting hydroxyl- to keto-radical (Smith and Ryan, 1962).

In response to follicle stimulating hormone (FSH) the thecal cells of the developing Graafian follicle secrete oestradiol, which produces a cyclical enhancement of the oestrogen effects on the reproductive organs, as well as regulating proliferation of the endometrium. Oestradiol also causes suppression of FSH production, a feedback mechanism which tends to give a self-regulating cycle, and at the mid cycle it stimulates a surge of production of luteinising hormone (LH) from the anterior pituitary gland with subsequent ovulation. The levels of prostaglandin $F_{2\alpha}$ in the follicular fluid rise during follicle development. Contraction of the smooth muscle fibres distributed through the ovary, in response to prostaglandin or catecholamines, may also be involved in rupture of the follicle. The regularity of the cycle is reinforced by ovulation and the production of progesterone from the corpus luteum.

The cyclical production of oestrogen under FSH influence affects the smooth muscle of the reproductive tract, tending to increase the conversion of myosin to actomyosin and also to increase high energy phosphate concentrations in parallel with an increase in the maximum working capacity of the myometrium. The intracellular water and sodium content of the muscle cells is increased disproportionately, raising the membrane potential. The muscle cells of the uterus and fallopian tubes then increase their tone and spontaneous electrical and mechanical activity and contract more readily in response to stimuli. Evidence is accumulating that myometrial prostaglandin metabolism is also facilitated. Under oestrogen influence the uterine sensitivity to stimulant drugs is increased, this response being accompanied by prostaglandin release and prevented by prostaglandin synthetase inhibitors.

The effects of oestrogen on the cervical mucus are to reduce its consistency and increase its volume. At mid cycle there is a copious flow of clear cervical mucus with a good spinnbarkeit, this being a measure of its elasticity. The reduced consistency of the mucus facilitates spermatozoal penetration by means of proteolytic enzymes in the spermatozoa heads. The spermatozoa are encouraged to move towards the uterus by the long, parallel, loosely bound glycoprotein molecules of the cervical mucus found at this time of the cycle.

In pregnancy the greatly increased production of oestrogen results in exaggeration of many oestrogen effects, though some are modified by the contemporaneous increase in progesterone influence. Oestrogen plays a part in the somatic, cardiovascular, fluid balance and metabolic changes of pregnancy. With progesterone it is involved in the suppression of ovulation and menstruation and in breast development. Increase in pelvic blood supply, softening of the pelvic connective tissue and uterine growth and increased functional capacity are oestrogen effects.

Synthetic Oestrogens

The synthetic oestrogens that have been used to any extent in clinical practice are stilboestrol, ethinyloestradiol and its 3-methyl ether, mestranol. These compounds are active when taken orally. Ethinyloestradiol is considerably more potent than stilboestrol, weight for weight, and probably a little more potent than mestranol. It is difficult to be dogmatic about the relative potency of ethinyloestradiol and mestranol, because the assessments have been carried out in terms of various animal functions, the relationship of which to the effects of the steroids in the human is uncertain. No completely relevant tests have been developed to assess properly the relative potency in humans of two similar synthetic oestrogens such as ethinyloestradiol and mestranol. The fact that similar amounts of these drugs are used in pharmaceutical preparations including the combined oral contraceptives suggests that their potency is similar. The relative effects of ethinyloestradiol and mestranol have been studied in the human endometrium (Delforge and Ferin, 1970), and based on this work Heinen (1971) has suggested that ethinyloestradiol is a little more active than mestranol.

A comprehensive review of the absorption, distribution and metabolism of mestranol and ethinyloestradiol has recently been presented by Helton and Goldzieher (1977).

Mestranol is mostly converted in the body to ethinyloestradiol (Warren and Fotherby, 1973; Bolt and Bolt, 1974), which probably passes into the target cells unchanged and acts on the oestradiol receptors at the cell nucleus.

Certain progestagens are said to have oestrogenic actions. It is often far from clear what this means. In addition, other steroids such as androgens, or gluco-corticoids in large doses, can be shown to have a weak effect on some pharma-cological tests generally believed to be characteristic of oestrogen activity. There are three possible explanations for this. Firstly, the substance may be relatively non-specific, its chemical structure being such that it can react to a limited degree with oestrogen receptors. Testosterone is an example. Secondly, the substance may be partially metabolised to a compound with oestrogen activity. For example, the 19-nortestosterone derivatives such as norethisterone may be metabolised to some extent to ethinyloestradiol (Brown and Blair, 1960). Thirdly, the pharmacological test in question may not be specific for oestrogen activity as usually defined. The mouse uterine weight test, for instance, is affected by many factors in addition to the anabolic effects of oestrogen.

PHARMACOLOGICAL ACTIONS OF OESTROGENS

Hypothalamus and Anterior Pituitary Gland

Ovulation can be inhibited by administration of synthetic oestrogens. Ethinyl-oestradiol and mestranol are more potent in this respect than other oestrogens such as stilboestrol (Goldzieher *et al.*, 1962).

Suppression of ovulation occurs because of reduced levels of gonadotrophin releasing factors produced in the hypothalamus. These factors are neurohumoral decapeptides which reach the pituitary gland through its portal blood supply. They are responsible for variations in the amount of gonadotrophins produced by the anterior pituitary, so regulating ovarian endogenous steroid production. In addition, there is some evidence (Gordon, H., personal communication, 1976) that exogenous oestrogen causes an elevation in plasma prolactin levels. Prolactin antagonises the effects of the releasing factors and could play a part in inhibiting gonadotrophin release.

Schally *et al.* (1968) demonstrated that whilst both oestrogens and progesta-gens depressed plasma LH levels in oophorectomised rats, simultaneous admini-stration of LH releasing factor and the two steroids elevated the depressed plasma LH to its original level. They concluded that the oral contraceptive steroids act mainly on the hypothalamus or on higher brain centres, rather than directly on the pituitary gland. Changes in FSH levels were found to be similar to the changes in LH values (McClintock and Schwartz, 1968). These authors and Guillemin (1972) suggested that FSH and LH may share a common releasing factor, but most workers attribute release of FSH and LH to separate factors.

The cyclical increase in plasma FSH is eliminated in women treated with mestranol in combination with a progestagen, and it is generally believed that the synthetic oestrogen component is responsible. Goldzieher *et al.* (1970) found that after seven years of such treatment basal FSH levels are reduced to 70% of control values, in addition to the abolition of the cyclical rise.

The reduction of levels of LH by oestrogens depends on the dose and on the oestrogen used. Jaffe and Midgley (1969) found that $20-50\,\mu g$ ethinyloestradiol produced elevations in LH levels; $100\,\mu g/day$ produced variable effects. Mestranol on the other hand produced marked suppression of LH levels. Several other authors have shown that the combined pill eliminates the mid cycle LH peak (Brown *et al.*, 1964; Thomas and Ferin, 1972). The actual reduction in gonadotrophin levels varies according to the amounts of oestrogen and progestagen in the mixture and to the duration of treatment. Goldzieher *et al.* (1970) found that after seven years' therapy with mestranol and norethynodrel the plasma LH levels were suppressed to 30% of control values with elimination of the mid cycle peak, but that the latter returned to normal within three months of stopping therapy. The maintenance of constant low levels of oestrogen with progesterone in the circulation alters the mechanism for controlling the gonadotrophin releasing factors (Briggs and Briggs, 1972) and hence the production of the appropriate gonadotrophins from the pituitary gland.

Increased levels of FSH releasing factor normally stimulate the anterior pituitary gland to produce FSH which in turn stimulates development of the Graafian follicle and the pre-ovulatory surge of 17β-oestradiol produced by its theca cells. Production of LH releasing factor, together with the rise in 17β-oestradiol, stimulates the anterior pituitary to produce the LH surge characteristically preceding ovulation. Synthetic oestrogens act primarily by suppressing the releasing factors thus inhibiting the rise in FSH and LH. Follicular development then does not occur and in consequence there is no rise in plasma oestradiol to stimulate further LH release. In the absence of a developed follicle and LH surge, ovulation does not occur.

Sequential oral contraceptive tablets contained only oestrogen in the first half of the cycle, and there was less reduction of the mid cycle LH peak. The oestrogen was usually adequate to reduce FSH production sufficiently for ovulation not to occur. Should the oestrogen dose, in the absence of exogenous progestagen, be insufficient to hold FSH secretion at a low level then a mature follicle may form and, in the presence of appropriate amounts of LH, ovulation may occur. This is one of the explanations of the slightly higher pregnancy rate that was found with sequential oral contraceptives.

Ovary

The abolition of FSH and LH peaks by oral contraceptives and the diminution in overall production of these gonadotrophins leads to reduced ovarian activity and failure of follicular maturation. Ovarian steroid production is diminished. The oestrogen and progestagen in the oral contraceptive serve to develop and maintain the uterus and other target organs, and withdrawal bleeding occurs at the end of the course of tablets. The oral contraceptive steroids inhibit ovarian follicle development and cause fibrosis of the stroma (Rock *et al.*, 1957; Zussman *et al.*, 1967; Ostergaard and Starup, 1968). Diminished FSH levels are responsible for the poor growth and absence of maturation of the follicle. The constant production of LH and FSH and the elimination of mid cycle peaks are primarily responsible for the failure to ovulate.

Endometrium

Oestrogen administration produces a proliferative endometrium. This means that the endometrium builds up from the basal cells remaining after menstruation by means of an increase in volume of both endometrial glands and stroma and by hypertrophy of the blood vessels, chiefly the branches of the spiral arterioles. The effect of individual oestrogens on the endometrium has not been studied extensively but ethinyloestradiol, 0.1 mg daily, gives glandular volume 100% larger and a stromal volume 50% larger than that in patients on the same dose of mestranol (Delforge and Ferin, 1970). Brosens and Pijnenborg (1976) did not confirm the difference in activities. They found that 0.05 or 0.1 mg daily of either compound would cause a reduction in the mitotic index in the endometrial glands, without affecting the height of the glandular epithelium. Prolonged cyclical administration of oestrogen in combination with a progestagen results in microtubular endometrial glands and a fibroblastic condensation of the stroma.

Cervical Mucus

The synthetic oestrogen used in sequential oral contraceptives, administered alone from Day 5 to 25 of the cycle, affects the mucus in such a way as to improve sperm penetration (Ansbacher and Campbell, 1971).

SYSTEMIC EFFECTS

Cardio-vascular System

Oestrogens have a significant effect both on the haemodynamics of the cardio-vascular system and on the constituents of blood itself. Increases in plasma volume, cardiac output and stroke volume have been found in women taking mestranol in doses of 75 and 100 μg (Walters and Lim, 1969, 1970; Lehtovirta, 1974a), the stroke volume change being due perhaps to a direct stimulant action on the myocardium. The consequent rise in blood pressure may be partly offset by an increase in venous distensibility which leads to a reduced peripheral venous flow (Goodrich and Wood, 1966), although a slight residual rise in mean and systolic blood pressure has been recorded with mestranol, 75 and 100 μg (Walters and Lim, 1969, 1970).

Increased oestrogen levels in pregnancy and in women on combined oral contraceptives are said to be responsible for a dilating effect on skin arterioles causing hyperaemia. Lim *et al.* (1970) infused oestrone (0.4 μg to 8 mg/min) or oestradiol (10 mg/min) intra-arterially for two minutes and found that this had no effect on peripheral blood flow. Lehtovirta (1974b) found that oestrogens cause an increase in peak blood flow and a diminished vascular resistance in the human forearm. The discrepancy between these two sets of results may be due to the fact that the intra-arterial infusion is an acute situation, while the action of oestrogens in pregnancy, in women on combined oral contraception and in the studies of Lehtovirta (1974b) are a response to chronic oestrogen influence.

Coagulation System

In the intact animal the coagulation system continuously causes a very slow intravascular formation of fibrin. Under physiological conditions this process is in equilibrium with the fibrinolytic system, which breaks down the small quantities of fibrin produced. The current concept of the coagulation mechanism, the cascade theory, is of a chain of processes involving all the coagulation factors in turn, culminating in the conversion of prothrombin to thrombin, which changes fibrinogen to fibrin. The process is shown in *Figure 2.3*. The system is essentially a biological amplifier and it is possible that stimulation at any one point in the chain can cause a cumulative acceleration of the processes with resultant clot formation. It is therefore possible that even small increases in the activity of

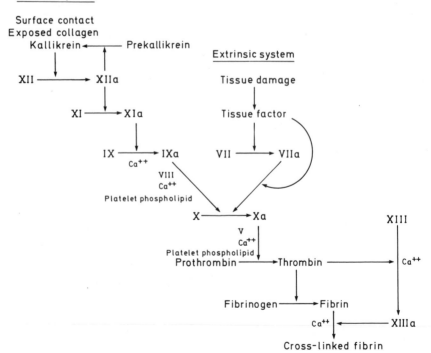

Figure 2.3 Cascade mechanism of blood coagulation (after Baugh and Hougie, 1977)

coagulation factors, supplemented by the exogenous and endogenous trauma of everyday life to the vascular tree and its contents, can lead to thrombosis. In addition oestrogens have been shown to diminish fibrinolytic activity.

Platelet Behaviour

Platelet aggregation precedes clot formation and oestrogens increase their tendency to aggregate, though not their adhesiveness. Oestrogen-containing oral contraceptives cause increased sensitivity of platelets to the aggregating effects of adenosine diphosphate (ADP) but not to those of nordrenaline. This is the same pattern as that observed in patients with atherosclerosis (Bolton *et al.,* 1968). Hampton (1970) reported that three patients taking the progestagen chlormadinone acetate, without any oestrogen had no abnormality in platelet behaviour, while the administration of oestrogens to men increased aggregation caused by ADP or noradrenaline. He also showed that the administration of oral contraceptives containing a synthetic oestrogen caused an increase in platelet mobility. Low density proteins appeared in the lecithin fraction of the plasma. These probably cause the abnormality in the electrophoretic behaviour of the platelets. Poller, Priest and Thomson (1969) found increased platelet aggregation in women on combined pills, but not in those taking chlormadinone acetate. These authors could find no increase in ADP induced aggregation.

Platelet adhesiveness is greatly increased following surgical trauma and in patients suffering from thrombosis, but there appears to be no unequivocal evidence of increased platelet adhesiveness in women taking oral contraceptives. Caspary and Peberdy (1965) suggested that adhesiveness was increased but other authors have been unable to detect any difference between female controls and those taking combined oral contraceptives (Hilden *et al.,* 1967). Hampton (1970) was unable to detect any effect on platelet adhesiveness in men treated with either synthetic or natural oestrogens. It is possible that changes in platelet adhesiveness are only seen in the few women who develop thrombosis whilst on oral contraceptives and as they form such a small proportion of the total number they would be difficult to detect. It seems doubtful if oestrogens are a significant factor in altering platelet behaviour and thus favouring the initiation of thrombosis.

Coagulation Factors

There are many reports suggesting that oral contraceptives, and particularly their oestrogen component, can cause increases in plasma coagulation factors. Poller and Thomson (1966) have shown that plasma factors VII and X are raised in pregnancy and they and Poller *et al.* (1968) reported raised plasma factors VII and X levels in women who had been taking oral contraceptives for more than three months. The length of time involved is important because Ygge *et al.* (1969) reported that there is no increase of these factors after one cycle, but only after two or three cycles. After two years of therapy factor VII levels are the same as those found in the third trimester of pregnancy. Daniel *et al.*

(1968) and Hakim *et al.* (1969) reported increased levels of factor IX in pregnancy, these becoming further elevated on the third day of the puerperium. The large doses of stilboestrol or hexoestrol used to suppress lactation caused marked increases in factor IX, but Elder *et al.* (1971) were unable to show any increase in factor IX levels in women on combined oral contraceptives for up to six months. Factor VIII levels showed no change after three months of oral contraceptive therapy, although they were significantly raised during the third trimester of pregnancy (Poller and Thomson, 1966). Sequential preparations produced the same changes in factor VII levels though factor X levels were not raised until after six months of treatment (Poller, 1970). It therefore seems clear that there are elevations of factors VII and X among patients on the oestrogen-containing oral contraceptives, but it is uncertain that these elevations are significant in causing thrombosis. Fibrinogen levels are slightly increased in subjects taking mestranol, $50-100\,\mu g$ daily (Hedlin, 1975). After the first cycle the values tend to return to normal. Fibrin degradation products are not increased.

Antithrombin III has been shown to be reduced by oral contraceptives containing ethinyloestradiol or mestranol, but not by conjugated equine oestrone (Greig and Notelowitz, 1975). Antithrombin III is believed to be the main antithrombin in plasma and serum and a reduction in this substance may be one of the precipitating factors in the development of thrombosis in pill takers. It may be that people with a tendency to have a low antithrombin III level before starting the pill are particularly at risk.

There is considerable disagreement in the literature as to the magnitude of the changes in the coagulation system and, in fact, as to whether or not any changes really occur. The reasons for the discrepancies are easy to see. The methods used to estimate the plasma activity of coagulation factors require much experience and are susceptible to imponderable variations in reliability, making it difficult to obtain consistent results from one laboratory to another. It is fairly easy to demonstrate changes produced by large doses of oestrogens, but alterations reputedly caused by the amounts of steroids in oral contraceptives are often so small that they correspond to differences of fractions of a second in coagulation times measured in the appropriate system. In our own work we found it easy to demonstrate that the large doses of stilboestrol or hexoestrol used to suppress lactation in postpartum women cause elevations in plasma factor IX (Hakim *et al.*, 1969), but like others, we were unable to detect any alterations in this factor with the small amounts of oestrogen in oral contraceptives (Elder *et al.*, 1971).

A major problem in work of this type arises from the need to store either the factor deficient plasma used in the estimations or the specimens of plasma from the patients. The small changes in activity sought occur over months, and if pre-treatment estimations are to be compared with tests undertaken three months later, either factor deficient plasma or patients' specimens must be stored for that time. Storage may be quite satisfactory when looking for the considerable abnormalities found in haemorrhagic diatheses, but deterioration may be sufficient to affect observations on the tiny changes found with oral contraceptives.

Experimental design can contribute something to the solution of these problems. A good example (*Figure 2.4*) is the work of Poller, Thomson *et al.* (1969). In serial studies on the same patients, these authors showed convincingly not only that factors VII and X levels were higher in patients on orthodox oral

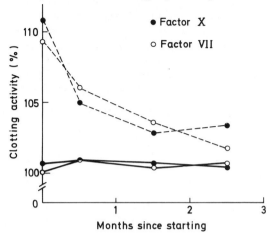

Figure 2.4 Factor VII and X assays during three months of chlormadinone administration. 'Pill' group expressed as percentage of mean control times. ———— Chlormadinone acetate group not having taken oral contraceptives previously. - - - - - - Group who had changed from 'combined pill' preparations to chlormadinone acetate (Poller, Thomson et al., 1969)

contraceptives, but also that the levels reverted to normal when the patients' therapy was changed to a low-dose continuous progesterone oral contraceptive.

Fibrinolytic State

Blood is constantly in a state of dynamic equilibrium between coagulation and fibrinolysis, and oestrogen-containing oral contraceptives may cause some fundamental changes in this equilibrium.

The overall tendency towards activation of the coagulation system is balanced by a tendency towards activation of the fibrinolytic system (Brehm, 1964). Increased levels of plasminogen have been found in patients on oestrogen-containing oral contraceptives (Brakman *et al.*, 1970; Peterson *et al.*, 1970; Hedlin, 1975). Increased fibrinolytic activity has been reported (Brakman *et al.*, 1970), measured by the euglobulin lysis time and by the spontaneous fibrinolytic activity and plasminogen levels (Hedlin, 1975). An intermediate product in the partial breakdown of fibrinogen and fibrin is a protein precipitated by cold, cryo-fibrinogen. Pindyck *et al.* (1970) found raised levels of this substance in the serum of women on oral contraceptives. Increased levels of α_2-macroglobulin (Horne *et al.*, 1970) and serum triglyceride (Barton *et al.*, 1970) have been reported among women on combined oral contraceptives. Both these factors tend to diminish fibrinolytic activity (Epstein *et al.*, 1970).

The significance of these facts becomes greater in the light of the findings of Åstedt *et al.* (1973). These authors studied coagulation factors and fibrinolytic activity in vein biopsies from women who had had a venous thrombosis whilst taking oral contraceptives six months previously. Although the coagulation factors were normal there was a reduction in fibrinolytic activity in the vein wall, an effect which could be attributed to ethinyloestradiol (Åstedt, 1971).

Thus in some already susceptible patients there may be a reduction in fibrinolysis which, together with raised clotting factors and altered platelet behaviour, may lead to an increase in coagulability. Daniel *et al.* (1967) and Jeffcoate *et al.* (1968) observed that oestrogen administration is associated with an increased incidence of venous thrombosis and embolism. This, taken in conjunction with the findings of Inman *et al.* (1970) that the incidence of thrombo-embolic phenomena in patients taking oral contraceptives is directly related to oestrogen dose, makes it clear that the marginal increases in coagulability are due to the oestrogen component.

Carbohydrate Metabolism

The effects of pregnancy on glucose tolerance and carbohydrate metabolism in general have been known for a long time, and it is not surprising that oral contraceptive steroids have a similar effect. This has been confirmed by many workers, but the extent and exact nature of these changes have not been precisely determined.

Methods of evaluation of carbohydrate metabolism vary from one study to another, and this makes comparison of results difficult. The oral glucose tolerance test is probably the best and certainly the most widely used index, despite the fact that variations due to absorption of glucose from the alimentary tract are difficult to control. Intravenous glucose tolerance tests have been used in an attempt to avoid this problem but these are also subject to quite marked day to day variation. A single postprandial blood sugar estimation is only about 70% accurate when used as a screening test for abnormal carbohydrate metabolism.

The other factor that makes it difficult to compare the results from different centres is the nature of the study. Some workers have studied the patients before, during and after oral contraceptive therapy while others have laid down arbitrary definitions of normality and then recorded the number of women on oral contraceptives who had normal carbohydrate metabolism. The former approach has clear advantages.

It is generally thought that the impairment of glucose tolerance brought about by oestrogen—progestagen preparations is primarily due to the oestrogen component (Goldman and Ovadia, 1969; Javier *et al.,* 1968; Pyörälä *et al.,* 1967). Spellacy *et al.* (1972) were unable to demonstrate significant changes in basal blood glucose or insulin levels in healthy women given doses of ethinyl-oestradiol or mestranol comparable to those in women on oral contraceptives. This does not exclude the possibility of changes in particularly susceptible women, but led Spellacy *et al.* (1970) to suggest that the changes in carbohydrate tolerance in women on a combined oral contraceptive are greater than those in women taking a sequential pill where most of the tablets contain oestrogen alone. The use of various sequential preparations has been studied in potential diabetics for up to two years (Goldzieher, 1970). At the beginning of pill use 27% of subjects had abnormal glucose tolerance tests, while after one year this had decreased to 6%, with 44% having 'borderline' abnormal tests. After two years there were no abnormal tests and 31% showed borderline abnormalities. There was thus an apparently beneficial effect of an oestrogen-containing oral contraceptive. These observations lead to the conclusion that the progestagen component of an oral contraceptive plays a distinct part in the changes in carbohydrate metabolism.

Oestrogen alone can cause resistance to insulin. Abnormalities of glucose tolerance are more common with mestranol than with ethinyloestradiol though variations in pancreatic islet cell reserve are of importance and have led to conflicting results.

Mean fasting plasma insulin levels vary during oral contraceptive therapy (Yen and Vela, 1968; Hazzard *et al.*, 1969). Spellacy *et al.* (1971) tested patients on a combined oral contraceptive pill before and after one year of therapy. During an oral glucose tolerance test there was significant elevation of plasma glucose and insulin levels in 41% of previously normal women. Three-quarters of these abnormal tests showed a borderline abnormality, and one-quarter were frankly abnormal. Serum growth hormone activity was also increased and it is thought that this might antagonise the activity of insulin in the tissues. Whether or not these changes are entirely due to oestrogen or whether the progestagens play small additional roles is still uncertain.

Wynn and Doar (1970) studied a group of 91 patients both before and during combined oral contraceptive therapy. They found that intravenous and oral glucose tolerance deteriorated in about one-quarter of patients during treatment, and that 13% of them developed chemical diabetes. Oral and intravenous glucose tolerance improved after stopping the contraceptive pill in 90% and 85% respectively of women tested both during and after therapy. The duration of pill consumption is important because, of 31 women on sequential pills for more than six years, 25% had abnormal oral glucose tolerance tests and of 31 women on combined pills for more than eight years, 77% had abnormal tests (Spellacy *et al.*, 1968).

The combined oral contraceptive pill increases the chance of abnormal carbohydrate metabolism developing, both in potential diabetics (Peterson *et al.*, 1966; Di Paola *et al.*, 1968) and in latent diabetics, such as women who have had abnormal carbohydrate metabolism during a pregnancy but who are currently normal (Javier *et al.*, 1968; Spellacy *et al.*, 1968). Despite a marked improvement in abnormal glucose tolerance on cessation of the pill there is evidence that 7% of women who have taken combined oral contraceptives for more than eight years develop permanently abnormal glucose tolerance (Spellacy *et al.*, 1970).

Lipid Metabolism

Free Fatty Acids

Plasma levels of free fatty acids are raised by the combined oral contraceptive pill, probably due to its oestrogen component (Wynn and Doar, 1969; Osman *et al.*, 1972). The elevation of free fatty acids may be partly responsible for hepatic formation and subsequent release of triglycerides into the bloodstream.

Triglycerides

There is considerable evidence to suggest that raised serum triglyceride levels can be caused by oestrogen-containing oral contraceptives (Barton *et al.*, 1970; Doar and Wynn, 1970; Goldzieher, 1970; Osman *et al.*, 1972), while after cessation of combined oral contraceptive therapy the mean fasting serum triglyceride levels fall significantly (Wynn and Doar, 1969). The elevation in levels appears to depend on the dose of oestrogen, and no rise is seen with 'progestagen only' preparations (Barton *et al.*, 1970; Spellacy *et al.*, 1975). No relationship has been found between the increases in plasma triglycerides, and age, parity, degree of obesity or a family history of diabetes.

Hazzard *et al.* (1969) thought that increased plasma insulin levels may stimulate endogenous hepatic triglyceride synthesis, and it has also been suggested that the altered carbohydrate metabolism due to the oral contraceptives causes raised fasting plasma-free fatty acid levels. These may increase hepatic formation and release of triglycerides into the bloodstream.

Ham and Rose (1969) suggest that diminished lipoprotein lipase activity may cause increased plasma levels of lipoprotein. The enzyme has an important role in the transport of lipids from the bloodstream across the vascular endothelium. Triglyceride uptake in adipose tissue is directly proportional to its lipoprotein lipase content (Garfinkel *et al.*, 1967), therefore subjects on oral contraceptive agents with diminished lipoprotein lipase activity may have a diminished capacity to clear circulating triglycerides from the plasma.

Low-dose progestagen administration does not have significant effects on plasma triglycerides in man but there seems no doubt that oestrogen affects triglyceride levels. Androgens appear to exert the opposite effect to that of oestrogens on lipoproteins (Furman *et al.*, 1958). Oral contraceptives suppress the hypophyseal gonadotrophic functions with a secondary decrease in the endogenous secretion of oestrogens from the ovaries, and this may produce changes in the lipid pattern similar to those found after the menopause. The progestagen used is important in that substances such as norethisterone acetate may oppose the action of the oestrogen administered. The 19-nortestosterone group of progestagens have varying degrees of androgenicity and oestrogenicity, and the interaction of these two factors is difficult to analyse.

Phospholipids; Lipoproteins; Cholesterol

Osman *et al.* (1972) have found that patients on a combined oral contraceptive show an increase in plasma total phospholipids, β-lipoproteins and in the β:α lipoprotein ratio. In contrast to the results of some earlier workers, Barton *et al.* (1970) found that plasma cholesterol levels were raised. Osman *et al.* (1972) found decreased cholesterol esterification. Barton *et al.* (1970) observed that there was an earlier and higher rise in cholesterol with 100 µg than with 50 µg of mestranol daily, suggesting that this change is oestrogen induced and dose dependent. The findings of Stokes and Wynn (1971) suggest that the response may also be affected by the amount of progestagen given in combination with the oestrogen.

Clinical Significance of the Lipid Changes

Raised serum triglyceride levels are associated with the development of clinical manifestations of atherosclerosis and may affect the fibrinolytic state (Epstein *et al.*, 1970). These facts, together with the alterations in platelet behaviour found by Bolton *et al.* (1968) to be associated with abnormal low density lipo-protein, suggest that the safety of long-term oral contraceptive therapy is still in doubt. There is considerable experimental and clinical evidence that athero-sclerosis in humans is associated with increased levels of plasma lipids and lipoproteins. The evidence depends largely on correlations of various strengths, and does not necessarily specify causal relationships. Thus, raised plasma lipids in the process of atherosclerosis may be coincidental rather than the specific cause of the condition. It is also unwise to assume that elevations of cholesterol or serum triglycerides from all causes are likely to have the same ultimate consequences in terms of production of atherosclerosis. The concept that use of oestrogen-containing oral contraceptives predispose to atherosclerosis may be unjustified.

Plasma Proteins

Oestrogens do not appear to have a significant effect on either free plasma or urinary amino acid levels (Zinneman *et al.*, 1965). A decrease in total serum protein and albumin has been reported by Doe *et al.* (1967) and an increase in α_2- and β-globulins by Settlage *et al.* (1970). The latter authors studied four groups of patients, one group taking a placebo, one taking a combined oral contraceptive (mestranol, $100\,\mu g$ and norethisterone, $2\,mg$), the third taking mestranol, $100\,\mu g$ alone, and the fourth taking $10\,mg$ of medroxyprogesterone actetate. The combined oral contraceptive caused a significant increase in β-globulin levels whilst the group on mestranol alone showed a significant decrease in albumin and increase in α_2- and β-globulins. Alterations in other serum proteins were not significant. These effects of oestrogens were confirmed by Briggs and Briggs (1971) who gave daily oral doses of 10, 20, 50 and $75\,\mu g$ of ethinyloestradiol. Concurrent administration of $1-3\,mg$ of norethisterone acetate with the $50\,\mu g$ daily dose of ethinyloestradiol had little extra effect on the serum proteins.

The lowered albumin concentration may be due to a decrease of total body albumin or it may represent an increase in total body water, perhaps associated with an increased binding of aldosterone.

Briggs (1974) administered ethinyloestradiol in daily doses of 30, 50 or $75\,\mu g$ from Day 5 to 28 of two cycles. He found that there were significant increases in plasma sex hormone binding globulin and ceruloplasmin, but signifi-cant decreases in plasma haptoglobulin, orosomucoid and albumin. These effects were thought to be due to direct changes induced in the liver cells by the oestro-gen. Addition of a progestagen made no difference except with norgestrel, when the protein levels tended to revert to the pre-treatment values.

Liver Function

There is no doubt that some women taking combined oral contraceptives have altered liver function (Ockner and Davidson, 1967), but in general these changes are slight and there is no reason to believe that they are of any consequence in a normal individual. They constitute a risk to patients with impaired liver function.

The liver function test most widely used to assess effects of oral contra-ceptives is bromsulphthalein retention and this has been found to be increased, albeit often transiently (Haller, 1970). The oestrogen component is thought to be responsible for these changes (Clinch and Tindall, 1969). The incidence of mild bromsulphthalein retention has been reported to vary between 10% and 50% in women taking oral contraceptives containing $100 \mu g$ of oestrogen (Tyler *et al.*, 1964; Larsson-Cohn and Stenram, 1965).

Plasma aminotransferase and alkaline phosphatase levels have been reported to be increased during administration of the combined pill. Alkaline phosphatase levels are raised in 12% of women. We found no changes in these enzymes in patients taking continuous progestagen oral contraceptives for up to nine months (Hawkins and Benster, 1977) and it is likely that the effect is due to oestrogen.

Oestrogen has been blamed for causing cholestatic jaundice, and a series of 40 such cases was described by Ockner and Davidson (1967). The conclusion that the oral contraceptive caused these cases of jaundice has been confirmed by the fact that the clinical features of the illness, as reported, have been constant: the jaundice occurs soon after starting therapy; recovery usually follows within a few weeks of stopping the drug; in those patients who have been restarted on similar therapy jaundice has usually recurred; and patients who have previously had idiopathic cholestatic jaundice in pregnancy are particularly susceptible.

The symptoms of this type of jaundice are anorexia, nausea, pruritis, pigmented urine and finally clinical jaundice. Plasma bilirubin is in the range of $3-10$ mg per 100 ml ($50-170 \mu mol/l$), and aspartate aminotransferase and alkaline phosphatase levels are raised. Electron microscopy findings are similar to those seen in other types of intrahepatic cholestasis, with dilatation of bile canaliculi, shortening and blunting of microvilli, bile stasis, and dilatation of the endoplasmic reticulum, which often lacks ribosomes (Larsson-Cohn and Stenram, 1965).

Water and Electrolytes

It is accepted that oestrogens cause a modest retention of salt and water. Although oestrogens have been reported to cause increases in circulating renin and plasma renin substrate, which might be expected to increase aldosterone secretion rate, it is by no means clear that this is the mechanism of salt retention. Good (1978) considers that the action of oestradiol in increasing peripheral venous distensibility leads to fluid retention, with an accompanying increase in intracellular hydration.

Ascorbic Acid

The administration of oestrogen to guinea-pigs results in a marked reduction of ascorbic acid in plasma and in the blood vessels (Saroja *et al.*, 1971). The dose of mestranol which was administered to the guinea-pigs was $50 \mu g$ and it must be stressed that this, in relation to the size of the animal, is an extremely large dose. These authors felt that, at least theoretically, these changes could lower the negative potential of the blood vessel walls and might therefore predispose to intravascular thrombosis. Oral contraceptives tend to reduce platelet ascorbic acid levels in women on low vitamin C diets. Again, in theory the reduction in ascorbic acid levels in the platelets may alter their negative electrical potential and this could contribute to an increased incidence of thrombo-embolic disease.

Urinary System

There is increased frequency of urinary tract infections among women on the combined pill. In a study of 107 non-pregnant women with asymptomatic bacteriuria, Asscher *et al.* (1969) found that the pill was used twice as often as in the control patients. The mechanism of this increase is uncertain. Silk and Perez-Varela (1970) have reported an increase in the bacterial growth rate in urine collected from ten oral contraceptive users compared with similar tests undertaken before the same women started the pill. This suggests that there may be some factor excreted in the urine enhancing bacterial growth.

Other workers have reported that the sex steroids induce dilatation of the ureters in non-pregnant women (Marshall *et al.*, 1966; Guyer and Delany, 1970). This suggestion has been refuted by Dure-Smith (1971) who pointed out that a history of previous urinary tract infections was a more likely cause. In large studies, Corriere *et al.* (1970) and Marchant (1972) were unable to demonstrate any anatomical changes due to oral contraceptives.

Whatever the mechanism there appears to be an increased incidence of urinary tract infections, and this is dependent on oestrogen dose (Royal College of General Practitioners' Oral Contraception Study, 1974).

Endocrine Effects

Cortisone Metabolism

Taliaferro *et al.* (1956) were the first to show that oestrogen administration causes a rise in total plasma cortisol. The main increase is in protein bound cortisol (Mills *et al.*, 1960) and is associated with an increase in corticosteroid binding globulin in the plasma (Musa *et al.*, 1967). Burke (1970) found that oral contraceptives containing 100 μg of mestranol increase plasma unbound and total cortisol. Total plasma cortisol is also increased with pills containing only 50 μg of mestranol or ethinyloestradiol but it is doubtful if the unbound cortisol level is then increased (Brien, 1975). The increased tissue exposure to unbound cortisone is at the most small and is only a minor factor in the metabolic changes produced by oral contraceptives.

In the absence of a capillary wall, cortisol bound to globulin may have access to hepatic cells in the liver sinusoids. An increase in the globulin-bound cortisol levels, reflecting the increased plasma total cortisone levels, could be responsible for causing increased protein synthesis.

Thyroid

Plasma protein bound iodine levels are raised in patients taking oestrogen-containing oral contraceptives (Alexander and Marmorston, 1961) and red cell triiodothyronine (T_3) uptake is decreased (Hollander *et al.*, 1963). These effects are probably due to changes in the binding proteins and do not imply altered thyroid function; ^{131}I uptake is unaffected. Similar changes in binding are seen in pregnancy, but they are then accompanied by an increased basal metabolic rate.

The alteration in protein bound iodine is reproduced by administration of ethinyloestradiol alone (Alexander and Marmorston, 1961). The reduction in red cell T_3 uptake is also probably due to oestrogen since it does not occur in response to medroxyprogesterone (Hollander *et al.*, 1963).

Pancreas

Two cases of acute pancreatitis, associated with gross hyperlipidaemia, have been reported as being due to combined oral contraception (Davidoff *et al.*, 1973). Both these women presented with abdominal pain and markedly raised serum amylase, triglyceride and cholesterol levels, perhaps due to oestrogen. The cause of pancreatitis in these cases is obscure; neither had gallstones. It has been suggested that in the presence of hyperlipidaemia, lipase in the blood vessels of the pancreas cause the triglyceride to break down within the chylomicrons, thus releasing fatty acids in excess. These might cause local capillary damage, leading to local release of enzymes, and hence pancreatitis.

Progesterone

Progesterone is a naturally occurring steroid hormone which is produced by the corpus luteum of the ovary, and the adrenal cortex, and during pregnancy by the placenta. Two of its main functions are the maintenance of a secretory endometrium during the post-ovulatory phase of the menstrual cycle and of a decidual reaction in the endometrium during pregnancy. During pregnancy it is also responsible for maintaining quiescence of the myometrium and is important in the development of the breasts.

Chemical Structure

Progesterone is a white crystalline solid which is freely soluble in lipids but only slightly soluble in water (12 μg/ml at 37.5 °C). It is a C-21 steroid, a derivative of

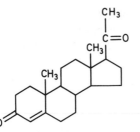

Figure 2.5 Structure of progesterone

pregnane, with a Δ^4-3-keto grouping in ring A, a 2 carbon atom side chain at position 17, and a ketone function at position 20 in the side chain. The ketone group in this side chain is present in both progesterone and the adrenal corticoids. In progesterone, in common with most other active natural steroids, positions 18 and 19 are methyl groups; progesterone also has a methyl group at position 21.

The structure of progesterone is shown in *Figure 2.5.*

Metabolism

Progesterone is synthesised from cholesterol in the corpus luteum, the adrenal cortex and the placenta. Two-thirds of the cholesterol is derived from the plasma and one-third is produced in the glands themselves (Davis and Plotz, 1956). In

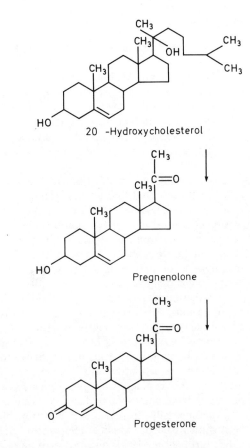

20 -Hydroxycholesterol

Pregnenolone

Progesterone

Figure 2.6 Synthesis of progesterone

all three tissues the position 17 side chain of cholesterol is oxidised to 20α-hydroxycholesterol and then to pregnenolone. Oxidation of the 3-hydroxy group of pregnenolone yields progesterone (*Figure 2.6*). In the ovary and placenta, progesterone is an end product, while in the adrenal cortex it is an intermediary in the production of corticoids, androgens and oestrogens.

Progesterone circulates in the plasma, 91% being bound to proteins such as albumin and orosomucoid. Disappearance of progesterone from the circulation is rapid, the routes of elimination being conjugation, metabolism and excretion, or deposition in fat. Conjugation is mainly to glucosiduronate and sulphate; this may be a transient intermediate step before deposition in fat or metabolism in the liver. Forty-seven to sixty-eight per cent of $4\text{-}^{14}C$ progesterone is excreted from the body within four days (Harkness and Fotherby, 1963). Some progesterone is metabolised to 20-dihydroprogesterone, or to pregnandione and pregnanolone, and then reduced at position 20 to form pregnanediol. More is hydroxylated to 17α-hydroxyprogesterone, a progesterone-like steroid with effects on the myometrium, endometrium and vaginal epithelium. It also provides a metabolic pathway for conversion to androstenedione, androgenic steroids and oestrogens. Finally, some progesterone is metabolised to corticosteroids.

Physiological Role of Progesterone

The systemic actions of progesterone include:

(1)   An overall catabolic effect;
(2)   Elevation of basal body temperature;
(3)   A hypnotic action;
(4)   Diminution of the secretion of pituitary gonadotrophins;
(5)   A decidual response of the endometrium;
(6)   A mild natriuretic and diuretic action.

The catabolic effect of progesterone was shown by Landau and Lugibihl (1967) who reported that administration of 50 mg progesterone per day to men resulted in an immediate increase in urinary nitrogen, together with a decrease in plasma concentrations of ten amino acids. These authors suggest that the effect occurs by enhancement of liver utilisation of both amino acids derived from exogenous protein and endogenous amino acids. Craft *et al.* (1970) suggested that there is an increase in amino acid utilisation during the luteal phase of the normal menstrual cycle.

The thermogenic action of progesterone is believed to be mediated by the hypothalamus. The rise in basal body temperature seen during the luteal phase of the menstrual cycle suggests ovulation. It is thought that progesterone from the corpus luteum formed in the ovary is responsible for this temperature rise. Follicular luteinisation begins in the theca interna cells during the stage of rapid growth before ovulation and this process is accelerated when the follicle ruptures. This explains why ovulation occurs very soon after the beginning of the rise in basal body temperature (Davis and Fugo, 1948; Doyle, 1951).

Experimentally, intramuscular injection of 5–10 mg progesterone daily has been shown to cause a rise in temperature of about 0.5 °C (Kappas and Palmer, 1963; Little *et al.*, 1974) and this may be due to a direct effect on the temperature regulating centre (Fischer, 1954).

Progesterone has a hypnotic action when given intravenously, and some of its metabolites have hypnotic effects greater than those of barbiturates. It has been suggested that as the rate of production of progesterone metabolites and secretion by the ovary can vary during the oestrous cycle they may be responsible, in part, for the mood and behavioural changes which occur during the menstrual cycle (Holzbauer, 1976).

Significant mood changes were not observed in men after the daily injection of 10 mg progesterone, but a decrease in autonomic activity as measured by more sluggish responses of skin conductance to sound stimuli, by a decreased variation in heart rate, and by an increased reaction time were found to occur. These findings are similar to those recorded in women immediately before menstruation. This supports the hypothesis that some features of 'pre-menstrual tension' are due to raised progesterone levels (Little *et al.*, 1974).

Progesterone has a direct inhibitory effect on the secretion of gonadotrophin releasing factors, and hence on release of LH, and to a lesser extent FSH. This prevents further follicular maturation and ovulation whilst the corpus luteum is active.

Progesterone induces a secretory response in oestrogen-primed endometrium. This response is characterised histologically by the occurrence of subnuclear vacuolation in the cells of the endometrial glands, by increasing tortuosity and lengthening of the glands and by the increased production of mucus. The stroma becomes oedematous and there is a differentiation of the stromal connective tissue cells into the typical large rounded decidual cells. These have large nuclei, prominent nucleoli and contain glycogen and lipid. This decidual response facilitates implantation.

The action of progesterone on cervical secretion is to alter it from the clear, copious mucus of oestrogen domination. The mucus becomes opaque, thick and sticky, with diminished elasticity as measured by its spinnbarkeit.

In the vaginal epithelium progesterone causes a decrease in cornification with lowering of the karyopyknotic index and increased folding and clumping of exfoliated cells.

Progesterone affects renal regulation of water and electrolyte balance by interfering with the action of aldosterone at the renal tubular level. Administration of progesterone thus facilitates excretion of sodium, and to a lesser degree that of chloride, and in consequence has a mild diuretic effect. The renin-angiotensin system is then activated and aldosterone secretion increases to restore homeostasis. The effect of progesterone on urinary excretion of potassium is inconstant, probably because the tendency to retain potassium, due to antagonism of aldosterone, is counterbalanced by some release of intracellular potassium which is then excreted (Landau, 1973). It seems likely that the mild diuretic effects are responsible for the relief of premenstrual pelvic congestion and oedema that some women obtain with progestagen supplements. Mineralocorticoid effects of progesterone on the kidney (sodium and water retention) are only demonstrable by the use of very large doses in adrenalectomised subjects.

Consistent changes in plasma sodium, chloride, potassium or copper during the menstrual cycle have not been demonstrated. It has been claimed that serum calcium rises at the time of ovulation, and that the levels of inorganic phosphorus and phosphate ions are higher during menstruation. Serum iron has been found to be highest during the early luteal phase of the cycle (Zilva and Patston, 1966). It seems unlikely that in the normal menstrual cycle progesterone has any direct effect on the levels of these constituents of blood.

Role in Pregnancy

The main site of progesterone synthesis during pregnancy is the corpus luteum during the first trimester and the placenta during the second and third trimesters.

Total maternal plasma progesterone concentration rises steadily during pregnancy, typical values being 10 ng/ml in the first trimester, 50 ng/ml in the second, and 100 ng/ml in the third trimester.

Progesterone is involved, with oestrogen, in the preparation of the endometrium for implantation, and then in the maintenance of the decidual reaction. During pregnancy progesterone reduces the excitability of the myometrial cell membrane, inducing a state of electrical and mechanical quiescence in the myometrial smooth muscle. The ability of bands of myometrial cells to conduct propagated electrical impulses accompanied by a wave of contraction is impaired. These electrophysiological effects are accompanied by changes in intracellular electrolytes. Progesterone reduces intracellular sodium in human myometrium (Hawkins and Nixon, 1961), while, under the influence of large amounts of progesterone such as are produced in pregnancy, intracellular potassium is increased (Kumar and Barnes, 1964). Progesterone decreases the potassium exchange across the cell membrane (Wagatsuma *et al.,* 1967) and this may be the mechanism by which hyperpolarisation of the membrane and subsequent quiescence of the myometrium is mediated. Reduction in tone of smooth muscle in other sites, such as the large bowel and the urinary tract is also due to progesterone. The effect is particularly evident in pregnancy when large amounts of the hormone are produced. In breast development, progesterone influences primarily alveolar growth.

SYNTHETIC PROGESTAGENS

Chemical Structure

Hydroxyprogesterone Derivatives

Esterification of the 17α-hydroxyl group of progesterone produces hydroxyprogesterone hexanoate, an active compound with progestational properties. Further modifications of this compound at position 6 enhance its activity. As one of the pathways of catabolism of hydroxyprogesterone involves hydroxylation at position 6, the addition of a methyl group or a chlorine radical at this position prolongs its action and enhances its progestational effect. The addition of an α-methyl group at position 6 gives medroxyprogesterone, which has increased progestational activity. Unsaturation between positions 6 and 7 gives megestrol. Substitution of a chlorine radical for the 6α-methyl group produces chlormadinone.

The chemical formulae of these compounds are shown in *Figure 2.7.*

19-Nortestosterone Derivatives

These steroids are used in many of the combined oral contraceptives. The removal of the methyl group from position 19 of testosterone results in the formation of 19-nortestosterone. This is much less androgenic than testosterone but possesses similar anabolic properties.

The first 19-nortestosterone derivative to be used as a progestagen in clinical trials was norethynodrel, which has a double bond between positions 5 and 10.

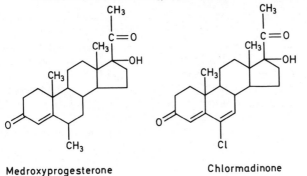

Medroxyprogesterone

Chlormadinone

Figure 2.7 Formulae of medroxyprogesterone and chlormadinone

The second was an isomer of norethynodrel, norethisterone (norethindrone) which has a double bond in the 4 to 5 position. Lynoestrenol (lynestrenol), in which there is no substitution at position 3, and ethynodiol diacetate, which has a hydroxy radical substituted for the ketone group at position 3 and is esterified with acetate groups at positions 3 and 17, are both highly effective progestational agents.

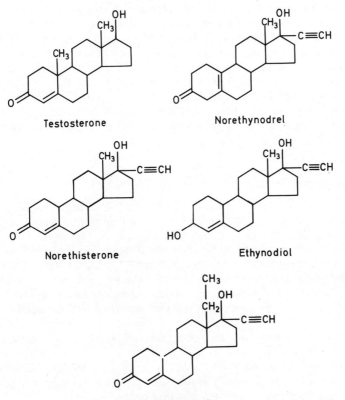

Testosterone

Norethynodrel

Norethisterone

Ethynodiol

Norgestrel

Figure 2.8 19-Nortestosterone derivatives with progestational activity

Norgestrel is a synthetic progestagen chemically related to the 19-nortesto-sterone derivatives. In bioassays in experimental animals for characteristic progestational effects such as pregnancy maintenance and delay of parturition in rats, norgestrel is qualitatively similar to, but much more potent than, progesterone. It is highly active when taken by mouth. This increased progestational activity may be because norgestrel is localised mainly in the target tissues, where it may block oestrogen receptor sites. There are *d* and *l* isomers of which only the *d*-isomer (levonorgestrel) is biologically active.

The chemical formulae of these 19-nortestosterone derivatives are shown in *Figure 2.8.*

Metabolism

The metabolism of synthetic progestagens varies considerably, not only between 17α-hydroxyprogesterone and 19-nortestosterone derivatives but also between individual compounds within the same group. The 19-nortestosterone deriva-tives are more slowly excreted than the 17α-hydroxyprogesterone derivatives (Fotherby *et al.,* 1968), although this does not appear to be due to delayed metabolism.

It has been considered that the 19-nortestosterone group of progestagens are converted to some extent into oestrogens. Norethynodrel, ethynodiol and lynoestrenol are converted to norethisterone, as the active metabolite (Fotherby, 1974a). Brown and Blair (1960) thought that the principle oestrogenic metabo-lite of norethisterone was ethinyloestradiol, a potent oestrogen. Fotherby *et al.* (1968) found that the proportions of norethisterone, lynoestrenol and norges-trel that were converted to phenolic compounds were 3.1%, 1.75% and 2% respectively. Recent work (Fotherby, 1974b) suggests that less than 1% and probably less than 0.1% of norgestrel is converted to oestrogens, and it is doubt-ful whether other 19-nortestosterone derivatives are converted to oestrogens to any extent.

Pharmacological Activity

Synthetic progestagens do not have all the effects of endogenous progesterone, and such properties as they do possess are present to varying degrees in different compounds. It is not easy to select suitable criteria for assessing the relative pharmacological potencies of the preparations used, and to depend on a single criterion is inadequate as this leads to confusing results. A potency ratio derived from one pharmacological test is not necessarily valid for another. Many of the criteria used in developing the synthetic progestagens have involved tests in animals, and it is generally accepted that these are not necessarily valid in humans.

Some of the indices of progestagen potency which may be used in humans are:

(1) Production of subnuclear vacuolation in the endometrium following a five day course of progestagen given to oestrogen-primed women with secondary amenorrhoea or amenorrhoea following oophorectomy.
(2) The production of a mid or late secretory endometrium in similar women following a ten day course of progestagen.

(3) Withdrawal bleeding following a five day course in women with secondary amenorrhoea.
(4) Inhibition of ovulation in normal women indicated by suppression of the luteal elevation of urinary pregnanediol excretion (Swyer *et al.,* 1960; Swyer and Little, 1962) or of plasma progesterone level, by absence of a luteal rise in basal body temperature and by endometrial biopsy.
(5) Postponement of menstruation in normal women given a 20 day course of progestagen starting from Day 20 of the cycle.
(6) Depression of the karyopyknotic index in the vaginal smear.
(7) An increase in viscosity and loss of spinnbarkeit of cervical mucus.

The most practical of these tests is (5) the postponement of menstruation test. The rationale for this test is that bleeding which normally follows withdrawal of progesterone can be prevented by an effective dose of a progestagen. The test, modified to produce valid dose-response relationships, is described by Swyer *et al.* (1960).

A standard dose of mestranol, 100 μg, is added to all the varying doses of progestagens. This is necessary to make the oestrogen environment constant and to prevent breakthrough bleeding.

The results of the relative potencies of various progestagens as assessed by postponement of menstruation are shown in *Table 2.1*. The ED50 dose is arrived at in the following manner: the progestagen is taken from Day 20 of the menstrual cycle for 20 days; if menstruation is postponed until after the end of the course the result is positive, and the dose of progestagen is halved for the next cycle; should bleeding occur during the 20 day course the result is negative,

Table 2.1 ACTIVITY OF ORAL PROGESTAGENS IN WOMEN, ASSESSED BY POST-PONEMENT OF MENSTRUATION. EFFECTIVE DOSES FOR 50% OF WOMEN (ED50) (AFTER SWYER AND LITTLE, 1962)

Drug	No. of observations	ED50 (mg/day)
Norethisterone (norethindrone)	89	4.25
Norethisterone acetate	51	10.5
Norethynodrel	16	20
Norethynodrel + mestranol (Enovid)	28	5.3
Medroxyprogesterone (Provera)	4	>10
Medroxyprogesterone + mestranol	21	22.5
Megestrol acetate	30	>10
Megestrol acetate + mestranol	51	1.8
Melengestrol acetate	17	>10
Melengestrol acetate + mestranol	16	2.5
17α-vinyl-19-nortestosterone (SC4641)	12	>10
17α-vinyl-19-nortestosterone + mestranol	13	7
21-fluoro,Δ^6,6-methylprogesterone acetate (SC10230)	4	< 2.5
Ethynodiol diacetate	9	> 4
Ethynodiol diacetate + mestranol	32	1.5
Quingestrone acetate (Gestovis)	7	>20
Quingestrone acetate + mestranol	22	<10
Quingestrone	1	>50
Quingestrone + mestranol	4	>25
Dydrogesterone	9	>20
Dydrogesterone + mestranol	4	>10

and the dose doubled for the next cycle. By suitable adjustment the 50% effective dose (ED50) can be estimated by interpolation. The test may be made more accurate and economical by using the Robbins—Monro procedure as described by Hawkins (1964).

Norgestrel has also been assessed, with and without the addition of mestranol. Without oestrogen its effectiveness is only moderate but with added mestranol the approximate ED50 is 0.125 mg. This indicates at least ten times greater potency than the next two most active substances, ethynodiol diacetate with mestranol and megestrol acetate with mestranol (*Table 2.1*).

The validity of animal experiments such as delay in parturition and the effects on the endometrium in assessing the potency of a particular progestagen in the human is open to question, and conclusions based on simple tests like delay of menstruation and metabolic studies in women are more likely to give meaningful answers. Even in the human there are differences between the assessment of the relative potency of progestagens assessed by different tests. Rudel (1970) reported that a study of menstrual delay caused by 20-day courses of progestagens showed that norethisterone was three times more potent than ethynodiol diacetate. Ferin (1972), using the deposition of glycogen in endometrial glandular cells as his criterion, reported that norethisterone, ethynodiol diacetate and lynoestrenol had similar potencies, but that these were two to four times less than that of norgestrel.

CLINICAL PHARMACOLOGY OF PROGESTAGENS

Hypothalamus and Anterior Pituitary Gland

Progestagens depress the production of LH, but have no effect on FSH levels. Schally *et al.* (1968) demonstrated that, while progestagens as well as oestrogens depress plasma LH levels in oophorectomised rats, simultaneous administration of LH releasing factor with the two steroids restored the depressed plasma LH level to its original level. They concluded that the oral contraceptive steroids act mainly on the hypothalamus or higher brain centres, reducing endogenous production of releasing factors, rather than directly on the pituitary gland.

The 19-nortestosterone derivative dydrogesterone in doses of 2.0 mg daily was found by Jaffe and Midgley (1969) to abolish the mid cycle LH peak, whilst FSH levels remained normal. In doses of 0.35—0.5 mg daily neither group of progestagens will regularly inhibit ovulation. This is consistent with the fact, demonstrated by Orr and Elstein (1969), that a typical mid cycle ovulatory peak of LH that was high enough to be associated with ovulation occurred when patients were taking chlormadinone acetate, 0.5 mg daily. Similar patterns of LH excretion were observed with daily doses of chlormadinone, 0.5 mg, or norethisterone, 1 mg by Diczfalusy *et al.* (1969).

Ovulation is suppressed in less than 50% of cycles by the administration of a progestagen such as chlormadinone acetate, 0.5 mg (Zañartu *et al.*, 1968). Moghissi (1972) studied 11 patients who had received norethisterone, 0.35 mg, quingestanol acetate, 0.5 mg, or norgestrel, 75 μg, and found presumptive evidence of ovulation in nine. Zañartu *et al.* (1974) observed direct evidence of ovulation at laparotomy in 60% of patients on both continuous and pre-coital regimens of progestagens. It is clear that suppression of ovulation is not a consistent effect of small doses of progestagens.

Intermediate doses of progestagens such as norethynodrel, 5 mg, were used to inhibit ovulation in the first oral contraceptives. Oestrogens were added merely to regulate the cycle before their potency in suppressing ovulation was fully appreciated. Similar doses of 5–10 mg of norethisterone inhibit ovulation but these doses are no longer used in current oral contraceptives.

Large doses of progestagens such as norethisterone oenanthate, 200 mg, given as intramuscular depot injections cause inhibition of ovulation (Howard *et al.*, 1975). Two weeks after injection, blood levels in these patients can be as high as 8000 ng/ml, falling to low levels only 10–12 weeks after injection. After ten weeks ovulation, as measured by the levels of oestrogens and progesterone, can occur. It is unlikely that a single injection of a progestagen such as medroxyprogesterone acetate, 150 mg, or norethisterone oenanthate 200 mg, will lead to long-term pituitary suppression and subsequent amenorrhoea, but repeated injections at three monthly intervals, or two injections within three months, can suppress the pituitary for a prolonged period of time.

Ovary

In women taking small doses of progestagens the structure of the corpus luteum seems to be normal, but luteal function, as indicated by pregnanediol excretion, is impaired by the administration of either norgestrel (Eckstein *et al.*, 1972) or norethisterone. The 17α-hydroxyprogesterone derivatives do not affect luteal function as measured in this way.

It is suggested that preferential concentration of progestagens in the genital tract under the influence of oestrogens may be explained by oestrogen-induced variations of receptor or binding sites. The decrease in the deposition of synthetic progestagens in the genital tract during the luteal phase may be due to competition with endogenous progesterone for binding sites in the target tissues. Some of the qualitative and quantitative morphological and biochemical differences in the endometrial response to progesterone, when compared to a synthetic progestagen, could be due to the higher affinity of these receptor binding proteins for the synthetic steroid. The contraceptive effect of *d*-norgestrel, which is effective in a dose seven times lower than chlormadinone acetate, could be partly explained by its preferential deposition in the endometrium.

Endometrium

Effects vary according to the type of progestational agent used and the duration of its administration.

The 19-nortestosterone compounds alter the development of the endometrial stroma and glands. The stroma is excessively vascularised, is oedematous and has the cellular appearance of decidua, contrasting with the glands, which are atrophic with an absence of mucus secretion. Klopper (1970) suggested that the unprepared endometrium is the one tissue in the body which is able to resist implantation and that overcoming this resistance by hormonal changes is an essential feature of the ovarian cycle. It is possible that synthetic progestagens do not mimic the action of the corpus luteum in this respect and so although the endometrium appears secretory, it is able to resist the implantation of the ovum. Another theory suggested by Klopper (1970) is that the 19-nortestosterone derivatives cause an inadequate secretory activity of the endometrium which then fails to maintain the blastocyst so that it cannot implant. With sufficiently small doses of progestagens a normal secretory endometrium is achieved, suggesting the occurrence of ovulation. Increasing the dose leads to a progressive reduction in glandular secretion and tortuosity (Rudel, 1970). This author suggested that the progestagen-induced glandular suppression reflects either interference with oestrogen action at the target organ, or with the production of oestrogen. The anti-oestrogenic effect of progestagens can be estimated clinically by studying the inhibition of glandular development. This was found to be directly related to progestagen dose (Rudel *et al.*, 1967). Norethisterone is one of the most potent of the compounds studied.

Radioactive levonorgestrel is highly selectively deposited in the endometrium. This selectivity is significantly lower during the luteal phase and may be related to the degree of oestrogen stimulation of the endometrium during the follicular phase of the cycle (Zaldívar and Gallegos, 1971). Tritium-labelled chlormadinone acetate shows an affinity for the mucus-producing epithelia of the genital tract, but there is also a marked concentration in abdominal subcutaneous fat (Gallegos *et al.*, 1970).

Prolonged exposure to progestagens can cause dilated endometrial sinusoids (Maqueo *et al.*, 1970), but this effect is not related to the appearance of breakthrough bleeding. Three-quarters of the women who took 5 mg norethisterone daily for five years showed absence of proliferation of the endometrium.

Fallopian Tube

The effects of progestational steroids on the human oviduct have not been studied very much, but it is possible that this is one of their sites of action. Preliminary studies (Oberti *et al.*, 1974) on the effects of progestagens on the tubal epithelium indicate a reduction in the numbers and in the height of the microvilli of the cilia, which could affect the transport of ovum and sperm within the tube. Recent work on the tubal epithelium microstructure two to six hours after ingestion of clogestone acetate, 1, 2 or 3 mg, or levonorgestrel, 75 or 150 μg, suggested that the effects on the numbers and size of microvilli and of the cilia are minimal (Elder *et al.*, unpublished data). The muscular motility, measured *in vitro*, of both medial and lateral parts of the tube are unaltered 1 and 12 hours after the ingestion of clogestone acetate, 2 mg. *dl*-Norgestrel, 150 μg, causes an increase in frequency and decrease in amplitude of contractions 12 hours after ingestion (Elder *et al.*, 1977).

Chlormadinone acetate has been shown to have an effect on sperm transport, as Zañartu *et al.* (1968) were unable to find any spermatozoa in the fallopian tubes between 12 and 20 hours after intercourse in ten patients. The fact that chlormadinone acetate concentration in the genital tract was greatest in the fallopian tubes and cervical mucus (Gallegos *et al.*, 1970) suggests these as two possible sites of contraceptive action.

Cervical Mucus

Progestagens act on the cervical mucus to make it more tenacious and difficult for sperm penetration to take place (Jackson, 1961; Martínez-Manautou *et al.*, 1967; Swyer and Little, 1968; Zañartu *et al.*, 1968). These changes in cervical mucus are associated with alterations in the nature and concentration of protein, which increases markedly after ovulation (Elstein, 1970). Norgestrel, 0.075 mg taken daily, increases the sialic acid concentration of cervical mucus and there is a highly significant reduction in the ability of sperms to penetrate this mucus (Eckstein *et al.*, 1972). Sialic acid contributes to strong cross-linkages between the glycoprotein fibrils of cervical mucus, and so reduces the ability of the proteolytic enzymes within the spermatozoa to break them down.

Both the 17-acetoxy progestagens and the 19-nortestosterone progestagens change the typical oestrogen-induced characteristics of cervical mucus which occur at mid cycle, and which are essential for the activity of spermatozoa. Giner-Velázquez *et al.* (1966) showed that chlormadinone acetate, 0.5 mg daily, caused increased viscosity, decreased spinnbarkeit, increased cellularity and inhibition of crystallisation in the mucus. Swyer and Little (1968), Lebech *et al.* (1969) and Moghissi and Marks (1971) found that chlormadinone and megestrol acetate in doses of 0.25 and 0.5 mg, and norgestrel, 0.025 mg to 0.1 mg, altered the cervical mucus in the way described by Giner-Velázquez *et al.* (1966). Norgestrel (Roland, 1968), medroxyprogesterone and chlormadinone (Chang, 1967) induce biochemical changes in the mucus which may prevent capacitation of spermatozoa. Boettcher (1974) suggests that progestagens in the mucus may act directly on respiration and motility of spermatozoa.

Any effect of progestagen in currently available combined pills on penetration of spermatozoa seems to be counterbalanced by the oestrogen component (Ansbacher and Campbell, 1971).

SYSTEMIC EFFECTS

Cardio-vascular System

Progestagens have little significant action on the cardio-vascular system, or on coagulation mechanisms.

Although slight upward trends in blood pressure have been found with patients taking chlormadinone (Hawkins and Benster, 1977), prolonged administration of small doses of ethynodiol diacetate, norgestrel or norethisterone have been reported to be associated with reductions in blood pressure (Spellacy and Birk, 1974; Hawkins and Benster, 1977).

Poller, Thomson *et al.* (1969) have demonstrated that plasma factors VII and X are not affected by chlormadinone acetate, 0.5 mg taken daily, and neither this drug nor norethisterone, 0.35 mg daily, affect plasma IX levels (Elder *et al.*, 1971). Factors VII and X were unchanged in patients taking norethisterone, 0.35 mg daily, or megestrol acetate, 0.5 mg daily in oil (Poller *et al.*, 1972; Hawkins, 1973). Briggs (1974) has shown that women taking ethinyloestradiol, 0.05 mg, and norethisterone, 1 mg, had factor VII levels raised to 120% of normal control values. When the medication was changed to ethinyloestradiol and norgestrel these values returned to normal. This suggests that norgestrel antagonises the action of ethinyloestradiol in this respect. As the coagulation factors are synthesised in the liver, the site of the antagonism may be oestrogen receptors in the cytoplasm of the liver cells, or perhaps transport of oestrogen to the cell nuclei may be affected.

Many women have now used progestagen-only oral contraceptives and there have been no reports of significant effects on coagulation factors or of associated thrombosis or embolism (Rinehart, 1975; Hawkins and Benster, 1977).

Carbohydrate Metabolism

The changes in carbohydrate metabolism caused by the combined oral contraceptives are a reduction in glucose tolerance, and raised plasma insulin and pyruvate levels. Most authors in the last few years have attributed these alterations to the oestrogen component. On the other hand, the effects may be due to the combined action of oestrogen and progestagen, and it has been thought that the 19-nortestosterone derivatives have an effect on carbohydrate metabolism that is greater than that produced by either the 17α-hydroxyprogesterone derivatives or the oestrogen component (Spellacy *et al.*, 1973). Using parenteral medroxyprogesterone acetate in doses of 150 mg monthly, Gershberg *et al.* (1969) found that carbohydrate metabolism in latent and overt diabetics was altered after three months. This dose is much larger than that used in oral contraceptives, and the affected individuals were already at risk. It is therefore not surprising to find that chlormadinone acetate, 0.5 mg daily (Larsson-Cohn *et al.*, 1969), norethisterone acetate, 0.35 mg daily (Di Paola *et al.*, 1968), ethynodiol diacetate, 0.5 mg daily (Goldman *et al.*, 1971) or megestrol acetate, 0.5 mg daily (Spellacy *et al.*, 1973) have no effects on carbohydrate metabolism.

The use of a combined pill containing 4 mg of megestrol has no significant effect on carbohydrate metabolism. Wynn *et al.* (1974) have shown that a combined pill containing norgestrel, 150 μg, and only 30 μg of ethinyloestradiol has no effect on glucose tolerance or on pyruvate levels, though there is a small increase in insulin secretion.

Lipid Metabolism

Fasting serum triglyceride levels are unaltered in women taking chlormadinone acetate, 0.5 mg daily (Barton *et al.*, 1970). Norethisterone causes a rise in serum triglyceride levels, but norgestrel, despite being a 19-nortestosterone derivative, causes no significant rise even when in combination with an oestrogen.

Serum cholesterol levels are also unaltered by the 17α-hydroxyprogesterone derivative, chlormadinone acetate (Barton *et al.*, 1970). Norethisterone causes a dose-dependent rise in serum cholesterol levels. Norgestrel, 150 μg, given in combination with ethinyloestradiol, 30 μg, reduces serum cholesterol levels from the normal control values (Wynn *et al.*, 1974).

Liver Function

Combined oral contraceptives cause alterations in biochemical parameters related to the liver (Ockner and Davidson, 1967) but in general these changes are slight and there is no reason to suppose that they are of any consequence in a normal individual. They may constitute a risk to patients with impaired liver function.

Electron microscopic studies by Martínez-Manautou *et al.* (1970) of liver biopsies of women treated with chlormadinone acetate, 0.5 mg daily, showed mild vacuolation of the endoplasmic reticulum, presence of a few small fat vacuoles and slightly increased variability in shape and size of mitochondria, some of which contained crystalloid inclusions. The cell nuclei, the bile canaliculi, the Kupfer cells and the glycogen deposits were all normal.

Fundamentally the liver seems unaffected by progestagens. Mild impairment of bromsulphthalein excretion of up to 10% has been reported to occur in 10–50% of women taking combined oral contraceptives containing 2 or 4 mg of norethisterone (Larsson-Cohn and Stenram, 1965). Other workers have found that progestagens alone do not affect liver function and can be used in cases of previous liver pathology even if this was associated with the pill or pregnancy (Rinehart, 1975). This view is supported by the findings of Briggs (1974), at least in respect to norgestrel, and by Hawkins and Benster (1977). The decreased levels of haptoglobin, orosomucin and albumin caused by oestrogens are restored to normal when the patient takes norgestrel in combination with the oestrogen.

Protein and Amino Acid Metabolism

It has been suggested that there is an increase in amino acid utilisation during the luteal phase of the normal menstrual cycle (Craft *et al.*, 1970) presumably due to progesterone (Craft and Wise, 1969). In women receiving combined oral contraceptives there is a similar increase in amino acid utilisation, and these authors suggest that the synthetic progestagens are primarily responsible for altered metabolism of the amino acids and the negative nitrogen balance. Landau and Lugibihl (1967) suggest that this catabolic effect occurs by the enhancement of liver utilisation of amino acids from exogenous protein and endogenous amino acids, together with an increased synthesis of urea. The mechanism by which this is mediated is not known. The net loss of urinary nitrogen is enhanced by increasing the protein intake which in turn enlarges the amino acid pool. The intensity of the catabolic process induced by progesterone is positively related to the size of the amino acid pool. Catabolism induced by 50 mg of intramuscular progesterone markedly reduced the plasma concentration of ten amino acids: threonine, proline, glycine, alanine, lysine, arginine, ornithine, citrulline, cystine, and serine. The levels of valine, tyrosine, methionine, isoleucine and leucine were also reduced by 10–15%.

Dale and Spivey (1971) studied three groups of women, one using intramuscular medroxyprogesterone acetate, 150 mg every three months, the second using oral contraceptives in the form of mestranol, 0.1 mg, and ethynodiol diacetate, 1 mg, for 21 days, whilst the third was a control group. The oestrogen-progestagen group showed an increase in α_1-, α_2- and β-globulins but a decreased total protein and albumin fraction when compared with the control group, whilst the group using intramuscular medroxyprogesterone acetate showed an increase in both albumin and globulin after three months. After 24 months the oral contraceptive group showed a decrease in albumin from the value obtained during the first three months, but this was the only significant difference in any of the groups over the complete period of the study.

Endocrine Systems

Low doses of progestagens have little or no effect on thyroid function (Rinehart, 1975), or on plasma cortisol levels (Burke, 1970; Brien, 1975). Women having intramuscular medroxyprogesterone have plasma levels of progesterone, oestradiol, testosterone and unbound corticosteroids which are normal for the follicular phase of the cycle (Briggs and Briggs, 1972).

Body Weight

Watson and Robinson (1965) measured body weight daily in 28 women for a period of 68 days under constant conditions. Weight increased steadily throughout the premenstrual phase, reaching a maximum during the first day or two of menstruation. Thereafter there was a fall to the lowest levels, which were recorded during the early follicular phase of the cycle, with a small rise at ovulation. It is suggested that these changes are associated with the cyclical changes in progesterone levels but no mechanism has been demonstrated and the effect is probably due to oestrogen. Kudzma *et al.* (1972) showed a small gain in body weight and sodium retention during a menstrual cycle and a pill cycle in four women. This response also is probably due to oestrogen, acting without enough progesterone to compensate by diuresis and natriuresis. Klein and Carey (1957) failed to find any change in either sodium balance or in body weight during the cycle, although it is the experience of many women that they feel heavier and bloated during the premenstrual phase of the cycle.

REFERENCES

ALEXANDER, R.W. and MARMORSTON, J. (1961). Effect of two synthetic estrogens on the level of serum protein-bound iodine in men and women with atherosclerotic heart disease. *J. clin. Endocr. Metab.*, **21**, 243–251

ANSBACHER, R. and CAMPBELL, C. (1971). Cervical mucus sperm penetration in women on oral contraception or with an IUD *in-situ*. *Contraception*, **3**, 209–217

ASSCHER, A.W., SUSSMAN, M., WATERS, W.E., EVANS, J.A.S., CAMPBELL, H., EVANS, K.T. and WILLIAMS, J.E. (1969). The clinical significance of asymptomatic bacteriuria in the non-pregnant woman. *J. infect. Dis.*, **120**, 17–21

ÅSTEDT, B. (1971). Low fibrinolytic activity of veins during treatment with ethinyl oestradiol. *Acta obstet. gynec. scand.*, **50**, 279–283

ÅSTEDT, B., ISACSON, S., NILSSON, I.M. and PANDOLFI, M. (1973). Thrombosis and oral contraceptives. Possible predisposition. *Br. med. J.*, iv, 631–634

BARTON, G.M.G., FREEMAN, P.R. and LAWSON, J.P. (1970). Oral contraceptives and serum lipids. *J. Obstet. Gynaec. Br. Commonw.*, **77**, 551–554

BAUGH, R.F. and HOUGIE, C. (1977). Biochemistry of blood coagulation. In *Recent Advances in Blood Coagulation*, number 2, p. 2. Ed. Poller, L., Churchill Livingstone, Edinburgh

BOETTCHER, B. (1974). A possible mode of action of progestagen-only oral contraceptives. *Contraception*, **9**, 123–129

BOLT, H.M. and BOLT, W.H. (1974). Pharmacokinetics of mestranol in man in relation to its oestrogenic activity. *Eur. J. clin. Pharmac.*, **7**, 295–305

BOLTON, C.H., HAMPTON, J.R. and MITCHELL, J.R.A. (1968). Effect of oral contraceptive agents on platelets and plasma phospholipids. *Lancet*, **i**, 1336–1341

BRAKMAN, P., SOBRERO, A.J. and ASTRUP, T. (1970). Effects of different systemic contraceptives on blood fibrinolysis. *Am. J. Obstet. Gynec.*, **106**, 187–192

BREHM. H. (1964). Circulation, blood coagulation and clinical observations during hormonal suppression of ovulation. *Int. J. Fert.*, **9**, 45–56

BRIEN, T.G. (1975). Cortisol metabolism after oral contraceptives: total plasma cortisol and the free cortisol index. *Br. J. Obstet. Gynaec.*, **82**, 987–991

BRIGGS, M. (1974). Effect of oral progestogens on oestrogen induced changes in serum protein. *The Second International Norgestrel Symposium. Some Metabolic Considerations of Oral Contraceptive Usage*, pp 35–41. Excerpta Medica, Amsterdam

BRIGGS, M.H. and BRIGGS, M. (1971). Effects of oral ethynyloestradiol on serum proteins in normal women. *Contraception*, **3**, 381–386

BRIGGS, M.H. and BRIGGS, M. (1972). Plasma hormone concentrations in women receiving steroid contraceptives. *J. Obstet. Gynaec. Br. Commonw.*, **79**, 946–950

BROSENS, I.A. and PIJNENBORG, R. (1976). Comparative study of the estrogenic effect of ethinyloestradiol and mestranol on the endometrium. *Contraception*, **14**, 679–685

BROWN, J.B. and BLAIR, H.A.F. (1960). Urinary oestrogen metabolites of 19-nor-ethisterone and its esters. *Proc. R. Soc. Med.*, **53**, 433

BROWN, P.S., WELLS, M. and CUNNINGHAM, F.J.(1964). A method for studying the mode of action of oral contraceptives. *Lancet*, **ii**, 446–447

BURKE, C.W. (1970). The effect of oral contraceptives on cortisol metabolism. *J. clin. Path.*, **23**, supplement 3, 11–18

CASPARY, E.A. and PEBERDY, M.(1965). Oral contraception and blood platelet adhesiveness. *Lancet*, **i**, 1142–1143

CHANG, M.C. (1967). Effects of progesterone and related compounds on fertilization, transportation and development of rabbit eggs. *Endocrinology*, **81**, 1251–1260

CLINCH, J. and TINDALL, V.R. (1969). Effects of oestrogens and progestogens on liver function in the puerperium. *Br. med. J.*, **i**, 602–605

CORRIERE, J.N., WALLACH, E.E., MURPHY, J.J. and GARCIA, C.R. (1970). Effect of anovulatory drugs on the human urinary tract and urinary tract infections *Obstet. Gynec., N.Y.*, **35**, 211–216

CRAFT, I.L. and WISE, I. (1969). Oral contraceptives and plasma amino-acids. *Nature, Lond.*, **222**, 487–488

CRAFT, I.L., WISE, I.J. and BRIGGS, M.H. (1970). Oral contraceptives and amino-acid utilization. *Am. J. Obstet. Gynec.*, **108**, 1120–1125

DALE, E. and SPIVEY, S.H. (1971). Serum proteins of women utilising combination oral or long-acting injectable progestational contraceptives. *Contraception*, **4**, 241–251

DANIEL, D.G., CAMPBELL, H. and TURNBULL, A.C. (1967). Puerperal thrombo-embolism and suppression of lactation. *Lancet*, **ii**, 287–289

DANIEL, D.G., BLOOM, A.L., GIDDINGS, J.C., CAMPBELL, H. and TURNBULL, A.C.

(1968). Increased IX levels in puerperium during administration of diethyl-stilboestrol. *Br. med. J.*, i, 801–803

DAVIDOFF, F., TISHLER, S. and ROSOFF, C. (1973). Marked hyperlipidaemia and pancreatitis associated with oral contraceptive therapy. *New Engl. J. Med.*, **289**, 552–555

DAVIS, M.E. and FUGO, N.W. (1948). The cause of physiologic basal temperature changes in women. *J. clin. Endocr. Metab.*, **8**, 550–563

DAVIS, M.E. and PLOTZ, E.J. (1956). The excretion of neutral steroids in the urine of normal non-pregnant and pregnant women. *Acta endocr., Copnh.*, **21**, 254–258

DELFORGE, J.P. and FERIN, J. (1970). A histometric study of two oestrogens; ethinyl-estradiol and its 3-methyl-ether derivative (mestranol); their comparative effect upon the growth of human endometrium. *Contraception*, **1**, 57–72

DICZFALUSY, E., GOEBELSMANN, U., JOHANNISSON, E., TILLINGER, K.G. and WIDE, L. (1969). Pituitary and ovarian function in women on continuous low dose progestogens; effect of chlormadinone acetate and norethisterone. *Acta endocr., Copnh.*, **62**, 679–693

DI PAOLA, G., PUCHULU, F., ROBIN, M., NICHOLSON, R. and MARTI, M. (1968). Oral contraceptives and carbohydrate metabolism. *Am. J. Obstet. Gynec.*, **101**, 206–216

DOE, R.P., MELLINGER, G.T., SWAIM, W.R. and SEAL, U.S. (1967). Estrogen dosage effects on serum proteins: a longitudinal study. *J. clin. Endocr. Metab.*, **27**, 1081–1086

DOAR, J.W.H. and WYNN, V. (1970). Serum lipid levels during oral contraceptive and glucocorticoid administration. *J. clin. Path.*, **23**, supplement 3, 55–61

DOYLE, J.B. (1951). Exploratory culdotomy for observation of tubo-ovarian physiology at ovulation time. *Fert. Steril.*, **2**, 475–484.

DURE-SMITH, P. (1971). Urinary tract dilation and oral contraceptives. *Br. med. J.*, i, 230

ECKSTEIN, P., WHITBY, M., FOTHERBY, K., BUTLER, C., MUKHERJEE, T.K., BURNETT, J.B.C., RICHARDS, D.J. and WHITEHEAD, T.P. (1972). Clinical and laboratory findings in a trial of norgestrel, a low-dose progestagen only contraceptive. *Br. med. J.*, iii, 195–200

ELDER, M.G., HAKIM, C.A. and HAWKINS, D.F. (1971). Plasma factor IX levels and oral contraception. *J. Obstet. Gynaec. Br. Commonw.*, **78**, 277–279

ELDER, M.G., MYATT, L. and CHAUDHURI, G. (1977). The effects of clogestone and norgestrel on the spontaneous activity of the fallopian tube. *Int. J. Fert.*, **23**, 61–64

ELSTEIN, M. (1970). The proteins of cervical mucus and the influence of progestagens. *J. Obstet. Gynaec. Br. Commonw.*, **77**, 443–456

EPSTEIN, S.E., ROSING, D.R., BRAKMAN, P., REDWOOD, D.R. and ASTRUP, T. (1970). Impaired fibrinolytic responses to exercise in patients with Type IV hyperlipoproteinaemia. *Lancet*, ii, 631–633

FERIN, J. (1972). The effects of progesterone on the uterovaginal tract. In *Pharmacology of the Endocrine System and Related Drugs: Progesterone, Progestational Drugs and Antifertility Agents*, volume I, pp. 441–456. Ed. Tausk, M., section 48, International Encyclopedia of Pharmacology and Therapeutics. Pergamon, Oxford

FISCHER, R.H. (1954). Progesterone metabolism III. Basal body temperature as an index of progesterone production and its relationship to urinary pregnanediol. *Obstet. Gynec., N.Y.*, **3**, 615–626

FOTHERBY, K. (1974a). Metabolism of synthetic steroids by animals and man. *Acta endocr., Copnh.*, supplement 185, 119–147

FOTHERBY, K. (1974b). Metabolism of 19-norsteroids to oestrogenic steroids. *The Second Norgestrel Symposium. Some Metabolic Considerations of Oral Contraceptive Usage*, pp 30–34. Excerpta Medica, Amsterdam

FOTHERBY, K., KAMYAB, S., LITTLETON, P. and KLOPPER, A.I. (1968). Metabolism of synthetic progestational compounds in humans. *J. Reprod. Fert.*, supplement 5, 51–61

FURMAN, R.H., HOWARD, R.P., NORCIA, L.N. and KEATY, E.C. (1958). The influence of androgens, estrogens and related steroids on serum lipids and lipoproteins. *Am. J. Med.*, **24**, 80–97

GALLEGOS, A.J., GONZÁLEZ-DIDDI, M., MERINO, G. and MARTÍNEZ-MANAUTOU, J. (1970). Tissue localization of radioactive chlormadinone acetate and progesterone in the human. *Contraception*, **1**, 151–161

GARFINKEL, A.S., BAKER, N. and SCHOTZ, M.C. (1967). Relation of lipoprotein lipase activity to triglyceride uptake in adipose tissue. *J. Lipid Res.*, **8**, 274–280

GERSHBERG, H., ZORRILLA, E., HERNANDEZ, A. and HULSE, M. (1969). Effects of medroxyprogesterone acetate on serum insulin and growth hormone levels in diabetics and potential diabetics. *Obstet. Gynec., N.Y.*, **33**, 383–389

GINER-VELÁZQUEZ, J., CASASOLA, J., ROJAS, B.A. and MARTÍNEZ-MANAUTOU, J. (1966). *Rev. de Invest. Clinica del Instituto Nacional de la Nutricion, Mexico*, **18**, 195. Cited by Martínez-Manautou, J. (1971) in *Control of Human Fertility. Proceedings of the Fifteenth Nobel Symposium held May 27–29, 1970 at Södergarn, Lidingö, Sweden*, p. 58. Ed. Diczfalusy, E. and Borell, U. Wiley, New York

GOLDMAN, J.A., ECKERLING, B., ZUKERMAN, Z. and MANNHEIMER, S. (1971). Blood glucose and plasma insulin levels with ethynodiol diacetate oral contraceptive. *J. Obstet. Gynaec. Br. Commonw.*, **78**, 255–260

GOLDMAN, J.A. and OVADIA, J.L. (1969). The effect of estrogen on intravenous glucose tolerance in women. *Am. J. Obstet. Gynec.*, **103**, 172–178

GOLDZIEHER, J.W. (1970). An assessment of the hazards and metabolic alterations attributed to oral contraceptives. *Contraception*, **1**, 409–445

GOLDZIEHER, J.W., KLEBER, J.W., MOSES, L.E. and RATHMACHER, R.P. (1970). A cross-sectional study of plasma FSH and LH levels in women using sequential combination, or injectable steroid contraceptives over long periods of time. *Contraception*, **2**, 225–248

GOLDZIEHER, J.W., MOSES, L.E. and ELLIS, L.T. (1962). Study of norethindrone in contraception. *J. Am. med. Ass.*, **180**, 359–361

GOOD, W. (1978). Water relations of the ovarian cycle. *Br. J. Obstet. Gynaec.*, **85**, 63–69

GOODRICH, S.M. and WOOD, J.E. (1966). The effect of estradiol-17β on peripheral venous distensibility and velocity of venous blood flow. *Am. J. Obstet. Gynec.*, **96**, 407–412

GREIG, H.B.W. and NOTELOWITZ, M. (1975). Natural oestrogens and anti-thrombin III levels. *Lancet*, **i**, 412–413

GUILLEMIN, R. (1972). Physiology and chemistry of the hypothalamic releasing factors for gonadotrophins: a new approach to fertility control. *Contraception*, **5**, 1–19

GUYER, P.B. and DELANY, D. (1970). Urinary tract dilatation and oral contraceptives. *Br. med. J.*, iv, 588–590

HAKIM, C.A., ELDER, M.G. and HAWKINS, D.F. (1969). Plasma factor IX levels in patients given hexoestrol or stilboestrol to suppress lactation. *Br. med. J.*, 4, 82–84

HALLER, J. (1970). A review of the long term effects of hormonal contraceptives. *Contraception*, 1, 233–251

HAM, J.M. and ROSE, R. (1969). Platelet adhesiveness and lipoprotein lipase activity in controls and in subjects taking oral contraceptives. *Am. J. Obstet. Gynec.*, 105, 628–631

HAMPTON, J.R. (1970). Platelet abnormalities induced by the administration of oestrogens. *J. clin. Path.*, 23, supplement 3, 75–80

HARKNESS, R.A. and FOTHERBY, K. (1963). The metabolism of progesterone in man. Extraction and separation by countercurrent distribution of the metabolites in urine. *Biochem. J.*, 88, 308–314

HAWKINS, D.F. (1964). Observations on the application of the Robbins–Munro process to sequential toxicity assays. *Br. J. Pharmac. Chemother.*, 22, 392–402

HAWKINS, D.F. (1973). Rischio tromboembolico contracessione steroidea. In *Atti del 1° Seminario Internazionale Problemi Medici e Sociali del Controllo della Fecondita, Genova, 3–5 Marzo 1972*, pp. 201–209. Ed. Pescetto, G. and DeCecco, L. Minerva Medica, Turin

HAWKINS, D.F. and BENSTER, B. (1977). A comparative study of three progestagens (chlormadinone acetate, megestrol acetate and norethisterone) as oral contraceptives. *Br. J. Obstet. Gynaec.*, 84, 708–713

HAWKINS, D.F. and NIXON, W.C.W. (1961). The influence of oestrogen and progesterone on the electrolytes of the human uterus. *J. Obstet. Gynaec. Br. Commonw.*, 68, 62–67

HAZZARD, W.R., SPIGER, M.J., BAGDADE, J.D. and BIERMAN, E.L. (1969). Studies on the mechanism of increased plasma triglyceride levels induced by oral contraceptives. *New Engl. J. Med.*, 280, 471–474

HEDLIN, A.M. (1975). The effect of oral contraceptive estrogen on blood coagulation and fibrinolysis. *Thromb. Diath. haemorrh.*, 33, 370–378

HEINEN, G. (1971). The discriminating use of combination and sequential preparations in the hormonal inhibition of ovulation. *Contraception*, 4, 393–400

HELTON, E.D. and GOLDZIEHER, J.W. (1977). The pharmacokinetics of ethynyl estrogens. *Contraception*, 15, 255–284

HILDEN, M., AMRIS, C.J. and STARUP, J. (1967). The haemostatic mechanism in oral contraception. *Acta obstet. gynec. scand.*, 46, 562–571

HOLLANDER, C.S., GARCIA, A.M., STURGIS, S.H. and SELENKOW, H.A. (1963). Effect of an ovulatory suppressant on the serum protein-bound iodine and the red cell uptake of radioactive tri-iodothyronine. *New Engl. J. Med.*, 269, 501–504

HOLZBAUER, M. (1976). Physiological aspects of steroids with anaesthetic properties. *Med. Biol.*, 54, 227–242

HORNE, C.H.W., HOWIE, P.W., WEIR, R.J. and GOUDIE, R.B. (1970). Effect of combined oestrogen–progestagen oral contraceptives on serum levels of α_2 macroglobulin, transferin, albumin and IgG. *Lancet*, i, 49–50

HOWARD, G., WARREN, R.J. and FOTHERBY, K. (1975). Plasma levels of norethisterone in women receiving norethisterone oenanthate intramuscularly. *Contraception,* 12, 45–52

INMAN, W.H.W., VESSEY, M.P., WESTERHOLM, B. and ENGELUND, A. (1970). Thrombo-embolic disease and the steroidal content of oral contraceptives, a report to the Committee on Safety of Drugs. *Br. med. J.,* ii, 203–209

JACKSON, M.H. (1961). Observations on the use of certain orally active progestogens for the control of fertility in women. *Proc. R. Soc. Med.,* 54, 984–987

JAFFE, R.B. and MIDGLEY, A.R. (1969). Current status of human gonadotrophin radioimmunoassay. *Obstetl gynec. Surv.,* 24, 200–213

JAVIER, Z., GERSHBERG, H. and HULSE, M. (1968). Ovulatory suppressants, estrogens and carbohydrate metabolism. *Metabolism,* 17, 443–456

JEFFCOATE, T.N.A., MILLER, J., ROOS, R.F. and TINDALL, V.R. (1968). Puerperal thromboembolism in relation to the inhibition of lactation by oestrogen therapy. *Br. med. J.,* iv, 19–25

JENSEN, E.V. and JACOBSON, H.I. (1962). Basic guides to the mechanism of estrogen action. *Recent Prog. Horm. Res.,* 18, 387–414

KAPPAS, A. and PALMER, R.H. (1963). Selected aspects of steroid pharmacology. *Pharmac. Rev.,* 15, 123–167

KLEIN, L. and CAREY, J. (1957). Total exchangeable sodium in the menstrual cycle. *Am. J. Obstet. Gynec.,* 74, 956–967

KLOPPER, A. (1970). Developments in steroidal hormonal contraception. *Br. med. Bull.,* 26, 39–44

KUDZMA, D.J., BRADLEY, E.M. and GOLDZIEHER, J.W. (1972). A metabolic balance study of the effects of an oral steroid contraceptive on weight and body composition. *Contraception,* 5, 31–37

KUMAR, D. and BARNES, A.C. (1964). Studies on human myometrium during pregnancy, VI. Tissue progesterone profile of the various compartments in the same individual. *Am. J. Obstet. Gynec.,* 92, 717–719

LANDAU, R.L. (1973). The metabolic influence of progesterone. In *Handbook of Physiology, Section 7, Endocrinology, Vol. II, Female Reproductive System. Part 1,* pp. 573–589. Ed. Greep, R.O. American Physiological Society, Washington

LANDAU, R.L. and LUGIBIHL, K. (1967). The effect of progesterone on plasma amino acids in man. *Metabolism,* 16, 1114–1122

LARSSON-COHN, U. and STENRAM, U. (1965). Jaundice during treatment with oral contraceptive agents. *J. Am. med. Ass.,* 193, 422–426

LARSSON-COHN, U., TENGSTRÖM, B. and WIDE, L. (1969). Glucose tolerance and insulin response during daily continuous low dose oral contraceptive treatment. *Acta endocr., Copnh.,* 62, 242–250

LEBECH, P.E., SVENDSEN, P.A., OSTERGAARD, E. and KOCH, F. (1969). The effects of small doses of megestrol acetate on the cervical mucus. *Acta obstet. gynec. scand.,* 48, supplement 3, 22–25

LEHTOVIRTA, P. (1974a). Haemodynamic effects of combined oestrogen/progestagen oral contraceptives. *J. Obstet. Gynaec. Br. Commonw.,* 81, 517–525

LEHTOVIRTA, P. (1974b). Peripheral haemodynamic effects of combined oestrogen/progestogen oral contraceptives. *J. Obstet. Gynaec. Br. Commonw.,* 81, 526–534

LIM, Y.L., LUMBERS, E.R., WALTERS, W.A.W. and WHELAN, R.F. (1970). Effects of oestrogens on the human circulation. *J. Obstet. Gynaec. Br. Commonw.*, **77**, 349–355

LITTLE, B.C., MATTA, R.J. and ZAHN, T.P. (1974). Physiological and psychological effects of progesterone in man. *J. nerv. ment. Dis.*, **159**, 256–262

McCLINTOCK, J.A. and SCHWARTZ, N.B. (1968). Changes in pituitary and plasma follicle stimulating hormone concentrations during the rat estrous cycle. *Endocrinology*, **83**, 433–441

MAQUEO, M.T., RICE-WRAY, E., GORODOVSKY, J. and GOLDZIEHER, J.W. (1970). The effect of contraceptive steroids on endometrial sinusoids and the failure of these changes to correlate with breakthrough bleeding or systemic vascular effects. *Contraception*, **2**, 283–288

MARCHANT, D.J. (1972). Effects of pregnancy and progestational agents on the urinary tract. *Am. J. Obstet. Gynec.*, **112**, 487–498

MARSHALL, S., LYON, R.P. and MINKLER, D. (1966). Ureteral dilatation following use of oral contraceptives. *J. Am. med. Ass.*, **198**, 782–783

MARTÍNEZ-MANAUTOU, J., AZNAR-RAMOS, R., BAUTISTA-O'FARRELL, J. and GONZÁLEZ-ANGULO, A. (1970). The ultrastructure of liver cells in women under steroid therapy. *Acta endocr., Copenh.*, **65**, 207–221

MARTÍNEZ-MANAUTOU, J., GINER-VELÁZQUEZ, J., CORTÉS-GALLEGOS, V., AZNAR, R., ROJAS, B., GUITTÉRREZ-NÁJAR, A and RUDEL, H.W. (1967). Daily progestagen for contraception: a clinical study. *Br. med. J.*, **ii**, 730–732

MILLS, I.H., SCHEDL, H.P., CHEN, P.S. and BARTTER, F.C. (1960). The effect of estrogen administration on the metabolism and protein binding of hydrocortisone. *J. clin. Endocr. Metab.*, **20**, 515–528

MOGHISSI, K.S. (1972). Morphologic changes in the ovaries of women treated with continuous microdose progestagens. *Fert. Steril.*, **23**, 739–744

MOGHISSI, K.S. and MARKS, C. (1971). Effects of microdose norgestrel on endogenous gonadotrophic and steroid hormones, cervical mucus properties, vaginal cytology and endometrium. *Fert. Steril.*, **22**, 424–434

MUSA, B.U., DOE, R.P. and SEAL, U.S. (1967). Serum protein alterations produced in women by synthetic estrogens. *J. clin. Endocr. Metab.*, **27**, 1463–1469

OBERTI, C., DABANCENS, A., GARCIA-HUIDOBRO, M., RODRIGUEZ-BRAVO, R. and ZANARTU, J. (1974). Low dosage oral progestagens to control fertility. II. Morphological modifications in the gonad and oviduct. *Obstet. Gynec., N.Y.*, **43**, 285–294

OCKNER, R.K. and DAVIDSON, C.S. (1967). Hepatic effects of oral contraceptives. *New Engl. J. Med.*, **276**, 331–334

ORR, A.H. and ELSTEIN, M. (1969). Luteinizing hormone levels in plasma and urine in women during normal menstrual cycles and in women taking combined oral contraceptives or chlormadinone acetate. *J. Endocr.*, **43**, 617–624

OSMAN, M.M., TOPPOZADA, H.K., GHANEM, M.H. and GUERGIS, F.K. (1972). The effect of an oral contraceptive on serum lipids. *Contraception*, **5**, 105–118

OSTERGAARD, E. and STARUP, J. (1968). Occurrence and function of corpora lutea during different forms of oral contraception. *Acta endocr., Copnh.*, **57**, 386–394

PETERSON, R.A., KRULL, P.E., FINLEY, P. and ETTINGER, M.G. (1970). Changes in antithrombin III and plasminogen induced by oral contraceptives. *Am. J. clin. Path.*, **53**, 468–473

PETERSON, W.F., STEEL, M.W. and COYNE, R.V. (1966). Analysis of the effect of ovulatory suppressants on glucose tolerance. *Am. J. Obstet. Gynec.,* **95**, 484–488

PINDYCK, J., LICHTMAN, H.C. and KOHL, S.G. (1970). Cryofibrinogenaemia in women using oral contraceptives. *Lancet,* **i**, 51–53

POLLER, L. (1970). Relation between oral contraceptive hormones and blood clotting. *J. clin. Path.,* **23**, supplement 3, 67–74

POLLER, L., PRIEST, C.M. and THOMSON, J.M. (1969). Platelet aggregation during oral contraception. *Br. med. J.,* **iv**, 273–274

POLLER, L., TABIOWO, A. and THOMSON, J.M. (1968). Effects of low-dose oral contraceptives on blood coagulation. *Br. med. J.,* **iii**, 218–219

POLLER, L. and THOMSON, J.M. (1966). Clotting factors during oral contraception: further report. *Br. med. J.,* **ii**, 23–25

POLLER, L., THOMSON, J.M., TABIOWO, A. and PRIEST, C.M. (1969). Progesterone oral contraception and blood coagulation. *Br. med. J.,* **i**, 554–556

POLLER, L., THOMSON, J.M. and THOMAS, P.W. (1972). Effects of progestogen oral contraception with norethisterone on blood clotting and platelets. *Br. med. J.,* **iv**, 391–393

PYÖRÄLA, K., PYÖRÄLA, T. and LAMPINEN, V. (1967). Sequential oral contraceptive treatment and intravenous glucose tolerance. *Lancet,* **ii**, 776–777

RINEHART, W. (1975). Minipill. A limited alternative for certain women. *Population Reports,* series A, no. 3, 53–67

ROCK, J., GARCIA, C.R. and PINCUS, G. (1957). Synthetic progestins in the normal human menstrual cycle. *Recent Prog. Horm. Res.,* **13**, 323–339

ROLAND, M. (1968). Norgestrel-induced cervical barrier to sperm migration. *J. Reprod. Fert.,* supplement 5, 173–177

ROYAL COLLEGE OF GENERAL PRACTITIONERS (1974). *Oral Contraceptives and Health. An interim report from the oral contraception study of the Royal College of General Practitioners,* pp. 61–62. Pitman Medical, London

RUDEL, H.W. (1970). Antifertility effects of low-dose progestin. *Fedn Proc. Fedn Am. Socs. exp. Biol.,* **29**, 1228–1231

RUDEL, H.W., LEBHERZ, T., MAQUEO-TOPETE, M., MARTÍNEZ-MANAUTOU, J. and BESSLER, S. (1967). Assay of the anti-oestrogenic effects of progestagens. *J. Reprod. Fert.,* **13**, 199–203

SAROJA, N., MALLIKARJUNESWARA, V.R. and CLEMETSON, C.A.B. (1971). Effect of estrogens on ascorbic acid in the plasma and blood vessels of guinea pigs. *Contraception,* **3**, 269–277

SCHALLY, A.V., CARTER, W.H., SAITO, M., ARIMURA, A. and BOWERS, C.Y. (1968). Studies on the site of action of oral contraceptive steroids. I. Effect of anti-fertility steroids on plasma LH levels and on the response to luteinizing hormone releasing-factor in rats. *J. clin. Endocr. Metab.,* **28**, 1747–1755

SETTLAGE, D.F., NAKAMURA, R.M., DAVAJAN, V., KHARMA, K. and MISHELL, D.R. (1970). A quantitative analysis of serum proteins during treatment with oral contraceptive steroids. *Contraception,* **1**, 101–114

SILK, M. and PEREZ-VARELA, M.R. (1970). Effect of oral contraceptives on urinary bacterial growth rate. *Invest. Urol.,* **8**, 239–241

SMITH, O.W. and RYAN, K.J. (1962). Estrogen in the human ovary. *Am. J. Obstet. Gynec.,* **84**, 141–153

SPELLACY, W.N. and BIRK, S.A. (1974). The effects of mechanical and steroid contraceptive methods on blood pressure in hypertensive women. *Fert. Steril.,* **25**, 467–470

SPELLACY, W.N., BUHI, W.C. and BIRK, S.A. (1972). The effect of estrogens on carbohydrate metabolism: glucose, insulin, and growth hormone studies on one hundred and seventy one women ingesting premarin, mestranol and ethinylestradiol for six months. *Am. J. Obstet. Gynec.*, **114**, 378–390

SPELLACY, W.N., BUHI, W.C. and BIRK, S.A. (1975). Effects of norethindrone on carbohydrate and lipid metabolism. *Obstet. Gynec., N.Y.*, **46**, 560–563

SPELLACY, W.N., BUHI, W.C., BIRK, S.A. and McCREARY, S.A. (1971). Studies of ethynodiol diacetate and mestranol on blood glucose and plasma insulin. *Contraception*, **3**, 185–194

SPELLACY, W.N., BUHI, W.C., SPELLACY, C.E., MOSES, L.C. and GOLDZIEHER, J.W. (1968). Carbohydrate studies of long term users of oral contraceptives. *Diabetes*, **17**, supplement 1, 344–345

SPELLACY, W.N., BUHI, W.C., SPELLACY, C.E., MOSES, L.C. and GOLDZIEHER, J.W. (1970). Glucose, insulin and growth hormone studies in long term users of oral contraceptives. *Am. J. Obstet. Gynec.*, **106**, 173–182

SPELLACY, W.N., NEWTON, R.E., BUHI, W.C. and BIRK, S.A. (1973). Carbohydrate and lipid studies during six months treatment with megestrol acetate. *Am. J. Obstet. Gynec.*, **116**, 1074–1078

STOKES, T. and WYNN, V. (1971). Serum-lipids in women on oral contraceptives. *Lancet*, **ii**, 677–680

SWYER, G.I.M. and LITTLE, V. (1962). Clinical assessment of orally active progestagens. *Proc. R. Soc. Med.*, **55**, 861–863

SWYER, G.I.M. and LITTLE, V. (1968). Clinical assessment of relative potency of progestagens. *J. Reprod. Fert.*, supplement 5, 63–68

SWYER, G.I.M., SEBOK, L. and BARNS, D.F. (1960). Determination of the relative potency of some progestogens in the human. *Proc. R. Soc. Med.*, **53**, 435

TALIAFERRO, I., COBEY, F. and LEONE, L. (1956). Effect of diethylstilboestrol on plasma 17-hydroxycorticosteroid levels in humans. *Proc. Soc. exp. Biol. Med.*, **92**, 742–744

TAYLOR, R.W. (1974). The mechanism of action of oestrogen in the human female. *J. Obstet. Gynaec. Br. Commonw.*, **81**, 856–866

THOMAS, K. and FERIN, J. (1972). Suppression of the mid cycle LH surge by a low dose mestranol–lynestrenol oral combination. *Contraception*, **6**, 1–16

TYLER, E.T. (1964). Current status of oral contraception. *J. Am. med. Ass.*, **187**, 562–565

WAGATSUMA, T., SULLIVAN, W.J. and KUMAR, D. (1967). The mechanism of action of progesterone in human myometrium, III. *In vitro* progesterone effects on potassium flux in human myometrium. *Am. J. Obstet. Gynec.*, **98**, 1050–1056

WALTERS, W.A.W. and LIM, Y.L. (1969). Cardiovascular dynamics in women receiving oral contraceptive therapy. *Lancet*, **ii**, 879–881

WALTERS, W.A.W. and LIM, Y.L. (1970). Haemodynamic changes in women taking oral contraceptives. *J. Obstet. Gynaec. Br. Commonw.*, **77**, 1007–1012

WARREN, R.J. and FOTHERBY, K. (1973). Plasma levels of ethinyloestradiol after administration of ethinyloestradiol or mestranol to human subjects. *J. Endocr.*, **59**, 369–370

WATSON, P.E. and ROBINSON, M.F. (1965). Variations in body-weight of young women during the menstrual cycle. *Br. J. Nutr.*, **19**, 237–248

WYNN, V., ADAMS, P., OAKLEY, N. and SEED, M. (1974). Metabolic investigations in women taking 30 μg ethinyloestradiol plus 150 μg d-norgestrel. *The Second International Norgestrel Symposium. Some Metabolic Considerations of Oral Contraceptive Usage*, pp. 47–57. Excerpta Medica, Amsterdam

WYNN, V. and DOAR, J.W.H. (1969). Some effects of oral contraceptives on carbohydrate metabolism. *Lancet*, **ii**, 761–765

WYNN, V. and DOAR, J.W.H. (1970). Effects of oral contraceptives on carbohydrate metabolism. *J. clin. Path.*, **23**, supplement 3, 19–36

YEN, S.S.C. and VELA, P. (1968). Effects of contraceptive steroids on carbohydrate metabolism. *J. clin. Endocr. Metab.*, **28**, 1564–1570

YGGE, J., BRODY, S., KORSAN-BENGTSEN, K. and NILSSON, L. (1969). Changes in blood coagulation and fibrinolysis in women receiving oral contraceptives. *Am. J. Obstet. Gynec.*, **104**, 87–98

ZALDÍVAR, A. and GALLEGOS, A.J. (1971). Metabolism and tissue localisation of (14–15^{3}H) d-norgestrel in the human. *Contraception*, **4**, 169–182

ZAÑARTU, J., PUPKIN, M., ROSENBERG, D., GUERRERO, R., RODRIGUEZ-BRAVO, R., GARCIA-HUIDOBRO, M. and PUGA, J.A. (1968). Effect of oral continuous progestagen therapy in micro-dosage on human ovary and sperm transport. *Br. med. J.*, **ii**, 266–269

ZAÑARTU, J., DABANCENS, A., OBERTI, C., RODRIGUEZ-BRAVO, R. and GARCIA-HUIDOBRO, M. (1974). Low-dosage oral progestagens to control fertility. *Obstet. Gynec., N.Y.*, **43**, 87–96

ZILVA, J.F. and PATSTON, V.J. (1966). Variations in serum-iron in healthy women. *Lancet*, **i**, 459–462

ZINNEMAN, H.H., MUSA, B. and DOE, R.P. (1965). Changes in plasma and urinary amino acids following estrogen administration to males. *Metabolism*, **14**, 1214–1219

ZUSSMAN, W.V., FORBES, D.A. and CARPENTER, R.J. (1967). Ovarian morphology following cyclic norethindrone-mestranol therapy. *Am. J. Obstet. Gynec.*, **99**, 99–105

3 Combined Oral Contraceptives

COMPOSITION OF PREPARATIONS

Oestrogens

The oestrogen component of the combined pill is either ethinyloestradiol or its 3-methyl ether derivative mestranol (*Table 3.1*). The dose of oestrogen used was often 100 μg until the possible association between the use of oestrogen-containing oral contraceptives and thrombo-embolism was established. The Committee on Safety of Medicines in Great Britain then advised that 50 μg should be the dose of oestrogen used. The value of this reduction in dose has been reinforced by the confirmation that other metabolic side-effects of the combined pill are dependent on oestrogen dose. More recently preparations have been marketed containing only 20–30 μg of oestrogen (Eugynon 30, Loestrin 20, Loestrin 1.5/30, Lo-ovral, Microgynon 30, Ovamin 30, Ovran 30, Ovranette and Zorane 1.5/30 and 1/20) in combination with the most potent progestagen available, norgestrel, or with norethisterone. Brevicon, Modicon, Neocon and Ovcon 35 contain 35 μg of ethinyloestradiol. More preparations contain ethinyloestradiol than mestranol, because of its reputedly greater effectiveness. Seventy to eighty per cent of mestranol is converted in the body into ethinyloestradiol.

There are still some oral contraceptives available that contain more than 50 μg of oestrogen. These are Conovid (Enovid), Conovid E (Enovid-E), Demulen, Norinyl 1+80, Norquen, Oracon, Oracon-28, Ortho-novin 1/80 (Ortho-novum 1/80), Ortho-novin 2 mg, and Ovulen 1 mg (Ovulen-21 and -28).

Progestagens

The 19-nortestosterone derivatives are the more commonly used type of progestagens, norethisterone (norethindrone) being the most popular. Preparations containing norethisterone are Anovlar 21 (4 mg), Gynovlar 21 (3 mg), Norlestrin 2.5 mg, Ortho-novin (Ortho-novum) 2 mg, Loestrin 1.5/30 and Zorane 1.5/30. Brevicon, Con-Fer, Loestrin 20, Minovlar, Minovlar ED, Neocon, Norinyl-1, Normyl 1/28 and 1/50, Norlestrin 1/50, Ovcon 50, Orlest 21, Ortho-novin 1/50 and 1/80 (Ortho-novum 1/50 and 1/80) and Zorane 1/50 and 1/20, all contain 1 mg of norethisterone or its acetate. Brevinor (Ovysmen)

Table 3.1 COMPOSITION OF COMBINED OESTROGEN–PROGESTAGEN ORAL CONTRACEPTIVES

U.K. proprietary name	U.S. proprietary name	Oestrogen component		Progestagen component	
ANOVLAR 21	—	Ethinyloestradiol	50 µg	Norethisterone acetate	4 mg
BREVINOR (see OVYSMEN)	—	Ethinyloestradiol	35 µg	Norethisterone	0.5 mg
CON-FER	NORLESTRIN Fe 1 mg	Ethinyloestradiol	50 µg	Norethisterone acetate	1 mg
CONOVA 30	—	Ethinyloestradiol	30 µg	Ethynodiol diacetate	2 mg
CONOVID	ENOVID 5	Mestranol	75 µg	Norethynodrel	5 mg
CONOVID-E	ENOVID E	Mestranol	100 µg	Norethynodrel	2.5 mg
DEMULEN	—	Mestranol	100 µg	Ethynodiol diacetate	0.5 mg
DEMULEN 50	—	Ethinyloestradiol	50 µg	Ethynodiol diacetate	0.5 mg
EUGYNON 30 (see OVRAN 30)	—	Ethinyloestradiol	30 µg	Levonorgestrel	0.25 mg
EUGYNON 50	—	Ethinyloestradiol	50 µg	Levonorgestrel	0.25 mg
GYNOVLAR 21	—	Ethinyloestradiol	50 µg	Norethisterone acetate	3 mg
LOESTRIN 20	LOESTRIN 1/20	Ethinyloestradiol	20 µg	Norethisterone acetate	1 mg
MICROGYNON 30 (OVRANETTE)	—	Ethinyloestradiol	30 µg	Levonorgestrel	0.15 mg
MINILYN	—	Ethinyloestradiol	50 µg	Lynoestrenol	2.5 mg
MINOVLAR	—	Ethinyloestradiol	50 µg	Norethisterone acetate	1 mg
MINOVLAR ED	—	Ethinyloestradiol	50 µg	Norethisterone acetate	1 mg
NORIMIN	—	Ethinyloestradiol	35 µg	Norethisterone	1 mg
NORINYL–1	NORINYL 1 + 50/21	Mestranol	50 µg	Norethisterone	1 mg
NORINYL 1/28	NORINYL 1 + 50/28	Mestranol	50 µg	Norethisterone	1 mg
NORINYL–2	—	Mestranol	100 µg	Norethisterone	2 mg

		Estrogen		Progestogen	
NORLESTRIN	NORLESTRIN 2.5 21	Ethinyloestradiol	50 µg	Norethisterone acetate	2.5 mg
ORLEST 21	NORLESTRIN 1.0 21	Ethinyloestradiol	50 µg	Norethisterone acetate	1 mg
ORTHO-NOVIN 1/50	ORTHONOVUM 1/50	Mestranol	50 µg	Norethisterone	1 mg
ORTHO-NOVIN 1/80	ORTHONOVUM 1/80	Mestranol	80 µg	Norethisterone	1 mg
ORTHO-NOVIN 2 mg	ORTHONOVUM 2	Mestranol	100 µg	Norethisterone	2 mg
OVAMIN 30	—	Ethinyloestradiol	30 µg	Ethynodiol diacetate	2 mg
OVRAN	OVRAL	Ethinyloestradiol	50 µg	Levonorgestrel	0.25 mg
OVRAN 30 (see EUGYNON 30)	—	Ethinyloestradiol	30 µg	Levonorgestrel	0.25 mg
OVRANETTE (MICROGYNON 30)	LO-OVRAL	Ethinyloestradiol	30 µg	Levonorgestrel	0.15 mg
OVULEN 50	DEMULEN	Ethinyloestradiol	50 µg	Ethynodiol diacetate	1 mg
OVULEN 1 mg	—	Mestranol	100 µg	Ethynodiol diacetate	1 mg
OVYSMEN (see BREVINOR)	—	Ethinyloestradiol	35 µg	Norethisterone	0.5 mg
—	BREVICON, MODICON	Ethinyloestradiol	35 µg	Norethisterone acetate	0.5 mg
—	LOESTRIN 21 1.5/30	Ethinyloestradiol	30 µg	Norethisterone acetate	1.5 mg
—	NEOCON	Ethinyloestradiol	35 µg	Norethisterone	1 mg
—	NORQUEN	Ethinyloestradiol	80 µg	Norethisterone acetate	2 mg
—	ORACON	Ethinyloestradiol	100 µg	Dimethisterone	25 mg
—	OVCON 35	Ethinyloestradiol	35 µg	Norethisterone	0.4 mg
—	OVCON 50, ZORANE 1/50	Ethinyloestradiol	50 µg	Norethisterone	1.0 mg
—	ZORANE 1.5/30	Ethinyloestradiol	30 µg	Norethisterone acetate	1.5 mg
—	ZORANE 1/20	Ethinyloestradiol	20 µg	Norethisterone acetate	1 mg

and Brevicon (Modicon) contain only 0.5 mg, and Ovcon 35 only 0.4 mg of norethisterone.

Other 19-nortestosterone derivatives used are ethynodiol, lynoestrenol, norethynodrel, and norgestrel. Ethynodiol diacetate is used in a dose of 0.5 mg in Demulen 50; Ovamin contains 2 mg; Ovulen 1 mg and Ovulen 50 each contain 1 mg lynoestrenol, 2.5 mg, is in Lyndiol 2.5 mg and Minilyn. Norethynodrel is in the two preparations related to the original contraceptive pill tried out 20 years ago, Conovid (5 mg) and Conovid E (2.5 mg). Norgestrel, of which only the *d*-isomer (levonorgestrel) is active, is used in the small dose of 0.25 mg in Eugynon 30 and 50, and in Ovral, Ovran and Ovran 30. This dose has been reduced to 0.15 mg of *dl*-norgestrel or 0.075 mg of levonorgestrel in the preparations Microgynon 30 and Ovranette.

The recently available combined oral contraceptives containing a 17α-hydroxyprogesterone derivative, megestrol, were Serial 28 (1 mg) and Volidan 21 (4 mg). These have been withdrawn from the market in Great Britain and the United States of America because of the association of megestrol with an increased incidence of breast lumps in beagles. Dimethisterone, a 17β-hydroxy-progesterone derivative, is used in Oracon.

Certain preparations contain 21 active pills and seven placebo tablets. In Great Britain these are Con-Fer, which contains seven tablets of ferrous fumarate 75 mg, and Minovlar ED, which contains seven inert lactose tablets. In the United States of America there are a number of similar preparations, denoted by the suffix '-28'.

Mode of Action

The mode of action of the combined pill is threefold: inhibition of ovulation, effects on the endometrium, and effects on the cervical mucus. The principal mode of action is inhibition of ovulation. With currently available pills with a low content of steroid, there seems to be no effect on spermatozoal penetration in cervical mucus (Ansbacher and Campbell, 1971).

Inhibition of Ovulation

Klopper (1970) suggested that the hypothalamic centres are unable to differen-tiate between naturally occurring steroids and those in oral contraceptives. Patients taking oral contraceptives maintain constant low plasma levels of oest-radiol and progesterone, similar to those found in the proliferative phase of the cycle (Briggs and Briggs, 1972; Kjeld *et al.,* 1976) and this may alter the mecha-nism controlling the gonadotrophin releasing factors and hence the release of the appropriate gonadotrophins from the pituitary gland. Production of FSH and LH is then minimal and the peaks of secretion necessary for ovulation to take place are abolished. Cargille and Ross (1968) showed that plasma FSH peaks are reduced in women treated with Enovid E, while Taymor (1964), Brown *et al.* (1964) and Thomas and Ferin (1972) found that combined oral contraceptives eliminate the mid cycle LH peak. The actual reduction in gonado-trophin levels varies according to the amounts of progestagen and oestrogen mixture administered and the duration of treatment.

The oestrogen in the oral contraceptive is responsible for reducing the FSH levels. The dose is important, because although 80 μg of ethinyloestradiol will inhibit ovulation the same daily dose of mestranol alone is inadequate for this purpose (Eckstein *et al.*, 1961; Jackson *et al.*, 1968). The effective dose of oestrogen depends on the amount and type of progestagen with which it is combined.

The pre-ovulatory LH surge is thought to be triggered off by rapidly rising plasma oestrogen, the major component of which is 17β-oestradiol secreted by the theca interna cells of the developing follicle. By suppressing the levels of oestradiol to those of the mid follicular phase of the menstrual cycle, the oral contraceptive steroids eliminate the normal mid cycle 17β-oestradiol peak, and consequently the peak of LH secretion.

Long-term studies by Goldzieher (1970a) showed that seven years of combined oral contraceptive therapy suppressed plasma FSH levels to 70% and LH levels to 20–30% of control values, as well as eliminating the mid cycle peaks. The difference between follicular and luteal phase levels of FSH and LH was preserved. Three months after stopping the combined pill the gonadotrophin levels were again within the normal range.

The abolition of FSH and LH peaks and the diminution in their overall production leads to minimal ovarian activity and failure of follicular maturation. Ovarian steroid production is reduced to levels consistent with the early follicular phase. The exogenous oestrogen and progestagen serve to develop and maintain the uterus and other target organs and thus withdrawal bleeding occurs at the end of the course of tablets. Further evidence of the effectiveness of the combination of oral contraceptive steroids in inhibiting ovulation has come from findings at laparotomy. No corpora lutea were present in women on various preparations (Rock *et al.*, 1957; Ostergaard, 1964; Ostergaard and Starup, 1968). There is also good evidence that there is atresia of the follicles and fibrosis of the stroma (Zussman *et al.*, 1967) in women taking combined oral contraceptives. The cyclical use of oral contraceptives prevents not only ovulation and corpus luteum formation but also inhibits maturation of follicles, which remain quiescent and undergo atresia. Diminished FSH levels are responsible for this minimal follicular growth and absence of maturation.

CLINICAL MANAGEMENT

Initial Prescription

An adequate history should be taken and a complete physical examination performed before prescribing the combined oral contraceptive pill. Menstrual and obstetric histories should be recorded. Questions relating to the patient's past medical history are necessary with particular reference to possible episodes of thrombosis or embolism, hypertension, liver disease, abnormal carbohydrate metabolism and depression. The patient should be examined with particular attention to detecting hypertension, heart disease or gynaecological disorders, and a cervical smear should be taken for cytological examination. If the patient has any history suggesting that she might be a potential or latent diabetic an oral glucose tolerance test should be performed; if she has been jaundiced liver function tests should be carried out.

Should there be no medical contra-indications then the combined oral contraceptive pill can be prescribed. Administration should commence on Day 5 of the next menstrual cycle, and one tablet taken daily for the next 21 days. The tablet should be taken at approximately the same time each day. The actual time is not important but regular consumption of the pill is useful as an *aide-mémoire* and is necessary to inhibit the natural cyclical hormonal pattern consistently. This is especially important with the low-dose preparations when even a few hours' lapse may alter the blood levels of gonadotrophins and allow ovulation to occur. If a tablet is forgotten, it should be taken as soon as possible the next day, in addition to that day's tablet taken at the usual time; additional contraceptive precautions are advisable.

After completing the course of 21 tablets the patient should not take tablets for the next seven days and then, irrespective of the presence or absence of vaginal bleeding, she should recommence the next cycle of 21 pills. The patient should in general not require additional protection during the first pill cycle but many practitioners advise extra precautions. It is possible to commence oral contraception a few days later than Day 5 of the menstrual cycle. The patient can discard the appropriate number of pills, or, if she takes the full 21 day course, menstruation will tend to adjust to correspond with the 'pill cycle' over the first month or two. Because ovulation may have taken place before or soon after commencement of pill therapy, contraceptive protection must then not be assumed until the second cycle of pills.

It is important that if preparations (Con-Fer and Minovlar ED) which contain seven placebo tablets are prescribed the need to take them in the correct sequence is explained.

At the time of the initial prescription patients may be warned of the possible occurrence of mild side-effects such as nausea, weight gain and mastalgia. They should be told that these symptoms, if they occur, usually disappear progressively over the first three cycles, and that they should not stop taking the pill unless symptoms are severe. The patients should also be told that any slight or moderate vaginal bleeding during a course of tablets should be ignored, and that they should continue to take the pill. Failure to inform patients of this is one of the commonest causes of patient failure with the combined oral contraceptives. Breakthrough bleeding towards the end of the course is commonest during the early cycles of therapy and tends to resolve spontaneously. If intermenstrual bleeding or other side-effects persist then a change of preparation may be necessary after three cycles.

There is undoubtedly a psychological element in the aetiology of mild symptoms that occur soon after starting a combined pill. Garcia (1974) gave either an oestrogen, a progestagen, an oestrogen—progestagen combination or a placebo to women who had been fitted with an intra-uterine device. They were not told that these preparations had any contraceptive effect. During the first three months he found that the group taking the placebo had the highest incidence of mild clinical side-effects. During the second three months the group on the combined pill had the highest residual incidence of mild side-effects.

Which Preparation Should Be Prescribed Initially?

For the reliable patient who will take her pills regularly it is probably wisest to start with one of the low-dose preparations containing only 30 μg of oestrogen.

The patient should be warned about breakthrough bleeding and spotting which occur in between 10 and 15% of patients (Garcia, 1974). If these symptoms persist then a higher dose preparation is necessary. Dickey and Dorr (1969) suggested that oral contraceptives could be divided into predominantly oestrogenic and predominantly progestagenic groups, and that the cause of their side-effects was a relative excess or deficiency of oestrogen or progestagen. There is little scientific evidence for such a theory.

There are certain clinical guide lines to correct prescription which should be followed. For example, a woman who had a large weight gain during a previous pregnancy undoubtedly needs a low-dose pill. A young woman who has scanty periods should not be given a strongly progestagenic pill containing 4 mg norethisterone such as Anovlar as this may be more likely to induce post-pill amenorrhoea. A woman who has been depressed should be on a low-dose pill if possible and not on one that contains a high dose of progestagen.

The preparation most likely to be satisfactory is the one that suits the patient's next door neighbour, sister or mother!

Subsequent Management

Once the patient is established on a suitable oral contraceptive she should be encouraged not to change. An initial check-up should be carried out after three to six months. Details of the menstrual cycle and of any side-effects should be reviewed. The patient should be weighed and her blood pressure recorded.

A repeat oral glucose tolerance test should be carried out on any patient who previously had a factor in her history suggesting a potential for developing diabetes mellitus, even though the 'pre-pill' test was normal. Liver function tests should be repeated in any patient who has a past history of jaundice.

Thereafter, visits may be annual, and the same procedure is repeated. Cervical cytology should be performed annually. In the absence of symptoms there is no reason to stop the pill at any time for a 'rest'. This has not been shown to have any beneficial effects and the risk of pregnancy is considerable even when the patient is advised about alternative contraception.

Changing Pills

The patient should be encouraged to put up with mild side-effects such as nausea, mastalgia or breakthrough bleeding for a short time, as these are so common during the first few cycles and will probably disappear. A change of preparation should be contemplated if unwanted effects are severe and prolonged. A woman who has developed considerable nausea or acute weight gain may benefit from a pill containing less oestrogen. Chronic weight gain suggests the need for a lower dose preparation to reduce the water-retaining and anabolic effects of the steroids.

Scanty periods whilst on the pill reflect an endometrium that has become atrophic because of the effects of the combination of oestrogen and progestagen, with an excessive dominance of particularly the 19-nortestosterone progestagens. This reduction in bleeding has become much less common as the dose of steroids in the combined pill has been progressively reduced. It does not necessarily herald post-pill amenorrhoea although the state of the endometrium may be a minor factor in the aetiology of this condition. Very scanty periods are not an absolute indication to change preparations. On the other hand the cautious practitioner may well decide to use a pill with a lower progestagen content in the young woman whose future fertility is of great importance.

When a progressive diminution in menstrual flow proceeds to amenorrhoea lasting more than two months some physicians feel there is a significant risk of post-pill amenorrhoea, and discontinue the oral contraceptive until menstruation returns. Although barrier methods may be advised meanwhile, a proportion of unwanted pregnancies arise from this procedure. Should menstruation not return, or the situation recur with a pill of different composition, full investigation for the causes of post-pill amenorrhoea should be conducted.

Persistent breakthrough bleeding necessitates a change to a higher dose of cyclical steroids. Initially the progestagen content should be increased and the oestrogen content kept at $50\,\mu g$ or below. Breakthrough bleeding is due to an oestrogen effect unbalanced by adequate progestagen or to a dose of the combined steroids which is inadequate to maintain endometrial development.

Depression and loss of libido are sometimes alleviated by changing to a pill containing less progestagen but these symptoms may be helped by any change of composition of the pill. The mode of action may involve a reduction in circulating 5-hydroxytryptamine due to induced alterations in tryptophan metabolism. Pyridoxine supplements sometimes help.

The more subtle variations in symptomatology are less likely to be affected by changing from one preparation to another and are more likely to be affected by the psychological impact of the change itself.

THE FAILURES – OUTCOME OF PREGNANCY

It has been assumed for years that in the rare event of a patient taking an oestrogen–progestagen oral contraceptive becoming pregnant, the pregnancy, confinement and the baby are all normal. In the Royal College of General Practitioners' Oral Contraception Study (1976) there were 102 women who continued taking the pill after conception and went to term. Only one baby had congenital abnormalities; one other had a congenital dislocation of the hip. There is thus no suggestion of any teratogenic effect in this study but it does not exclude the possibility of causation of low-incidence abnormalities.

There is reason to believe that the administration of an oestrogen–progestagen complex in the first trimester as an 'oral pregnancy test' may be associated with the production of a small number of congenitally abnormal babies (Gal *et al.*, 1967; Nora and Nora, 1973; Janerich *et al.*, 1974; Greenberg *et al.*, 1975; Nora and Nora, 1975; Janerich *et al.*, 1977). There is some evidence of an even smaller risk with respect to inadvertent pregnancy occurring in patients taking oral contraceptives. Janerich *et al.* (1974) studied case records of 108 patients who had delivered babies with limb reduction defects in New York State. Six had become pregnant whilst taking a combined pill and in each case the affected child was male. Only one patient in a matched control series of 108 mothers with normal babies had become pregnant on the pill. Nora and Nora (1975) found a similar correlation between limb and associated vertebral cardiac, gastro-intestinal and renal anomalies. Janerich *et al.* (1977) found only two infants whose mothers had continued to take the pill after conception amongst 104 infants with congenital heart disease.

What then is the risk to a woman who becomes pregnant whilst taking a combined oral contraceptive that her baby will be abnormal? Judging from the Royal College of General Practitioners' (1976) report the risk is under 2% and does not differ significantly from the risk in any pregnancy. In these circumstances we would not feel that in Great Britain there is a case for terminating the pregnancy under the Abortion Act, 1967, which specifies 'a substantial risk that if the child were born it would suffer from such physical or mental abnormalities as to be seriously handicapped' as a legal ground for therapeutic abortion. In Great Britain, the physician must now bear in mind the provisions of the Congenital Disabilities (Civil Liability) Act, 1976, but this specifies that the physician is not answerable if he took reasonable care having due regard to the 'then received professional opinion applicable to the particular class of case'. In the absence of a demonstrable difference in prognosis for the baby of a patient who becomes pregnant on the pill, it should be accepted as customary practice to advise continuation of the pregnancy.

STOPPING THE PILL

Pregnancy

In general, the time women take to conceive after ceasing oral contraception is a little longer than that after ceasing other contraceptive procedures (Vessey *et al.,* 1978). Nonetheless, including those who have secondary amenorrhoea due to the pill, and those with other undiagnosed causes of infertility, 80% of non-parous and 90% of parous women will have conceived within one year of stopping the pill (Goldheizer, 1970a; Royal College of General Practitioners' Oral Contraception Study, 1974). The duration of previous oral contraceptive therapy has no general effect on the return of fertility sufficient to be reflected in statistics on an unselected population. It has been suggested that fertility is enhanced in some women after stopping the pill because of a rebound increase in gonadotrophin levels once the inhibiting effect of the contraceptive steroids is removed. There is no valid evidence to substantiate this.

There is often a delay of a few days and sometimes of a few weeks in the resumption of spontaneous menstruation. This is commonly associated with late or absent ovulation in the first cycle and it is not unusual for several menstrual cycles to occur before ovulation is resumed.

Secondary amenorrhoea is an occasional sequel to the use of the combined pill, particularly after prolonged administration. Many cases resolve spontaneously in a few months but amenorrhoea persisting more than a year after stopping the pill may not be amenable to therapy with clomiphene or gonadotrophins (Shearman, 1975).

Most authorities feel that pregnancy occurring after stopping the pill is no more likely to end in abortion than pregnancy occurring at any other time (Peterson, 1969; Robinson, 1971). The Royal College of General Practitioners' Oral Contraception Study (1974) found that in women who stopped the pill specifically to become pregnant, 13% of the subsequent pregnancies ended in abortion. The overall incidence of spontaneous abortion in Great Britain is 10—15%. When the pill was stopped for another reason, for example symptomatic side-effects or a medical contra-indication such as hypertension, the incidence of abortion was 30%. This may be primarily attributable to the conditions predisposing to cessation of oral contraception, but doubtless some of the pregnancies were unwanted and abortion was induced.

There is to date no valid evidence that oral contraceptives can cause any alterations in the patient's chromosomes or in those of the fetus in subsequent pregnancies, although there have been a number of studies directed to this issue. On the basis of general population statistics, the incidence of stillbirth, multiple births or fetal congenital abnormalities in subsequent pregnancies does not seem to be increased among previous pill users. On the other hand, conception within a month or two of ceasing to take oral contraceptives can give rise to uncertainty of the maturity of the pregnancy and complicate the management of a high-risk pregnancy. Ultrasonic dating of the pregnancy in the first trimester may reduce the chance of error. Until accurate measurements of this type are widely available patients with predictable high-risk situations are well advised to use barrier contraception until there is evidence of regular ovulatory cycles. Otherwise there is a distinct risk that premature labour may be induced unexpectedly and a perinatal death can result. This may be the factor that led to neonatal jaundice being reported as being associated with previous maternal use of oral contraceptives. The association has not been confirmed in a subsequent study where this effect was controlled (Gould *et al.*, 1974).

It has been suggested in New York State that there may be an association between the recent use of oral contraceptives and congenital limb reduction defects. The work is based on retrospective surveys with all their difficulties, including that of the biased recall of mothers of abnormal babies. Limb reduction defects are a relatively rare malformation whose incidence in New York State (0.25 per 1000 births in 1973) has been rising in parallel with increased use of oral contraceptives. Janerich *et al.* (1974) found that an increased proportion of mothers of babies with the defect had discontinued oral contraception in the cycle immediately before conception compared with control series. This may be linked with the 'aging ovum' situation. Ovulation may be delayed in the first cycle and conception late in the cycle has been linked with congenital abnormalities (Cross, 1961; Iffy, 1963; Hertig and Shea, 1967). The association has not been confirmed in Great Britain (Royal College of General Practitioners' Oral Contraception Study, 1976). There might be a case for advising 'high-risk' patients to avoid conception in the first one or two post-pill cycles; at least this would make it easier for the obstetrician to assess the maturity of the pregnancy accurately.

Surgery

Major surgery alters the coagulation—fibrinolytic system in favour of coagulation, and so does the oestrogen-containing pill. During surgery there is venous stasis, particularly in the deep veins of the leg, and this together with the increased coagulation tendency, increases the risk of thrombosis occurring during the operation and of postoperative thrombo-embolism. Oral contraception should be stopped six weeks before elective major surgery. Stopping the combined pill is unnecessary before minor procedures such as laparoscopy or dilation and curettage. Emergency surgery is carried out on many women on the combined pill with no ill effects. Where surgery is urgent and there are no additional factors predisposing to thrombosis and no postoperative complications, anticoagulation is not advised, but intravenous infusions of dextran (molecular weight 70 000) in a dose of 500 ml/24 h for two days during and after the operation and the use of elastic stockings will minimise the risk of thrombus formation. Early ambulation should be encouraged and a careful watch kept for the development of deep vein thrombosis. Patients with postoperative pelvic infection, with its risk of pelvic vein thrombosis should have both antibiotic and anticoagulant therapy with low-dose subcutaneous heparin or warfarin.

The Over 40's

Although oral contraceptives are more commonly used by younger women, there are now many users of the pill who are over 40 years of age. The advantages of continuing after this age are that it is an easy and effective contraceptive method to which the individual may have become accustomed. The disadvantages are that as the woman gets older so the risks of metabolic side-effects rise. In particular, the risks of thrombo-embolism (Inman and Vessey, 1968) and coronary thrombosis (Mann *et al.,* 1975) rise significantly. The greater the number of years for which the patient has taken the pill, the greater the risk of developing many of the complications such as diabetes mellitus, hypertension and gallstones.

It is reasonable to continue the pill in this age group if the patient does not smoke, is not obese, hypertensive or hyperlipidaemic, and feels strongly that the benefits to her outweigh the increased risks. If a combined pill containing 50 µg or more of oestrogen is being used it is advantageous to try changing to a preparation with only 30 µg of oestrogen. Pregnancy in this age group also carries increased risks but as fertility is declining other methods of contraception are relatively more effective. The patient may wish to continue to take the pill until the age when the menopause normally occurs. Whether or not she has ceased to menstruate may be determined by stopping the pill, with use of a barrier contraceptive as a temporary precaution.

The Menopause

Once the menopause has been reached the advantages of continuing to take a low-oestrogen pill for some time are that it prevents the changes that occur due to the reduction of endogenous oestrogen production. The vasomotor instability, atrophic vaginitis, atrophy of the breasts, general depression and loss of libido associated with the menopause may not occur if administration of the pill is continued. Oestrogen administration must be commenced during the first six years of the menopause in order to prevent a small and currently unpredictable number of women developing irreversible bone decalcification. If oestrogens are given within two months of bilateral oophorectomy bone changes do not occur, while administration during the first three years after the menopause leads to a significant improvement in the mineral content of bone (Aitken *et al.,* 1973).

The disadvantages of providing menopausal hormone replacement therapy by means of the combined oral contraceptives are the increased risk of metabolic side-effects, deep venous thrombosis, pulmonary embolism and coronary thrombosis, attributed principally to the oestrogen component. For this reason it has been suggested that oestrogens other than ethinyloestradiol, oestradiol valerate for example, should be used, but there is no good evidence that these oestrogens convey any less risk.

If the combined pill is to be used to attenuate the effects of the menopause it is essential that clinical examinations with urine testing and blood pressure measurements are carried out every six months; annual glucose tolerance tests are desirable.

Before menstruation has ceased, the use of oestrogens alone, even cyclically, to relieve climacteric symptoms is not uncommonly followed by menstrual irregularity. A combined pill does not usually have this effect unless there is underlying uterine pathology. Furthermore, cyclical administration of oestrogen combined with a progestagen should minimise the chance of development of endometrial hyperplasia or carcinoma.

After the menopause it is our experience that the development of bleeding with continuous administration of oestrogen alone is rare in the absence of uterine pathology, provided that the dose is sufficiently small (ethinyloestradiol $10-30\,\mu g$ daily). Retrospective studies have indicated an association between the effects of certain oestrogens, particularly conjugated oestrone, and the subsequent development of endometrial carcinoma (Ziel and Finkle, 1976). These studies were poorly controlled and factors such as the dose and duration of therapy and the presence or absence of obesity were not adequately considered. It has previously been suggested that the direct protective effect of progestagens and the cyclical bleeding induced by a combined pill render it unlikely to cause endometrial hyperplasia or carcinoma.

There would appear to be no good case for using the combined pill as replacement therapy after the menopause, because of its metabolic side-effects. On the other hand low-oestrogen pills administered cyclically may occasionally be the answer when oestrogen alone fails to resolve menopausal symptoms. We have seen a few cases where loss of libido appeared to respond to this manoeuvre.

CLINICAL SIDE-EFFECTS OF THE COMBINED PILL

Clinical evidence indicates that the incidence and intensity of some side-effects of combined oral contraceptive pills are proportional to the dose of drug ingested. The dose of oestrogen in the combined pills is usually $50\,\mu g$ of either ethinyloestradiol or mestranol. The pharmacological and biological activities of the progestagens vary so that assessing a preparation on the basis of the actual weight of progestagen is misleading. Side-effects attributed by some to oestrogen excess are nausea, headaches, dizziness, fluid retention and hence acute weight gain, breast congestion, hypertension, and mucus discharge. Symptoms sometimes attributed to progestagens are progressive weight gain, tiredness, depression and decreased libido. Side-effects related to relative progestagen excess are said to increase with prolonged treatment (Dickey and Dorr, 1969). If patients present with obvious side-effects relating to excess of steroid then the pill may be altered to one with less oestrogen or less progestagen according to the side-effects. According to Dickey and Dorr (1969) an indication of progestagen requirements is the length of menstruation: amenorrhoea and hypomenorrhoea being signs of excessive progestagen administration and hypermenorrhoea indicating a relative lack of progestagen.

Effect on Lactation

Combined oral contraception, initiated whilst a patient is breast-feeding her baby, may inhibit or suppress lactation. In addition it is possible that steroid metabolites pass into breast-milk and could perhaps affect the baby. Most authorities consider that alternative contraception should be used until such time as breast-feeding is discontinued. Fertility is much reduced during lactation and barrier methods or a low-dose progestagen should give adequate protection.

Irregular Bleeding

Menstrual cycles are usually regular with combined oral contraceptives and were better still with sequential preparations. There is considerable variation between patients and also between preparations, depending on their hormone content. The contraceptives containing a relatively high dose of progestagen tend to produce an atrophic endometrium and there is a low incidence of breakthrough bleeding. The 20 μg and 30 μg oestrogen pills give a higher incidence of breakthrough bleeding than most combined pills. When low doses of both oestrogen and progestagen are used, cycles of amenorrhoea followed by breakthrough bleeding can occur, perhaps related to occasional ovulatory cycles. Sequential tablets produced a marked proliferative response due to the administration of oestrogen alone for 16 days, and a short secretory phase when the progestagen was added. In general the administration of higher dose and strongly progestagenic combined preparations will reduce or remove the problem of breakthrough bleeding.

Breakthrough bleeding is commoner during the first few cycles of use, with an incidence of anything from 10 to 15% during the first cycle, reducing to about 5% during the third and subsequent cycles. If a patient has been taking an oral contraceptive for some time without breakthrough bleeding and then develops intermenstrual bleeding, this must not be attributed to the oral contraceptive before a diagnostic curettage has been carried out to exclude organic causes. Out-patient curettage (Holt, 1970) is sometimes appropriate.

Headache

This can be due to several factors. If it occurs during the treatment cycle it is possibly due to oestrogen excess; during the pill-free interval it may be due to progestagen withdrawal or fluctuations in oestrogen levels (Heber, 1974).

The oral contraceptives may also precipitate typical migraine. Grant (1968) found an association between the occurrence of headaches and the degree of development of endometrial arterioles, postulating that this may be evidence of a generalised vascular change related to the oestrogen/progestagen ratio. Migrainous headaches may precede cerebro-vascular accidents occurring in association with oral contraception.

Hypertension

It is established that an increase in blood pressure, albeit minor in most cases, can develop in a small proportion of women on combined oral contraceptives (Laragh *et al.,* 1967; Woods, 1967; Loudon and Burton, 1969; Laragh, 1971; Crane *et al.,* 1971). In the majority of women who develop this relatively rare side-effect, the blood pressure returns to normal if the pill is discontinued. Chidell (1970) found that approximately 1% of normotensive patients became mildly hypertensive whilst on the pill, but that the elevated blood pressure returned to normal soon after the oral contraceptive was stopped. The Royal College of General Practitioners' Oral Contraception Study (1974) confirmed the 1% incidence in the first year but found that by the fifth year of use hypertension was likely to be two to three times more common than this. The likelihood of hypertension was directly related to the age of the patient but not to her parity. Other workers have found an incidence as high as 18% (Saruta *et al.,* 1970), and Weir *et al.* (1971) reported that 50 out of 66 patients had a mean rise in systolic blood pressure of 6.6 mm Hg but that there was no rise in diastolic blood pressure. Although the mean increases in blood pressure are small a few patients have developed significant hypertension whilst on combined oral contraceptives. One such case has been reported (Zech *et al.,* 1975) in whom malignant hypertension with irreversible renal failure followed combined oral contraceptive therapy. In interpreting such reports the natural history of essential hypertension must be borne in mind. This is a disease with a strong familial element, and there are well authenticated cases in whom a transient cause of hypertension has precipitated the development of progressive hypertension in previously normotensive individuals. It is desirable to recheck the blood pressure of all women starting on a combined pill within a few months, and to monitor the blood pressure of patients with a relevant family history closely, even though Weir *et al.* (1971) were unable to demonstrate that the incidence of hypertension due to combined oral contraceptives was related to a family history of the disease.

The onset of hypertension is sometimes associated with the carpal tunnel syndrome and has been thought to be due to the oestrogen component of the combined oral contraceptive (Sabour and Fadel, 1971). Weir *et al.* (1970) and Crane *et al.* (1971) found a rise in plasma renin substrate concentration in some women on the combined oral contraceptive. They thought that this was probably an oestrogen effect causing increased hepatic synthesis of the renin substrate. In the same women Weir *et al.* (1970) found a drop in plasma renin concentration and no consistent response in plasma aldosterone levels. None of the women in this small prospective study had developed hypertension. Despite raised plasma renin substrate concentrations, elevations of plasma renin and hypertension need not occur. These findings conflict with those of Newton *et al.* (1968) who recorded raised levels of plasma renin with an increased production of angiotensin, which normally feeds back to reduce the levels of renin. This feedback mechanism may be defective in patients who develop hypertension whilst on oestrogen-containing pills (Saruta *et al.*, 1970). Diffuse intravascular coagulation leading to intrarenal microthrombi obstructing the renal vessels has also been suggested as a possible cause of pill induced hypertension (Brown *et al.*, 1973). Neither the incidence of hypertension nor the duration of therapy necessary to produce hypertension in susceptible women is known, and the exact mechanism involved in its production is also.uncertain. It may be that the oestrogen stimulus to hepatic production of plasma renin substrates plays a part.

Crane *et al.* (1971) have another theory of the pathogenesis of hypertension due to oral contraceptives. They suggest that both the oestrogen which causes increased aldosterone production, and the synthetic progestagen which suppresses endogenous progesterone, encourage the retention of sodium and water. Recent evidence from the Royal College of General Practitioners' Oral Contraception Study (1974) suggests that norethisterone adds to any hypertensive effect of oestrogen.

The conclusion that can be drawn is that, as approximately 1% of patients may develop hypertension in their first year on the pill, all women commencing oral contraception should have their blood pressure checked at regular intervals, initially after three months and if normal then every six or twelve months.

In a study of 47 patients with a past history of pre-eclamptic toxaemia of pregnancy, Chidell (1970) was unable to demonstrate an association between the use of oral contraceptives and hypertension.

Leg Aches and Cramps

Some patients report aching in the calves and other leg muscles, which they associate with taking an oral contraceptive. Grant (1969) has found an association between this complaint and stromal condensation round endometrial sinusoids, suggesting that a similar phenomenon occurs in the leg veins. The symptom promotes anxiety about the potential for thrombosis, particularly if the patient has varicose veins. In the latter instance she should be sent for treatment of the veins. Otherwise, changing to a pill with a lower oestrogen content sometimes appears to relieve the symptoms. If the aches persist and attempts to reassure the patient are not completely successful, it may be as well to change to another method of contraception, even though the primary reason may merely be the anxieties of the physician and his patient.

Urinary Tract Infections

There is a slightly increased incidence of urinary infections in patients taking oral contraceptives; in most cases these infections are asymptomatic (Royal College of General Practitioners' Oral Contraception Study, 1974; Tagahashi and Loveland, 1974). The incidence of asymptomatic bacteriuria in oral contraceptive users has been found to be about 2.4%; annual screening by culture of a mid-stream urine may be considered desirable.

Skin Conditions

The Royal College of General Practitioners' Oral Contraception Study (1974) showed small increases in the incidence of photosensitivity, rosacea, eczema, chloasma, erythema multiforme and erythema nodosum in patients taking combined oral contraceptives. If a patient develops one of these conditions whilst taking the pill, or a previous skin condition is exacerbated, it is reasonable to discontinue this form of contraception.

The porphyrias are commonly thought to be 'oestrogen-sensitive'. The diagnosis may be suggested by a reaction to an oestrogen-containing oral contraceptive.

Acne or a tendency to develop sebaceous cysts may be relieved by oestrogen-containing oral contraceptives.

Other Disorders

The incidence of some other disorders was noted to be increased in the Royal College of General Practitioners' Oral Contraception Study (1974). Virus infections such as chicken-pox, gastro-enteritis, herpes simplex and rubella were a little more common in women using oral contraceptives. There were small increases in incidence of epilepsy, brachial neuritis and Raynaud's disease, but the numbers of cases of these conditions were small. There was an increase in the reporting of new cases of gallstones after three years of use of oral contraception, and this seemed to be related to dose of progestagen rather than oestrogen. The incidence of 'wax in the ears', of benign ovarian neoplasms and of rheumatoid arthritis (Wingrave, 1978) tends to be reduced in oral contraceptive patients.

Wearers of contact lenses may find that with some oral contraceptives fluid retention can distort the cornea causing difficulty in retaining the lenses and disturbance of vision.

PSYCHOLOGICAL SIDE-EFFECTS

The desire to reproduce has a very deep-seated emotional basis and the feeling of sterility which the use of oral contraceptives can induce in some women may well lead to a loss of femininity and libido, and to emotional confusion. In other patients, by removing the fear of pregnancy and by diminishing the incidence of menstrual symptoms, oral contraception can have a beneficial effect on a woman's psyche.

Physical effects of the pill which may give rise to beneficial psychological changes include a significant reduction in menstrual blood loss (Nilsson and Solvell, 1967) and of the symptoms associated with premenstrual tension (Goldzieher *et al.*, 1962; Moos, 1968). Dysmenorrhoea is also relieved in many patients (Rice-Wray *et al.*, 1962). These effects, together with the high contraceptive effectiveness of the combined pill can result in a feeling of freedom and reduced anxiety.

Physical side-effects that have an adverse effect on a woman's psychological adjustment to this form of contraception include nausea, headaches, lethargy and depression.

Nausea   This is frequently attributed to the combined oral contraceptive pill. Large doses of oestrogens undoubtedly cause nausea, but it is debatable whether the small doses of oestrogen currently used in combined oral contraceptives can cause significant nausea. The psychological effects of taking oral medication are sufficient to induce nausea during the first few months, and as the patient becomes accustomed to taking pills this symptom disappears (Garcia, 1974).

Loss of Libido   It has been suggested that this is due to the low oestrogen and high progestagen content of some preparations (Grant and Mears, 1967; Nilsson *et al.,* 1967). In contrast, prospective studies by Nilsson and Solvell (1967) showed an unchanged level of libido, while other studies indicate increased libido (Ryder and Westoff, 1966). Increased coital frequency is partly due to the convenience of this method of contraception, and the almost complete removal of the fear of pregnancy.

Incidence of Psychological Side-effects

The incidence of psychiatric symptoms is similar to that of somatic side-effects and in many cases symptoms are so intense that oral contraception is discontinued (Nilsson *et al.,* 1967). Frequency of psychiatric side-effects is not related to the patient's age, parity, marital status or social class. Women with a previous history of psychiatric or emotional problems in association with pregnancy report more psychiatric symptoms with oral contraceptives (Herzberg *et al.,* 1971).

It has been estimated that depression and neurasthenic symptoms occur in 10–20% of women who start using oral contraceptives (Nilsson and Solvell, 1967; Nilsson *et al.,* 1967). These symptoms tend to diminish after a period of three months and it was suggested that after six months the study group as a whole did not have more psychological symptoms than before beginning treatment (Cullberg *et al.,* 1969). The Royal College of General Practitioners' Oral Contraception Study (1974) found no increase in the incidence of *severe* depression in pill takers.

Mode of Action

The mode of action of the combined oral contraceptive pill in producing psychological symptoms may involve some endocrine and neural factors. Pincus *et al.* (1958) suggested that only a very small proportion of the side-effects of the pill have a physical basis, but there are some established physiological effects of oral contraceptives which may react on the functioning of the hypothalamus. These are the increase in plasma protein bound iodine, an increase in plasma cortisol due, at least in part, to increased binding of cortisol in subjects taking oestrogen-containing preparations, and a decrease in production of 17-hydroxycorticosteroids. The variation in the physiological effects may in part account for the variation in psychological effects when relatively fixed doses of combined preparations are taken by large numbers of women. It is certain that at least some will be taking a dose that is either too high or too low for their ideal requirements. The fact that side-effects tend to be most evident during the first few cycles of therapy suggests that anxiety caused by the taking of a new drug may underly many of the symptoms reported. The production of a functional deficiency of pyridoxine may also play a part in producing depression in some women (Larsson-Cohn, 1975).

Failure to Take the Pill

A patient who is afraid of taking pills, or of drugs in general, or simply an absent-minded person, may forget to take the pill, while an obsessional, responsible individual will be much less likely to forget. The fact that women who take the pill carry the responsibility of contraception may have a varying effect upon their attitudes. This form of contraception and the responsibility for it may have been forced upon her by her husband. The woman may become subconsciously hostile, and may manifest this by irregular taking of the pill (Zell and Crisp, 1964). Immature women who have a tendency to acting out and who avoid taking responsibilities are also prone to forget their oral contraceptives (Bakker and Dightman, 1964). This forgetfulness is enhanced by the presence of discord between husband and wife, and by conflicting attitudes towards sexuality. Ziegler *et al.* (1968) argued that the continuation of using oral contraceptives is related to the attitude of responsibility and they showed that wives who continue to take the pill are more responsible than their husbands. In addition it has been noted that the rejection rates for the intra-uterine device and the oral contraceptive pill are similar (Moos, 1968).

DRUG INTERACTION

Mumford (1974) suggested that there was a relative increase in the pregnancy rate among women taking both combined oral contraceptives and the anti-tuberculosis drug, rifampicin, or barbiturates.

Since then occasional cases of apparent interaction between a wide variety of commonly prescribed drugs and the oral contraceptive steroids have been described. In some instances there seems to be a reduction in the contraceptive efficacy while in other circumstances the contraceptive steroids may modify the metabolism or pharmacological action of another drug.

Breakthrough bleeding is a warning sign of reduced contraceptive efficacy. This is because the enzymes for the contraceptive steroid metabolism have been activated by the other drug, leading to their more rapid breakdown and lower than adequate blood levels. The possibility that there is some pathological cause for breakthrough bleeding in a woman who has been on the pill for some time without this symptom, must also be kept in mind.

The following drugs may possibly reduce contraceptive efficacy, as measured by an increased incidence of breakthrough bleeding or pregnancy:

(1) amidopyrine (aminophenazone);
(2) phenacetin;
(3) anticonvulsants such as phenytoin and primidone;

(4) antibiotics such as ampicillin, chloramphenicol, rifampicin and sulpha-methoxypyridazine;

(5) phenobarbitone;

(6) sedatives such as chlordiazepoxide, chlorpromazine and meprobromate;

(7) vasoconstrictors, such as dihydroergotamine.

Oral contraceptives may alter the dose required of the following groups of drugs:

(1) anticoagulants;

(2) tricyclic antidepressants;

(3) corticosteroids;

(4) insulin or oral hypoglycaemic agents.

POST-PILL AMENORRHOEA

Post-pill amenorrhoea may be defined as the absence of spontaneous menstruation two months or more after ceasing to take a combined oral contraceptive. It is a serious condition for those desiring pregnancy; of those in whom the amenorrhoea persists for 12 months, more than half will remain infertile in spite of treatment (Shearman, 1975). The combined pill prevents the release of gonadotrophin releasing factors from the hypothalamus, thereby inhibiting cyclical stimulation of the ovary by the pituitary gonadotrophins. It seems that, in some women, the inhibition persists long after administration of exogenous hormone ceases. It has been suggested that the incidence of post-pill amenorrhoea is higher amongst young patients who do not have a well established menstrual cycle and also amongst those with scanty and infrequent menstruation. The possible increase in incidence of post-pill amenorrhoea may be due to the increased use of the combined pill amongst progressively younger girls and its incorrect use to 'regulate the cycle' in patients with irregular and infrequent periods.

The evidence that the combined oral contraceptive causes secondary amenorrhoea in some women is strong. A highly significant relationship between the use of oral contraceptives and the subsequent development of secondary amenorrhoea has been shown (Shearman and Smith, 1972; Shearman, 1975). The effect occurs more commonly in young women of unproven fertility (Friedman and Goldfien, 1969), women who had late onset of the menarche (Evrard *et al.*, 1976) and in those with previous menstrual irregularities (Golditch, 1972).

The incidence of post-pill amenorrhoea is difficult to establish. A figure of 0.2% of pill users has been suggested (Golditch, 1972) but no criteria as to the definition of amenorrhoea were given. An incidence as high as 2.6% has been recorded in the Royal College of General Practitioners' Oral Contraception Study (1974). This figure is based on a definition of one or more missed periods. Shearman (1971) found that less than 1% of oral contraceptive users had more than six months of post-pill amenorrhoea.

There is sometimes an association between oral contraception and galactorrhoea (Shearman and Smith, 1972; Shearman, 1975) but the occurrence of milk secretion with secondary amenorrhoea suggests a cause other than the pill. Marshall *et al.* (1976) found that 14 out of 24 patients with amenorrhoea after stopping the pill had causes for this such as premature ovarian failure, pituitary tumours or polycystic ovarian disease. Haesslein and Lamb (1976) found 17% of pituitary tumours in patients whose amenorrhoea persisted for two years. It is clear from this evidence that radiology of the skull with coned views or tomograms of the pituitary fossa should be carried out to exclude a tumour and serial basal serum LH levels should be estimated to differentiate an ovarian from a pituitary or hypothalamic lesion. Serum prolactin levels are often high in cases of amenorrhoea and galactorrhoea of pituitary origin.

Post-pill amenorrhoea usually resolves spontaneously. Drew and Stifel (1968) found that 95% of women with post-pill amenorrhoea had menstruated spontaneously within 12–18 months of stopping the pill. Although the incidence of post-pill amenorrhoea is probably increasing, particularly amongst young women, there is no need to treat these cases for at least a few months. If investigations to exclude a pituitary tumour or hyperprolactinaemia are negative an expectant policy should be pursued for at least six months, unless pregnancy is urgently desired.

The normal multiparous woman who has a stable menstrual cycle and normal fertility reverts readily to normal menstrual function after ceasing to take the contraceptive steroids. When it occurs, secondary amenorrhoea after combined oral contraceptives is probably due to continuing suppression of the normal hypothalamic gonadotrophin releasing systems. It would be reasonable to suppose that drugs capable of stimulating gonadotrophins would be an effective remedy. Clomiphene has been used in most cases. It is believed to block the inhibiting effect of oestrogen on gonadotrophin secretion, the resulting gonadotrophin release stimulating ovulation. Many authors have reported successful returns of ovulation and menstruation after clomiphene treatment (Shearman, 1968; Marshall *et al.*, 1976), but only 35 out of 61 patients in Shearman's (1975) series responded by ovulating.

Gonadotrophins in the form of human menopausal gonadotrophin containing FSH and LH (Pergonal), followed by HCG (Shearman, 1968) or as human pituitary gonadotrophin (Shearman, 1975) have also been used quite successfully. Patients with high prolactin levels may respond to bromocriptine treatment.

Nonetheless, it must be borne in mind that of Shearman's (1975) 61 patients with post-pill amenorrhoea of 12 months' duration, only 26 became pregnant after treatment with clomiphene and/or gonadotrophins. Regular treatment should not be instituted unless pregnancy is desired, because clomiphene tends to become less effective with continued use and administration of the gonadotrophins constitutes an expensive and potentially risky treatment which is unjustified merely to produce menstruation.

Absence of withdrawal bleeding during oral contraceptive therapy is not necessarily predictive of the development of amenorrhoea. It is usually due to atrophy of the endometrial glands, with inactive epithelium and minimal secretion. The stroma becomes dense and inactive, whilst the development of arterioles is almost completely suppressed. This does not relate to the onset of secondary amenorrhoea on stopping the pill unless the individual is particularly susceptible to this complication. In most cases the endometrial changes are reversible and menstruation will recur on cessation of oral contraceptive therapy.

CONTRA-INDICATIONS

RISKS OF THROMBOSIS AND EMBOLISM

The first important potential hazard of an oestrogen-containing oral contraceptive to receive publicity was thrombo-embolism (Jordan, 1961). Although the evidence for this association is still disputed (Goldzieher and Dozier, 1975) and despite the reduction in oestrogen dose, deep venous thrombosis and pulmonary embolus, together with cerebral and coronary thrombosis, are still commonly believed to be the major causes of mortality associated with the combined pill. In Great Britain the association between intake of oestrogen-containing oral contraceptives and thrombo-embolic phenomena is now generally accepted. In the United States of America acceptance is not so widespread. The evidence that the association is causal is in fact suggestive rather than conclusive. For these reasons, some of the more important studies will be reviewed here.

Oral Contraceptives and Plasma Coagulation Factors

There are reports suggesting that combined oral contraceptives increase the plasma levels of fibrinogen, and of factors V, VII, VIII, IX and X. In addition there are suggestions that the combined oral contraceptives cause changes in platelet adhesiveness and aggregation. All these changes reach a steady state after about nine months and there is no further cumulative effect thereafter (Poller *et al.*, 1971). There have been reports suggesting that combined oral contraceptives can interfere with the fibrinolytic processes, and finally, that they increase venous distensibility and predispose to stasis in the venous circulation.

Briggs (1974) showed that patients on ethinyloestradiol, $50\,\mu g$, and norethisterone, 1 mg, (Minovlar) had plasma factor VII levels that were 120% of the control values. When medication was changed to a combined pill containing the same oestrogen dose and norgestrel, 0.5 mg, the factor VII levels reverted to normal. A second group of patients who started with the pill containing norgestrel, and then changed to Minovlar, showed an increase in factor VII levels from 100 to 120%. This type of cross-over study is able to detect the small changes that occur in plasma coagulation factors due to combined oral contraceptives.

In almost all studies where positive changes in mean activity of coagulation factors have been demonstrated in association with steroid contraceptive administration, both the occurrence and the magnitude of the change varies considerably from patient to patient. In normal subjects the size of the changes in the factor concerned are small compared with patient to patient variation. If the statistically proven association between oral contraceptives and a small risk of deep venous thrombosis or pulmonary embolism is in fact mediated by changes in plasma coagulation factors, then it should be possible to demonstrate an association between patients with the highest levels or the most marked changes and the occurrence of thrombosis or embolism. So far, good evidence on this point is lacking.

The considerable delay between the first report of pulmonary embolism in a woman taking a combined oral contraceptive (Jordan, 1961) and the production of definitive studies, the public denials of an association whilst physicians were seeing such cases in clinical practice, and the even greater reluctance to accept the hypothesis in the United States of America (Katz, 1972), all suggest that vested interests were at work.

Vessey and Doll (1968) reported a ninefold increase in venous thrombosis or embolism, and Inman and Vessey (1968) reported an eightfold increase in deaths due to these causes, amongst women taking combined oral contraceptives. In Vessey and Doll's (1968) study the figures were derived from women admitted to hospital with deep venous thrombosis; those used by Inman and Vessey (1968) were obtained from death certificates. The control group in the former study was a population matched for age, parity and other factors, taken from hospital admissions for unrelated causes. Inman and Vessey (1968) also reported a small increase in the incidence of, and in the mortality from, cerebral thrombosis amongst women on combined oral contraceptives. Doll and Vessey (1970) summarised the work of Inman and Vessey (1968), Doll (1969) and Vessey and Doll (1969). They recorded a sixfold increase in incidence and an eightfold increase in mortality from deep venous thrombosis and pulmonary embolism. There was a sixfold increase in the incidence of cerebral thrombosis, and in mortality from this condition.

Goldzieher (1970b) pointed out that the incidence of idiopathic thrombosis or embolism is much lower in the Far East than in the Western world, where obesity, the use of tobacco, and a sedentary, stressful way of life are far more common. All these factors are known to have a significant influence in the production of thrombosis and embolism. In addition, according to Goldzieher (1970b), there has been an increase in fatal pulmonary embolism in women who have never used oral contraceptives. The data presented by Vessey and Inman (1973) would appear to confirm this, showing a higher mortality from thrombo-embolism in the years 1962 to 1975 than in 1953 to 1961. This makes it much more difficult to demonstrate a further increase in thrombosis and embolism directly due to combined oral contraceptives. Goldzieher (1970b) was critical of Vessey and Doll's (1968) report, in that it was small, retrospective and based on hospital admissions, thereby including uncontrolled variables. In the early studies one of these was smoking. Seltzer (1969) agreed with the statistical validity of the work from Great Britain but suggested that it showed an association, but not necessarily a causal relationship, between increased thrombosis and embolism and the use of combined oral contraceptives. Haller (1970) entered into this controversy by collecting six hospital studies from the United States of America involving a total of over 50 000 woman-years of oral contraceptive use. He calculated that 101 cases of thrombophlebitis would have been expected amongst this number of patients, and in practice only 28 cases of thrombophlebitis were observed. These conflicting views are further confused by the fact that the British authors refer to thrombo-embolism, that is, deep venous thrombosis with or without associated pulmonary embolism, whilst the American figures largely refer to thrombophlebitis. Although severe thrombophlebitis is frequently associated with silent deep venous thrombosis the conditions are not the same.

Epidemiological Studies and Their Defects

Goldzieher (1970a) quotes an annual incidence of thrombophlebitis requiring hospital admission in the United States of America and Canada of 0.91 per 1000 women, and an incidence in antenatal patients of 0.74 per 1000 women.

This latter figure is surprisingly low, and suggests that many of these patients are not admitted to hospital. These figures may be compared with an annual incidence of thrombophlebitis of 0.55 per 1000 women on combined oral contraceptives (Drill and Calhoun, 1968) and 0.56 per 1000 women on sequential preparations (Goldzieher, 1970a). Further variables are introduced by the fact that some authors use only hospital statistics, whereas others use those derived from the general population. In all these composite studies there is difficulty in getting constant criteria for an unbiased diagnosis.

Criticisms of the work of Drill and Calhoun (1968) are that the control population was studied under different circumstances and that the criteria for diagnosing thrombophlebitis were variable. The problem of under-reporting in clinical trials is self-evident, and in these studies this may be the case because many of them showed a high patient drop-out rate. More cases of thrombophlebitis might occur in those patients who failed to return for follow-up, or in those who were checked at infrequent intervals. In Goldzieher's (1970a) study the drop-out rate was unusually low, and the patients were checked every month.

A further important criticism of these studies is that in any population of women with thrombophlebitis, 80—90% of patients would be excluded from the analysis because factors predisposing to thrombophlebitis are demonstrated. Vessey and Doll (1968, 1969) eliminated 85% of patients because of predisposing factors and so the group studied amounted to approximately one patient per hospital per year. The use of hospital populations is always dangerous since the factors responsible for hospitalisation are likely to vary. The fact that Vessey and Doll's work (1968, 1969) was retrospective made it necessary to undertake the task of matching controls with the test patients. When the two groups were studied further it was found that of those admitted with thromboembolism, 36% had a history of previous thrombotic episodes, whilst only 4% of control subjects had a similar history. The investigators re-examined the data and excluded all patients with a previous history of thrombotic episodes, finding that the higher incidence of oral contraceptive use in those developing thrombosis or embolism persisted. This type of study proves that of those women developing thrombosis, a significantly greater number are on the pill. It does not prove that the pill causes the thrombosis. These doubts are expounded in a statistical analysis of trials to date (Goldzieher and Dozier, 1975).

Kay *et al.* (1969) have shown that oral contraceptive users are significantly more likely to be smokers, and particularly heavy smokers, than non-users, but this factor was not thought to cause a significant bias in the studies of Vessey and Doll.

It is possible that the ninefold increase in the incidence of thrombosis and embolism in pill users can be attributed to the increase in diagnosis of thromboembolic disease, which is more common than is generally realised. Morrell and Dunhill (1968) found pulmonary emboli in 52% of 263 autopsies if one lung was carefully examined. Routine examination of the other lung revealed pulmonary emboli in only 12% of cases. In approximately three-quarters of relevant cases the diagnosis would have been missed at a routine autopsy. Patients on oral contraceptives dying of anything suggesting a pulmonary embolus would be expected to have a careful autopsy. In a so-called control patient having a routine autopsy or even no autopsy, the presence of a small pulmonary embolism may well be missed.

Sartwell *et al.* (1969) carried out a study in the United States of America similar in design to the British epidemiological studies using hospital patients but with the criteria for diagnosis clearly defined. Again, 90% of the initial cases of thrombosis and embolism were discarded because of other predisposing factors. The risk of thrombosis was approximately four times as high in patients using combined oral contraceptives as in non-users. In contrast to Doll and Vessey's (1970) study there was no increase in risk with increasing age and no relation to duration of pill use. Sartwell *et al.* (1969) found an increase in cerebral vascular accidents; the British workers recorded a sixfold increase in conditions believed to be due to cerebral thrombosis. In the study of Sartwell *et al.* (1969) it was shown that there was a significantly increased risk of thrombosis and embolism among pill users in New York and Philadelphia; there was no significant increase in Baltimore, Washington or Pittsburgh. It is possible that this is due to differences in population characteristics, but it is more likely to be due to sampling variation.

A recent study by the Collaborative Drug Surveillance Program, Boston (1973), confirmed the findings of Inman and his colleagues but it is open to similar criticisms; the work involved small numbers of patients, collected from 24 hospitals, and it was retrospective. Badaracco and Vessey (1974) followed up the original 42 women with thrombosis and embolism reported on in 1969. They found that the risk of recurrence of thrombo-embolism during pregnancy or the puerperium was the same whether or not they had been on the pill. Thrombosis unassociated with pregnancy was four times commoner in those who had not taken the pill, indicating some inherent predisposition to coagulation in this group. It is debatable whether or not the pill merely precipitates thrombosis in an already predisposed person, but Badaracco and Vessey (1974) suggest that it has a more specific aetiological role.

A prospective study involving 23 000 women on combined oral contraceptives and 23 000 matched controls has recently been published (Royal College of General Practitioners' Oral Contraception Study, 1974). This suggests that the incidence of thrombosis and embolism amongst women on combined oral contraceptives is six times higher and that the incidence of death from these causes is three times higher, than in the control group. The risks of the combined pill may be artificially reduced in this study by the fact that the control group had twice the incidence of previous venous thrombo-embolic disease and cerebral vascular accidents than the oral contraceptive users before entering the study. This illustrates the difficulty in any study that is not randomised. A control group, even if it can be accurately matched for all the different factors studied, is inherently different from the study group, because of the process of self selection.

Jick *et al.* (1969) reported a threefold increase in thrombo-embolic disorders among women with blood groups A, B or AB compared with those of blood group O. Lower levels of antithrombin III are thought to be responsible for this (Fagerhol *et al.*, 1971).

In conclusion, it must be borne in mind that although combined oral contraceptives may predispose to venous thrombosis and embolism, the deficiencies of the various studies suggest that the case is not yet proven. The risk of the contraceptive method must be balanced against the very low risk of an unwanted pregnancy due to method failure, and must be assessed against the relative risks of other everyday activities. Even with full oestrogen dose preparations (greater than 50 µg of ethinyloestradiol or mestranol), the increased risk of thrombo-embolic consequences is sufficiently small in women under 30 that it may be discounted except in patients who are otherwise predisposed to these conditions. Goldzieher (1970b) says that when the father of a household buys a motorboat he introduces a risk of sudden death into the family which is ten times greater than that claimed to be associated with the mother taking combined oral contraceptives.

Effect of Oestrogen Dose

Combined oral contraceptives contain either ethinyloestradiol or mestranol, which is converted in part to ethinyloestradiol in the body. Recent studies have suggested that these substances are of approximately equal potency in the human (Goldzieher *et al.*, 1975a, b and c). The effects of the added progestagen cannot be ignored, and as these are as yet undetermined, this creates some doubts about the conclusions reached.

Inman *et al.* (1970) suggested that there was a higher risk of thrombosis and embolism with combined preparations containing 100 or more µg of oestrogen. The population at risk was derived from sales figures of the various preparations. Consideration of the type and amount of progestagen led to confusing results. Despite these criticisms, the study was accepted and as a result the oestrogen dose was reduced to 50 µg or less. Subsequently further evidence was presented which suggests that a reduction in oestrogen dosage below 100 µg reduces the risk of thrombosis or embolism (Drill and Calhoun, 1972). Concurrent with a reduction in oestrogen dosage, there has been a reduction in the amount of progestagen in many preparations, but the progestagen used varies, making comparisons between different pills difficult. It has been suggested that norgestrel minimises many of the oestrogen-induced biochemical changes (Briggs and Briggs, 1976) and so the use of a low-dose oestrogen (30 µg) preparation plus norgestrel might be advantageous.

Effect of Age

Women over the age of 35 are subject to five times the risk of death from pulmonary embolism or cerebral thrombosis than younger women, in relation to an abortion or a confinement (Arthure *et al.*, 1975). Similar considerations apply to women taking combined oral contraceptives containing 100 µg or more of oestrogen (Inman and Vessey, 1968). These authors estimated that the risk of death from pulmonary embolism and cerebral thrombosis in women over 35 years of age to be 39 per million users per annum. This is nearly three times the figure for women aged 20–34 years. A recent prospective study in Australia found that although women over 40 had a higher incidence of thrombosis than younger women on the pill, this risk was still lower than that in non-users, taking into account the increased hazards of pregnancy in this age group (Grounds, 1974).

It has been suggested that combined oral contraceptives should not be prescribed for women with varicose veins. Although varicosities of the lower limbs may cause a tendency to venous stasis and trauma to the varicose vessels to occur, the risk of thrombosis on the pill is tiny, provided the varicosities are not extensive or complicated by thrombophlebitis. If there are extensive varicosities or thrombophlebitis is present then there is a risk of deep venous thrombosis and a combined pill should not be prescribed.

Coronary Thrombosis

The suggestion has been made that oral contraceptives can, very rarely, cause coronary thrombosis. The pathology of arterial occlusion differs from that of venous thrombosis and pulmonary embolism. The fast and variable blood flow through an artery makes it unlikely that occlusive thrombosis will occur, unless lesions of the arterial wall which reduce the flow considerably already exist. This contrasts with the venous circulation where increased coagulability or minor trauma may suffice to cause clot formation. It follows that with an arterial thrombosis the primary cause is much more likely to be pathology in the vessels than the effect of a drug on coagulation factors. One of the factors which seriously affect coronary artery status is heavy smoking and some emphasis has recently been given to the synergism between smoking and oral contraception in predisposing to myocardial infarction amongst older women.

Comhaire *et al.* (1971) studied 148 cases of thrombosis and embolism occurring during the use of oral contraception. 70% of the episodes of venous thrombosis with or without pulmonary embolism, occurred within four months of starting oral contraceptives. In contrast 50% of cases of arterial thrombosis involving both cerebral and coronary arteries occurred after more than eight months of oral contraceptive use. In addition, venous thrombosis commonly occurred in women who had had no children or one child, while arterial occlusions were common among women of higher parity, allowing for age. This suggests a different pathological mechanism for the two types of thrombosis.

Inman *et al.* (1970) thought that the incidence of coronary thrombosis was related to the dose of oestrogen in the oral contraceptive but Oliver (1970) observed that other factors such as hypertension, obesity, hyperlipidaemia and smoking were equally important. It is interesting that 9 out of 11 of Oliver's (1970) cases of myocardial infarction in women taking the pill smoked 10 or more cigarettes daily. Fischer and Mosbech (1971) found that in Denmark during the years 1967 and 1968, only 15% of 54 women aged 30–44 years who died of myocardial infarction were taking oral contraceptives. It was estimated then that 15% of all women of childbearing age were taking oral contraceptives, and it must be concluded that in Denmark there was no association between these drugs and death from myocardial infarction. On the other hand Mann *et al.* (1975) suggested that in women over 40 the risk of coronary thrombosis was increased fivefold if they were taking combined oral contraceptives. In the person already at risk because of other factors such as hyperlipidaemia, obesity and particularly smoking, the combined pill may be an additional factor in the aetiology of coronary thrombosis (Jain, 1976).

Cerebral Thrombosis

The initial reports of an association between combined oral contraceptive usage and cerebral thrombosis were based on such small numbers that no particular weight can be attached to them (Inman and Vessey, 1968; Vessey and Doll,

1968, 1969). A study of strokes in young women reported in 1973 and 1975 (Collaborative Group for the Study of Stroke in Young Women) indicated that the relative risks for oral contraceptive users when compared with matched controls of both haemorrhagic and thrombotic strokes were significantly increased. Deficiencies of this study are the large difference in incidence of stroke from one reporting centre to another, presumably due to diagnostic bias, a large drop-out rate and insufficient attention to details which might bias the results such as the relative incidence of sickle cell disease among the negroes in the study. There was an excessive number of low income women who smoked amongst those with strokes. The case is not proven, and again there is the difficulty of drawing valid conclusions from poorly matched groups. On the other hand there is evidence from prospective studies such as that of the Royal College of General Practitioners (1974) which supports the idea that there is an association between oral contraceptive use and thrombosis and embolism, particularly in older women.

Conclusion

The statistical evidence on the relationship of combined oral contraceptives to venous thrombo-embolism and coronary thrombosis is highly suggestive but the results of further very large scale prospective studies will be necessary before the case can be regarded as proven beyond doubt. Any such studies must carefully control all the variable factors, such as smoking, and the type of population from which figures are drawn, that is, a hospital or a general population, and they must clearly define the pathological lesions discussed. On the other hand the apparent relationship between the oestrogen content of contraceptive pills and the incidence of thrombo-embolic complications (Inman *et al.*, 1970), and the laboratory evidence that blood coagulability is increased provides presumptive evidence that this relationship is causal.

If the incidence of thrombosis and embolism and the increases in coagulation factors are dependent on the dose of oestrogen it is desirable to use oral contraceptive preparations with as low an oestrogen content as possible. For this reason, the Committee on Safety of Medicine in Great Britain and the Food and Drug Administration in the United States of America suggest that combined preparations containing $50\,\mu g$ or less of oestrogen should be used, to minimise the chance of thrombosis.

The combined pill should not in general be prescribed for patients who have had venous thrombosis, pulmonary embolism, coronary thrombosis or a cerebral vascular accident, or who have rheumatic heart disease or severe varicose veins of the lower limbs with associated thrombophlebitis. For this reason a full medical history must be taken before prescription. Caution should be exercised in the use of the combined pill in women over 40 years of age, especially those who smoke heavily, are obese, or who have a strong family history of coronary thrombosis. We know of no clear evidence that the pill is contra-indicated in patients with haemoglobinopathies such as sickle cell trait or disease.

RISK OF DIABETES MELLITUS

The steroids in the combined oral contraceptives, when given for a long time, can cause an alteration in carbohydrate metabolism, known as 'steroid diabetes'.

This can occur when large doses of corticosteroids are given for a short time, or during pregnancy. The chance of a previously normal person developing chemical diabetes whilst on the pill is small, and if it does occur it is usually reversible. After a number of years of continuous combined oral contraceptive therapy a small proportion of women may become chemical diabetics. The risk of this happening is greater if the person is already a potential or latent diabetic. A potential diabetic is a person who has a family history of diabetes mellitus, or who has a history containing risk factors such as previous large babies — birth weight greater than 10 lb (4.5 kg) — glycosuria or unexplained perinatal mortality. A latent diabetic is defined as a person who has abnormal carbohydrate metabolism during steroid administration or during pregnancy, but who reverts to normal once the 'steroid stress' is over.

Both oestrogens (Javier *et al.*, 1968) and progestagens (Gershberg *et al.*, 1969; Spellacy *et al.*, 1973; Tuttle and Turkington, 1974) have been cited as causes of the altered carbohydrate metabolism seen in some women on the combined oral contraceptive pill. Oestrogens alone can cause resistance to insulin and abnormalities of glucose tolerance are more common with mestranol than with ethinyloestradiol. Variation of the pancreatic islet cell reserve is an important factor and may lead to conflicting results. The dose of oestrogens used in these studies was the same as in the current range of combined oral contraceptives, 50 μg, but the doses of progestagens used were very much higher than those in the combined pill. Oestrogens are likely to be primarily responsible for the altered carbohydrate tolerance but the possible potentiating effect of combination with a progestagen must not be forgotten.

Many other factors predispose to the development of abnormal carbohydrate metabolism in association with oral contraception. Both intravenous and oral glucose tolerance deteriorates in about 25% of patients on the combined pill and 13% develop chemical diabetes (Wynn and Doar, 1970).

After one year of therapy Spellacy, Carlson *et al.* (1968) showed a significant elevation of glucose and insulin levels during an oral glucose tolerance test in 40% of previously normal women. Three-quarters of these tests bordered on abnormality, and the remainder were frankly abnormal. Serum growth hormone activity was also increased and it is thought that this might antagonise the activity of insulin on the tissues. These changes may either be directly due to oestrogen, progestagen or both, or they may be secondary to increased levels of other hormones such as cortisol. There is evidence that 77% of women who have taken oral contraceptives for more than eight years have an abnormal oral glucose tolerance test (Spellacy, Buhi *et al.*, 1968), but Wynn and Doar (1970) have shown a marked improvement in abnormal glucose tolerance on ceasing to take the pill.

Age

The effect of this factor is doubtful, because some authors have found that there is no correlation between the incidence of abnormal carbohydrate metabolism caused by oral contraception and age (Wynn and Doar, 1969) while others have found that the incidence of abnormal carbohydrate metabolism induced by the combined oral contraceptive pill increases with advancing age (Spellacy, Carlson *et al.*, 1968).

Parity

No relationship between parity and abnormal carbohydrate metabolism due to oral contraceptives has been shown.

Obesity

This is well known to be associated with impaired glucose tolerance. Doar and Wynn (1970) investigated oral glucose tolerance and the use of oral contraception in matched groups of women who did not have diabetes, subdivided by weight. The risk factors were obesity and use of combined oral contraceptives, each of which caused a slight impairment of glucose tolerance. The combination of these two factors could lead to a more abnormal oral glucose tolerance test.

Family History of Diabetes

There is a difference of opinion regarding the effect of oral contraceptives on potential diabetics with a family history of diabetes or a personal history of a large baby, because Wynn and Doar (1969) were unable to find impaired oral glucose tolerance, but on the other hand Spellacy, Buhi *et al.* (1968) found that women who had had a baby weighing over 9 lb (4.1 kg) had slightly impaired intravenous glucose tolerance whilst taking a combined pill daily and Di Paola *et al.* (1968) also found an increased incidence of abnormal carbohydrate metabolism among potential diabetics on oral contraceptives.

Latent Diabetes

There is a positive relationship between latent diabetics with a history of abnormal carbohydrate metabolism during a previous pregnancy, and the induction of carbohydrate intolerance by oral contraceptives (Javier *et al.*, 1968; Spellacy, Carlson *et al.*, 1968) as many as 50% of patients being affected. Reversal of the carbohydrate intolerance to normal once the pill has stopped is thought to be the general rule, but the time taken for this is proportional to the duration of combined oral contraceptive therapy, and the degree of abnormality of glucose tolerance. Szabo *et al.* (1970) studied five latent diabetics who all developed abnormal glucose tolerance on oral contraceptives; only one showed improvement within a few months of stopping the pill.

Conclusion

Only strictly controlled long-term prospective studies will determine the true incidence, severity and reversibility of the changes in carbohydrate metabolism.

It is interesting to note that the incidence of abnormal carbohydrate metabolism in reports from Great Britain is higher than that from the United States of America. This, as we have seen, applies also to the incidence of thromboembolism, and it applied more than ten years ago to the simpler side-effects of oral contraceptives such as nausea, weight gain, and menstrual irregularities. These differences on different sides of the Atlantic may be due to the different populations studied and to socio-economic factors such as diet. Lack of uniformity of clinical criteria and variation in techniques of collecting data must introduce many imponderables into these studies. Care must therefore be taken when assessing and comparing results.

All women on the pill should have their urine tested for sugar six-monthly.

Those who are on the combined pill for five or more years, should have an oral glucose tolerance test performed, and preferably repeated every two years.

The potential diabetic has exhibited some potentially diabetic trait or has a family history of the disease. A proportion of these women will become latent, and then frank diabetics, and the combined pill could accelerate this process. If alternative contraceptive procedures prove unacceptable to such patients, it is reasonable to give them low-oestrogen combined oral contraceptives for a limited number of years. At the same time a programme of weight control and annual oral glucose tolerance tests should be instituted. If there is any sign of the condition proceeding to a latent diabetic state, then use of the combined pill should be stopped.

Latent diabetes should, at least until further evidence is available, be regarded as a contra-indication to the use of combined oral contraception. The continued use of the combined pill in these patients can precipitate overt diabetes mellitus at an earlier age than it would otherwise have occurred (Adams and Oakley, 1972).

In *overt diabetics*, combined oral contraceptives can be used with caution. They already have diabetes, and there is no evidence that the combined pill worsens the prognosis or makes control more difficult although the insulin requirement may be increased a little. Pregnancy is more likely to increase the rate of development of diabetes than the oral contraceptive steroids. If the pill is used, exceptionally careful control of the diabetic state is desirable.

The progestagen-only pill seems safe to prescribe to potential, latent and overt diabetics. It should be the only oral contraceptive prescribed to latent diabetics, and should be given consideration in the management of the other two categories.

The use of combined pills containing norgestrel may alter this assessment of the overall situation; Wynn *et al.* (1974) have suggested that this progestagen can produce a normal glucose tolerance test.

RISK OF LIVER DAMAGE

There is no doubt that women taking combined oral contraceptives have altered results in many protein and enzyme estimations because of effects on the liver (Ockner and Davidson, 1967). In general these changes are slight and there is no reason to assume that they are of any consequence in a normal individual. The changes include significant increases in amylase, β-glucuronidase, transferrin, ceruloplasmin, transcortin, sex hormone binding globulin, plasminogen and fibrinogen (Briggs and Briggs, 1976). Changes in the hormone binding globulins have widespread effects and this ripple effect, starting from changes in liver biochemistry, is responsible for many of the alterations in metabolism induced by the combined pill. In a healthy individual there is no evidence that the pill or the biochemical changes consequent on its use cause damage to the liver. There is a risk to those patients whose liver function is already impaired. Patients with a history of jaundice should have their liver function investigated before commencing oral contraceptive therapy and reviewed after three months on the pill.

The oestrogen component of the pill seems to be responsible for many biochemical alterations, as oestrogens can cause changes in the rate of synthesis and secretion of proteins such as binding globulins, ceruloplasmin and transferrin which are manufactured by the liver.

Oestrogens can also cause cholestasis, resulting in jaundice, anorexia and pruritus. This is similar to the clinical picture of 'recurrent jaundice of late pregnancy'. This completes the description of this disease; it needn't be recurrent, it needn't produce jaundice, it needn't occur late in pregnancy, and now the patient need not even be pregnant! There have been many reports of cholestatic jaundice developing within the first few weeks of starting therapy with combined oral contraceptives. The typical symptoms of this type of jaundice are anorexia, nausea, pruritus, pigmented urine and finally clinical jaundice. Some patients may only get pruritus, if the condition is mild. Plasma bilirubin is in the range 3—10 mg/100 ml (50—170 μmol/l) and alkaline phosphatase levels are increased. Electron microscopic findings are similar to those of other types of intrahepatic cholestasis, with dilatation of bile canaliculae, shortening and blunting of microvilli, bile stasis and swelling of the endoplasmic reticulum which often lacks ribosomes (Larsson-Cohn and Stenram, 1965).

The first case of cholestatic jaundice due to the pill was reported in 1962, and in 1967 a series of 40 cases was described by Ockner and Davidson (1967). Several oral contraceptives employ 17α-alkyl-substituted steroids, and these compounds have been shown by Sherlock (1968) to be capable of causing cholestasis. The implication that the combined oral contraceptive causes this type of jaundice has been confirmed by the fact that the clinical features of the illnesses reported have been consistent; that the jaundice usually occurs soon after starting therapy; that recovery usually follows within a week or two of stopping the drug; and that in those patients who have been restarted on similar therapy jaundice has usually recurred. Finally, many of the women who develop jaundice on the pill have previously suffered from cholestatic jaundice or pruritus of pregnancy.

Cessation of the oral contraceptive usually results in complete remission of the condition within a few weeks. As oestrogens seem to be the aetiological link between the clinical picture just described and cholestatic jaundice of pregnancy, anyone with a history of jaundice or pruritus in pregnancy should avoid oral contraceptives containing oestrogens (Hargreaves, 1970), as should patients with established liver disease. A past history of infective hepatitis or jaundice of unknown aetiology is not a contra-indication to oral contraceptives provided liver function is normal. It is probable that the low-dose progestagen preparations do not affect hepatic function.

The Boston Collaborative Drug Surveillance Program (1973) has confirmed statistically what some practitioners have already suspected, that there is an association between taking combined oral contraceptives and young women developing gallstones. Various combined oral contraceptives have been shown to increase the percentage saturation of cholesterol in bile, and this predisposes to gallstone formation (Bennion *et al.,* 1976). This increase in percentage saturation may be due to a rise in cholesterol turnover or to a decrease in the bile acids and phospholipids which maintain the solubility of cholesterol in bile. Large doses of oestrogens given to rats have been shown to produce both changes (Kritchevsky *et al.,* 1961; Davis and Kern, 1974), but caution must be exercised in extrapolating from this experimental situation to that pertaining in humans.

At present it would be wise not to prescribe the combined pill for women who have gallstones, or have a history of cholecystitis. Also, the association should be remembered when young women on combined oral contraceptives present with pain in the right hypochondrium.

Benign tumours of the liver were described by Baum *et al.* (1973) in seven users of oral contraceptives and over 100 similar cases have since been reported.

In contrast, using several major data sources, Vessey *et al.* (1977) were only able to identify a single case of a benign liver tumour in a woman of reproductive age in Great Britain over the last few years. It seems from comparison with the report of Edmondson *et al.* (1976) that these tumours are more common in the United States of America.

HYPERTENSION

Uncomplicated benign essential hypertension or hypertension under treatment are not absolute contra-indications to combined oral contraception, though it may be felt that the increased hazards of myocardial infarction in such patients justify advising alternative contraceptive procedures. Hypertensive patients over 35 who have a high blood cholesterol are at particular risk; if they are obese and smoke heavily as well we consider the risk to be prohibitive.

If an oral contraceptive is prescribed for a hypertensive patient, blood pressure should be monitored in succeeding weeks and months, the pill being discontinued if there is any exacerbation.

PSYCHOLOGICAL CONTRA-INDICATIONS

The pill causes psychological effects of varying degrees of severity. The only one that may constitute a relative contra-indication to the prescription of the pill is depression.

Depression has been attributed to the low oestrogen and high progestagen content of some combined preparations (Grant and Mears, 1967). A positive relationship between the degree of depression and the monoaminoxidase activity estimated in the endometrium has been described. It may be that the activity of this enzyme in the nervous system is also affected (Grant and Pryse-Davies, 1968). Altered tryptophan metabolism leading to a functional deficiency of pyridoxine, a co-enzyme in the production of 5-hydroxytryptamine, may be another factor causing depression (Larsson-Cohn, 1975). Consequently it has been suggested that pyridoxine be given to women with a history of depression who are taking oral contraceptives (Winston, 1969) and even that the pill may be contra-indicated in such patients (British Medical Journal, 1969). In Spain a combined oral contraceptive containing 25 mg pyridoxine is marketed under the name Cicloseguer.

Pills with a relatively high progestagen content can cause depression of varying degrees, but any combined pill may cause depression in women. This psychological side-effect is often coupled with lethargy and loss of libido. A woman with a history of depression is more at risk and the pill should be avoided in these patients. When it is necessary to use oral contraception the lowest dose of preparation should be prescribed together with pyridoxine.

CARCINOGENESIS

To date there is no evidence that the combined pill causes cancer of any form. Nevertheless, as with any other medication, it may be another 20 years before it can be stated with certainty that there is no risk whatsoever.

Breast

Large doses of oestrogens when given to specific strains of mice can produce mammary tumours. Oestrogens also potentiate the development of mammary tumours, initiated by polycyclic carcinogens, in mice (Kaslaris and Jull, 1962).

In the human there is an association between ovarian function and breast carcinoma. Both pregnancy (MacMahon and Cole, 1969) and bilateral oophorectomy (Feinlieb, 1968) are associated with a lower incidence of breast carcinoma. This is due to an interruption of normal cyclical ovarian function at some time between the ages of 20 and 40 (Feinlieb, 1968). In addition to oestrogens the ovary produces androgens, and the possible effects of these on the aetiology of breast carcinoma cannot be ignored. The Boston Collaborative Drug Surveillance Program (1973) and the Royal College of General Practitioners (1974, 1977) have suggested that the continued use of combined oral contraceptive therapy reduces the incidence of benign breast tumours and that the progestagen may be an important factor. Fibro-adenomata are thought to be induced by cyclical hormonal changes and the substitution of a constant hormonal environment by the use of oral contraception may be the process responsible. There is no evidence to date to suggest that combined oral contraceptive therapy causes breast carcinoma.

It is usually said that patients with carcinoma of the breast, even if this has been apparently successfully treated, should not take combined oral contraceptives as the tumour might be 'oestrogen-sensitive'. It is now no longer considered that the progress of breast carcinoma is accelerated by pregnancy, and it may be that oral contraceptives are also without influence. On the other hand if the patient is taking the pill, rapid progress or recurrence of a breast carcinoma is likely to be blamed on this, and combined oral contraceptives are probably best avoided.

Cervix

Melamed *et al.* (1969) suggested that there was a greater prevalence of carcinoma *in situ* in women on oral contraceptives compared to those using diaphragms. What was in fact shown by these authors is that women who prefer the pill as a contraceptive are, for a variety of reasons, more prone to develop abnormal cervical cytology. It is clear that in any study, careful matching for age at first coitus, age at first pregnancy, socio-economic status, and prevalence of the malignancy under consideration must be carefully equated before any conclusions can be drawn implicating a contraceptive method. In a controlled study, Boyce *et al.* (1972) matched patients for age, ethnic background, age at first coitus, age at first pregnancy, and socio-economic status. Patients with cervical carcinoma had not used oral contraceptives to any greater extent than control patients. This has been confirmed in another recent study (Sandmire *et al.*, 1976).

It is also worth bearing in mind that as with thrombosis and embolism, the incidence of cervical carcinoma and of breast cancer appears to be increasing in the population, and it is therefore very much harder statistically to implicate any single aetiological factor. It is nevertheless desirable that all women taking oral contraceptives should have cervical smears taken before starting and at intervals thereafter, and that they should be instructed in self-examination of the breasts.

Endometrium

It has been suggested that individuals with a late menopause are more prone to develop endometrial carcinoma, which is thought to be due to prolonged exposure of the endometrium to endogenous oestrogens.

When the possible involvement of oestrogens in endometrial carcinoma is considered, the potential protective effect of progestational therapy must also be taken into account. It is known that endometrial carcinoma can regress under the influence of large doses of progestational agents. If physiological oestrogen production is among the factors which predispose to genital tract or other malignancy, it has been suggested that cyclic progestational exposure, as, for example, during oral contraceptive therapy, might have some prophylactic value (Leis, 1966).

As with the other malignancies, there is no valid evidence to date that combined oral contraceptive therapy causes endometrial carcinoma.

Malignant Melanoma

This condition is said to be a contra-indication to oral contraception. This is related to the belief that recurrences are precipitated by pregnancy, though the evidence for this is slender, and to the fact that skin pigmentation sometimes increases in women taking oral contraceptives.

Hodgkin's Disease

It has been said that oral contraceptives are contra-indicated in this condition. Some physicians feel that oral contraception is the only reliable way of preventing pregnancy during chemotherapy. Cyclical or continuous administration of a pill with a high progestagen content can be a useful manoeuvre for attenuating menstrual loss in young women who have been rendered anaemic and thrombocytopenic by chemotherapy.

REFERENCES

ADAMS, P.W. and OAKLEY, N.W. (1972). Oral contraceptives and carbohydrate metabolism. *Clin. Endocr. Metab.*, **1**, 697–720

AITKEN, J.M., HART, D.M. and LINDSAY, R. (1973). Oestrogen replacement therapy for prevention of osteoporosis after oophorectomy. *Br. med. J.*, **iii**, 515–518

ANSBACHER, R. and CAMPBELL, C. (1971). Cervical mucus sperm penetration in women on oral contraception or with an IUD *in situ. Contraception*, **3**, 209–217

ARTHURE, H., TOMKINSON, J., ORGANE, Sir G., LEWIS, E.M., ADELSTEIN, A.M. and WEATHERALL, J.A.C. (1975). Report on confidential enquiries into maternal deaths in England and Wales, 1970–72. *D.H.S.S. Rep. Hlth. Soc. Subj.*, No. 11. Her Majesty's Stationery Office, London

BADARACCO, M.A. and VESSEY, M.P. (1974). Recurrence of venous thrombo-embolic disease and use of oral contraceptives. *Br. med. J.*, **i**, 215–217

BAKKER, C.B. and DIGHTMAN, C.R. (1964). Psychological factors in fertility control. *Fert. Steril.,* **15**, 559–567

BAUM, J.K., HOLTZ, F., BOOKSTEIN, J.J. and KLEIN, E.W. (1973). Possible association between benign hepatomas and oral contraceptives. *Lancet,* **ii**, 926–929

BENNION, L.J., GINSBERG, R.L., GARNICK, M.B. and BENNETT, P.H. (1976). Effects of oral contraceptives on the gall bladder bile of normal women. *New Engl. J. Med.,* **294**, 189–192

BOSTON COLLABORATIVE DRUG SURVEILLANCE PROGRAM (1973). Oral contraceptives and venous thromboembolic disease, surgically confirmed gall bladder disease and breast tumours. *Lancet,* **i**, 1399–1404

BOYCE, J.G., LU, T., NELSON, J.H. and JOYCE, D. (1972). Cervical carcinoma and oral contraception. *Obstet. Gynec., N.Y.,* **40**, 139–146

BRIGGS, M. (1974). Effect of oral progestagens on estrogen induced changes in serum protein. *The Second International Norgestrel Symposium. Some Metabolic Considerations of Oral Contraceptive Usage,* pp. 35–41. Excerpta Medica, Amsterdam

BRIGGS, M.H. and BRIGGS, M. (1972). Plasma hormone concentrations in women receiving steroid contraceptives. *J. Obstet. Gynaec. Br. Commonw.,* **79**, 946–950

BRIGGS, M.H. and BRIGGS, M. (1976). Clinical and biochemical investigations of an ultra-low-dose combined type oral contraceptive. *Curr. med. Res. Opin.,* **3**, 618–623

BRITISH MEDICAL JOURNAL (1969). Leading article. Oral contraception and depression. *Br. med. J.,* **iv**, 380–381

BROWN, C.B., ROBSON, J.S., THOMSON, D., CLARKSON, A.R., CAMERON, J.S. and OGG, C.S. (1973). Haemolytic uraemic syndrome in women taking oral contraceptives. *Lancet,* **i**, 1479–1481

BROWN, P.S., WELLS, M. and CUNNINGHAM, F.J. (1964). A method for studying the mode of action of oral contraceptives. *Lancet,* **ii**, 446–447

CARGILLE, C.M. and ROSS, G.T. (1968). Oral contraceptives and follicle stimulating hormone. *Lancet,* **i**, 924–925

CHIDELL, M.P. (1970). Oral contraceptives and blood pressure. *Practitioner,* **205**, 58–64

COLLABORATIVE GROUP FOR THE STUDY OF STROKE IN YOUNG WOMEN (1973). Oral contraception and increased risk of cerebral ischaemia or thrombosis. *New Engl. J. Med.,* **288**, 871–878

COLLABORATIVE GROUP FOR THE STUDY OF STROKE IN YOUNG WOMEN (1975). Oral contraceptives and stroke in young women. *J. Am. med. Ass.,* **23**, 718–722

COMHAIRE, F., VANDEWEGHE, M. and VERMEULEN, A. (1971). Vascular incidents and oral contraceptives. Arterial versus venous thromboembolism. A statistical study. *Contraception,* **3**, 301–312

CRANE, M.G., HARRIS, J.J. and WINSOR, W. (1971). Hypertension, oral contraceptive agents and conjugated oestrogens. *Ann. intern. Med.,* **74**, 13–21

CROSS, R.G. (1961). Prevention of anencephaly and foetal abnormalities by a preconceptional regimen. *Lancet,* **ii**, 1124

CULLBERG, J., GELLI, M.G. and JONSSON, C.-O. (1969). Mental and sexual adjustments before and after six months' use of an oral contraceptive. *Acta psychol. scand.,* **45**, 259–276

DAVIS, R.A. and KERN, F. (1974). Effect of ethinyl oestradiol and bile salts on

84   *Combined Oral Contraceptives*

cholesterol excretion: a possible mechanism of gallbladder disease. *Clin. Res.,* **22**, 356A

DICKEY, R.P. and DORR, C.H. (1969). Oral contraceptives – selection of the proper pill. *Obstet. Gynec., N.Y.,* **33**, 273–287

DI PAOLA, G., PUCHULU, F., ROBIN, M., NICHOLSON, R. and MARTI, M. (1968). Oral contraceptives and carbohydrate metabolism. *Am. J. Obstet. Gynec.,* **101**, 206–216

DOAR, J.W.H. and WYNN, V. (1970). Serum lipid levels during oral contraceptive and glucocorticoid administration. *J. clin. Path.,* **23**, supplement 3, 55–61

DOLL, R. (1969). Recognition of unwanted drug effects. *Br. med. J.,* **ii**, 69–76

DOLL, R. and VESSEY, M.P. (1970). Evaluation of rare adverse effects of systemic contraceptives. *Br. med. Bull.,* **26**, 33–38

DREW, F.L. and STIFEL, E.N. (1968). Secondary amenorrhoea among young women entering religious life. *Obstet. Gynec., N.Y.,* **32**, 47–51

DRILL, V.A. and CALHOUN, D.W. (1968). Oral contraceptives and thrombo-embolic disease. *J. Am. med. Ass.,* **206**, 77–84

DRILL, V.A. and CALHOUN, D.W. (1972). Oral contraceptives and thrombo-embolic disease. II. Estrogen content of oral contraceptives. *J. Am. med. Ass.,* **219**, 593–596

ECKSTEIN, P., WATERHOUSE, J.A.H., BOND, G.M., MILLS, W.G., SANDILANDS, D.M. and SHOTTON, D.M. (1961). The Birmingham oral contraceptive trial. *Br. med. J.,* **ii**, 1172–1178

EDMONDSON, H.A., HENDERSON, B. and BENTON, B. (1976). Liver-cell adenomas associated with use of oral contraceptives. *New Engl. J. Med.,* **294**, 470–472

EVRARD, J.R., BUXTON, B.H. and ERIKSON, D. (1976). Amenorrhoea following oral contraception. *Am. J. Obstet. Gynec.,* **124**, 88–91

FAGERHOL, M.K., ABILDGAARD, U. and KORNSTAD, L. (1971). Antithrombin III concentration and ABO blood groups. *Lancet,* **ii**, 664–665

FEINLIEB, M. (1968). Breast cancer and artificial menopause: a cohort study. *J. natn. Cancer Inst.,* **41**, 315–329

FISCHER, A. and MOSBECH, J. (1971). Mortality due to coronary occlusion in young women with respect to oral contraceptives as a possible etiological factor. *Ugeskr. Leag.,* **132/52**, 2480–2482

FRIEDMAN, S. and GOLDFIEN, A. (1969). Amenorrhoea and galactorrhoea following oral contraceptive therapy. *J. Am. med. Ass.,* **210**, 1888–1891

GAL, I., KIRMAN, B. and STERN, J. (1967). Hormonal pregnancy tests and congenital malformations. *Nature, Lond.,* **216**, 83

GARCIA, C-R. (1974). The side effects of oral contraceptives: can the patient be reassured? *The Second International Norgestrel Symposium. Some Metabolic Considerations of Oral Contraceptive Usage,* pp. 65–71. Excerpta Medica, Amsterdam

GERSHBERG, H., ZORRILLA, E., HERNANDEZ, A. and HULSE, M. (1969). Effects of medroxyprogesterone acetate on serum insulin and growth hormone levels in diabetics and potential diabetics. *Obstet. Gynec., N.Y.,* **33**, 383–389

GOLDITCH, I.M. (1972). Post contraceptive amenorrhoea. *Obstet. Gynec., N.Y.,* **39**, 903–908

GOLDZIEHER, J.W. (1970a). Oral contraceptives: a review of certain metabolic effects and an examination of the question of safety. *Fedn. Proc. Fedn. Am. Socs. exp. Biol.,* **29**, 1220–1227

GOLDZIEHER, J.W. (1970b). An assessment of the hazards and metabolic alterations attributed to oral contraceptives. *Contraception,* **1**, 409–445

GOLDZIEHER, J.W. and DOZIER, T.S. (1975). Oral contraceptives and thrombo-embolism: a reassessment. *Am. J. Obstet. Gynec.*, **123**, 878–914

GOLDZIEHER, J.W., MOSES, L.E. and ELLIS, L.T. (1962). Study of norethindrone in contraception. *J. Am. med. Ass.*, **180**, 359–361

GOLDZIEHER, J.W., MAQUEO, M., CHENAULT, C.B. and WOUTERSZ, T.B. (1975a). Comparative studies of the ethinyl estrogens used in oral contraceptives. I. Endometrial response. *Am. J. Obstet. Gynec.*, **122**, 615–618

GOLDZIEHER, J.W., PENA, A., CHENAULT, C.B. and CERVANTES, A. (1975b). Comparative studies of the ethinyl estrogens used in oral contraceptives. III. Effect on plasma gonadotrophins. *Am. J. Obstet. Gynec.*, **122**, 625–636

GOLDZIEHER, J.W., PENA, A., CHENAULT, C.B. and WOUTERSZ, T.B. (1975c). Comparative studies of the ethinyl estrogens used in oral contraceptives. II. Anti-ovulatory potency. *Am. J. Obstet. Gynec.*, **122**, 619–624

GOULD, S.R., MOUNTROSE, U., BROWN, D.J., WHITEHOUSE, W.L. and BARNARDO, D.E. (1974). Influence of previous oral contraception and maternal oxytocin infusion on neonatal jaundice. *Br. med. J.*, **iii**, 228–230

GRANT, E.C.G. (1968). Relation between headaches from oral contraceptives and development of endometrial arterioles. *Br. med. J.*, **iii**, 402–405

GRANT, E.C.G. (1969). Venous effects of oral contraceptives. *Br. med. J.*, **iv**, 73–77

GRANT, E.C.G. and MEARS, E. (1967). Mental effects of oral contraceptives. *Lancet*, **ii**, 945–946

GRANT, E.C.G. and PRYSE-DAVIES, J. (1968). Effect of oral contraceptives on depressive mood changes and on endometrial monoamine oxidase and phosphatases. *Br. med. J.*, **iii**, 777–780

GREENBERG, G., INMAN, W.H.W., WEATHERALL, J.A.C. and ADELSTEIN, A.M. (1975). Hormonal pregnancy tests and congenital malformations. *Br. med. J.*, **ii**, 191–192

GROUNDS, M. (1974). Anovulants: thrombosis and other associated changes. *Med. J. Aust.*, **ii**, 440–446

HAESSLEIN, H.C. and LAMB, E.J. (1976). Pituitary tumors in patients with secondary amenorrhoea. *Am. J. Obstet. Gynec.*, **125**, 759–765

HALLER, J. (1970). A review of the long-term effects of hormonal contraceptives. *Contraception*, **1**, 233–251

HARGREAVES, T. (1970). Oral contraceptives and liver function. *J. clin. Path.*, **23**, supplement 3, 1–10

HEBER, K.R. (1974). A flexible low dosage system of oral contraception. *Contraception*, **10**, 241–250

HERTIG, A.T. and SHEA, S.M. (1967). Human trophoblast: normal and abnormal. *Am. J. clin. Path.*, **47**, 249–268

HERTZBERG, B.N., DRAPER, K.C., JOHNSON, A.L. and NICOL, G.C. (1971). Oral contraceptives, depression and libido. *Br. med. J.*, **iii**, 495–500

HOLT, E.M. (1970). Out-patient diagnostic curettage. *J. Obstet. Gynaec. Br. Commonw.*, **77**, 1043–1046

IFFY, L. (1963). The time of conception on fetal monstrosities. *Gynaecologia*, **156**, 140–142

INMAN, W.H.W. and VESSEY, M.P. (1968). Investigations of deaths from pulmonary, coronary and cerebral thrombosis and embolism in women of child-bearing age. *Br. med. J.*, **ii**, 193–199

INMAN, W.H.W., VESSEY, M.P., WESTERHOLM, B. and ENGELUND, A. (1970).

Thromboembolic disease and the steroidal content of oral contraceptives; a report to the Committee on Safety of Drugs. *Br. med. J.,* ii, 203–209

JACKSON, J.L., SPAIN, W.T. and PAYNE, H. (1968). The antiovulatory dose of ethinyl estradiol. A titration study. *Fert. Steril.,* 19, 649–653

JAIN, A.K. (1976). Cigarette smoking, use of oral contraceptives and myocardial infarction. *Am. J. Obstet. Gynec.,* 126, 301–307

JANERICH, D.T., DUGAN, J.M., STANDFAST, S.J. and STRITE, L. (1977). Congenital heart disease and prenatal exposure to exogenous sex hormones. *Br. med. J.,* i, 1058–1060

JANERICH, D.T., PIPER, J.M. and GLEBATIS, D.M. (1974). Oral contraceptives and congenital limb reduction defects. *New Engl. J. Med.,* 291, 697–700

JAVIER, Z., GERSHBERG, H. and HULSE, M. (1968). Ovulatory suppressants, estrogens, and carbohydrate metabolism. *Metabolism,* 17, 443–456

JICK, H., SLONE, D., WESTERHOLM, B., INMAN, W.H.W., VESSEY, M.P., SHAPIRO, S., LEWIS, G.P. and WORCESTER, J. (1969). Venous thromboembolic disease and ABO blood type. A co-operative study. *Lancet,* i, 539–545

JORDAN, W.M. (1961). Pulmonary embolism. *Lancet,* ii, 1146–1147

KASLARIS, E. and JULL, J.W. (1962). The induction of tumours following the direct implantation of four chemical carcinogens into the uterus of mice and the effect of strain and hormones thereon. *Br. J. Cancer,* 16, 479–483

KATZ, J.H. (1972). *Experimentation with Human Beings,* pp. 736–793. Russell Sage Foundation, New York

KAY, C.R., SMITH, A. and RICHARDS, B. (1969). Smoking habits of oral contraceptive users. *Lancet,* ii, 1228–1229

KJELD, J.M., PUAH, C.M. and JOPLIN, G.F. (1976). Changed levels of endogenous sex steroids in women on oral contraceptives. *Br. med. J.,* ii, 1354–1356

KLOPPER, A. (1970). Redevelopments in steroidal hormonal contraception. *Br. med. Bull.,* 26, 39–44

KRITCHEVSKY, D., STAPLE, E., RABINOWITZ, J.L. and WHITEHOUSE, M.W. (1961). Differences in cholesterol oxidation and biosynthesis in liver of male and female rats. *Am. J. Physiol.,* 200, 519–522

LARAGH, J.H. (1971). The pill, hypertension and the toxaemias of pregnancy. *Am. J. Obstet. Gynec.,* 109, 210–213

LARAGH, J.H., SEALEY, J.E., LEDINGHAM, J.G.G. and NEWTON, M.A. (1967). Oral contraceptives: renin, aldosterone and high blood pressure. *J. Am. med. Ass.,* 201, 918–922

LARSSON-COHN, U. (1975). Oral contraceptives and vitamins: a review. *Am. J. Obstet. Gynec.,* 121, 84–90

LARSSON-COHN, U. and STENRAM, U. (1965). Jaundice during treatment with oral contraceptive agents. *J. Am. med. Ass.,* 193, 422–426

LEIS, H.P. (1966). Endocrine prophylaxis of breast cancer with cyclic estrogen and progesterone. *Int. Surg.,* 45, 496–503

LOUDON, N.B. and BURTON, J.L. (1969). Oral contraceptives and blood pressure. *Lancet,* ii, 217

MACMAHON, B. and COLE, P. (1969). Endocrinology and epidemiology of breast cancer. *Cancer, N.Y.,* 24, 1146–1150

MANN, J.I., VESSEY, M.P., THOROGOOD, M. and DOLL, R. (1975). Myocardial infarction in young women with special reference to oral contraceptive practice. *Br. med. J.,* ii, 241–245

MARSHALL, J.C., REED, P.I. and GORDON, H. (1976). Luteinising hormone secretion in post oral contraceptive amenorrhoea: evidence for a hypothalamic feedback abnormality. *Clin. Endocr.*, **5**, 131–143

MELAMED, M.R., KOSS, L.G., FLEHINGER, B.J., KELISKY, R.P. and DUBROW, H. (1969). Prevalence rates of uterine cervical carcinoma *in situ* for women using the diaphragm or contraceptive oral steroids. *Br. med. J.*, **iii**, 195–200

MOOS, R.H. (1968). Psychological aspects of oral contraceptives. *Archs Gen. Psychiat.*, **19**, 87–94

MORRELL, M.T. and DUNNILL, M.S. (1968). The post-mortem incidence of pulmonary embolism in a hospital population. *Br. J. Surg.*, **55**, 347–352

MUMFORD, J.P. (1974). Drugs affecting oral contraceptives. *Br. med. J.*, **ii**, 333–334

NEWTON, M.A., SEALEY, J.E., LEDINGHAM, J.G.G. and LARAGH, J.H. (1968). High blood pressure and oral contraceptives. *Am. J. Obstet. Gynec.*, **101**, 1037–1045

NILSSON, A., JACOBSON, L. and INGEMANSON, C.A. (1967). Side-effects of an oral contraceptive with particular attention to mental symptoms and sexual adaptation. *Acta obstet. gynec. scand.*, **46**, 537–556

NILSSON, L. and SOLVELL, L. (1967). Clinical studies on oral contraceptives: a randomized, double blind, crossover study of 4 different preparations. *Acta obstet. gynec. scand.*, **46**, Supplement 8, 1–31

NORA, J.J. and NORA, A.H. (1973). Birth defects and oral contraceptives. *Lancet*, **i**, 941–942

NORA, A.H. and NORA, J.J. (1975). A syndrome of multiple congenital anomalies associated with teratogenic exposure. *Archs envir. Hlth*, **30**, 17–21

OCKNER, R.K. and DAVIDSON, C.S. (1967). Hepatic effects of oral contraceptives. *New Engl. J. Med.*, **276**, 331–334

OLIVER, M.F. (1970). Oral contraceptives and myocardial infarction. *Br. med. J.*, **ii**, 210–213

OSTERGAARD, E. (1964). Inhibition of ovulation observed at laparotomy in patients treated with 6-dehydro-6-methyl-17α-acetoxyprogesterone (DMAP). *Int. J. Fert.*, **9**, 25–28

OSTERGAARD, E. and STARUP, J. (1968). Occurrence and function of corporea lutea during different forms of oral contraception. *Acta endocr., Copenh.*, **57**, 386–394

PETERSON, W.F. (1969). Pregnancy following oral contraceptive therapy. *Obstet. Gynec., N.Y.*, **34**, 363–367

PINCUS, G., ROCK, J. and GARCIA, C.R. (1958). Effects of certain 19 nor-steroids upon reproductive processes. *Ann. N.Y. Acad. Sci.*, **71**, 677–690

POLLER, L., THOMSON, J.M., TABIOWO, A. and PRIEST, C.M. (1969). Progesterone oral contraception and blood coagulation. *Br. med. J.*, **i**, 554–556

POLLER, L., THOMSON, J.M. and THOMAS, W. (1971). Oestrogen/progestagen oral contraception and blood clotting: a long-term follow-up. *Br. med. J.*, **iv**, 648–650

RICE-WRAY, E., SCHULZ-CONTRERAS, M., GUERRERO, I. and ARANDA-ROSELL, A. (1962). Long term administration of norethindrone in fertility control. *J. Am. med. Ass.*, **180**, 355–358

ROBINSON, S.C. (1971). Pregnancy outcome following oral contraceptives. *Am. J. Obstet. Gynec.*, **109**, 354–358

ROCK, J., GARCIA, C.R. and PINCUS, G. (1957). Synthetic progestins in the normal human menstrual cycle. *Recent Prog. Horm. Res.*, **13**, 323–339

ROYAL COLLEGE OF GENERAL PRACTITIONERS' ORAL CONTRACEPTION STUDY (1974). *Oral contraceptives and health. An interim report from the oral contraception study of the Royal College of General Practitioners.* Pitman Medical, London

ROYAL COLLEGE OF GENERAL PRACTITIONERS' ORAL CONTRACEPTION STUDY (1976). The outcome of pregnancy in former oral contraceptive users. *Br. J. Obstet. Gynec.*, **83**, 608–616

ROYAL COLLEGE OF GENERAL PRACTITIONERS' ORAL CONTRACEPTION STUDY (1977). Effect on hypertension and benign breast disease of progestagen component in combined oral contraceptives. *Lancet*, **i**, 624

RYDER, N.B. and WESTOFF, C.F. (1966). Use of oral contraception in the United States, 1965. *Science, N.Y.*, **153**, 1199–1205

SABOUR, M.S. and FADEL, H.E. (1971). Hypertension and the oral contraceptives. A report of 19 patients. *Int. J. Gynecol. Obstet.*, **9**, 129–132

SANDMIRE, H.F., AUSTIN, S.D. and BECHTEL, R.C. (1976). Carcinoma of the cervix in oral contraceptive steroid and IUD users and non-users. *Am. J. Obstet. Gynec.*, **125**, 339–343

SARTWELL, P.E., MASI, A.T., ARTHES, F.G., GREENE, G.R. and SMITH, H.E. (1969). Thromboembolism and oral contraceptives: an epidemiological case-control study. *Am. J. Epidemiology*, **90**, 365–380

SARUTA, T., SAADE, G.A. and KAPLAN, N.M. (1970). A possible mechanism for hypertension induced by oral contraceptives. *Archs intern. Med.*, **126**, 621–626

SELTZER, C.C. (1969). Thromboembolic disorders and oral contraceptives. An editorial viewpoint. *J. Am. med. Ass.*, **207**, 1152

SHEARMAN, R.P. (1968). Investigation and treatment of amenorrhoea developing after treatment with oral contraceptives. *Lancet*, **i**, 325–326

SHEARMAN, R.P. (1971). Prolonged secondary amenorrhoea after oral contraceptive therapy. Natural and unnatural history. *Lancet*, **ii**, 64–66

SHEARMAN, R.P. (1975). Secondary amenorrhoea after oral contraceptives – treatment and follow up. *Contraception*, **11**, 123–132

SHEARMAN, R.P. and SMITH, I.D. (1972). Statistical analysis of relationship between oral contraceptives, secondary amenorrhoea and galactorrhoea. *J. Obstet. Gynaec. Br. Commonw.*, **79**, 654–656

SHERLOCK, S. (1968). Drugs and the liver. *Br. med. J.*, **i**, 227–229

SPELLACY, W.N., BUHI, W.C., SPELLACY, C.E., MOSES, L.C. and GOLDZIEHER, J.W. (1968). Carbohydrate studies in long-term users of oral contraceptives. *Diabetes*, **17**, supplement 1, 344–345

SPELLACY, W.N., CARLSON, K.L., BIRK, S.A. and SCHADE, S.L. (1968). Glucose and insulin alterations after one year of combination-type oral contraceptive treatment. *Metabolism*, **17**, 496–501

SPELLACY, W.N., NEWTON, R.E., BUHI, W.C. and BIRK, S.A. (1973). Carbohydrate and lipid studies during six months' treatment with megestrol acetate. *Am. J. Obstet. Gynec.*, **116**, 1074–1078

SZABO, A.J., COLE, H.S. and GRIMALDI, R.D. (1970). Glucose tolerance in gestational diabetic women during and after treatment with a combination-type oral contraceptive. *New Engl. J. Med.*, **282**, 646–650

TAKAHASHI, M. and LOVELAND, D.B. (1974). Bacteriuria and oral contraceptives: routine health examination of 12 076 middle-class women. *J. Am. med. Ass.*, **227**, 762–765

TAYMOR, M.L. (1964). Effect of synthetic progestins on pituitary gonadotrophin excretion. *J. clin. Endocr. Metab.,* **24**, 803–807

THOMAS, K. and FERIN, J. (1972). Suppression of the mid cycle LH surge by a low dose mestranol/lynestrenol oral combination. *Contraception,* **6**, 1–16

TUTTLE, S. and TURKINGTON, V.E. (1974). Effects of medroxyprogesterone acetate on carbohydrate metabolism. *Obstet. Gynec., N.Y.,* **43**, 685–692

VESSEY, M.P. and DOLL, R. (1968). Investigation of relation between use of oral contraceptives and thromboembolic disease. *Br. med. J.,* **ii**, 199–205

VESSEY, M.P. and DOLL, R. (1969). Investigation of relation between the use of oral contraceptives and thromboembolic disease: a further report. *Br. med. J.,* **ii**, 651–657

VESSEY, M.P. and INMAN, W.H.W. (1973). Speculations about mortality trends from venous thromboembolic disease in England and Wales and their relation to the pattern of oral contraceptive usage. *J. Obstet. Gynaec. Br. Commonw.,* **80**, 562–566

VESSEY, M.P., KAY, C.R., BALDWIN, J.A., CLARKE, J.A. and MACLEOD, I.B. (1977). Oral contraceptives and benign liver tumours. *Br. med. J.,* **i**, 1064–1065

VESSEY, M.P., WRIGHT, N.H., McPHERSON, K. and WIGGINS, P. (1978). Fertility after stopping different methods of contraception. *Br. med. J.,* **i**, 265–267

WEIR, R.J., TREE, M. and FRASER, R. (1970). Effect of oral contraceptives on blood pressure and on plasma renin, renin substrate and corticosteroids. *J. clin. Path.,* **23**, supplement 3, 49–54

WEIR, R.J., BRIGGS, E., MACK, A., TAYLOR, L., BROWNING, J., NAISMITH, L. and WILSON, E. (1971). Blood pressure in women after one year of oral contraception. *Lancet,* **i**, 467–470

WINGRAVE, S.A. (1978). Reduction in incidence of rheumatoid arthritis associated with oral contraceptives. Royal College of General Practitioners' Oral Contraception Study. *Lancet,* **i**, 569–571

WINSTON, F. (1969). Oral contraceptives and depression. *Lancet,* **ii**, 377

WOODS, J.W. (1967). Oral contraceptives and hypertension. *Lancet,* **ii**, 653–654

WYNN, V., ADAMS, P., OAKLEY, N. and SEED, M. (1974). Metabolic investigations in women taking 30 µg ethinyloestradiol plus 150 µg d-norgestrel. *The Second International Norgestrel Symposium. Some Metabolic Considerations of Oral Contraceptive Usage,* pp. 47–57. Excerpta Medica, Amsterdam

WYNN, V. and DOAR, J.W.H. (1969). Some effects of oral contraceptives on carbohydrate metabolism. *Lancet,* **ii**, 761–765

WYNN, V. and DOAR, J.W.H. (1970). Effects of oral contraceptives on carbohydrate metabolism. *J. clin. Path.,* **23**, supplement 3, 19–36

ZECH, P., RIFLE, G., LINDNER, A., SASSARD, J., BLANC-BRUNAT, N. and TRAEGER, J. (1975). Malignant hypertension with irreversible renal failure due to oral contraceptives. *Br. med. J.,* **iv**, 326–327

ZELL, J.R. and CRISP, W.E. (1964). A psychiatric evaluation of the use of oral contraceptives – a study of 250 private patients. *Obstet. Gynec., N.Y.,* **23**, 657–661

ZIEL, H.K. and FINKLE, W.D. (1976). Association of estrone with the development of endometrial carcinoma. *Am. J. Obstet. Gynec.,* **124**, 735–740

ZIEGLER, F.J., ROGERS, D.A., KRIEGSMAN, S.A. and MARTIN, P.L. (1968). Ovulation suppressors, psychological functioning and marital adjustment. *J. Am. med. Ass.,* **204**, 849–853

ZUSSMAN, W.V., FORBES, D.A. and CARPENTER, R.J. (1967). Ovarian morphology following cyclic norethindrone-mestranol therapy. *Am. J. Obstet. Gynec.*, **99**, 99–105

4 Other Hormonal Contraceptive Procedures

SEQUENTIAL ORAL CONTRACEPTIVES

Sequential preparations contained an oestrogen in all 21 or 22 tablets and a progestagen in either the last five to seven tablets (Norquen, Oracon, Oracon 28, Ortho-Novum SQ, Serial 28) or in the last 15 tablets (Ovanon). Some manufacturers included a placebo to be taken from Days 21 to 28 to maintain continuity of pill taking. The amount of oestrogen in these preparations was higher than in the conventional combined pill, usually being between 75 and 100 μg. The amount of progestagen was the same as in some combined pills.

The chief mode of action of sequential pills was inhibition of ovulation. Oestrogen, which was the sole component of the first 7 or 14 pills, suppressed FSH releasing factor and so reduced FSH secretion and inhibited follicle development. A daily intake of 80 μg of ethinyloestradiol alone will effectively suppress ovulation (Jackson et al., 1968) but levels of 50 μg are less effective. Despite their higher oestrogen content ovulation occurred more frequently with sequential than with conventional combined preparations. This is because of the absence of a progestagen with its inhibitory effect on the LH levels in the first half of the cycle and on the peak in LH secretion associated with ovulation. The absence of the other contraceptive effects of a progestagen on the endometrium and cervical mucus at this time also contributed to the higher failure rate of the sequential preparations. It was for this reason that in some sequential pills the progestagen was commenced after seven days.

There are few clinical indications for using sequential preparations in preference to the standard combined pills. Sequential pills were originally introduced because the hormone administration approximates to the normal pattern and cycle control is good. They enjoyed a period of popularity in the late 1960s and it was recently estimated that 500 000 American women were taking them. Realisation of the higher failure rate caused their popularity to wane in Great Britain with the result that no preparations are currently marketed here. They may be helpful for short term use in patients who require a lot of oestrogen, that is, women who develop amenorrhoea or very scanty withdrawal bleeding, depression, or loss of libido whilst taking the standard combined preparations. The larger dose of oestrogen may cause side-effects such as nausea and fluid retention. One report (Silverberg and Makowski, 1975) suggests that the use of sequential oral contraceptives by young women may predispose to the development of endometrial carcinoma before the age of 40 and that this may be due to synthetic oestrogen unopposed by progestagen. With the introduction of the more effective and medically safer low-dose combined pills containing only 30 μg of oestrogen and reduced amounts of progestagen, side-effects such as loss of libido and depression are much less common and the role of sequential preparations in contraceptive practice becomes very small.

The use-effectiveness of the sequential preparations was extensively studied by Sturtevant and Wait (1970). They collected data from several trials involving 5952 women studied for 59 492 cycles. The preparation contained 100 μg of ethinyloestradiol with 25 μg dimethisterone added from Days 16–21. They concluded that the failure rate was approximately 1 per 100 woman-years. Other authors have recorded failure rates of over 2 per 100 woman-years. Most authorities are agreed that sequential pills had a higher failure rate than combined oral contraceptives.

The risks of oestrogen-dependent metabolic complications such as venous thrombosis, pulmonary embolism, abnormal carbohydrate metabolism and biliary cholestasis were higher with sequential preparations. The incidence of endometrial carcinoma, though very small, may also be increased in sequential pill users. In general the higher risks of pregnancy and of side-effects outweigh any advantage of sequential oral contraceptives with respect to control of the menstrual cycle. The three sequential preparations which were available in the United States of America were recently withdrawn from the market.

LONG-ACTING ORAL CONTRACEPTION

Quinestrol, which is the 3-cyclo-pentyl ether of ethinyloestradiol, is an oestrogen which has prolonged activity in both animals and man as a result of storage in and subsequent release from the body fat. After its release it is metabolised, chiefly to conjugates of ethinyloestradiol. Quingestanol acetate, the 3-cyclopentyl-ether of norethynodrel acetate, is a progestagen with similar biological actions to norethisterone acetate.

A combination of these two steroids has been used as a long-acting oral contraceptive. A single dose of quinestrol, 2 mg, is given, preferably on Day 1 of the first menstrual cycle of treatment only. On Day 22, a combined dose of 2 mg quinestrol and 5 mg quingestanol is given. Subsequently the combined preparation is taken every four weeks without regard to bleeding. Postpartum patients are given the combination of drugs 4–6 weeks after delivery and the dose is repeated every four weeks.

Mode of Action

Effects on the Ovary

Wedge resections of the ovaries were carried out by Guiloff *et al.* (1970) on nine patients who had received the medication for more than one year. There was no effect on primordial follicles; a few developing follicles and an occasional cystic follicle were seen. There were no fresh corpora lutea. It appears that ovarian action is inhibited in the later stages of follicular maturation.

Effects on the Endometrium

A secretory response is produced earlier and a proliferative response later in the cycle. This is the reverse of the normal physiological response and of that seen with sequential regimes. Ninety-three per cent of biopsies obtained from Days 4–10 of the cycle showed early secretory changes. In a few cases there were either more advanced secretory changes or only proliferative changes. Of specimens taken one day after the dose most showed only proliferative changes but a few showed active secretion possibly indicating ovulation had occurred (Guiloff *et al.*, 1970). Reversal of the state of the endometrium is probably a secondary mode of action of this oral contraceptive preparation.

Use Effectiveness

A regimen of 2 mg quinestrol and 5 mg quingestanol has been studied by Guiloff *et al.* (1970) in 719 patients for 7441 cycles; 220 patients completed one year. Many were grand multiparae and the patient population was highly fertile, with a mean of 5.7 previous pregnancies. Twenty-five pregnancies occurred, an overall failure rate of 4.0 per 100 woman-years. Six of these patients became pregnant during the first cycle of therapy, having received only quinestrol. The pregnancy rate after the first cycle was 3.1 per 100 woman-years.

Maqueo-Topete *et al.* (1969) used the same preparation and recorded an overall pregnancy rate of 1.5 per 100 woman-years. With 2.5 mg of quingestanol acetate and 2.0 mg quinestrol a failure rate of 1.9 was found when 303 women were studied for 2493 cycles (Larranaga and Bergman, 1970). In this study all the pregnancies occurred during the first cycle, while in another series pregnancies occurred after 19, 22, 25 and 28 months of treatment, respectively.

Quinestrol is stored in fat and it is possible that obese patients liberate the steroid at a different rate from women of average weight. However, the average weight of those who became pregnant did not differ from those who did not become pregnant.

Menstruation

Withdrawal bleeding occurs 5–20 days after the combined dose has been taken (Guiloff *et al.*, 1970). Larranaga and Berman found that the interval was more predictable, being 6–13 days, and that predictability increased with more prolonged use of the method. Sixty-six per cent of cycles are between 26 and 33 days (Guiloff *et al.*, 1970). Using half the dose of quingestanol acetate, 72% of patients have cycle lengths between 26 and 33 days (Larranaga and Berman, 1970).

Duration of menstrual flow is usually normal, varying from three to six days, but occasionally patients are troubled with prolonged and heavy bleeding. This is commoner in the postpartum patient (Guiloff *et al.*, 1970) and continues for a few cycles. After this the chance of menorrhagia occurring in any individual is no higher than in women who have not had a recent pregnancy.

Spotting occurs in 7–10% of patients and breakthrough bleeding in 7–18% (Guiloff *et al.*, 1970, Larranaga and Berman, 1970). Increasing duration of therapy in the same population leads to a reduction in the incidence of spotting and breakthrough bleeding.

Side-effects

Nausea and vomiting are common side-effects occurring in from 21% (Guiloff *et al.*, 1970) to 29% of patients. As with the conventional combined oral contraceptives the frequency of these side-effects diminishes after the first few cycles until only about 7% of patients are affected (Guiloff *et al.*, 1970). Headaches were found to occur frequently in the first cycle (Larranaga and Berman, 1970) but other workers have reported that as few as 1% of patients had headaches (Maqueo-Topete *et al.*, 1969). Eliciting the incidence of as subjective a side-effect as headache depends very much on the psychological outlook of the subjects and the nature of the questions put by the observer. Leucorrhoea, another subjective side-effect that is difficult to measure, affects between 25% (Maqueo-Topete *et al.*, 1969) and 84% (Larranaga and Berman, 1970) of women starting to use the preparation. Complaints of both headache and leucorrhoea decrease with increasing use of the long-acting oral preparation, but it is not clear whether or not this is due to the most severely affected women discontinuing use. Lactation is reduced in as many as 78% of patients (Guiloff *et al.*, 1970).

Conclusion

It seems that quinestrol–quingestanol has a failure (pregnancy) rate of the same order as that found with other contraceptives but gives rise to menstrual irregularity and a moderately high rate of subjective side-effects, at least during the first few cycles of treatment. The mode of action probably resembles that of the conventional combined oral contraceptive together with a reversal of the endometrial phase. The metabolic side-effects, which have not been studied, are also likely to be the same. Quinestrol has been shown to cause a prolonged increase in plasma coagulation factors VII and X, and also of plasminogen and antiplasmin (Howie *et al.*, 1970). The main advantage is a reduction in pill taking. A large prospective study will be necessary before any conclusions can be made about the acceptability of quinestrol–quingestanol as a method of contraception. A dose of 2.5 mg quingestanol acetate seems to be as effective in preventing pregnancy as 5 mg.

CONTINUOUS PROGESTAGEN ORAL CONTRACEPTION

The metabolic effects that have been attributed to oestrogens led research workers to try out progestagens alone as contraceptive agents. Rudel *et al.* (1965) suggested that effective contraception with progestagens was possible without inhibition of ovulation. The progestational agents that have been used as low-dose contraceptives are of two groups, the 17-acetoxyprogesterone and the 19-nortestosterone derivatives. The former group includes chlormadinone, medroxyprogesterone, megestrol and clogestone, while the latter group includes norethynodrel, norethisterone (norethindrone), *d*-norgestrel, ethynodiol diacetate and lynoestrenol.

The first progestagens used on a continuous basis for contraception were chlormadinone acetate and norethisterone. Martínez-Manautou *et al.* (1966) attempted to find a dose of chlormadinone acetate which when administered continuously would not inhibit ovulation but would be an effective contraceptive. After considerable experience it seemed that 0.5 mg was an appropriate daily dose.

Rudel and Kincl (1966) reported the first use of norethisterone as a continuous daily progestagen-only pill. No real protection against pregnancy was provided by 0.2 mg per day, but 0.5 or 1.0 mg daily gave reasonably effective contraception.

Therapeutic Ratio

The basic problem with the continuous progestagen oral contraceptives so far available is one of obtaining an acceptably low failure (pregnancy) rate without an unacceptably high incidence of irregular vaginal bleeding. The effectiveness of these preparations in preventing pregnancy is dose-related. For example, in one study Martínez-Manautou and Giner Velazquez (1969) found that the pregnancy rate (Pearl index) of 0.5 mg chlormadinone acetate daily was 4 per 100 woman-years, while that of 0.3 mg daily was 8 per 100 woman-years; the relationship of pregnancy rate to dose has also been demonstrated with norgestrel (Foss *et al.*, 1968; Tyler, 1968; Tejuja *et al.*, 1974), megestrol acetate (Avendaño *et al.*, 1970; *Table 4.1*) and ethynodiol diacetate (Zañartu *et al.*, 1974).

As the dose of progestagen increases, so the incidence of breakthrough bleeding and irregular cycles also increases. This has been documented by Tyler (1968) and Tejuja *et al.* (1974) with norgestrel and by Avendaño *et al.* (1970; *Table 4.1*) with megestrol, and has been confirmed in many unpublished pilot

Table 4.1 MEGESTROL ACETATE AS A LOW-DOSE PROGESTAGEN ORAL CONTRACEPTIVE. RATES PER 100 WOMAN-YEARS (AVENDAÑO *et al.*, 1970)

Dose (daily)	Pregnancies	Intermenstrual bleeding	Other side-effects
250 mg	14.3	19.3	7.0
500 mg	4.4	32.9	22.9

studies with other compounds. Zañartu (personal communication) encourages his patients to accept an irregular cycle as an insurance against pregnancy; some sceptics have suggested that the mode of action of preparations with a high incidence of breakthrough bleeding is as a deterrent to intercourse!

Mode of Action

Ovulation

Ovulation is not suppressed in more than 50% of cycles by chlormadinone acetate, 0.5 mg (Zañartu *et al.*, 1968). Moghissi (1972) studied 11 patients who had received norethisterone, 0.35 mg, quingestanol acetate, 0.3 mg, or *dl*-nor-gestrel, 0.075 mg, and found presumptive evidence of ovulation in nine of them. Zañartu *et al.* (1974) observed direct evidence of ovulation at laparoscopy in 73% of patients on continuous or pre-coital regimes of various progestagens. It is clear therefore that inhibition of ovulation is not the primary mode of action of these contraceptive regimes.

Pituitary Gland

It seems that pituitary gonadotrophic function is not markedly suppressed by chlormadinone, 0.5 mg daily, because mid cycle peaks of LH high enough to be associated with ovulation have been demonstrated (Orr and Elstein, 1969). Similar patterns of LH excretion occur with continuous megestrol acetate (Mason *et al.*, 1967) and with norgestrel (Foss *et al.*, 1968). In patients in whom interference with the mechanisms stimulating ovulation does occur, it is thought that suppression of ovulation is due to reduction of the mid cycle LH peak, though as Diczfalusy *et al.* (1969) have pointed out, it is often difficult to be certain that ovulation has really occurred.

Corpus Luteum

The structure of the corpus luteum in these patients seems to be normal but the luteal function of progesterone production may be impaired by the administra-tion of norgestrel since pregnanediol excretion is reduced during the secretory phase of the cycle (Eckstein *et al.*, 1972). Chlormadinone seems to have no effect upon the excretion of pregnanediol or oestrogens. The 19-nortestosterone derivatives seem to be more likely to affect luteal function than the 17-acetoxy-progesterones.

Endometrium

Klopper (1970) suggested that the unprepared endometrium is the one tissue in the body which is able to resist implantation and that overcoming this resistance by hormonal changes is an essential feature of the ovarian cycle. It is possible that synthetic progestagens do not mimic the action of the corpus luteum in this respect and so although the endometrium appears secretory, it is able to resist the implantation of the ovum. Another theory of Klopper's (1970) is that the 19-nortestosterone derivatives cause inadequate secretory activity of the endo-metrium which fails to maintain the blastocyst until such time as implantation is complete. When small doses of progestagens are administered daily a normal secretory endometrium is achieved, suggesting the occurrence of ovulation and the secretion of endogenous progesterone. As the dose is increased there is a progressive reduction in glandular secretion and tortuosity (Rudel, 1970). The fact that increasing doses of the 19-nortestosterone derivatives are more effec-tive than the 17-acetoxyprogesterone derivatives in diminishing the normal secretory response is shown in *Table 4.2* (Martínez-Manautou, 1971). Rudel (1970) suggested that the progestagen-induced glandular suppression reflects

Table 4.2 LOW-DOSE PROGESTAGEN CONTRACEPTIVE THERAPY ENDOMETRIAL
PATTERN (MARTÍNEZ-MANAUTOU, 1971)

	Chlormadinone acetate (µg/day)				Norethisterone (µg/day)			Megestrol acetate (µg/day)	
	250 %	300 %	400 %	500 %	250 %	300 %	500 %	250 %	500 %
Normal secretory	59.6	51.5	37.2	29.8	30.0	25.7	9.7	39.6	39.1
Irregular secretory	29.2	25.8	41.8	33.4	36.3	34.9	26.9	37.5	52.2
Irregular	5.6	6.4	10.6	15.0	11.2	17.4	34.2	14.6	6.5
Inactive	1.1	4.2	2.6	9.9	17.5	14.4	13.4	0.0	0.0
Proliferative	4.5	12.1	7.8	11.9	5.0	7.6	15.8	8.3	2.2
Number of biopsies	89	141	153	1468	81	195	82	48	46

either interference with oestrogen action at the target organ or with production
of oestrogen. Inhibition of glandular development is directly related to progestagen dosage; norethisterone is one of the most potent, in this respect, of the
compounds studied. Both levonorgestrel (Zaldivar and Gallegos, 1971) and
chlormadinone have been shown to have an affinity for the mucus-producing
epithelia of the genital tract, levonorgestrel being highly specific in its deposition in the endometrium. The interference with the usual cyclic development
of the uterine lining (Maruffo *et al.*, 1974) and atrophic changes in the glands
may render the endometrium unsuitable for the implantation of a fertilised
ovum.

Cervical Mucus

The 17-acetoxyprogestagens and the 19-nortestosterone derivatives alter cervical
mucus, reducing penetration by spermatozoa. Hostility to spermatozoa is also
reflected by reduced or absent motility (Boettcher, 1974). The latter observation
is not always consistent in that in some cases motile spermatozoa are seen in cervical mucus, though none were found in washings of the fallopian tubes carried
out at laparotomy (Zañartu *et al.*, 1968) or in the endometrial cavity (Rowland,
1968).

Mears *et al.* (1969) felt that increased viscosity of cervical mucus was not
always associated with contraceptive effectiveness. It has also been pointed out
(Hawkins, 1974) that an action on cervical mucus cannot possibly be the
primary mode of action of low-dose progestagens in preventing pregnancy as
these preparations do not prevent ectopic gestation (Bonnar, 1974; Hawkins,
1974; Bergsjø *et al.*, 1974; Beral, 1975). If the cervical mucus changes constitute
a significant barrier to the passage of spermatozoa it would be expected that the
tubal pregnancy rate in these women would be lower than in the overall population.

Fallopian Tube

Zañartu *et al.* (1968) were unable to find any spermatozoa in the fallopian tubes
at hysterectomy conducted between 12 and 20 hours after intercourse in ten

patients taking chlormadinone acetate, 0.5 mg, daily. The fact that the concentration of radioactive chlormadinone acetate in the genital tract was high in the fallopian tubes suggests that this could be a site of contraceptive action (Gallegos *et al.*, 1970). If the incidence of ectopic gestation is in fact increased by low-dose progestagens, this also points to an effect on tubal motility.

It is therefore possible that the oviduct is one of the sites of action of the progestational steroids. The effect of clogestone acetate in varying doses on the epithelial microstructure has been studied by Oberti *et al.* (1974). The microvilli and cilia appeared to be reduced in number and size, but similar electron microscopic studies of the effects of both clogestone and norgestrel have failed to show any consistent effect on the tubal epithelium (Elder, unpublished observations). The muscular motility of the medial, lateral or both segments of the tube may be directly affected by progestagens. Coutinho *et al.* (1973) have suggested that tubal motility is increased thus accelerating passage of the ovum and allowing less time for fertilisation or development of a fertilised ovum within the tube. On the other hand reduced ability of the tube to transport the ovum, spermatozoa or fertilised ovum could result in failure of implantation. Whilst ingestion of clogestone, 2 mg, had no effect on human fallopian tube motility subsequently studied *in vitro, dl*-norgestrel, 0.15 mg, significantly increased the frequency but diminished the amplitude of fallopian tube contractions (Elder *et al.*, 1977).

Conclusion

The endometrium is probably the primary site of contraceptive action of low-dose progestagens. Apart from the histologically demonstrable endometrial changes caused by these preparations, the fact that the higher the incidence of irregular bleeding the lower is the pregnancy rate suggests an endometrial mode of action.

Although progestagens undoubtedly affect the nature of cervical mucus, it is doubtful if this is a principal site of their contraceptive action, because the tubal pregnancy rate in women on these pills is the same or higher than that in the general population at risk.

Altered tubal motility or diminution in numbers of epithelial cells affecting the time the fertilised ovum spends in the tube may contribute to the contraceptive effect.

CLINICAL USE OF CONTINUOUS LOW-DOSE PROGESTAGENS

The principal differences between low-dose progestagen and combined oral contraceptives are the higher failure rate, the increased incidence of abnormal menstruation and the absence of metabolic side-effects of the low-dose progestagens. The higher failure rate limits the population for whom the low-dose progestagens are advisable. Progestagens alone are not suitable for the patient who is very anxious to avoid pregnancy. Because of the higher rate of irregular bleeding they are unsuitable for those patients who find this socially or culturally unacceptable. They are not suitable for forgetful patients or those who find swallowing a pill objectionable. They may be ineffective in patients with a malabsorption syndrome.

Conversely, they are suitable for patients who wish to space their pregnancies, and who would not find it disastrous if they were to become pregnant sooner than expected. They are suitable for patients who are lactating, because there is no inhibition of milk production, and these patients are not very likely to conceive. Only traces of the steroids are found in breast-milk, and these are of no consequence to the infant. Progestagens can induce small changes in the relative concentrations of lipids, lactose and protein in the milk, but again these effects are too small to be of any consequence.

Finally, low-dose progestagens are suitable for patients who desire oral contraception but who are unable to take oestrogen-containing pills because of their metabolic side-effects. This group includes patients with previous thromboembolism or liver disease and latent diabetics. There is no evidence that low-dose progestagens affect the coagulation mechanism, liver function, or glucose tolerance. On the other hand, Spellacy *et al.* (1975) have shown that despite normal carbohydrate metabolism, norethisterone 0.35 mg daily, does affect the peripheral activity of insulin in such a way that higher circulating levels are required to maintain normal glucose homeostasis.

All the low-dose progestagens must be taken every day, and should be ingested at a constant time of day. They are available in packs which provide a mnemonic. In our opinion the actual time is not important provided it is approximately the same each day. We feel that in this way regular blood levels are more likely to be achieved, reducing the risk of failure and of disturbance of menstruation. Martínez-Manautou (1971) has also suggested that with *d*-norgestrel a well maintained blood level is important. In a recent study of 17α-acetoxy -6β,11β-dichloro-19-norpregna-4,6-diene-3,20-dione the use of morning and evening doses of 0.2 mg was compared with daily doses of 0.35 mg in the hope that the former regimen would provide a more constant blood level. In fact no difference in the incidence of bleeding problems or failures was found (McEwen *et al.*, 1977).

Most of the progestagens used in the combined pills have been tested at one time or another as low-dose progestagen oral contraceptives. The 17-acetoxyprogesterone derivatives used have been chlormadinone and megestrol. Both these compounds when administered chronically to beagle bitches have induced breast tumours. Despite the facts that beagles are very prone to develop breast tumours and that the doses used in the experiments were very high, the Food and Drug Administration in the United States of America and the Committee on Safety of Medicines in Great Britain advised withdrawal of these preparations from the market.

The only low-dose progestagens available now are 19-nortestosterone derivatives. These are norethisterone, 0.35 mg, *dl*-norgestrel, 0.075 mg, levonorgestrel, 0.03 mg, ethynodiol diacetate, 0.35 mg, lynoestrenol, 0.5 mg, and quingestanol acetate, 0.3 mg.

FAILURES WITH LOW-DOSE PROGESTAGEN; PREGNANCY RATES

Principal Causes of Failure

These are fairly evenly divided between method and patient failures (*see Table 4.3*). Method failure implies failure of the progestagens, when taken as directed,

Table 4.3 LOW-DOSE PROGESTAGEN ORAL CONTRACEPTION. NET PREGNANCY RATES PER 100 WOMAN-YEARS (±s.e.) IN WOMEN WHO AGREE TO USE THE PREPARATION FOR A COMPLETE YEAR (HAWKINS AND BENSTER, 1977)

	Megestrol acetate, 0.5 mg in oil (108 cases)	*Norethisterone, 0.35 mg (160 cases)*	*Chlormadinone acetate, 0.5 mg (125 cases)*
Method failure	5.1 ± 2.5	3.5 ± 2.2	1.6 ± 1.1
Patient failure	4.1 ± 2.0	4.9 ± 1.9	5.8 ± 2.2
Ectopic gestation*	0.9 ± 0.9	−	0.8 ± 0.8

*Both method failures

to prevent pregnancy, the effects on the genital tract having been insufficient to prevent fertilisation and implantation. Occasionally they can be due to malabsorption such as occurs with a gastro-intestinal upset at the mid cycle; patients should be warned to take additional precautions in such an event. Method failures occur more frequently during the first few months of use (*see Table 4.4*).

Table 4.4 LOW-DOSE PROGESTAGEN ORAL CONTRACEPTION. METHOD FAILURE PREGNANCIES' INCLUDING ECTOPIC GESTATION. NET LIFE TABLE RATES (±s.e.) FOR WOMEN WHO AGREE TO USE THE PREPARATION FOR A COMPLETE YEAR (HAWKINS AND BENSTER, 1977)

	Megestrol acetate, 0.5 mg in oil	*Norethisterone, 0.35 mg*	*Chlormadinone acetate, 0.5 mg*
0–3 months	3.1	2.1	1.6
4–6 months	2.0	0.8	0.8
7–9 months	0.9	0	0
10–12 months	0	0.6	0
13–24 months	(2 pregnancies)	(No pregnancies)	(No pregnancies)

Patient failure is caused by the patient forgetting to take the tablet and possibly even by her taking it at varying times of the day. Patient failures are a more important cause of pregnancy with low-dose progestagens than with combined pills and contribute heavily to the increased failure rate with the former preparations. All those who have worked extensively with low-dose progestagens agree that the omission of a single pill at the mid cycle can result in conception. This is presumably because ovulation is not in general inhibited by the progestagen and the contraceptive effect on the rest of the genital tract is transient. With an orthodox combined pill, provided sufficient pills have been taken to prevent ovulation, the omission of one dose does not matter.

Patient failure pregnancies are strongly associated with poor motivation. Regrettably, this defect tends to manifest itself at the mid cycle (Lehfeldt, 1959). In *Table 4.5* it will be noted that patient failures with megestrol and norethisterone occurred during the first six months of use with all three progestagens. The pregnancies with chlormadinone during the second six months of use were associated with newspaper publicity to the effect that the drug caused breast lumps in beagles. It is likely that in general poorly motivated patients tend to be eliminated from a study population during the first six

Table 4.5 LOW-DOSE PROGESTAGEN ORAL CONTRACEPTION. PATIENT FAILURE
PREGNANCIES, INCLUDING ECTOPIC GESTATION. NET LIFE TABLE RATES (±s.e.)
FOR WOMEN WHO AGREE TO USE THE PREPARATION FOR A COMPLETE YEAR
(HAWKINS AND BENSTER, 1977)

	Megestrol acetate, 0.5 mg in oil	*Norethisterone, 0.35 mg*	*Chlormadinone acetate, 0.5 mg*
0–3 months	1.9	4.3	0.8
4–6 months	2.2	0.6	1.8
7–9 months	0	0	1.6
10–12 months	0	0	1.6
13–24 months	(No pregnancies)	(3 pregnancies, 1 of them ectopic)	(No pregnancies)

months; they complain of complications which are considered to justify discontinuation of the contraceptive method and a few become pregnant. Patients continuing to take a progestagen up to a year are better motivated and pregnancies are then few.

Failure Rates

The efficiency of low-dose progestagen preparations as contraceptives is debatable. Both the progestagen used and its dose are important in attaining maximum efficiency.

Reported total pregnancy rates using chlormadinone acetate, 0.5 mg daily, varied between 1.7 (Christie, 1969), 2.1 (Martínez-Manautou *et al.*, 1967), 9.5 (Butler and Hill, 1969) and 12 (Mears *et al.*, 1969) per 100 woman-years, respectively. This large variation is probably related as much to the design of the trials as to the patients studied. Exclusion of unreliable patients and inadequate follow-up can easily distort the results. Apart from variations attributable to dose, the patient population studied and the environment seem to have an influence. Mears *et al.* (1969) found considerably higher failure rates for chlormadinone, norethisterone and norgestrel in Yugoslavia than those reported by workers in other environments; Hawkins and Benster (1977) found high failure rates for chlormadinone, megestrol acetate and norethisterone in West London.

Some pregnancy rates which have been reported for currently available preparations are summarised in *Table 4.6*. The total failure rate for low-dose progestagen probably lies between 2 and 10 per 100 woman-years and differs little from that now recognised to apply to intra-uterine devices. They therefore provide a suitable contraceptive for those who merely wish to delay a pregnancy and for women desiring oral contraception who are unable to take a combined preparation. Low-dose progestagens used alone cannot be recommended to a woman who desires maximum protection against pregnancy or for whom pregnancy is firmly contra-indicated.

Ectopic Gestation

It has been reported that the incidence of ectopic gestation is increased in women taking low-dose progestagens (Bergsjø *et al.*, 1974; Bonnar, 1974; Smith

Table 4.6 EFFECTIVENESS OF LOW-DOSE PROGESTAGEN ORAL CONTRACEPTIVES IN SELECTED CLINICAL TRIALS, 1970–1977 (MODIFIED FROM RINEHART, 1975)

Author, date and daily dose.	Number of patients	Number of months studied	Number of pregnancies — Total	Number of pregnancies — Method failure	Use-effectiveness — Failures per 100 woman-years**
ETHYNODIOL DIACETATE					
Zanartu et al., 1974, (0.25 mg)	363	2 959	39	27	10.9
Zanartu et al., 1974, (0.5 mg)	180	2 230	19	8	4.3
LYNOESTRENOL					
Prsić and Kočović, 1973	274	2 702	2	1	0.9
Voerman, 1973	4 731	37 405	29	19	0.9
NORETHISTERONE (NORETHINDRONE) (0.35 mg)					
Hawkins and Benster, 1977	200	2 130	14	5	7.9
Keifer, 1973	151	2 141	3	1	1.7
Larsson-Cohn, 1973, (0.3 mg)	221	4 083		1	1.4
Lawson and Bradshaw, 1972	503	2 555	5	1	2.0
McQuarrie et al., 1972	318	3 453	7	6	2.4
NORGESTREL*					
Eckstein et al., 1972, (dl, 0.075 mg)	144	1 781	3	1	2.0
Ferrari et al., 1973, (d, 0.0375 mg)	565	4 273	9	4	2.5
Foss, 1971, (dl, 0.05 mg)	242	4 278	13	3	3.6
Hernandez-Torres, 1970, (dl, 0.075 mg)	290	2 767	4	1	1.7
Kesserü et al., 1972, (d, 0.03 mg)	643	5 713	19	5	4.0
Korba and Paulson, 1974, (dl, 0.075 mg)	2 202	29 006	53	26	2.4
Rice-Wray et al., 1972, (d, 0.03 mg)	167	2 019	4	0	2.6
Scharff, 1973, (d, 0.03 mg)	1 969	15 393	55	12	4.3
QUINGESTANOL ACETATE (0.3 mg)					
Jubhari et al., 1974	382	3 208	6	3	2.9
Maqueo et al., 1972	400	4 370	12	7	3.3
Moggia et al., 1973	1 148	11 892	43	15	4.3
Rubio et al., 1972	181	2 489	4	4	1.9

*Doses of dl-norgestrel which are twice as large as doses of levonorgestrel (d-norgestrel) have the same pharmacological activity
**Pearl's index

et al., 1974; Beral, 1975). We found rates for ectopic gestation which were merely consistent with the view that the progestagens prevent intra-uterine pregnancy but not tubal pregnancy (Hawkins, 1974). It has been suggested that ectopic gestation is less likely to occur in failures from lynoestrenol than in those associated with other progestagens (Liukko and Erkkola, 1976).

In any event, when a patient taking a low-dose progestagen complains of pelvic pain investigation should be prompt. The other symptoms of ectopic gestation — delayed menstruation and intermenstrual bleeding, resemble low-dose progestagen side-effects. This, together with the knowledge that the patient is taking a contraceptive, can lead to a delay in diagnosis.

SIDE-EFFECTS

Menstrual Irregularities

The main side-effects of the low-dose progestagens are irregular menstrual cycles and intermenstrual bleeding. The duration of the first cycle varies widely from patient to patient. Irregular short cycles are more frequent during the first few months of therapy.

dl-norgestrel, 0.075 mg, commonly produces shortening of the cycle in the early months: 21% of cycles are of less than 17 days' duration (Eckstein *et al.,* 1972). With increasing duration of therapy the cycle has been found to become more regular with chlormadinone or norethisterone, but not with megestrol (Hawkins and Benster, 1977). The apparent improvement may partly be due to the fact that as the trial continues those women with troublesome short cycles have dropped out leaving those with more regular cycles in the study.

Prolonged cycles can also occur and as many as one-fifth of the patients can have a cycle length of more than 35 days (Hernandez-Torres, 1970). Long cycles are more common as the duration of therapy increases. Amenorrhoea for more than 60 days is relatively uncommon but occurs in the first year of use in 2–5% of patients (Hawkins and Benster, 1977). It creates anxiety in some women who think they might have an early pregnancy. Repeated pregnancy tests and examinations may be required to dispel this notion, in view of the gynaecologist's inability to diagnose a pregnancy of less than six weeks' maturity accurately. Of ten such patients studied by Hawkins and Benster (1977) menstruation returned spontaneously within two or three months of discontinuing the progestagen in seven, after taking a combined oestrogen–progestagen pill in two and after a diagnostic curettage in the remaining patient. Four of these patients subsequently had intra-uterine devices fitted; four others became pregnant.

The duration of the first menstrual period is often increased, particularly with chlormadinone. Thereafter the mean duration of menstrual flow is normal or slightly increased, but variability is considerable. In many trials there are roughly equal numbers of women complaining of increased and decreased flow. The incidence of menstrual irregularities is not much affected by the particular progestagen used. It must be remembered that comparison of the results of menstrual irregularities from one trial to another is difficult because of different definitions and the very subjective nature of the assessment of menstrual flow.

The magnitude of the problem of poor control of the menstrual cycle when using these progestational agents must not be underestimated. Eighty-six per cent of users of continuous quingestanol complained of menstrual irregularities (Jubhari *et al.*, 1974) while 58% of withdrawals from a study of norgestrel (Eckstein *et al.*, 1972) were due to poor cycle control. Hawkins and Benster (1977) found that 33% of women on chlormadinone acetate, 0.5 mg, or megestrol acetate, 0.5 mg, in oil discontinued the progestagen because of bleeding problems, whilst the corresponding figure for norethisterone, 0.35 mg, was only 23 per 100 woman-years.

The problem with low-dose continuous progestagens is that they may be really effective only when a dose is employed which causes a high incidence of menstrual irregularity. This difficulty tends to restrict use of the preparations to patients for whom combined oral contraceptives are contra-indicated.

Other Side-effects

Excessive weight gain, nausea, headache and defective libido, are not serious problems. Their incidence is lower than with the combined pill. A significant proportion of patients taking quingestanol in fact report an increase in their libido and some women taking low-dose progestagens report relief of pre-menstrual tension and dysmenorrhoea. Hernandez-Torres (1970) found instances of weight gain of more than 5 lb (2.3 kg), headache and nausea or vomiting in only 6%, 5% and 2% of cycles respectively, with the use of 75 μg mestranol. Heinen (1971) recorded higher incidences; headaches occurring in 12% and nausea in 17% of patients, but these symptoms occurred in only 1.6% and 2% respectively of all cycles. Bernstein and Seward (1972) recorded nausea in only 3% of patients. Zañartu *et al.* (1974) did not find these symptoms a problem in a large series of patients taking clogestone, norgestrel or ethynodiol diacetate. Hawkins and Benster (1977) found such symptoms uncommon with chlormadinone, megestrol or norethisterone.

Neither coagulation mechanisms nor carbohydrate metabolism are altered by the administration of chlormadinone acetate, norethisterone or norgestrel. This is in contrast to the well known effects of oestrogen-containing oral contraceptives on both blood coagulation and carbohydrate metabolism. Eckstein *et al.* (1972) studied many biochemical variables in patients before and after taking *dl*-norgestrel, 0.075 mg, and they found that the values were all normal except for significantly reduced serum cholesterol and globulin levels. No explanation for this can be offered, but it is worth contrasting these findings with those of Wynn *et al.* (1966) who found that oestrogen-containing pills raised the level of serum cholesterol in proportion to the duration of administration, but that oestrogen and norgestrel combinations could reduce serum cholesterol (Wynn *et al.*, 1974). Low-dose progestagens do not produce any consistent changes in the usual tests of liver function or thyroid function.

Low-dose progestagens have no consistent effect on blood pressure. Sporadic cases of women who have become hypertensive whilst taking progestagens are probably coincidental. We found only one such patient in a study of 557 patients involving 4500 woman-months of use of chlormadinone, megestrol or norethisterone. The series included 22 women with hypertension or other major cardiovascular disorders none of whom deteriorated.

The labelling of commercial preparations of progestagens usually mentions history of liver disease, thrombophlebitis or varicose veins as contra-indications. This is purely precautionary and there is no evidence that this form of contraception has any effect on such patients. Our study included 23 women with a history of liver disease (226 woman-months of use), 95 women with varicose veins (973 woman-months) and 15 with a history of thrombophlebitis (140 woman-months) and none had any deterioration or recurrence.

Six of our patients were found to have small fibro-adenomata of the breast whilst taking low-dose progestagens; two others developed corpus luteum cysts of the ovary. We regard this as a normal incidence for patients of reproductive age. Martínez-Manautou (1971) concluded that chlormadinone does not increase the incidence of breast tumours.

Of 158 patients taking progestagens whom we studied by vaginal cytology for one to two years none developed dysplasia or carcinoma *in situ* of the cervix. The incidence of these problems in a large series of women taking chlormadinone was not increased (Martínez-Manautou, 1971).

There have been no reports of any increase of birth defects in patients becoming pregnant whilst taking low-dose progestagens. Of 18 patients in our series who conceived whilst taking a progestagen and in whom the pregnancy continued, all had normal babies. The incidence of defects was not unusual in the series of 96 pregnancies conceived on chlormadinone studied by Martínez-Manautou (1971).

CONCLUSION

Compared with the combined pill the continuous progestagen preparations used so far have a higher rate of pregnancy and cause more menstrual irregularities resulting in a higher discontinuation rate. No other undesirable metabolic side-effects have been reported and this will ensure that these preparations have some place in current contraceptive practice. They are particularly suitable for patients who are informed about their properties, and who wish to postpone their next pregnancy rather than to secure maximum protection against conception. They are useful in helping to prevent conception during prolonged lactation. In malnourished populations a rapid cessation of lactation after commencement of the combined oral contraceptive early in the puerperium can lead to severe malnutrition, gastro-enteritis and death of the infant, and low-dose progestagens started postpartum may be particularly applicable.

DEPOT HORMONAL CONTRACEPTION

There are two modes of depot hormonal contraception. One is the intramuscular injection of hormones which are slowly released from the injection site, and the other is the insertion of a silicone polymer ring into the vagina, or capsules beneath the skin, from which hormones are released. Recently intra-uterine devices which release hormones have been studied; these are considered in Chapter 9 (p. 172).

The injectable hormone preparations contain either a progestagen alone or a combination of oestrogen and progestagen. The progestagen preparations employ medroxyprogesterone acetate in an aqueous suspension or norethisterone oenanthate. They have been given intramuscularly in doses of 150 mg and 100 mg respectively, the depot lasting for 12 weeks.

The combined oestrogen–progestagen preparation that has been used in this way contains algestone acetonide (previously known as dihydroxyprogesterone acetophenide), 150 mg, and oestradiol oenanthate, 10 mg, repeated every 28 days.

INTRAMUSCULAR PROGESTAGEN DEPOTS

Mode of Action

The mode of action is similar to that of continuous low-dose oral progestagen preparations. This is an excessive progestagen effect on the endometrium, making it atrophic and difficult for implantation to take place should conception occur, an effect on the cervical mucus making penetration of spermatozoa difficult and probably also inhibition of ovulation.

Goldzieher *et al.* (1970) found that immediately before each three-monthly injection of 150 mg medroxyprogesterone acetate FSH levels were normal and LH levels depressed to 65% of control levels. Jeppsson and Johansson (1976) did not find the reduction in plasma LH. The administration of progestagen appears to lead to inhibition of the peak of LH production at mid cycle, but a random sampling technique does not provide an accurate reflection of the gonadotrophin levels throughout the month. The ovaries continue to produce oestradiol in amounts similar to the early follicular phase of the normal menstrual cycle (Mishell *et al.*, 1972). These facts suggest that ovulation is commonly suppressed.

Preliminary studies using 200 mg norethisterone oenanthate (Howard *et al.*, 1975) suggest that ovulation is in general inhibited by this substance, although in one subject ovulation probably occurred between eight and ten weeks after the injection.

The duration of action of medroxyprogesterone acetate and norethisterone differs significantly. The peak serum level of medroxyprogesterone acetate after injection has been reported to be 10–25 ng/ml at 5–20 days after the injection, decreasing to 5–10 ng/ml by 30 days after injection; Jeppsson and Johansson (1976) observed a similar pattern of serum levels but found the actual values to be considerably lower. Detectable levels can still be found 185 days after injection (Kirton and Cornette, 1974). Using 200 mg of norethisterone oenanthate Howard *et al.* (1975) found that peak serum levels of 8 ng/ml were reached about ten days after injection, but that by 98–112 days the levels were undetectable. As the norethisterone oenanthate depot has a shorter life the resumption of normal menstruation and the return of fertility seems to be more prompt. After more than 7 injections the rate of decline of blood levels of norethisterone gets slower in some patients (Fotherby *et al.*, 1978).

Ceasing three-monthly administration of depot medroxyprogesterone acetate led to a resumption of normal periods within one year in 87.5% of patients who had received one injection but in only 52.9% of patients who had received four injections (Scutchfield *et al.*, 1971). Similar results were recorded by Gardner and Mishell (1970) who found that only 50% of women who discontinued depot medroxyprogesterone acetate had resumed normal cycles within six months of the last injection. The other 50% had irregular bleeding which tended to become regular within 15 months. Three of the patients had not resumed normal ovulation 18 months after stopping the depot injections. The findings of Tyler *et al.* (1970) were similar in that in only one-third of patients given between one and three injections had ovulation restarted within six months. Nearly all of their patients ovulated within one year of the last injection.

Delay in return of ovulation after stopping treatment is a major drawback to the use of medroxyprogesterone acetate but, from the limited data available, there is no significant delay with norethisterone oenanthate (Howard, G. *et al.*, personal communication). Most women prefer a method of contraception that is immediately reversible, but for the woman who has completed her family, or for one who is not desirous of pregnancy for years the delay in return of ovulation is probably acceptable.

Use Effectiveness

With medroxyprogesterone acetate, 150 mg every three months, Tyler *et al.* (1970) recorded no pregnancies in a study of 350 women over a period of four years; Scutchfield *et al.* (1971) recorded one pregnancy, a rate of 0.23 per 100 woman-years; and Dodds (1975) found only one pregnancy, attributed to being three weeks late for an injection, in 1883 women with 38 599 woman-months of treatment. Zañartu (1968) employed a six-monthly injection of between 200 mg and 1000 mg of medroxyprogesterone acetate for a total of 30 900 woman-months. Method failure pregnancies were 1.1 per 100 woman-years. Data accumulated from many sources by Rinehart and Winter (1975) gave an average pregnancy rate of 0.3 per 100 woman-years, but this may be an underestimate.

Intramuscular medroxyprogesterone, 150 mg, is effective in preventing pregnancy for four months after a confinement (Sharp and MacDonald, 1973). Lactation is not affected in women who are breast-feeding. Used postpartum, medroxyprogesterone can prolong postpartum bleeding, but this can be managed with a cyclical combined oestrogen and progestagen oral contraceptive. The onset of the first menstrual period is often delayed.

McDaniel and Pardthaisong (1974) used 400 mg of medroxyprogesterone acetate six-monthly, supplemented by 40 μg oral ethinyloestradiol every four weeks. There was one accidental pregnancy in 26 women; the gross cumulative pregnancy rate over five years was 3.2 per 100 woman-years. Rinehart and Winter's (1975) review suggests that failure rates with the six-monthly regimen are higher than with three-monthly injections.

There is little data available on the use effectiveness of norethisterone oenanthate, but Chinnatamby (1971) recorded an extremely low failure rate. In our series of 160 patients studied for 1070 cycles using 200 mg doses there have been only three pregnancies. These women conceived at 107, 109 and 126 days, respectively, after the last injection. Since the time between injections has been reduced to 70 days, there have been no pregnancies (Howard, personal communication). The failure rates received by Rinehart and Winter (1975) vary from 0 to 14.8 per 100 woman years.

Side-effects

With medroxyprogesterone acetate menstruation tends to become irregular, often proceeding to amenorrhoea. Tyler *et al.* (1970) found that the time required for ten episodes of bleeding varied between 153 and 425 days. The interval between cycles and the duration of bleeding is extremely variable from episode to episode, as it is between patients, and intermenstrual spotting is common. This variability in vaginal bleeding accounts for a drop-out rate of 17% from one trial after 18 months (Scutchfield *et al.*, 1971) and 19% after 12 months in another (Dodds, 1975). The latter author noted that the amount of blood loss decreased and the interval between menstrual periods increased with each succeeding injection. Amenorrhoea can also be a problem with medroxy-progesterone acetate, episodes of five or more months being recorded (Tyler *et al.*, 1970). As the dose or frequency of these injections increases so does the incidence of amenorrhoea, which may occasionally become permanent. In Dodds' (1975) study using 150 mg doses all 709 patients followed up had resumed normal menstruation within ten months of ceasing the injections and 40 out of 60 women who wanted a pregnancy conceived within 18 months of discontinuation.

Bleeding patterns with norethisterone oenanthate are more regular, according to preliminary data (Howard, personal communication). In 313 patients studied for 3503 cycles there was considerable variation in the duration of menstrual bleeding. After three or more injections amenorrhoea becomes more common.

Bleeding problems such as a greater variation between cycle lengths and episodes of heavy bleeding are probably due to variations in progestagen levels caused by irregular release from the depot. Amenorrhoea is probably due to greater pituitary suppression than that produced by continuous oral progestagen preparations. Due to varying release rates the duration of effectiveness is uncertain and there may be times when the blood and tissue levels of the progestagen cease to influence the endometrium.

Provided other gynaecological causes are excluded, irregular vaginal bleeding can be treated by the administration of cyclical oestrogens. Even so, the incidence of irregular vaginal bleeding is high with large doses of progestagen, 61% of patients having either irregular or heavy bleeding or amenorrhoea after one injection of 400 mg of medroxyprogesterone acetate (McDaniel and Pardthaisong, 1974).

Many women having medroxyprogesterone acetate injections notice weight gain. Average increases range from 1.4 lb (0.6 kg) to 9 lb (4.1 kg) in clinical studies (Rinehart and Winter, 1975).

Tyler *et al.* (1970) found that the side-effects of medroxyprogesterone included nervousness (4.6%), nausea (3.4%), headache (2.1%), feeling of bloatedness (1.7%) and breast tenderness (1.3%). These are low incidences considering the subjective nature of the symptoms.

There seems to be no increase in the incidence of breast nodules or in the size of the breasts with the use of medroxyprogesterone acetate (McDaniel and Pardthaisong, 1972, 1973). Despite this the use of other 17α-hydroxyprogesterone acetate derivatives, such as chlormadinone and megestrol, has been discouraged by the Federal Drug Administration in the United States of America and by the Committee on the Safety of Medicines in Great Britain because of the increased incidence of breast nodules produced by these hormones in beagles. The 19-nortestosterone derivatives such as norethisterone do not seem to have the same effect.

It has been claimed that the use of medroxyprogesterone injections is associated with an increased incidence of carcinoma *in situ* of the cervix but the evidence is entirely inconclusive.

Metabolic Complications

No significant changes in blood pressure, fasting blood sugar, blood urea nitrogen, or prothrombin time were noted by Tyler *et al.* (1970) during therapy with intramuscular medroxyprogesterone acetate.

Other workers have noted changes in carbohydrate metabolism in patients on depot progestagens. Gershberg *et al.* (1969) found that medroxyprogesterone acetate, 150 mg, caused impairment of the glucose tolerance of overt diabetics, with increased fasting levels of growth hormone and diminished hormone response to insulin. Latent diabetics developed impaired glucose tolerance after three months. Tuttle and Turkington (1974) studied 18 women on 400 mg of depot medroxyprogesterone six-monthly. Although only one patient had an impaired glucose tolerance test, the progestagen caused a significant increase in both fasting and three-hour levels of plasma insulin, and an increase in serum growth hormone levels at three hours. This evidence suggests that medroxyprogesterone in this dose can be diabetogenic, presumably because of the very high blood levels that occur soon after injection.

Preliminary data on ten women studied with intravenous glucose tolerance tests before, and 2 and 12 weeks after, injection of 200 mg norethisterone oenanthate suggest that there is no effect on carbohydrate metabolism or on the blood coagulation mechanism. Prothrombin time and plasma factor VII and X levels are unchanged (Howard *et al.*, 1977). Intramuscular progestagen regimens are best avoided in latent diabetics until more information is available.

Conclusions

For the average individual in a Western country, depot progestagen preparations have a limited use because of the high incidence of irregular vaginal bleeding, and the slight risks of permanent amenorrhoea. The administration of cyclical oestrogen progestagen preparations to regulate vaginal bleeding constitutes an additional risk factor. Most women using contraception in Great Britain request an immediate return to the fertile state on discontinuation and this may not happen for many months after using intramuscular progestagen.

Certain categories of women are suitable for depot progestagens: intelligent women who are unable to manage with other methods, but who understand the risks involved; women who require temporary contraception while waiting for their husbands' sperm counts to become negative after vasectomy and those who have had rubella vaccination; and various psychiatric patients, including drug addicts, who seem to have a dichotomy between their desire to prevent pregnancy and their ability to employ the usual contraceptive methods, and in whom an intra-uterine device is contra-indicated. Finally, depot progestagens provide an effective, acceptable and simple method of contraception for the underdeveloped world, which can be easily administered by paramedical personnel. The intramuscular injection of a depot progestagen provides a reliable method whose administration is the responsibility of physician, district nurse, or other trained person.

COMBINED OESTROGEN–PROGESTAGEN INJECTIONS

These preparations are sometimes used because they result in better control of the menstrual cycle than the injection of a progestagen alone. The steroids that have been used are algestone acetophenide, 150 mg, and oestradiol oenanthate, 10 mg, or norgestrel, 25 mg, and oestradiol hexahydrobenzoate, 5 mg, given together as monthly injections. These compounds were chosen because their activity within the body lasts for approximately three weeks. The first injection is given on Day 8 of the menstrual cycle, and repeated every 28 days.

Mode of Action

The mode of action of these combinations of steroids are the same as those of combined oral contraceptive tablets, including inhibition of ovulation and secondary progestagen effects which make the cervical mucus less easily penetrated by spermatozoa and the endometrium too advanced in its secretory phase for implantation to occur.

Suppression of ovulation is due to the inhibitory effects of both hormones on the production of gonadotrophin releasing factors, resulting in low FSH levels which cause failure of the follicle to develop and low LH levels which fail to stimulate ovulation.

Use Effectiveness

No pregnancies were reported by Tyler *et al.* (1970) in a study involving 615 patients for 516 woman-years of use, in which algestone acetophenide, 150 mg and oestradiol oenanthate, 10 mg, were employed. Using the same combination of steroids Creasey *et al.* (1970) in a small study of 38 women for 353 cycles reported no pregnancies. Using norgestrel, 25 mg, and oestradiol hexahydrobenzoate, 5 mg, De Souza and Coutinho (1972) in a study of 50 women for 550 cycles also found no pregnancies.

The effectiveness of the combination of oestrogen and progestagen seems, from these studies, to differ little from that of oral combinations. The groups of patients studied are not sufficiently large to give an accurate comparison.

Side-effects

In contrast with oral combinations, the method shares with progestagen injections the disadvantage that menstrual irregularity commonly develops. The average duration of menstrual bleeding was increased in the study of Tyler *et al.* (1970) from 4.7 days to 6.6 days. Before the combined hormone injection 88%

of women had a menstrual cycle of 22–30 days; during therapy this dropped to 75%. Other authors have found a higher incidence of menstrual irregularities. Creasey *et al.* (1970) noted in their small study that this occurred in women who had had five or more injections. The reason for the irregular bleeding is probably irregular absorption of the hormones from the depot site.

The incidence of other side-effects, such as depression, breast tenderness and nausea was high, being 43%, 43% and 31% respectively (Tyler *et al.*, 1970). These figures were obtained in response to direct leading questions and were not spontaneous complaints from the patient. This may be a factor in increasing the recorded incidence of side-effects but it is likely that the underlying incidence of genuine side-effects is moderately high. This view has been confirmed by Creasey *et al.* (1970).

Metabolic Complications

These have not been evaluated. It can be assumed that they are the same as the combined pill, but the fact that the steroids used in two of the trials were algestone acetophenide and oestradiol oenanthate means that their metabolic effects, primarily on the liver, may differ from those of the 19-nortestosterone-derived progestagens and ethinyloestradiol or mestranol used in the combined pill.

It is unlikely that this method will be acceptable to the majority of contraceptive users. The main disadvantage seems to be the need for monthly injections and the inferior menstrual cycle control compared to the combined oral preparations. If the injection can be carried out by the patient herself or by a community nurse visiting the home, then there is scope for the method to be used by some patients, particularly those who wish reliable contraception, but do not like swallowing tablets.

OTHER DEPOT PREPARATIONS

These consist of silicone polymer impregnated with progestagens such as norgestrel, norethisterone acetate, megestrol acetate or medroxyprogesterone acetate and used as vaginal rings or subcutaneous capsules.

Vaginal Rings

These are usually 60–80 mm in diameter and 7–10 mm thick, being made of polysiloxane. The first progestagen to be used in this way was medroxyprogesterone acetate in doses of between 50 and 400 mg; the rings were 75 mm in diameter. Other progestagens which have been incorporated into the same base are chlormadinone acetate (Henzl *et al.*, 1973), norethisterone and norgestrel (Mishell *et al.*, 1975). The optimum dose of progestagen and the length of time that the ring should be left *in situ* have not yet been determined.

Mode of Action

Significant amounts of progestagen are absorbed from the rings into the blood stream. Mishell and Lumkin (1970) found that 27 mg of medroxyprogesterone acetate has been absorbed during a three-week insertion period. Mishell *et al.* (1975) found that 18–32 mg of norgestrel, depending on the amount of steroid used, were lost from the ring during the three-week interval. Blood levels of levonorgestrel after insertion of intravaginal Silastic rings containing 50 mg of *dl*-norgestrel reached a peak of 5 ng/ml between the first and fourth day after insertion (Stanczyk *et al.*, 1975). These levels were similar to plasma levels found two hours after the oral ingestion of 250 μg *dl*-norgestrel (Victor *et al.*, 1975). Thereafter the levels decreased steadily to reach zero after about 30 days. Initial blood levels are higher if the dose of progestagen in the ring is increased but the total duration of an adequate circulating level of steroid is no greater (Stanczyk *et al.*, 1975). The levels of circulating progestagen are sufficient to inhibit ovulation in most cycles. Using raised plasma progesterone levels as an index of ovulation, Mishell *et al.* (1975) found that ovulation occurred in one-sixth of cycles when the ring contained 50 mg of norethisterone or 10 mg norgestrel. When the dose was doubled there were no ovulatory cycles with either hormone. This inhibitory effect on ovulation, as measured by depression of plasma oestradiol and progesterone to 'early follicular' levels has been confirmed by Victor *et al.* (1975) using rings containing 50 mg of norgestrel. The progestagens may also have their characteristic effects on the cervical mucus making it difficult or impossible for spermatozoa to penetrate.

Use Effectiveness

The present studies concerned with the rate of absorption of progestagen and the effects on ovulation have been too small to draw any conclusions about the effectiveness of these rings. No pregnancies were recorded. From the evidence of blood levels of norgestrel (Victor *et al.*, 1975; Stanczyk *et al.*, 1975) and the resultant inhibition of ovulation with rings containing norgestrel or other closely related compounds (R2323; 13-ethyl-17-hydroxy-18,19-dinor-17α-pregna-4,9,11-trien-20yn-3-one; Johansson *et al.*, 1975) it is probable that the failure rate in large scale studies will be similar to that found with oral progestagens.

Side-effects

The earlier rings were stiff and there was a problem with discomfort and vaginal ulceration due to pressure (Mishell and Lumkin, 1970). These symptoms were probably due to the inclusion of a spring within the substance of the ring to prevent dislodgement. With the use of thicker and softer rings, the need for a spring has disappeared, as have these side-effects.

The incidence of irregular vaginal bleeding is quite high. Intermenstrual bleeding occurred in one-third of cycles when the ring contained 50 mg of norgestrel but this reduced to one-quarter of cycles when the dose of norgestrel was increased to 100 mg. With 100 mg medroxyprogesterone acetate there was intermenstrual bleeding in 17% of cycles (Mishell *et al.*, 1975). Irregular bleeding was an even greater problem when norethisterone 50 and 100 mg were used. Absence of withdrawal bleeding after removal of the ring was not a problem with the use of medroxyprogesterone acetate 100 mg but did occur after 10–15% of cycles in which rings containing 50–100 mg of norgestrel were used (Mishell *et al.*, 1975).

An offensive odour due to absorption of blood into the ring has been found to be a slight problem in about one-tenth of cycles in which norgestrel was used in the ring. It did not happen when medroxyprogesterone acetate was used (Mishell *et al.*, 1975). This difference is difficult to explain. On the evidence available medroxyprogesterone acetate seems to be slightly better in reducing the incidence of bleeding whilst the ring is *in situ* and it is associated with a lower incidence of amenorrhoea after the removal of the ring. This may be due to a more constant absorption of the steroid. As the administration of large doses of the 17-acetoxyprogestagens is suspected of being associated with breast lumps, it is unlikely that this hormone will be widely acceptable even if use is permitted. It seems therefore that if progestagen-containing rings are to be introduced into practice, it will be with the 19-nortestosterone progestagens.

More recently a Silastic vaginal device containing chlormadinone acetate has been tested. Ovulation occurs in the presence of the device but when thin tubing was used as the ring blood levels of chlormadinone were higher than those found after the oral administration of 0.5 mg of the steroid, daily (Henzl *et al.*, 1973). It is possible that the blood levels of chlormadinone are more constant with a vaginal device than with oral administration.

The disadvantages of this method of contraception are those of any continuous progestagen administration, a fairly high pregnancy rate and poor control of the menstrual cycle. In the case of subcutaneous capsules, surgical removal is needed to stop therapy. In a small highly motivated group of patients there may be a place for such contraception. There may also be a place for it in the underdeveloped countries where patients need contraception but cannot be relied upon to take tablets regularly and where other methods are unacceptable.

Subcutaneous Implants

Silastic capsules 20–30 mm in length and having a wall thickness of about 0.5 mm have been used as a depot from which progestagens may be released slowly into the blood stream.

Megestrol acetate, 23–33 mg per capsule, was the first progestagen to be used in this way. Using four Silastic capsules inserted subcutaneously, pregnancy rates of 10–16 per 100 woman-years were recorded (Coutinho *et al.*, 1970; Croxatto *et al.*, 1971). Spotting and breakthrough bleeding occurred in 30–34% of the early cycles. Using a higher dose of megestrol acetate within five capsules inserted subcutaneously in the forearm Coutinho *et al.* (1972) recorded only a single pregnancy in 1440 cycles observed for up to 15 months but Croxatto *et al.* (1971) found a pregnancy rate of 6.0 per 100 woman-years.

Progestagens of the 19-nortestosterone group such as norethisterone acetate and levonorgestrel have also been used. Croxatto *et al.* (1975) compared the use of capsules 20 mm in length containing 20–30 mg of either megestrol acetate, levonorgestrel or norethisterone. The release rates were: megestrol acetate,

13–17 µg/(cm/day), levonorgestrel 3–5 µg/(cm/day), norethisterone acetate 11 µg/(cm/day). Six capsules of megestrol seemed to be the most effective, giving a pregnancy rate of 3.2 per 100 woman-years. The number of capsules inserted was greater than with the other two progestagens and the release of megestrol from the capsule was faster. The results with the 19-nortestosterone derivatives were not good but this may have been due to an inadequate dose or an inadequate rate of release. In a small study using norethisterone acetate in capsules of varying size and wall thickness the most effective seemed to be a capsule 22 mm long with a wall thickness of 0.59 mm giving a release rate of 128 µg/24 hours for about ten months (Jeyaseelan *et al.*, 1977). The overall pregnancy rate in this study was 9.2 per 100 woman-years, confirming that the results with 19-nortestosterone derivatives are inferior as yet to those obtained with megestrol. Further studies of different doses seem to be necessary. There is evidence that the incidence of ectopic gestation is increased in pregnancies resulting from the failure of subcutaneous Silastic implants containing progestagens (Tatum and Schmidt, 1977).

Cycle control is initially poor and with the use of megestrol, intermenstrual bleeding occurred in 25–34% of cycles during the first three months of use (Croxatto *et al.*, 1975). The incidence of irregular bleeding increased with increasing dose of progestagen used.

The long-term use of megestrol implants has no demonstrable effect on the coagulation mechanism as measured by platelet counts and adhesiveness, clotting time, prothrombin time, partial thromboplastin time, prothrombin consumption test, thromboplastin generation time, euglobulin lysis time, plasma fibrinogen or plasma factors II, V, VII and X, X and VIII (Lira *et al.*, 1975).

Although a 17-acetoxy-progestagen, megestrol seems to be the most effective in Silastic implants at present. The fact that it has been taken off the market in the United States of America and Great Britain means that it will not become an accepted method in the developed countries. It is therefore difficult to justify its use in underdeveloped countries. The disadvantages of depot contraception are those of any continuous progestagen administration, a fairly high pregnancy rate and poor control of the menstrual cycle, at least initially. With subcutaneous capsules surgical removal is needed to stop the therapy. There is probably a place for this method in underdeveloped countries where patients need contraception but cannot be relied upon to take tablets regularly and other methods are unacceptable. It seems essential that an appropriate dose of a 19-nortestosterone derivative be defined as soon as possible.

POSTCOITAL CONTRACEPTION

Hormonal contraceptives which will be effective in preventing pregnancy if administered within a few hours after intercourse have been developed from two different points of view. The patient who has been, perhaps unwillingly, the subject of an isolated episode of sexual intercourse which is unlikely to be repeated, may need medication which will prevent her becoming pregnant in consequence. Administration of fairly large doses of oestrogen have been employed for this purpose. The other group of patients for whom a postcoital pill would appear suitable are those who would like a manoeuvre which can be repeated *ad libitum*, but cannot predict when intercourse will occur and do not wish to take synthetic steroids regularly when they may not need them. The use of a progestagen contraceptive pill to be taken after intercourse has been studied with this type of patient in mind.

Oestrogens

In 1926 it was observed that injection of oestrogen two days after copulation in rats and mice caused a rapid reappearance of oestrus and failure of pregnancy (Parkes and Bellerby, 1926). Oestrogens alter the passage of ovum and spermatozoa, prevent implantation and act as an abortifacient. Emmens (1970) reviewed much of the animal work; a range of compounds with oestrogenic or oestrogen antagonist activity are effective in preventing pregnancy when administered postcoitally in rodents, and some have been shown to be active in primates. Oestrogens, either stilboestrol, 50 mg, or ethinyloestradiol, 0.5–2 mg daily, for up to six days were found in a careful study by Morris and van Wagenen (1966) to be effective in preventing pregnancy in women who had had an episode of unprotected intercourse.

The mode of action of these large doses of oestrogen is probably by delaying transport of the ovum within the fallopian tube (Pincus and Kirsch, 1936), and by preventing implantation of the blastocyst. Apart from tending to inhibit the secretory change in the endometrium, oestrogen reduces endometrial carbonic anhydrase and this may prevent implantation by impairing the removal of carbon dioxide produced by the conceptus.

The administration of high doses of oestrogen after intercourse seems to act as an effective contraceptive (Shearman, 1973). Kuchera (1974) studied 1217 women given 25 mg stilboestrol twice a day for five days starting within 72 hours of intercourse and there were no pregnancies. Seventy per cent of the women had had intercourse within three days of the expected date of ovulation. Half the patients had nausea, but in many this only persisted for one day, while there were only low incidences (1–2%) of headaches and dizziness. An antiemetic drug is usually needed to prevent nausea and vomiting with high doses of oestrogens. The results of other studies using oestrogens for a postcoital contraceptive regime are summarised in *Table 4.7*.

Table 4.7 OESTROGENS AS POSTCOITAL CONTRACEPTIVES (MODIFIED FROM RINEHART, 1976)

		Number of cases	*Failures*		
			Pregnancies	*%*	*Reference*
Stilboestrol	25–50 mg/day × 5	524	4	0.8	Haspels and Andriesse (1973)
	50 mg/day × 4	107	0	0	Hall (1974)
	50 mg/day × 4–5	150	3	2.0	Coe (1972)
	50 mg/day × 5	80	1	1.2	Sparrow (1974)
	50 mg/day × 5	247	4	1.6	Massey *et al.* (1971)
	50 mg/day × 5	1217	0	0	Kuchera (1974)
Ethinyloestradiol	1 mg/day × 5	32	0	0	Döring (1971)
	2–5 mg/day × 3–5	133	2	1.5	Lehfeldt (1973)
	2–5 mg/day × 5	1418	10	0.7	Haspels and Andriesse (1973)

If the use of high doses of oestrogen is to be effective it is important that treatment is initiated soon after intercourse, preferably within 24 hours and certainly within 72 hours, and that it is taken for the prescribed time, usually five days, despite nausea. It is also important to repeat the dose should vomiting occur. The Food and Drug Administration in the United States of America approved the use of stilboestrol as a postcoital contraceptive in 1973, but only as an emergency measure. Its routine use as a contraceptive is undesirable because of the symptomatic side-effects and the risks of thrombosis and embolism that are associated with high doses of oestrogens. Nonetheless, Szontágh and Kovács (1969) have given postcoital dienoestrol as a regular contraceptive and found it effective. Its use is contra-indicated in patients with a history of thrombosis, embolism, disease of the liver or heart, or hypertension.

The delayed appearance of carcinoma of the vagina has been reported in the female children of mothers treated with stilboestrol in high doses during pregnancy (Herbst et al., 1971). Because the stilboestrol was given later in the pregnancy and for a longer period of time than postcoital oestrogen it has been claimed that the oncogenic risk to the fetus is irrelevant to postcoital use (Rinehart, 1976). Despite the fact that relevant data in humans are lacking it is prudent to exclude the presence of an established pregnancy before the use of postcoital stilboestrol because of the risk of teratogenicity in an existing conceptus.

The use of large doses of stilboestrol and its selection as a postcoital contraceptive is surprising because of its common side-effects such as nausea, vomiting and mastalgia, and because it may cause congenital abnormalities if the pregnancy continues. Teratogenesis has not been reported with ethinyloestradiol, which is also effective as a postcoital contraceptive (Haspels and Andriesse, 1973). Ethinyloestradiol may be used orally, preferably starting within 24 hours of the episode of intercourse and giving 5 mg daily for five days. Alternatively, oestradiol benzoate, 30 mg daily, can be given intramuscularly for five days. Intramuscular preparations of conjugated oestrogens have also been used. The intramuscular route may be valuable if vomiting is a problem with oral preparations.

Ectopic Pregnancy

When postcoital oestrogens fail to prevent pregnancy the incidence of ectopic pregnancy has been reported to be one in ten (Morris and van Wagenen, 1973). This rate is sufficiently high as to suggest that not only do postcoital oestrogens fail to prevent ectopic gestation but also that they tend to slow the passage of the ovum through the fallopian tube (Smythe and Underwood, 1975) and make extra-uterine implantation more likely.

Progestagens

These steroids also have a postcoital antifertility effect. They have been tested as postcoital contraceptives used regularly as a primary contraceptive manoeuvre.

Quingestanol acetate, a long-acting progestagen, is the 3-cyclopentyl-enol-ether of norethisterone acetate. Rubio et al. (1970) found that less than 0.5 mg taken within 24 hours of coitus was ineffective as a contraceptive, but that

0.8 mg taken after every act of coitus completely prevented pregnancy in 200 women studied during 1004 cycles. The mean rate of coitus in these women was 10.6 times per month. Three-quarters of the patients maintained their normal menstrual cycle of between 26 and 33 days. The duration of the menstrual flow was similar to that of pre-treatment menses, but one-quarter of the patients had some intermenstrual bleeding. Other workers (Mischler, 1974; Moggia *et al.*, 1974) have used 0.8, 1.5 or 2.0 mg doses of quingestanol acetate.

Levonorgestrel was used postcoitally in a study of 4631 women over 41 802 months with an average coital frequency of 8.0 per month by Kesserü *et al.* (1973). The recorded failure rates using doses of 150, 250, 300 and 400 μg norgestrel after intercourse were 45.2, 6.8, 4.9 and 3.5 pregnancies per 100 woman-years, respectively. The commonest side-effect was disturbance of menstruation. The number of patients withdrawing from this trial for unknown reasons varied between 10% and 17% in the subgroups, and this high withdrawal rate may have concealed a higher pregnancy rate.

Clogestone acetate, a 17α-acetoxyprogesterone derivative, has been used immediately pre-coitally in doses of 0.6 mg. One of the sites of action of this compound is the cervical mucus, in which progestational changes take place within 4–6 hours of the administration of a single dose of 1.0 mg.

Clogestone acetate, 1.0 mg, has also been used at the time of intercourse or up to four hours after intercourse. Only preliminary studies have been carried out but despite encouraging reports from South America and South Africa, the results in Great Britain were sufficiently poor that the trial was stopped. Further trials using 2 mg have also been abandoned due to unacceptably high pregnancy rates. In many of these patients menstruation became irregular, normal menstrual cycles occurring in only 62% of patients, short cycles (<24 days) in 23% and long cycles (>36 days) in 15% of patients.

Oestrogen–Progestagen Combinations

Yuzpe, Thurlow, Ramzy and Leyshon (1974) gave a single dose of 0.1 mg ethinyloestradiol and 1.0 mg *dl*-norgestrel to women after single episodes of intercourse, but had three pregnancies in 143 cases. There were no pregnancies in a further series of 243 cases given a second dose 12 hours after the first (Yuzpe, Thurlow and Lancee, 1974).

A small trial of regular use of dienoestrol, 2.5 mg, with ethynodiol diacetate, 0.2 mg, as a postcoital pill resulted in one pregnancy in 35 women over a total of 284 cycles (Szontágh and Kovács, 1969).

Ethical and Legal Implications

Evading the relatively philosophical question of whether or not the prevention of early development of the conceptus is abortion, and subject in Great Britain to the conditions of the Abortion Act 1967, ethical considerations remain. It is surprising that therapeutic trials with agents such as stilboestrol which has a reputed teratogenic potential (Herbst *et al.*, 1971; Herbst *et al.*, 1972) and related drugs whose teratogenic potential is unknown should be permitted in environments where abortion cannot be guaranteed in the event of failure. The possibility must be envisaged of legal proceedings against a physician who was not in a position to form a judgment in advance as to whether or not the conditions of the Abortion Act will eventually be satisfied. Physicians in Great Britain who feel that 'in good faith' is a fair defence against actions for negligence would do well to consider the implications of the Congenital Disabilities (Civil Liability) Act, 1976, on the rights of the unborn child. To be sued many years later, perhaps in one's retirement, by a teenage girl with adenocarcinoma of the vagina would be poor recompense for 'helping out' her mother, possibly when a student, with stilboestrol as a postcoital contraceptive.

Oestrogen given in sufficient dose and in time is effective as a postcoital contraceptive after a single act of unprotected intercourse, although the ethical and legal implications are unresolved. The side-effects of oestrogens preclude their use as a regular postcoital contraceptive. The progestagens can be used but the increasing incidence of menstrual disorders as coital frequency increases, and the high failure rate, makes them unsuitable at the present time. Further research into their mode of action and into the best progestagen and its optimum dose are necessary.

The use of insertion of a copper intra-uterine device as a postcoital contraceptive is considered in Chapter 10 (p. 211).

CONCLUSION

There is a clear moral justification for the employment of a postcoital contraceptive procedure to relieve the anxiety of the rape victim that she might have become pregnant. Whether or not such an approach to the problem of the woman who has willingly had a single episode of unprotected intercourse and fears pregnancy is justified, is a matter for the individual to decide. Certainly many young women, uncommitted to sexual intercourse and hence unprovided with contraceptive protection, might well react differently in provocative circumstances if they could be certain that a safe way of preventing pregnancy would be available the following day. In this day and age fear of pregnancy, to be terminated by either an abortion or a confinement, is still a deterrent to intercourse in unsophisticated young women. The development of a postcoital contraceptive which conveys no ill-effects might well be conducive to promiscuity in such women.

A postcoital contraceptive pill which is sufficiently innocuous that it can be employed as a primary method of contraception could be useful for the woman whose need for protection is infrequent, irregular or unpredictable. It is to be hoped that further studies will lead to a really effective agent of this type, and provide a convenient means of contraceptive which reduces the intake of synthetic steroids to the minimum necessary to achieve the object.

REFERENCES

AVENDAÑO, S., TATUM, H.J., RUDEL, H.W. and AVENDAÑO, O. (1970). A clinical study with continuous low doses of megestrol acetate for fertility control. *Am. J. Obstet. Gynec.*, **106**, 122–127

BERAL, V. (1975). An epidemiological study of recent trends in ectopic pregnancy. *Br. J. Obstet. Gynaec.*, **82**, 775–782

BERGSJØ, P., LANGENGEN, H. and AAS, J. (1974). Tubal pregnancies in women using progestagen-only contraception. *Acta obstet. gynec. scand.*, **53**, 377–378

BERNSTEIN, G.S. and SEWARD, P. (1972). Daily chlormadinone acetate as an oral contraceptive. *Contraception*, **5**, 369–388

BOETTCHER, B. (1974). A possible mode of action of progestagen-only oral contraceptives. *Contraception*, **9**, 123–131

BONNAR, J. (1974). Progestagen-only contraception and tubal pregnancies. *Br. med. J.*, **i**, 287

BUTLER, C. and HILL, H. (1969). Chlormadinone acetate as oral contraceptive: a clinical trial. *Lancet*, **i**, 1116–1119

CHINNATAMBY, S. (1971). A comparison of the long-acting contraceptive agents norethisterone oenanthate and medroxyprogesterone acetate. *Aust. & N.Z.J. Obstet. Gynaecol.*, **11**, 233–236

CHRISTIE, G.A. (1969). Chlormadinone acetate as oral contraceptive. *Lancet*, **i**, 1262.

COE, B.B. (1972). The use of diethylstilbestrol as a post-coital contraceptive. *J. Am. Coll. Hlth Ass.*, **20**, 286

CONGENITAL DISABILITIES (CIVIL LIABILITY) ACT (1976). Her Majesty's Stationery Office, London

COUTINHO, E.M., MAIA, H. and XAVIER DA COSTA, R. (1973). The effect of a continuous low dose progestin on tubal and uterine motility. *Int. J. Fert.*, **18**, 161–166

COUTINHO, E.M., MATTOS, C.E.R., SANT'ANNA, A.R.S., FILHO, J.A., SILVA, M.C. and TATUM, H.J. (1970). Long-term contraception by subcutaneous silastic capsules containing megestrol acetate. *Contraception*, **2**, 313–321

COUTINHO, E.M., MATTOS, C.E.R., SANT'ANNA, A.R., FILHO, J.A., SILVA, M.C. and TATUM, H.J. (1972). Further studies on long term contraception by subcutaneous silastic capsules containing megestrol acetate. *Contraception*, **5**, 389–393

CREASY, R.K., HILLIG, J.A. and MORRIS, J.A. (1970). Physiologic control of conception with an intramuscular progestagen-oestrogen: clinical experience. *Contraception*, **1**, 271–278

CROXATTO, H.B., DÍAZ, S., ATRIA, P., CHEVIAKOFF, S., ROSATTI, S. and ODDÓ, H. (1971). Contraceptive action of megestrol acetate implants in women. *Contraception*, **4**, 155–167

CROXATTO, H.B., DÍAZ, S., QUINTEROS, E., SIMONETI, L., KAPLAN, R., LEIXELARD, P. and MARTINEZ, C. (1975). Clinical assessment of subdermal implants of megestrol acetate, d-norgestrel and norethindrone as long term contraceptive in women. *Contraception*, **12**, 615–628

DE SOUZA, J.C. and COUTINHO, E.M. (1972). Control of fertility by monthly injections of a mixture of norgestrel and a long-acting oestrogen. *Contraception*, **5**, 395–399

DICZFALUSY, E., GOEBELSMANN, U., JOSANNISSON, E., TILLINGER, K.G. and WIDE, L. (1969). Pituitary and ovarian function in women on continuous low dose progestogens; effect of chlormadinone acetate and norethisterone. *Acta endocr. Copenh.*, **62**, 679–693

DODDS, G.H. (1975). The use of sterile medroxyprogesterone acetate suspension as a contraceptive during a three year period. *Contraception*, **11**, 15–23

DÖRING, G.K. (1971). Morning-after-pill: die postkoitale hormonelle Schwanger-schaftsverhütung. *Dt. Ärtzebl.,* **35**, 2395–2396

ECKSTEIN, P., WHITBY, M., FOTHERBY, K., BUTLER, C., MUKHERJEE, T.K., BURNETT, J.B.C., RICHARDS, D.J. and WHITEHEAD, T.P. (1972). Clinical and laboratory findings in a trial of norgestrel, a low-dose progestogen-only contraceptive. *Br. med. J.,* **iii**, 195–200

ELDER, M.G., MYATT, L. and CHAUDHARI, G. (1977). The effects of clogestone and norgestrel on the spontaneous activity of the fallopian tube. *Int. J. Fert.,* **23**, 61–64

EMMENS, C.W. (1970). Postcoital contraception. *Br. med. Bull.,* **26**, 45–50

FERRARI, A., MEYRELLES, J.C., SARTORETTO, N.N. and SOARESFILHO, A. (1973). The menstrual cycle in women treated with *d*-norgestrel, 37.5 micrograms, in continuous administration. *Int. J. Fert.,* **18**, 133–140

FOSS, G.L. (1971). Experience with norgestrel in continuous microdosage. In *Current Problems in Fertility,* pp. 139–144. Ed. Ingelman-Sundberg, A. and Lunell, N.O. Plenum, New York

FOSS, G.L., SVENDSEN, E.K., FOTHERBY, K. and RICHARDS, D.J. (1968). Contraceptive action of continuous low doses of norgestrel. *Br. med. J.,* **iv**, 489–491

FOTHERBY, K., HOWARD, G., SHRIMANKER, K., ELDER, M.G. and BYE, P. (1978). Plasma levels of norethisterone after single and multiple injections of norethisterone oenanthate. *Contraception,* **18**, 1–6

GALLEGOS, A.J., GONZÁLEZ-DIDDI, M., MERINO, G. and MARTÍNEZ-MANAUTOU, J. (1970). Tissue localization of radioactive chlormadinone acetate and progesterone in the human. *Contraception,* **1**, 151–161

GARDNER, J.M. and MISHELL, D.R. (1970). Analysis of bleeding patterns and resumption of fertility following discontinuation of long-acting injectable contraceptive. *Fert. Steril.,* **21**, 286–291

GERSHBERG, H., ZORRILLA, E., HERNANDEZ, A. and HULSE, M. (1969). Effects of medroxyprogesterone acetate on serum insulin and growth hormone levels in diabetics and potential diabetics. *Obstet. Gynec., N.Y.,* **33**, 383–389

GOLDZIEHER, J.W., KLEBER, J.W., MOSES, L.E. and RATHMACHER, R.P. (1970). A cross-sectional study of plasma FSH and LH levels in women using sequential, combination or injectable steroid contraceptives over long periods of time. *Contraception,* **2**, 225–248

GUILOFF, E., BERMAN, E., MONTIGLIO, A., OSORIO, R. and LLOYD, C.W. (1970). Clinical study of a once-a-month oral contraceptive: quinestrol—quingestanol. *Fert. Steril.,* **21**, 110–118

HALL, M.N. (1974). Use of the "morning-after pill" in a college student health service. *J. Am. Coll. Hlth Ass.,* **22**, 395–396

HASPELS, A.A. and ANDRIESSE, R. (1973). The effect of large doses of estrogens post coitum in 2000 women. *Eur. J. Obstet. Gynec. reprod. Biol.,* **3**, 113–117

HAWKINS, D.F. (1974). Progestogen-only contraception and tubal pregnancies. *Br. med. J.,* **i**, 387

HAWKINS, D.F. and BENSTER, B. (1977). A comparative study of three progestogens used as oral contraceptives. *Br. J. Obstet. Gynaec.,* **84**, 708–713

HEINEN, G., RINDT, W., YEBOA, J. and UMLA, H. (1971). Hormonal contraception with 0.5 mg chlormadinone acetate by continuous administration. *Contraception,* **3**, 45–53

HENZL, M.R., MISHELL, D.R., VELAZQUEZ, J.G. and LEITCH, W.E. (1973). Basic studies for prolonged progestogen administration by vaginal devices. *Am. J. Obstet. Gynec.*, **117**, 101–106

HERBST, A.L., KURMAN, R.J., SCULLY, R.E. and POSKANZER, D.C. (1972). Clear-cell adenocarcinoma of the genital tract in young females. *New Engl. J. Med.*, **287**, 1259–1264

HERBST, A.L., ULFELDER, H. and POSKANZER, D.C. (1971). Adenocarcinoma of the vagina: association of maternal stilbestrol therapy with tumor appearance in young women. *New Engl. J. Med.*, **284**, 878–881

HERNANDEZ-TORRES, A. (1970). Preliminary evaluation of fertility control with continuous microdose norgestrel. *Adv. Planned Parenthood*, **5**, 125–130

HOWIE, P.W., MALLINSON, A.C., PRENTICE, C.R.M., HORNE, C.H.W. and McNICOL, G.P. (1970). Effect of combined oestrogen-progestogen oral contraceptives, oestrogen and progestogen on antiplasmin and antithrombin activity. *Lancet*, **ii**, 1329–1332

HOWARD, G., MYATT, L. and ELDER, M.G. (1977). The effects of intramuscular norethisterone oenanthate used as a contraceptive on intravenous glucose tolerance and on blood coagulation factors VII and X. *Br. J. Obstet. Gynaec.*, **84**, 618–621

HOWARD, G., WARREN, R.J. and FOTHERBY, K. (1975). Plasma levels of norethisterone in women receiving norethisterone oenanthate intramuscularly. *Contraception*, **12**, 45–52

JEPPSSON, S. and JOHANSSON, E.D.B. (1976). Medroxyprogesterone acetate, estradiol, FSH and LH in peripheral blood after intramuscular administration of Depo-Provera to women. *Contraception*, **14**, 461–469

JEYASEELAN, S., TAKKAR, D., BHUYAH, U.N., LAUMAS, K.R. and HINGORANI, V. (1977). Local tissue response to silastic implant containing norethisterone acetate in women. *Contraception*, **15**, 39–51

JOHANSSON, E.D.B., LUUKKAINEN, T., VARTIAINEN, E. and VICTOR, A. (1975). The effect of progestin R 2323 released from vaginal rings on ovarian function. *Contraception*, **12**, 299–307

JUBHARI, S., LANE, M.E. and SOBRERO, A.J. (1974). Continuous microdose (0.3 mg) quingestanol acetate as an oral contraceptive agent. *Contraception*, **9**, 213–219

KEIFER, W.(1973). A clinical evaluation of continuous norethindrone (0.35 mg). *A Clinical Symposium on 0.35 mg Norethindrone; Continuous Regimen Low-dose Oral Contraceptive*, pp. 9–14. Ortho Pharmaceutical, Raritan, New Jersey

KESSERÜ, E., LARRAÑAGA, A., HURTADO, H. and BENAVIDES, G. (1972). Fertility control by continuous administration of *d*-norgestrel, 0.03 mg. *Int. J. Fert.*, **17**, 17–27

KESSERÜ, E., LARRAÑAGA, A. and PARADA, J. (1973). Post coital contraception with *d*-norgestrel. *Contraception*, **7**, 367–379

KIRTON, K.T. and CORNETTE, J.C. (1974). Return of ovulatory cyclicity following an intramuscular injection of medroxyprogesterone acetate. *Contraception*, **10**, 39–45

KLOPPER, A. (1970). Developments in steroidal hormonal contraception. *Br. med. Bull.*, **26**, 39–44

KORBA, V.D. and PAULSON, S.R. (1974). Five years of fertility control with microdose norgestrel; an updated clinical review. *J. reprod. Med.*, **13**, 71–75

KUCHERA, L.K. (1974). Post coital contraception with diethyl stilbestrol — updated. *Contraception*, **10**, 47–54

LARRANAGA, A. and BERMAN, E. (1970). Clinical study of a once-a-month oral contraceptive: quinestrol-quinestanol. *Contraception*, **1**, 137–148

LARSSON-COHN, U. (1973). Continuous microdose norethindrone vs. combined oral contraceptives. *A Clinical Symposium on 0.35 mg Norethindrone; Continuous Regimen Low-dose Oral Contraceptive*, pp. 4–8. Ortho Pharmaceutical, Raritan, New Jersey

LAWSON, J.P. and BRADSHAW, F.R. (1972). Experience with norethisterone 0.35 mg as an oral contraceptive — a preliminary report. *Curr. med. Res. Opin.*, **1**, 53–61

LEHFELDT, H. (1959). Willful exposure to unwanted pregnancy (WEUP). Psychological explanation for patient failures in contraception. *Am. J. Obstet. Gynec.*, **78**, 661–665

LEHFELDT, H. (1973). Choice of ethinyl estradiol as a postcoital pill. *Am. J. Obstet. Gynec.*, **116**, 892–893

LIRA, P., RIVERA, L., DIAZ, S. and CROXATTO, H.B. (1975). Study of blood coagulation in women treated with megestrol acetate implants. *Contraception*, **12**, 639–644

LIUKKO, P. and ERKKOLA, R. (1976). Low-dose progestogens and ectopic pregnancy. *Br. med. J.*, **ii**, 1257

McDANIEL, E.B. and PARDTHAISONG, T. (1972). Changes in breast size during prolonged use of contraceptive injections. *J. med. Ass. Thai.*, **55**, 294–297

McDANIEL, E.B. and PARDTHAISONG, T. (1973). Incidence of breast nodules in women receiving multiple doses of medroxyprogesterone acetate. *J. biosoc. Sci.*, **5**, 83–88

McDANIEL, E.B. and PARDTHAISONG, T. (1974). Use effectiveness of six-month injections of DMPA as a contraceptive. *Am. J. Obstet. Gynec.*, **119**, 175–180

McEWEN, J.A., JOYCE, D.N., TOTHILL, A.U. and HAWKINS, D.F. (1977). Early experience in contraception with a new progestogen. *Contraception*, **16**, 339–349

McQUARRIE, H.G., HARRIS, J.W., ELLSWORTH, H.S., STONE, R.A. and ANDERSON, A.E. (1972). The clinical evaluation of norethindrone in cyclic and continuous regimens. *Proceedings of the Ninth Annual Meeting of the American Association of Planned Parenthood Physicians, Excerpta Medica International Congress Series No. 246*, pp. 124–130. Excerpta Medica, Amsterdam

MAQUEO, M., MISCHLER, T.W. and BERMAN, E. (1972). The evaluation of quingestanol acetate as a low dose oral contraceptive. *Contraception*, **6**, 117–125

MAQUEO-TOPETE, M., BERMAN, E., SOBERON, J. and CALDERON, J.J. (1969). A pill-a-month contraceptive. *Fert. Steril.*, **20**, 884–891

MARTÍNEZ-MANAUTOU, J. (1971). Low level progestogens. *Control of Human Fertility, Proceedings of the 15th Nobel Symposium, Södergarn, Lidingö, Sweden, May 27–29, 1970*, pp. 53–67. Ed. Diczfalusy, E. and Borell, U. Wiley, New York

MARTÍNEZ-MANAUTOU, J. and GINER-VELÁZQUEZ, J. (1969). *IX Reunión Anual de la Sociedad Mexicana de Nutrición y Endocrinología, San José, Purúa, Mexico*, p. 263. Cited by Martínez-Manautou, J. (1971), *q.v.*

MARTÍNEZ-MANAUTOU, J., GINER-VELÁZQUEZ, J., CORTES-GALLEGOS, V., AZNAR, R., ROJAS, B., GUITTEREZ-NAJAR, A. and RUDEL, H.W. (1967). Daily progestogen for contraception: a clinical study. *Br. med. J.*, **ii**, 730–732

MARTÍNEZ-MANAUTOU, J., GINER-VELÁZQUEZ, J., CORTES-GALLEGOS, V., CASASOLA, J., AZNAR-RAMOS, R. and RUDEL, H.W. (1966). Fertility control with microdoses of progestogen. In *Proceedings of the sixth Pan–American Congress of Endocrinology, Mexico City, October 10–15, 1965,* pp. 157–165. Ed. Gual, C. Excerpta Medica, Amsterdam
MARUFFO, C.A., CASAVILLA, F., VAN NYNATTEN, B. and PEREZ, V. (1974). Modifications of the human endometrial fine structure induced by low-dose progestogen therapy. *Fert. Steril.,* **25**, 778–787
MASON, B.A., COX, H.J.E., MASON, D.W. and GRANT, V. (1967). Clinical and experimental studies with low doses of megestrol acetate. *Postgrad. med. J.,* **43**, supplement, 45–48
MASSEY, J.B., GARCIA, C-R. and EMICH, J.P. Jr. (1971). Management of sexually assaulted females. *Obstet. Gynec., N.Y.,* **38**, 29–36
MEARS, E., VESSEY, M.P., ANDOLŠEK, L. and OVEN, A. (1969). Preliminary evaluation of four oral contraceptives containing only progestogens. *Br. med. J.,* **ii**, 730–734
MISCHLER, T.W., BERMAN, E., RUBIO, B., LARRANAGA, A., GUILOFF, E. and MOGGIA, A.V. (1974). Further experience with quingestanol acetate as a postcoital oral contraceptive. *Contraception,* **9**, 221–225
MISHELL, D.R., KHARMA, K.M., THORNEYCROFT, I.H. and NAKAMURA, R.M. (1972). Estrogenic activity in women receiving an injectable progestogen for contraception. *Am. J. Obstet. Gynec.,* **113**, 372–376
MISHELL, D.R. and LUMKIN, M.E. (1970). Contraceptive effect of varying dosages of progestogen in silastic vaginal rings. *Fert. Steril.,* **21**, 99–103
MISHELL, D.R., LUMKIN, M. and JACKAMICZ, T. (1975). Initial clinical studies of intravaginal rings containing norethindrone and norgestrel. *Contraception,* **12**, 253–260
MOGGIA, A., BEAUQUIS, A., FERRARI, F., TORRADO, M.L., ALONSO, J.L., KOREMBLIT, E. and MISCHLER, T. (1974). The use of progestogens as post-coital oral contraceptives. *J. reprod. Med.,* **13**, 58–61
MOGGIA, A., MISCHLER, T., BEAUQUIS, A., ZARATE, J., TORRADO, M., FERRARI, F. and KOREMBLIT, E. (1973). Evaluation of the contraceptive efficacy of quingestanol acetate in daily microdose and post coitum. *J. reprod. Med.,* **10**, 186–192
MOGHISSI, K.S. (1972). Morphologic changes in the ovaries of women treated with continuous microdose progestogens. *Fert. Steril.,* **23**, 739–744
MORRIS, J.M. and VAN WAGENEN, G. (1966). Compounds interfering with ovum implantation and development. *Am. J. Obstet. Gynec.,* **96**, 804–813
MORRIS, J.M. and VAN WAGENEN, G. (1973). Interception: the use of post ovulatory estrogens to prevent implantation. *Am. J. Obstet. Gynec.,* **115**, 101–106
OBERTI, C., DABANCENS, A., GARCIA-HUIDOBRO, M., RODRIGUEZ-BRAVO, R. and ZANARTU, J. (1974). Low dosage oral progestogens to control fertility. II. Morphological modifications in the gonad and oviduct. *Obstet. Gynec., N.Y.,* **43**, 285–294
ORR, A.H. and ELSTEIN, M. (1969). Luteinizing hormone levels in plasma and urine in women during normal menstrual cycles and in women taking combined oral contraceptives or chlormadinone acetate. *J. Endocr.,* **43**, 617–624
PARKES, A.S. and BELLERBY, C.W. (1926). Studies on the internal secretions of

the ovary. II. The effects of injection of the oestrus producing hormone during pregnancy. *J. Physiol., Lond.,* **62**, 145–155

PINCUS, G. and KIRSCH, R.E. (1936). The sterility in rabbits produced by injections of oestrone and related compounds. *Am. J. Physiol.,* **115**, 219–228

PRISĆ, J. and KOĆOVIĆ, P.M. (1973). Low-dose lynestrenol as a contraceptive method. *Contraception,* **8**, 315–326

RICE-WRAY, E., BERISTAIN, I.I. and CERVANTES, E. (1972). Clinical study of a continuous daily microdose progestogen contraceptive – *d*-norgestrel. *Contraception,* **5**, 279–294

RINEHART, W. (1975). Minipill. A limited alternative for certain women. *Population Reports,* series A, number 3, 53–67

RINEHART, W. (1976). Postcoital contraception – an appraisal. *Population Reports,* series J, number 9, 141–154

RINEHART, W. and WINTER, J. (1975). Injectable progestagens – officials debate but use increases. *Population Reports,* series K, number 1, 1–16

ROLAND, M. (1968). Norgestrel-induced cervical barrier to sperm migration. *J. reprod. Fertil.,* supplement 5, 173–177

RUBIO, B., BERMAN, E., LARRANAGA, A. and GUILOFF, E. (1970). A new post coital oral contraceptive. *Contraception,* **1**, 303–314

RUBIO, B., MISCHLER, T.W. and BERMAN, E. (1972). Contraception with a daily low-dose progestogen: quingestanol acetate. *Fert. Steril.,* **23**, 668–671

RUDEL, H.W. (1970). Antifertility effects of low dose progestin. *Fedn Proc. Fedn Am. Socs exp. Biol.,* **29**, 1228–1231

RUDEL, H.W. and KINCL, F.A. (1966). The biology of anti-fertility steroids. *Acta endocr., Copnh.,* **51**, supplement 105, 1–45

RUDEL, H.W., MARTÍNEZ-MANAUTOU, J. and MAQUEO-TOPETE, M. (1965). The role of progestogens in the hormonal control of fertility. *Fert. Steril.,* **16**, 158–169

SCHARFF, H.J. (1973). Clinical experience with *d*-norgestrel in a continuous microdose. *Fertility and Sterility. Proceedings of the Seventh World Congress of Fertility and Sterility. Excerpta Medica International Congress Series No. 278,* pp. 900–901. Excerpta Medica, Amsterdam

SCUTCHFIELD, F.D., LONG, W.N., COREY, B. and TYLER, C.W. (1971). Medroxy progesterone acetate as an injectable female contraceptive. *Contraception,* **3**, 21–35

SHARP, D.S. and MACDONALD, H. (1973). Use of medroxyprogesterone acetate as a contraceptive in conjunction with early postpartum rubella vaccination. *Br. med. J.,* **iv**, 443–446

SHEARMAN, R.P. (1973). Post coital contraception: a review. *Contraception,* **7**, 459–476

SILVERBERG, S.G. and MAKOWSKI, E.L. (1975). Endometrial carcinoma in young women taking oral contraceptive agents. *Obstet. Gynec., N.Y.,* **46**, 503–506

SMITH, M., VESSEY, M.P., BOUNDS, W. and WARREN, J. (1974). Progestogen-only oral contraception and ectopic gestation. *Br. med. J.,* **iv**, 104–105

SMYTHE, A.R. and UNDERWOOD, P.B. (1975). Ectopic pregnancy after postcoital diethylstilbestrol. *Am. J. Obstet. Gynec.,* **121**, 284–285

SPARROW, M.J. (1974). Oestrogen interception: the morning-after pill. *N.Z. med. J.,* **79**, 862–864

SPELLACY, W.N., BUHI, W.C. and BIRK, S.A. (1975). Effects of norethindrone on carbohydrate and lipid metabolism. *Obstet. Gynec., N.Y.,* **46**, 560–563

STANCZYK, F.Z., HIROI, M., GOEBELSMANN, U., BRENNER, P.F., LUMKIN, M.E. and MISHELL, D.R., Jr.(1975). Radioimmunoassay of serum *d*-norgestrel in women following oral and intravaginal administration. *Contraception*, **12**, 279–298

STURTEVANT, F.M. and WAIT, R.B. (1970). High dose oestrogen sequential oral contraception. I. Effectiveness assessed by the Life Table technique. *Contraception*, **2**, 187–191

SZONTÁGH, F.E. and KOVÁCS, L. (1969). Post coital contraception with dienoestrol. *Medical Gynaecology and Sociology*, **4**, 36–37

TATUM, H.J. and SCHMIDT, F.H. (1977). Contraceptive and sterilization practices and extrauterine pregnancy: a realistic perspective. *Fert. Steril.*, **28**, 407–421

TEJUJA, S., SAXENA, N.C., CHOUDHURY, S.D. and MALHOTRA, U. (1974). Experience with 50 mcg and 75 mcg *dl*-norgestrel as a minipill in India. *Contraception*, **10**, 385–394

TUTTLE, S. and TURKINGTON, V.E. (1974). Effects of medroxyprogesterone acetate on carbohydrate metabolism. *Obstet. Gynec., N.Y.*, **43**, 685–692

TYLER, E.T. (1968). Studies of "mini' micro" contraceptive doses of a new progestogen. *Int. J. Fert.*, **13**, 460–465

TYLER, E.T., LEVIN, M., ELLIOT, J. and DOLMAN, H. (1970). Present status of injectable contraceptives: results of seven-years' study. *Fert. Steril.*, **21**, 469–481

VICTOR, A., EDQVIST, L-E., LINDBERG, P., ELAMSSON, K. and JOHANSSON, E.D.B. (1975). Peripheral plasma levels of *d*-norgestrel in women after oral administration of *d*-norgestrel and when using intravaginal rings impregnated with *d*-norgestrel. *Contraception*, **12**, 261–278

VOERMAN, J. (1973). Cited by Rinehart, W., *Population Reports*, series A, number 3, 53–67

WYNN, V., ADAMS, P., OAKLEY, N. and SEED, M. (1974). Metabolic investigations in women taking 30 μg ethinyl oestradiol plus 150 μg *d*-norgestrel. *The Second International Norgestrel Symposium. Some Metabolic Considerations of Oral Contraceptive Usage*, pp. 47–54. Excerpta Medica, Amsterdam

WYNN, V., DOAR, J.W.H. and MILLS, G.L. (1966). Some effects of oral contraceptives on serum lipid and lipoprotein levels. *Lancet*, **ii**, 720–723

YUZPE, A.A., THURLOW, H.J. and LANCEE, W.J. (1974). Post coital contraception-follow-on to a pilot study. Cited by Rinehart, W. (1976). *Population Reports*, series J, number 9, 141–154

YUZPE, A.A., THURLOW, H.J., RAMZY, I. and LEYSHON, J.I. (1974). Post-coital contraception – a pilot study. *J. reprod. Med.*, **13**, 53–58

ZALDIVAR, A. and GALLEGOS, A.J. (1971). Metabolism and tissue localisation of (14-15 3H)*d*-norgestrel in the human. *Contraception*, **4**, 169–182

ZAÑARTU, J. (1968). Long-term contraceptive effect of injectable progestagens: inhibition and reestablishment of fertility. *Int. J. Fert.*, **13**, 415–426

ZAÑARTU, J., DABANCENS, A., OBERTI, C., RODRIGUEZ-BRAVO, R. and GARCIA-HUIDOBRO, M. (1974). Low-dosage oral progestogens to control fertility. I. Clinical investigations. *Obstet. Gynec., N.Y.*, **43**, 87–96

ZAÑARTU, J., PUPKIN, M., ROSENBERG, D., GUERRERO, R., RODRIGUEZ-BRAVO, R., GARCIA-HUIDOBRO, M. and PUGA, J.A. (1968). Effect of oral continuous progestogen therapy in microdosage on human ovary and sperm transport. *Br. med. J.*, **ii**, 266–269

5 The Relative Effectiveness and Risks of Hormonal Contraception

Assessment of the real effectiveness of a contraceptive is always difficult because of the problem of separating method failure from patient failure. This problem is further complicated by patients who fail to use the method properly in order that there may be some risk attached to sexual intercourse. A couple doing this for their own pleasure may subconsciously feel that it is socially irresponsible and be reluctant to admit to it to an investigator.

The enthusiasm of the investigator is another important factor. This can encourage patients to attend regularly and ensure that they use the method properly, thereby reducing the failure rate. They can also be persuaded to put up temporarily with minor side-effects, which might otherwise have led to their dropping out from the study. An enthusiastic investigator will see that as few patients as possible are lost to follow-up, thereby ensuring the accuracy of the study.

Short periods of time during which a contraceptive is not used are usually excluded in assessing contraceptive efficiency, but the inclusion of such short periods in the assessment of extended use-effectiveness has been advocated by Tietze and Lewit (1968).

No method of contraception is without risk; pregnancies have even been reported after hysterectomy. Properly used, there is no doubt that the combined oral contraceptive is the most effective reversible procedure for preventing pregnancies, with a method failure rate of 0.5 per 100 woman-years at the most, and an overall failure rate of up to 2.5 per 100 woman-years. From these figures it seems that in terms of overall efficacy there is not all that much to choose between oral contraceptives, intra-uterine devices and mechanical methods. As the oral contraceptive is the only really new form of contraception, and as its long-term hormonal effects may take many years to be distinguished as clinical entities, it may not turn out to have the lowest morbidity.

Since the report by Inman *et al.* (1970), incriminating oestrogen doses of 100 μg or more as contributing to the causes of thrombosis and embolism, many combined pills contain only 50 μg or 30 μg of oestrogen. Apart from an increased risk of ovulation at the change-over period from a preparation containing a higher dosage of oestrogen to a lower dose, the failure rate seems to be approximately the same. The combined pill has a 'belt and braces' effect in that the primary action is inhibition of ovulation, but the progestational component also affects cervical mucus and the endometrium, thereby making pregnancy less likely should some pills be missed and ovulation occur.

127

Table 5.1 ANNUAL MORTALITY (ENGLAND AND WALES) FROM MYOCARDIAL INFARCTION, THROMBO-EMBOLIC DISEASE AND UNPLANNED PREGNANCY IN WOMEN USING ORAL CONTRACEPTIVES OR A DIAPHRAGM (MANN *et al.*, 1976)

	Mortality per 100 000 users per year Age 20–34	Age 35–44
Oral Contraceptive Users		
Myocardial infarction	1.1	8.1
Pulmonary and cerebral thrombo-embolism	1.3	3.4
Unplanned pregnancy	0.1	0.5
Total	2.5	12.0
Diaphragm Users		
Unplanned pregnancy	1.1	2.5

Much emphasis has recently been laid on the increased magnitude of these risks in women over 35. *Table 5.1*, from Mann *et al.* (1976), indicates the magnitude of the mortality associated with oral contraception in women aged 20–34, and 35–45 years, respectively. The hazards are compared with the risks of using a diaphragm, which are solely those of pregnancy if the barrier method fails. In women over 35 the mortality of oral contraception is five times that of younger women, and five times that in diaphragm users.

In addition, the added risk of oral contraceptives in cigarette smokers has been emphasised. Jain (1977) has shown that it is probable that the risks of oral contraception are increased by smoking, in all age groups. In women over 40 who are moderate or heavy smokers the risk of death associated with oral contraception is even greater than the potential mortality of the repeated pregnancies that might result if no contraception were used. The risks of myocardial infarction are summarised in *Table 5.2*, from the International Family

Table 5.2 ANNUAL MORTALITY (UNITED STATES OF AMERICA) FROM MYOCARDIAL INFARCTION IN ORAL CONTRACEPTIVE USERS; EFFECT OF HYPERTENSION, HIGH BLOOD CHOLESTEROL AND SMOKING

	Mortality per 100 000 users per year Age 30–39	Age 40–44
All women using oral contraception	15.1	50.4
Users without predisposing factors	3.0	10.2
Users with predisposing factors	40.0	134.1

Planning Digest (1977). The annual death rate for women over 40, with a predisposing factor such as hypertension, high blood cholesterol or smoking is 1 in 750 from myocardial infarction alone, if they use oral contraception.

The publicity given to venous thrombosis and embolism due to combined oral contraceptives makes it important to put the incidence of deaths from these causes in perspective, by comparing them to mortality figures from other hazards of everyday life. The risk of death from thrombosis or embolism and myocardial infarction due to oral contraceptives in women under 35 is less than that associated with accepted everyday activities such as riding in a car, and significantly less than the death rate associated with pregnancy or cancer (*Table 5.3*). The risks of oral contraceptives in the 'over 35' groups are much higher. If a woman has sexual intercourse, then she must accept a finite risk to her life, be it through pregnancy, abortion, or by the use of some method of contraception. This risk must be realised and accepted, but it should not be allowed to be perceived out of proportion.

Table 5.3 DEATH RATES FROM VARIOUS CAUSES PER 100 000 WOMEN OF CHILDBEARING AGE IN ENGLAND AND WALES IN 1973 (VESSEY AND DOLL, 1976)

	Age in Years	
	20–34	35–44
Associated with oral contraception	2.4	11.6
Cancer of the breast	2.6	25.3
Cancer of the cervix	0.9	4.9
Multiple sclerosis	0.5	1.4
Nephritis and nephrosis	0.8	2.0
Motor vehicle traffic accidents	5.9	4.6
Murder and manslaughter	1.2	1.0
Suicide	4.4	7.7
Deaths from all causes	52.8	155.2

More remote factors may offset the relation of oral contraceptives to their overall mortality. It is conceivable that deaths either in the home or on the streets, caused by a woman's diminished efficiency premenstrually, may be reduced by oral contraception. A reduction in unwanted pregnancies and their attendant social tensions may reduce the incidence of infanticide and battered babies. These are conjectures which are impossible to assess quantitatively, but are points in favour of oral contraception with its high patient acceptability.

There is as yet no evidence of general applicability of any increase in congenital abnormalities amongst the babies of women who have taken oral contraceptives before becoming pregnant.

Conventional oral contraception undoubtedly provides the surest and most convenient form of contraception available at the present time. The symptomatic side-effects, such as nausea and breakthrough bleeding, are minimal and can be reduced by choosing a combination of oestrogen and progestagen which appears appropriate for the individual patient. The silent and more important side-effects such as those on blood coagulation, on carbohydrate metabolism, and on the functioning of the hypothalamus have only recently been appreciated. Pills containing more than 50 µg of oestrogen cause sufficient alteration in the patient's basic physiology as to raise the possibility of potential hazards occurring over a long period of time. The low-dose oestrogen (30 µg) combined pill is likely to have a reduced incidence of oestrogen-dependent side-effects. The potential hazards of the conventional pill should be weighed against those of pregnancy and it is probable that its great efficacy in preventing ovulation outweighs its potential disadvantages.

Low-dose progestagen preparations certainly seem to be free from the metabolic side-effects attributed to the oestrogen component of the combined pill.

On the other hand, their overall failure rate is approximately the same as that for mechanical methods, at least 4 per 100 woman-years, so their use may be limited to those who can afford socially, economically and medically to have an unexpected pregnancy, and merely wish to delay the event.

The other method of hormonal contraception such as the oestrogen or progestagen postcoital pills, and depot injections of progestagen, with or without oestrogen, have not been evaluated for long enough to assess their efficacy and safety completely. It is unlikely that the postcoital progestagen pill carries any risk of death but its effectiveness needs to be ascertained. The depot injection preparations of progestagen may have long term side-effects such as the development of permanent amenorrhoea or abnormal carbohydrate metabolism, but the evidence for the occurrence of the latter is not strong.

REFERENCES

INMAN, W.H.W., VESSEY, M.P., WESTERHOLM, B. and ENGELUND, A. (1970). Thrombo-embolic disease and the steroidal content of oral contraceptives. A report to the Committee on Safety of Drugs. *Br. med. J.,* ii, 203–209

INTERNATIONAL FAMILY PLANNING DIGEST (1977). Pill is hazardous for smokers age 30 and up. Volume 3, number 1, 8–9

JAIN, A.K. (1977). Mortality risk associated with the use of oral contraceptives. *Stud. fam. Plann.,* 8, 50–54

MANN, J.I., INMAN, W.H.W. and THOROGOOD, M. (1976). Oral contraceptive use in older women and fatal myocardial infarction. *Br. med. J.,* ii, 445–447

TIETZE, C. and LEWIT, S. (1968). Statistical comparison of contraceptive methods: use-effectiveness and extended use-effectiveness. *Demography,* 5, 461–471

VESSEY, M.P. and DOLL, Sir R. (1976). Evaluation of existing techniques. Is 'the pill' safe enough to continue using? *Proc. R. Soc. B.,* 195, 69–80

Part II
Barrier Methods

6 Condoms, Diaphragms and Caps

A barrier method of contraception prevents spermatozoa from reaching the upper female genital tract. Diaphragms or cervical caps used alone can allow the passage of spermatozoa and so combination with a spermicide is essential to their effectiveness. The condom forms a more effective barrier if used properly and the risks of pregnancy are not significantly diminished further by the use of a spermicide. All barrier methods involve application of the contraceptive device before intercourse, and then its disposal or removal afterwards. This recurrent physical element, which must not be omitted if the method is to have any value, requires motivation. Motivation may be reinforced by the intrinsic advantages of the method, or by the disadvantages of other methods. It is preferable if it is the former factor that is operative. Without it the failure rate is quite high.

It is interesting to note that in a sample of physicians, none of whom recommended the use of condoms or diaphragms, 25% of their wives reported these as their method of contraception (Wassertheil-Smoller *et al.*, 1973).

CONDOMS

Historically the condom dates back to Roman times, when animal bladders were used for protection against venereal disease rather than as contraceptives. Linen sheaths were used in Italy in the 16th century for the same reasons. Other materials used in the manufacture of sheaths included silk and leather. They are now made of latex rubber, except for a few products which consist of plastic or animal membranes.

Condoms, protectives or sheaths come in all forms and colours. The basic condom as used in the Western world is a thin, stretchable latex film, produced by a two-stage dipping process. It is dried by heating and rolled off the glass mould with brushes before being dusted with talc. The condom is put on a metal mould and passed through an electrolyte bath, whilst 10—15 volts are applied between the mould and the wall of the bath. Holes or weak areas in the rubber allow the passage of current, denoting a faulty condom which is discarded. The condoms are then lubricated and packed, ready rolled, in a foil wrapper. Quality control also involves testing a sample of all the condoms by filling them with 300 ml of water to test for leaks and by distending them up to 28.3 litres with air. The minimum tensile strength of the latex film should be 200 kg/sq. cm, and the elongation at breaking point should be between 600 and 700%. These tests apply in Denmark, Great Britain, India, Sweden and the United States of America.

The dimensions of condoms vary from country to country, and are regulated in eight countries: Great Britain, Hungary, India, Israel, Japan, Norway, Sweden and the United States of America. The strength of a condom is related to its thickness, and a compromise thickness must be found which interferes as little as possible with sensation, but which does not allow the condom to burst under the stress of intercourse. In the United States of America the minimum allowable thickness is 0.04 mm, but in Japan condoms can be as thin as 0.03 mm, with no reported increase in defects. Thicker, washable condoms are available. These can be used several times but they are now unpopular because of the reduction of sensation they cause and the nuisance of cleaning and drying them. Most condoms have a teat end to catch the ejaculate, but some are plain ended. Some are not lubricated.

Other types of male protective include American or Grecian tips, which merely cover the glans penis, and various varieties which have corrugations or protuberances for additional clitoral or vaginal stimulation. The American or Grecian tips are extremely unreliable as they are easily dislodged during intercourse.

Recently, a plastic condom has been manufactured. The material is ethylene ethyl acrylate, 0.0254 mm thick, with a rubber ring sealed into the base to assist retention during intercourse. The advantage of this material over the rubber sheath is that it will store for indefinite periods, an important property in hot countries. Plastic has a greater degree of lubricity than rubber, and it transmits heat better so that sensation is improved. Simple equipment is all that is required to manufacture these sheaths because they are merely stamped out of sheets of the plastic material and heat-sealed at the seam. Preliminary results suggest that they are not always successful, because of leakage of seminal fluid through this sealed seam and around the rubber ring at the base.

Use of the Condom

The condom is a good contraceptive for stable couples having occasional intercourse. It is convenient during the few weeks after a confinement; many physicians prefer to wait several weeks before fitting a diaphragm or an intra-uterine device, and condoms, unlike hormonal contraceptives, do not interfere with lactation. The young person having casual intercourse for the first few times is unlikely to use any other contraceptive; the condom is easily available, with good results *if used properly*. Condoms also provide protection against venereal disease, an important consideration in a section of the population which has a high incidence of gonorrhoea.

On a regular basis the condom should be a good method for a couple in which the male assumes the dominant role in contraception. It is also a good method of contraception for couples in which the woman cannot or will not take the pill or use an intra-uterine device. These couples usually choose a barrier method. The one chosen depends on whether the male or female is the partner taking the initiative in contraception. This in turn depends on their individual personalities, their respective desires to prevent pregnancy and the extent of their sexual motivation.

The condom is the most commonly used contraceptive in Great Britain. Thirty-six per cent of contraceptive users employ it (Bone, 1973b). Among

Table 6.1 METHOD OF CONTRACEPTION CURRENTLY USED (OR LAST USED) BY 287 COUPLES TOGETHER WITH TOTAL USE AND FAILURE RATES IN 5 YEARS OF MARRIAGE (PEEL, 1972)

Method	Couples currently using or last using (%)	Total months of use	Pregnancies	Failure rate per 100 woman-years
Condom	33.5	3698	12	3.9
Oral contraceptive	31.7	2920	3	1.2
Withdrawal	21.6	1640	30	21.9
Diaphragm	3.1	497	3	7.2
Rhythm	5.2	461	13	33.9
Others	4.9	209	3	17.2

social classes 1 and 2 the proportion is 38%. Its use has declined from 41% for non-manual workers and 38% for manual workers who were first married in the years 1951 to 1955, to 30% and 33% respectively for those married between 1966 and 1970. This decrease has been accompanied by a decrease in coitus interruptus, and is probably due to the increasing use of oral contraception and intra-uterine devices. Peel (1972), in his study of the contraceptive practice of 500 randomly selected newly-married couples from Hull, found that 59% used the condom at one time or another, 48% had taken oral contraceptives and 41% had used coitus interruptus. The method of contraception currently used by these couples, together with total use and failure rates in the first five years of marriage, are shown in *Table 6.1*. Most couples who ceased to use the condom did so during the first year of marriage; after that its use was fairly constant. The condom users formed a consistent cross-section of the total sample divided on the basis of socio-economic status (Peel, 1972). Employment of condoms in the

Table 6.2 INTERNATIONAL USE OF BIRTH CONTROL METHODS (DALSIMER, *et al.*, 1973)

Country	Year of survey	Percentage of couples using birth control	Oral contraceptives	Intra-uterine devices	Condoms	Rhythm; withdrawal	Other
Developed							
Australia	1971	92	38	8	9	33	12
Great Britain	1970	87	22	5	37	33	14
Japan	1969	52	2	0	68	41	30
Sweden	1967	73	14	1	38	21	11
U.S.A.	1970	65	34	7	14	9	36
Developing							
Colombia	1971	18	55	31	3	–	11
Iran	1972	51	41	6	18	35	–
Jamaica	1972	42	26	14	41	12	7
Korea	1972	45	31	27	20	20	2
Panama	1972	46	59	15	4	13	9
Philippines	1972	33	24	9	6	61	–
Thailand	1972	40	60	23	5	5	8
Venezuela	1972	48	27	27	19	23	4

Figures for some countries exceed a total of 100 per cent because some patients use multiple methods and are therefore represented in more than one category.

United States of America has dropped from 27% of all couples practising contraception in 1955 to 18% in 1965 (Segal and Tietze, 1969), but in underdeveloped countries use is steadily increasing. The estimated number manufactured in nine major producing countries in 1968 was 2293 million, of which approximately 38% were sold in the United States of America, 36% in Japan and 13% in Great Britain. *Table 6.2* shows the incidence of condom use, compared to other methods, in several developing and developed countries.

Advantages and Disadvantages

The condom has several advantages. The first of these is its availability from many retail outlets such as chemists' and barbers' shops. In recent years slot-machines have been placed in public lavatories, public houses and dance halls. In Great Britain it is now the policy of the Government to distribute condoms from family planning clinics as part of a free comprehensive service. In many underdeveloped countries Government distribution supplements commercial outlets.

The second and most important advantage is freedom from side-effects. There are no metabolic problems, as encountered with the combined contraceptive pill, and no other medical side-effects of any significance.

There are other, important, medical advantages which have not yet been fully proven. The first of these is protection from some venereal disease. It is the impression of many venereologists that the condom used consistently offers protection against gonorrhoea. Regular use of the condom has been found to afford this protection (Barlow, 1977). Similar protection against contracting non-specific urethritis or syphilis does not seem to be provided.

Squamous carcinoma of the cervix can be considered as a sexually transmitted disease. This is not a new concept, but Singer (1974) has suggested that the development of malignancy may depend to some degree on the incorporation of sperm into the cervical cells at the time of active metaplasia. This occurs at some time during adolescence, during the first pregnancy and after cervical cautery for erosions (Singer, 1975). At these times the cells are capable of ingesting the sperm by phagocytosis. The incorporation of foreign DNA can set in motion events which lead to the cellular changes such as dysplasia and carcinoma *in situ*, which often terminate in invasive carcinoma of the cervix.

The role of herpesvirus hominis (herpes simplex) in the aetiology of cervical carcinoma is also uncertain (Poste *et al.,* 1974). It has been suggested that the virus causes malignancy by producing symptomless attacks of herpetic infection in the cervical epithelial cells, with the incorporation of virus particles within the developing cervical cells. Herpesvirus may live symbiotically in the male genital tract and thereby increase the potential of some men's spermatozoa for causing mutations once incorporated into the cervical epithelial cells (Singer, A., personal communication, 1975).

Any of these theories imply that the predisposition to cervical carcinoma is sexually transmitted and the risk of developing the disease will, at least in theory, be reduced by the constant use of a barrier method of contraception. This is particularly the case during adolescence, when the association of early intercourse and promiscuity with carcinoma *in situ* is most easily demonstrated.

Disadvantages of condoms are difficult to prove. One unwanted medical effect that has been recorded in a solitary case is peritonitis due to foreign body granulomata (Saxen *et al.,* 1963). The foreign body particles isolated from the peritoneal lesions were very similar in their physical characteristics to the starch in the condom lubricant and the suggestion was made that this was the cause of the numerous foreign body granulomata found.

Other disadvantages which have been cited include the care and timing necessary with the application of the condom. It must be put on before sexual contact as spermatozoa can be present in the pre-ejaculatory fluid. The teat end, if present, collects the spermatozoa and seminal fluid and so it should be compressed before application to exclude air. The condom must be applied to its full extent. Many couples include application of the condom as part of the ritual of sexual stimulation of the male by the female. This is conducive to correct use. The penis must be withdrawn soon after ejaculation to prevent leakage of spermatozoa and to prevent the condom from slipping off.

Another disadvantage is the loss of sensation. This does occur to some extent but in the young and sexually inexperienced the use of the condom may reduce the tendency to premature ejaculation, and it may prolong intercourse in the more mature couple to their mutual satisfaction. Advancement of rubber technology is such that the condom today is extremely thin, reducing loss of sensation to a minimum without diminishing safety. A very rare side-effect of the condom is an allergy due to the lubricant on the rubber. The allergy manifests itself as a local penile or vaginal skin irritation. Dry condoms, which can be lubricated with oil or a water soluble inert jelly, or skin condoms can be purchased. Most of the women who complain of dyspareunia allegedly due to the condom will be found to have either an infective vaginitis or a psychosexual problem. The need for the unlubricated or non-rubber condom is therefore small.

Finally, use of the condom puts the onus for contraception on the male. In a stable relationship, when the male has decided to undertake this responsibility, there should be no problem. In the situation of contraception in casual relationships, the male may be less responsible and less thoughtful of the long-term consequences of pregnancy. The more effective female methods of contraception available at present are designed for premeditated, regular, long-term use and are not suitable for intermittent casual use. The advent of a safe post-coital pill would alter this situation radically.

Failure Rate

The failure rate of the condom has been quoted in the past as anything from 5 to 15%. The studies on which these figures were based originated about 40 years ago in America and have no real bearing on the situation pertaining throughout the world today.

Accurate use-effectiveness figures for the condom are not easy to obtain because its main distribution is not through medical outlets. Some recent studies in Great Britain have yielded consistent results that show the condom to be an effective method of contraception. Peel (1969) in a study of 53 highly fertile couples of low social status who had completed their families, found a total failure rate over a period of three years of 3.1 per cent per 100 woman-years. There were four pregnancies in this study and three of these were due to admitted patient failure. Peel (1972) in his Hull family survey over a period of 308 woman-years of use found that there were 12 pregnancies of which five were method failures, with an overall failure rate of 3.9 per 100 woman-years. A third study carried out by John (1973) recorded an overall failure rate of 4.8 per 100 woman-years and a method failure rate of 0.4 per 100 woman-years. These results are summarised in *Table 6.3.* Although these studies are small,

Table 6.3 USE-EFFECTIVENESS RATES OF THE CONDOM, WHEN USED CONSISTENTLY (JOHN, 1973)

Author	Population studied	Total duration of risk (years)	Total preg-nancies	Method failure pregnancies	Total pregnancies per 100 woman-years	Method failure pregnancies per 100 woman-years
Peel (1969)	Highly fertile couples in Hull	127	4	1	3.1	0.8
Peel (1972)	Couples married in Hull 1965–1966	308	12	5	3.9	1.6
John (1973)	National Health Service patients of a Leicester-shire practice	248	12	1	4.8	0.4
Aggregate		683	28	7	4.1	1.0

they were well conducted and their results are in harmony. The overall failure rate of 4.1 per 100 woman-years and a method failure rate of 1.0 per 100 woman-years revealed that the condom, if properly used, is undoubtedly an effective contraceptive. In a much larger study involving 2057 couples Glass *et al.* (1974) recorded an overall failure rate of 4.0 per 100 woman-years, con-firming the results of the smaller studies quoted.

The commonest reason for failure is improper use. The number of preg-nancies attributable to faults in the rubber must be very small, and the claim that the sheath burst is one that must be treated with much suspicion.

Another reason for pregnancy is 'risk taking', meaning deliberate abstention from the usual contraceptive practice to heighten the excitement of intercourse. It is recognised that this does stimulate some couples. Peel (1972) felt that there was a higher incidence of 'risk takers' among condom users. The reasons for this are numerous. There are teenagers who omit contraception for the physical pleasure of taking a risk, to demonstrate that they do not care, or to demonstrate their virility. There is the male who feels aggressive and wishes to show his dominance over his female partner by impregnating her. There is the female who may wish for unprotected intercourse because she enjoys the physical pleasures of occasional risk taking. She does not like the security of a reliable contraceptive method, and will take risks whatever the outcome may be. Finally, there are females who desire unprotected intercourse, hoping to get pregnant so that they may seek attention for themselves in a maternal role.

Given that the condom is as effective as recent studies suggest, if couples really wish to prevent pregnancy and find that the method suits them, their motivation will ensure that the number of unwanted pregnancies will be very small.

DIAPHRAGMS

A rubber cap was first inserted into the vagina as a contraceptive in Germany in 1838. Use of this device spread to Holland and then to this country, hence the colloquial name of the 'Dutch cap'.

The diaphragm is a thin latex rubber dome attached to a circular metal spring base, which is covered with a rubber moulding before attachment of the diaphragm, to prevent its cutting through. The metal rim is either a tightly wound wire coil or a flat watch-spring. Most of the diaphragms currently made in Great Britain have a flat spring rim, whilst in the United States of America they are mainly of the wire cord rim variety. The reason for the geographical difference in manufacture of these two types is obscure. The evidence that diaphragms with particular types of spring are appropriate for women with corresponding pelvic anatomy is largely anecdotal; opinions have been reviewed by Wortman (1976). There is no obvious difference in degree of comfort. An advantage of the flat spring is that it will not bend into a figure-of-eight, as will the round wire spring. Diaphragms vary in size from 45 mm to 100 mm in diameter, in 5 mm increments. The rubber is thicker than that used for condoms and is rigorously tested to make sure that there are no holes.

Fitting

In order to ascertain the correct size of diaphragm for a patient, a bimanual pelvic examination must be performed. The size and position of the uterus and the state of the cervix are noted. Any other pelvic pathology is excluded, and a cervical smear taken. The examining fingers are then inserted as far as possible into the posterior fornix, and the distance to the pubic symphysis noted. This gives the approximate size of diaphragm needed, and the appropriate fitting ring or diaphragm can then be inserted. Most parous women need a 70, 75 or 80 mm size, but it may be necessary to try more than one size before getting the correct fit. When correctly in position the upper anterior edge of the diaphragm should be behind the pubic symphysis and the lower posterior edge should be in the posterior vaginal fornix. The diaphragm should slip easily into place, covering the cervix and fitting comfortably and closely against the vaginal walls. One rule is to use the largest size which will fit in this way without the patient being aware of its presence.

A diaphragm can be used irrespective of the position of the uterus, but severe laxity of the vaginal walls with prolapse predisposes to displacement. The Matrisalus or 'Bowbent' diaphragm has a spring the same shape as a Hodge pessary. It is said to provide a better fit for the woman with vaginal laxity, particularly cystocele.

The dome of the diaphragm covers the cervix and anterior vaginal wall, becoming adherent to them by the surface tension of tissue fluid. This fluid film becomes saturated with spermicide.

Once a correct fit has been obtained it is essential that the patient is shown how to apply spermicide to the diaphragm, how to insert it, how to verify that it is covering the cervix and how to remove it. This can be done by a trained nurse, demonstrating to the patient on a model, and by allowing the patient to practice on herself under supervision. Some women insert their diaphragms in a dorsal (supine) position with the knees drawn up, others kneel, bending forwards, and some stand up, putting one foot on a chair. It is usually advised that the diaphragm be inserted 'dome down', but some women find the devices easier to insert and more comfortable if inserted 'dome up'. Provided the fit is good in this position and use of the spermicide is liberal and consistent, diaphragms can be equally effective when used in this way if the spermicide-saturated fluid film is maintained over the cervix. Some women find it easy to remove their diaphragm by simply hooking an index finger under the rim from below. Others need to insinuate a finger between the diaphragm and the anterior vaginal wall and either hook the rim out or grasp it between finger and thumb.

During training by a nurse, two psychological problems may arise. The physician must be observant to detect the patient who dislikes – for any one of a number of deep-seated reasons – another woman observing or conducting manipulations at the introitus or penetrating the vagina. Secondly, he must be aware of the woman who cannot come to terms with her body to the extent of self-insertion of devices into body orifices. Pressure on such a patient to proceed can sometimes lead to a hysterical reaction.

It is our custom to give the patient a diaphragm to practice insertion and removal at home. We then see her a week later to check that she can achieve correct placement before she relies on the device for contraception. In addition, the fitting is checked – the anxiety and tension of a first visit can lead to unusually high tone in the pelvic musculature and underestimation of size.

Before intercourse the diaphragm should be smeared liberally on both sides with spermicidal cream and then inserted. After intercourse it should be left in position for at least six hours. Its principal mode of action is to prevent access of spermatozoa to the cervix. As spermatozoa can pass around the edges of the diaphragm, however good the fit, the spermicide is essential. A secondary action of the diaphragm is to retain a bolus of spermicide in the upper vagina which kills spermatozoa deposited in the posterior fornix.

Fitting should be checked after the patient has undergone a significant loss or gain in body weight, after an abortion or a confinement, and after any pelvic surgery.

Use of the Diaphragm

The extent of use of the diaphragm has never been very great but it remained relatively steady during the years 1951 to 1970. Among non-manual workers the figure has varied between 7% of contraceptive users married between 1951 and 1955 and 10% of those married between 1966 and 1970. It is a much less common method among manual workers, use being limited to 2–4% in the first year of marriage (Bone, 1973b). The overall current use of the diaphragm is

4%. Nineteen per cent of women users of contraception have had diaphragms at one time or another (Bone, 1973a). Peel (1970) recorded a similar rate in that 14% of people had at some time or another used the diaphragm; current diaphragm users amounted to 3.1% of his sample (Peel, 1972). Many diaphragm users try the condom as their second choice of contraceptive, probably because they prefer barrier methods. The use of the diaphragm is relatively constant among the upper social classes. These women are strongly motivated towards contraception, and are the dominant partners in initiating it. Some of them use the diaphragm because they are unable or unwilling to take oral contraceptives or use an intra-uterine device.

Diaphragms are unpopular in underdeveloped countries, where patients suffer from lack of privacy and washing facilities or motivation may be poor. There may also be shortages of clinical personnel for fitting and instruction, and of supplies of spermicides.

Advantages and Disadvantages

The main advantages of the diaphragm are that it is free from medical side-effects and that it is cheap. The diaphragm is washed and re-used and if kept in good condition will last for several years. Another advantage is that it puts the onus of responsibility for contraception on to the female who is more likely to bear the consequences of pregnancy in mind.

The disadvantages of the diaphragm are numerous. It must be fitted reasonably accurately and so it is of no use in the post-partum period whilst vaginal involution is still occurring. The diaphragm can be uncomfortable if the fitting is too tight. Should it be too loose, it will be ineffective. It is not suitable for women with anatomical abnormalities, such as cystocele or rectocele, considerable uterine prolapse, or a deficient perineum. Other vaginal abnormalities such as the presence of a septum or a cyst stop the diaphragm fitting properly.

Both the diaphragm and the associated spermicide must be inserted before coitus. This loss of spontaneity makes it an unacceptable method of contraception for many couples. It is an unsuitable method for couples having intercourse more than once during a 6–8 hour period, as a further application of spermicide is then necessary and the diaphragm must be removed and re-inserted. A few women have psychological difficulties or aesthetic objections to the use of diaphragms with spermicides.

The method is susceptible to failure due to women 'forgetting' to insert the diaphragm. Such forgetfulness tends to occur at mid cycle, and there is usually an underlying motivation towards pregnancy, however inconvenient (Lehfeldt, 1959).

Failure Rate

The use-effectiveness of the diaphragm has been easier to study than that of the condom and relatively consistent figures for overall failure rate of about 7% have been recorded (Peel, 1972). More recently Vessey and Wiggins (1974), in a large study over 5909 woman-years, recorded an overall failure rate of 2.4 per 100 woman-years. Although this study involved only established users, it does indicate the method effectiveness once the initial problems of fitting and acceptance of the method are overcome. Most of the patients were of the upper social classes, and all were married.

This low failure rate has been confirmed from the United States of America but in a very different population (Lane *et al.*, 1976). This study involved 2168 women, 80% of whom were under 30 years of age, 70% of whom were unmarried and many of whom were of low socio-economic status. The failure rate ranged from 1.9 per 100 woman-years during the first year of use in the under 18 year olds to 3.0 per 100 woman-years among the 30—34 year olds. Eighty per cent of women continued to use the diaphragm after one year.

The reasons for mechanical failure are poor fit, failure to use a spermicide or defects in the rubber. As diaphragms are designed to last for several years, proper cleaning is essential. The diaphragm should be washed and rinsed after use to remove all traces of soap. It should be kept in a cool place out of direct heat to prevent the rubber from perishing. Spermicides containing petroleum jelly or oils, greases or fats, such as those used in some soluble pessaries, cause rapid deterioration of the rubber and should not be used in conjunction with the diaphragm.

Side-effects are rare. Irritation due to a spermicide usually resolves on changing to another preparation; real rubber allergy is very rare. Infection is uncommon, possibly because of the antiseptic properties of the spermicide, but can result if the diaphragm is forgotten and left *in situ* for days.

VAULT AND CERVICAL CAPS

The vault cap is made of rubber which is thicker towards the rim and thinner in the centre. It adheres to the vaginal vault by suction, covering the cervix. Caps range in size from 50 to 74 mm in diameter. The cervix must not be elongated otherwise it will not be properly covered and for insertion the patient must be able to reach the cervix with her fingers. Vault caps are rarely used nowadays.

Cervical caps can be made of several materials such as rubber or plastic and are available in four sizes, from 22 to 31 mm, in diameter. The cap fits closely over the cervix, which protrudes into its concavity. This type of cap is suitable for a person with an elongated cervix but the cervix must be healthy to allow for close apposition and proper fitting. It is claimed that a cervical cap can be used effectively by a woman with prolapse (Wortman, 1976).

Vault and cervical caps must be used with spermicide applied to both sides.

Other types of cap include a Vimule, which is a combination cervical and vault cap in which the rim is thinned out and expanded. It is made of rubber or plastic, and is useful for women with some degree of vaginal prolapse. Vault caps are made in three sizes, from 45 to 51 mm in diameter. Cervical caps and Vimules usually have strings attached to them to facilitate removal.

Advantages and Disadvantages

The advantages of these caps are essentially the same as those of the diaphragm. They are cheap and relatively free from side-effects. The onus for contraception is on the female.

Disadvantages are that the cap cannot be used in patients in whom the cervix is anatomically unsuitable because of elongation, ectropion, lacerations or severe chronic cervicitis. The vault cap is not always suitable in cases of genital prolapse. Fitting can be difficult and the user must learn the proper technique. A spermicide must be used on all occasions and the cap must be left *in situ* for several hours after intercourse so that the spermicide can act. A vault cap may be dislodged during defaecation. Both types of cap may be dislodged during intercourse and become ineffectual. The use of vault and cervical caps is very limited in Great Britain and in other developed countries. They are not used in the underdeveloped countries. There are no up-to-date use-effectiveness figures available.

REFERENCES

BARLOW, D. (1977). The condom and gonorrhoea. *Lancet,* **ii**, 811–812.

BONE, M. (1973a, b). *Family planning services in England and Wales.* pp. 18 and 19 respectively. Her Majesty's Stationery. Office, London

DALSIMER, I.A., PIOTROW, P.T. and DUMM, J.J. (1973). Condom. An old method meets a new social need. *Population Reports*, series H, No. 1, 1–19

GLASS, R., VESSEY, M. and WIGGINS, P. (1974). Use-effectiveness of the condom in a selected family planning clinic population in the United Kingdom. *Contraception,* **10**, 591–598

JOHN, A.P.K. (1973). Contraception in a practice community. *Jl R. Coll. Gen. Pract.,* **23**, 665–675

LANE, M.E., ARCEO, R. and SOBRERO, A.J. (1976). Successful use of the diaphragm and jelly by a young population: report of a clinical study. *Fam. Plann. Perspect.,* **8**, 81–86

LEHFELDT, H. (1959). Wilful exposure to unwanted pregnancy (WEUP). Psychological explanation for patient failures in contraception. *Am. J. Obstet. Gynec.,* **78**, 661–665

PEEL, J. (1969). A male orientated fertility control experiment. *Practitioner,* **202**, 677–681

PEEL, J. (1970). The Hull family survey. I. The Survey couples, 1966. *J. biosoc. Sci.,* **2**, 45–70

PEEL, J. (1972). The Hull family survey. II. Family planning in the first 5 years of marriage. *J. biosoc. Sci.,* **4**, 333–346

POSTE, G., HAWKINS, D.F. and THOMLINSON, J. (1972). Herpesvirus hominis infection of the female genital tract. *Obstet. Gynec., N.Y.,* **40**, 871–890

SAXEN, L., KASSINEN, A. and SAXEN, E. (1963). Peritoneal foreign body reaction caused by condom emulsion. *Lancet,* **i**, 1295–1296

SEGAL, S.J. and TIETZE, C. (1969). Contraceptive technology: current and prospective methods. *Reports on Population/Family Planning,* October, 20

SINGER, A. (1974). Cancer of the cervix: a sexually transmitted infection? *Lancet,* **ii**, 41

SINGER, A. (1975). The uterine cervix from adolescence to the menopause. *J. Obstet. Gynaec. Br. Commonw.,* **82**, 81–99

VESSEY, M. and WIGGINS, P. (1974). Use-effectiveness of the diaphragm in a selected family planning clinic population in the United Kingdom. *Contraception,* **9**, 15–21

144 *Condoms, Diaphragms and Caps*

WASSERTHEIL-SMOLLER, S., ARNOLD, C.B., LERNER, R.C. and HEIMRATH, S.L. (1973). Contraceptive practices of wives of obstetricians. *Am. J. Obstet. Gynec.*, **117**, 709–715

WORTMAN, J. (1976). The diaphragm and other intravaginal barriers. A review. *Population Reports*, series H, 57–75

7 Spermicides

Until the newer female methods such as oral contraceptives and the intra-uterine device were developed, spermicides were an important method of fertility control. Now the use of vaginal pessaries, creams or foams is limited, because they are not very effective in preventing pregnancy and are not there-fore recommended by professional advisers. Their use is essential in conjunction with a diaphragm and has been advised in conjunction with a condom, although there is doubt if their use with the latter in fact improves efficacy. There is some evidence that vaginal spermicides can increase the efficacy of intra-uterine devices (Snowden and Williams, 1975) but this was not our experience with the M-device (Murdoch and Hawkins, 1969).

Pessaries or suppositories can have either a water-soluble or a wax base. They should be inserted at least 15 minutes before intercourse, to allow time for dissolution of the pessary and dispersion of the spermicide.

Creams have an emulsified fat base, which is insoluble in water. They tend to remain where they are put, rather than spreading out over the vaginal walls, and so care in insertion is vital if spermatozoa are to be prevented from passing through the cervical canal.

Jellies or pastes usually have a water-soluble base such as gelatin, which liquefies rapidly at body temperatures, allowing the active spermicidal ingredient to spread throughout the vagina. About 5 g should be used.

Foam tablets usually contain a bicarbonate of soda and acid mixture so that carbon dioxide is released when in contact with water. The foam conveys the spermicide throughout the vagina. Its appearance at the vulva may well cause sufficient amusement to the participants to distract from the matter in hand!

Foam aerosols. Ready-made foam can be injected into the vagina from a pressure can and, provided that it is inserted high enough into the vagina, dispersal of the spermicide occurs.

ACTION OF SPERMICIDES

The commonly used modern spermicides are surface active agents which attach themselves to spermatozoa and inhibit oxygen uptake. The surface tension of the cell wall is reduced, the osmotic balance is upset, and some spermatozoa are destroyed.

The agents include nonylphenoxypolyethoxyethanol (nonoxynol-9), *p*-di-isobutylphenoxypolyethoxyethanol, methoxypolyoxyethylene glycol, *p*-methanylphenylpolyoxythylene ether, and tri-isopropylphenoxypolyethoxyethanol.

Bactericidal agents were the first spermicides used, and they include mercuric and quinine derivatives, and ricinoleic acid and its compounds. They combine with sulphur and hydrogen bonds in the spermatozoa thereby disrupting their metabolism. Surfactants and bactericidal agents may have synergistic toxic effects on spermatozoa leading to more potent spermicidal action. The bactericidal agents are rarely used nowadays, because of their systemic toxicity.

PESSARIES, CREAMS AND PASTES

These are only really effective in conjunction with a barrier method. The history of spermicidal substances goes back very many years. In 1850 B.C. crocodile dung mixed with honey was inserted as a bolus into the vagina; in A.D. 200 pomegranate pulp or honey and cedarwood oil pessaries were described. In 1880 Rendell in London produced the first commercial pessary containing quinine as the spermicide. Several of the pessaries currently available, such as Orthoforms or Rendells, contain nonylphenoxypolyethoxyethanol. Contraceptive spermicidal jellies and creams include Duragel, Koromex jelly, Ortho-Gynol jelly, Preceptin Gel, Prentif Compound and Staycept jelly; Antemin cream, Conceptrol cream, Delfen cream, Duracreme, Immolin creme-jel, Koromex cream and Orthocreme. Both Preceptin jelly and Ortho-Gynol contain *p*-di-isobutylphenoxypolyethoxyethanol and ricinoleic acid.

Use-effectiveness figures are available for Preceptin jelly but they show wide variation. Finkelstein *et al.* (1954) reported a failure rate of 25 per 100 woman-years during the first six months of use, but as the patients gained experience, and as less well motivated patients left the study, this fell after a period of 14 months to 2.6 per 100 woman-years. Wolf *et al.* (1957) in a small study, recorded a failure rate of 0.13, while Wulff and Jonas (1956) obtained a rate of 9.5 per 100 woman-years.

Ortho-Gynol, which was originally designed to be used in conjunction with a diaphragm, was found to have failure rates of between 3.6 and 9.4 per 100 woman-years (Goldstein, 1943; Garvin, 1944) when used alone.

The range of use-effectiveness figures for Delfen cream, which contains nonylphenoxypolyethoxyethanol as a spermicide, is similar. Behne *et al.* (1956) recorded a method failure rate of 0.6 per 100 woman-years and a total failure rate of 4.2. Wolf *et al.* (1957) reported a failure rate of 5.5, while Dubrow and Kuder (1958) recorded a total failure rate of 7.6 per 100 woman-years. Rovinsky (1964) found a total failure rate of 9.1, but in those users claiming to have employed the method consistently this figure fell to 3.7 per 100 woman-years. He found that 5% of couples reported irritation and that more than 5% found some aesthetic objection to the method.

The spermicidal agent of Immolin creme-jel is methoxypolyoxyethylene glycol. Goldstein (1957) obtained a pregnancy rate of 2.0 per 100 woman-years after 1972 months of use, whilst Finkelstein and Goldberg (1959) found an overall pregnancy rate of 5.7 per 100 woman-years and a method failure rate of 3.2 per 100 woman-years.

Recently it has been suggested that the chemical spermicides Volpar or Lorophyn may be harmful as they contain mercury in the form of phenyl-mercuric acetate. The mercury may be absorbed but the exact extent of absorption and the significance of this is not clear. Volpar is no longer marketed in Great Britain.

FOAMS

Among the foams available at present are Emko and Delfen vaginal foams. These are aerosols containing nonylphenoxypolyethoxyethanol as the spermicidal agent.

The failure rate with Emko vaginal foam was found by Paniagua *et al.* (1961) to be as high as 29 per 100 woman-years in a trial in Puerto Rico. After one year's use this fell to 17 per 100 woman-years. The motivation and ability of the population studied to use the preparation properly seems doubtful.

Mears (1962) in a small study in Great Britain found a pregnancy rate of 9.7 per 100 woman-years. Failure rates of 3 per 100 woman-years (Carpenter and Martin, 1970) or 4 per 100 woman-years over 28 000 cycles (Bernstein, 1971) have been recorded among motivated groups. It seems clear that motivation and consistently correct technique are of paramount importance. Many patients cease to use the method because of the need for pre-coital application, the problems of using the applicator and physical irritation to both partners. The main advantage of the method is its simplicity. The main disadvantage is that in general it has a high failure rate.

C–FILMS

These are films 5 cm square and 80 μ thick with 67 mg of the spermicide nonyl-phenoxypolyethoxyethanol incorporated into them. They were designed with a view to being employed by either partner, being inserted into the vagina one hour before intercourse, or applied to the moistened glans penis before penetration. With the latter procedure, mechanical difficulties engendered by the heat of the moment can make it difficult for the average man to retain the film in place. The film is supposed to dissolve in aqueous fluids within 60 seconds but practical experience suggests times of up to five minutes.

Trials indicate that C-film has no significant effect on the vaginal bacteriology or moisture content, cervical cytology, or on the production of irritation of the penis or vagina. Lichtman *et al.* (1973) found that C-film was as effective as spermicidal vaginal foam in preventing the arrival and survival of the sperm in the cervical mucus. Ragab (1973) found that in 34 women with previously normal postcoital tests, application of C-film 15 minutes to 2 hours before intercourse resulted in the absence of motile sperms from the cervix and vagina in all patients. On the other hand, Guillebaud (1973) showed that 8 out of 38 women using C-film had motile spermatozoa in the cervical mucus although there were none in the posterior fornix of the vagina. This is probably due to the fact that the film was not inserted over the cervix. If this is the case it is a significant criticism of the technique.

Advantages and Disadvantages

The advantages of the method are that it provides a compact, neat and cheap way of inserting an adequate dose of effective spermicide into the vagina in a relatively non-messy form. The majority of patients in an acceptability study (Allan and Kennaby, 1974) considered C-film simple and convenient. There is some problem if the film becomes sticky and adheres to the inserting finger but this can be minimised by using talc on the finger and folding the film in four.

Women using C-film studied by Lichtman *et al.* (1973) thought the need for insertion some time before intercourse a major disadvantage – and they had only been asked to anticipate intercourse by 30 minutes. They found this a very different proposition from immediate pre-coital insertion.

The main disadvantage is that of the relatively high failure rate when a spermicide is used alone. Results of recent studies indicate failure rates of up to 62 per 100 woman-years (Smith *et al.*, 1974), equivalent to using no contraceptive at all. Frankman *et al.* (1975) have claimed that better results can be obtained with adequate instruction and 'reliable' use, with a pregnancy rate of only 9 per 100 woman-years. Despite detailed instructions, many women find insertion difficult and are uncertain about the optimum position of the film over the cervix (Lichtman *et al.*, 1973). Mild vaginal irritation is experienced by up to 20% of users.

The final concentration of the spermicide from C-film in the vagina is about 0.7%, close to the minimum inhibitory concentration for *N. gonorrhoea* (Cowan and Cree, 1973). C-film may thus interfere with the diagnosis of gonorrhoea whilst it is of doubtful prophylactic value against the disease.

GENERAL CONSIDERATIONS WITH SPERMICIDES

It seems from these studies that the real use-effectiveness rates of spermicidal preparations, used on their own, is in the region of 5–7 per 100 woman-years. In the hands of consistent, motivated users this figure undoubtedly falls. Inclusion in a clinical trial improves patient motivation and thereby helps to reduce failure rates of all contraceptive techniques. The wide range of rates recorded means that conclusions must not be formed on the basis of a single study. High failure rates can easily arise from improper explanation of technique to the patient and from the inclusion of poorly motivated persons. On the other hand, unreasonably low figures for method failure may be arrived at by calling these 'patient failures'.

Spermicides are simple and lack long-term side-effects. They must be inserted before intercourse and no douching should take place until a few hours afterwards. They have a high failure rate, the leakage from them can be messy, and they can give rise to chemical irritation.

The availability of spermicidal products encourages their use on the assumption that they are as effective as other methods. Experience of seeing women who have, without medical advice, purchased and employed spermicides in the belief that they are effective contraceptives and found themselves with an unwanted pregnancy, makes many gynaecologists feel that the preparations should not be freely available on the market. At least, advertising should be restricted to the use of spermicides in conjunction with barrier methods.

The view that spermicides used alone are 'better than nothing' is a confession of inadequacy, and responsible physicians should never advocate their use as a sole method of contraception.

REFERENCES

ALLAN, G. and KENNABY, D.R. (1974). An acceptability study of C-film. *Family Planning Research Unit Report No. 13*, University of Exeter

BEHNE, D., CLARK, F., JENNINGS, M., PALLIAS, V., OLSON, H., WOLF, L. and TYLER, E.T. (1956). Clinical effectiveness of a new vaginal contraceptive cream: a preliminary report. *West. J. Surg. Obstet. Gynec., 64*, 152–157

BERNSTEIN, G.S. (1971). Clinical effectiveness of an aerosol contraceptive foam. *Contraception, 3*, 37–43

CARPENTER, G. and MARTIN, G.J. (1970). Clinical evaluation of a vaginal contraceptive foam. *Advances in Planned Parenthood, Volume 5. Proceedings of the Seventh Annual Meeting of the American Association of Planned Parenthood Physicians, San Francisco, California, April 9–10. International Congress Series No. 207*, 170–175. Ed. Sobrero, A.J. and McKee, C. Excerpta Medica, New York

COWAN, M.E. and CREE, G.E. (1973). A note on the susceptibility of *N. gonorrhoea* to contraceptive agent Nonyl-P. *Br. J. ven. Dis., 49*, 65–66

DUBROW, H. and KUDER, K. (1958). Combined postpartum and family planning clinic. *Obstet. Gynec., N.Y., 11*, 586–590

FINKELSTEIN, R. and GOLDBERG, R.B. (1959). Evaluation of a new contraceptive cream-jel based on long-term usage. *Am. J. Obstet. Gynec., 78*, 657–660

FINKELSTEIN, R., GUTTMACHER, A. and GOLDBERG, R. (1954). Effectiveness of Preceptin. Study of its use as sole contraceptive agent in an urban clinic population. *Obstet. Gynec., N.Y., 4*, 217–221

FRANKMAN, O., RAABE, N. and INGEMANSSON, C.A. (1975). Clinical evaluation of C-film, a vaginal contraceptive. *J. int. med. Res., 3*, 292–296

GARVIN, O.D. (1944). Jelly alone versus diaphragm and jelly. *Hum. Fert., 9*, 73–76

GOLDSTEIN, L.Z. (1943). Jelly alone as a contraceptive in postpartum cases. *Hum. Fert., 8*, 43–47

GOLDSTEIN, L.Z. (1957). Control of contraception: the use-effectiveness of a new cream-gel. *Obstet. Gynec., N.Y., 10*, 133–139

GUILLEBAUD, J. (1973). Report on further post-coital C-film investigations. In *C-Film, Medical and Technical Data*, 42–48. Potter and Clarke, Croydon, Surrey

LICHTMAN, A.S., DAVAJAN, V. and TUCKER, D. (1973). C-film: a new vaginal contraceptive. *Contraception, 8*, 291–297

MEARS, E. (1962). Chemical contraceptive trial. II. *J. Reprod. Fert., 4*, 337–343

MURDOCH, D. and HAWKINS, D.F. (1969). M-213 – monthly net event rates. *IUD Performance Patterns. Vol. 2. July 1969. Tables and Charts Prepared for Investigators*, part 4, M213, 8. Ed. Bernard, R.P. Pathfinder Fund, Boston

PANIAGUA, M.E., VAILLANT, H.N. and GAMBLE, C.J. (1961). Field trial of a contraceptive foam in Puerto Rico. *J. Am. med. Ass., 177*, 125–129

RAGAB, M.I. (1973). Report on further post-coital investigations after use of

C-film. In *C-Film. Medical and Technical Data*, 49–54. Potter and Clarke, Croydon, Surrey

ROVINSKY, J.J. (1964). Clinical effectiveness of a contraceptive cream. *Obstet. Gynec., N.Y.*, **23**, 125–131

SMITH, M., VESSEY, M.P., BOUNDS, W. and WARREN, J. (1974). C-film as a contraceptive. *Br. med. J.*, **iv**, 291

SNOWDEN, R. and WILLIAMS, M. (1975). The United Kingdom Dalkon Shield trial: two years of observation. *Contraception,* **11**, 1–13

WOLF, L., OLSON, H.J. and TYLER, E.T. (1957). Observations on the clinical use of cream-alone and gel-alone methods of contraception. *Obstet. Gynec., N.Y.,* **10**, 316–321

WULFF, G. Jr. and JONAS, H.S. (1956). Conception control: a clinical evaluation of the Preceptin-gel method. *Am. J. Obstet. Gynec.,* **72**, 549–556

8 Coitus Interruptus; Periodic Abstinence

COITUS INTERRUPTUS

Coitus interruptus, or male withdrawal, is a very old, widespread, and at times effective method of contraception. Its use seems to have been responsible for the significant changes in birth rate which have occurred during critical times in the history of many developed countries. The historical origins of the method go back to the book of Genesis, in which Onan is said to have spilled his seed upon the ground to avoid impregnating his brother's wife. Onan was slain by God, presumably for this sin. Later, Jewish theological teaching and Mohammedan thinking proscribed the practice, as did the Christian church. The time when coitus interruptus became a widespread contraceptive technique is uncertain but since about A.D. 1700 there has been a decline in the average number of births per father in first marriages which remained only marriages (Peller, 1965).

Table 8.1 EUROPE'S RULING FAMILIES SINCE A.D. 1500. AVERAGE NUMBER OF BIRTHS IN FIRST MARRIAGES WHICH WERE ONLY MARRIAGES (PELLER, 1965)

Date of parents' marriage	Average births per father
1500–1549	5.6
1550–1599	6.1
1600–1649	6.0
1650–1699	6.1
1700–1749	5.7
1750–1799	4.9
1800–1849	4.7
1850–1899	4.5
1900–1920	3.4
1921–1925	2.9

These figures were collected from a study of 3000 male members of Europe's ruling families and the reduction is probably independent of contemporary contraceptive practices (*Table 8.1*). Hollingsworth (1965), in a study of 1900 members of British ducal families, found that the mean family size of dukes' sons fell from 5.6 during the years 1730 to 1779 to 2.4 during the years 1880 to 1939.

The only widely available methods of limiting family size during the 18th and 19th centuries were abstinence, coitus interruptus or abortion, and although the precise part played by each of these alternatives is obscure, it seems very probable that coitus interruptus was to a large extent responsible for this reduction in fertility. The reduction of the birth rate in Great Britain during the years of the depression in the 1920's and 1930's to 2.04 children per family must have been largely brought about by similar methods. More recently in Turkey the use of coitus interruptus has increased from 14.5% to 25.2% of couples practising contraception in the years between 1963 and 1968. This increase has been accompanied by a reduction in the average family size from 3.2 to 2.7 children. Coitus interruptus is also extremely common in eastern European countries in which the birth rate today is very low.

To what extent is coitus interruptus practised today? In Great Britain during the years 1967 to 1968, 27% of professional people and 52–53% of social classes 3, 4 and 5 said that they had used coitus interruptus at some time or another (Potts, 1973). The extent of current use is 4% for professional people and 12–19% among social classes 3, 4 and 5. Cartwright (1970a) found that coitus interruptus was used by 22% of couples whose contraceptive practices were male dominated, but by only 13% of those couples whose contraceptive practices were female dominated. Peel (1970) recorded similar figures in that 44% of couples had at one time or another used coitus interruptus and that 21.6% of couples were currently using the method. The failure rate during 1640 months of use was 21.9 per 100 woman-years (Peel, 1972). Over the five year period of this study there was only a slight reduction in overall use of the method, in contrast with a much greater reduction in the use of the condom or diaphragm.

There appear to be geographical and cultural variations in that withdrawal is not widely used in Asia (Muramatusu, 1967; Wyon and Gordon, 1971). It seems to be used more commonly in Latin America where up to one-quarter of couples employ withdrawal and this practice is second only to the rhythm method in overall popularity (Stycos, 1968).

Advantages and Disadvantages

The advantages of the method are that it involves no cost or appliances and it ensures complete privacy for the couple. The mortality is nil, apart perhaps from Onan. The pelvic congestion syndrome (Taylor, 1954) is often attributed to the use of coitus interruptus. It is alleged that this syndrome causes congestive dysmenorrhoea, leucorrhoea, and low backache. It is possible that these symptoms may be induced either organically or psychologically by failure to achieve orgasm, but it is difficult to prove or disprove these assertions. Provided orgasm can be achieved there is no reason why the method should cause any symptoms in the female, but there is no doubt that it demands concentration and self-control on the part of the male.

Those that cease using the method and present at a family planning clinic seeking an alternative include individuals who are dissatisfied sexually. This sample, which doctors come across, is therefore biased against the method. The majority, who are perfectly happy using coitus interruptus, will not be seen. Cartwright (1970b) found that of 311 women who had discontinued use of the method only 31% did so because they found it unpleasant.

Benign prostatic hypertrophy and various neuroses in males have been attributed to coitus interruptus, but again in the absence of adequate studies it is impossible to state any definite views one way or the other. The case is unproven.

Effectiveness

Accurate use-effectiveness studies for coitus interruptus are difficult to obtain, but in 1949 the Royal Commission on Population found that there was no significant difference in pregnancy rates between those who used appliances for contraception and those who did not. Peel (1972) recorded a pregnancy rate for non-appliance methods of 21.9 per 100 woman-years. A precise figure for use-effectiveness will never be obtained because the ability to practise coitus interruptus successfully varies from couple to couple and there can be no standardisation of the method.

One of the suggested reasons for failure of the method is that there are spermatozoa present in the pre-ejaculatory fluid. In most cases of failure, ejaculation has probably taken place before complete withdrawal of the penis.

Conclusion

What is the role of this method in the overall contraceptive scene? In present-day Great Britain it is a method which is diminishing in popularity and is at present largely confined to the lower social classes, partly because of ignorance of other methods, but principally because it is a method traditionally accepted by these groups as satisfactory. It seems to have played its part, along with abstinence and abortion, in effectively reducing the birth rate in Great Britain during the last two centuries and in developing countries at the present time. In the very overpopulated, underdeveloped countries which are being encouraged to move from having no family planning at all to the sophisticated methods of the late 20th century there may well be a place for coitus interruptus as a half-way house.

PERIODIC ABSTINENCE

The safe period or rhythm method is the only contraceptive technique that is available at present to strictly orthodox members of the Roman Catholic Church. Its failure rate has always been assumed to be high by gynaecologists who see the failures. As with coitus interruptus, it is extremely difficult to get accurate use-effectiveness figures. The use of rhythm birth control is declining as more Roman Catholics employ conventional contraception. In the United States of America use of the rhythm method dropped from 22% of couples practising contraception in 1955 to 6.7% in 1970. This trend has been followed in many other developed countries. Use of the rhythm method in the underdeveloped countries has been disappointing, both with regard to extent of use and to results. Many of the failures are undoubtedly due to inadequate instruction and to careless use of the safe period. Times in the menstrual cycle during which it is relatively safe to have unprotected intercourse occur before and after ovulation. It is usually assumed that spermatozoa can remain viable in the female genital tract for up to five days, though they are probably only capable of effecting fertilisation for two or three days. It is unlikely that an ovum will be fertilised more than 24 hours after release from the follicle.

The Pre-ovulatory Infertile Period

Recognition of this period is difficult and imprecise. It is usually calculated by means of a calendar based on previous menstrual cycles. Where these were short or irregular the calculation becomes very inaccurate. Due to the natural variation of a few days in even so-called regular cycles, the use of the pre-ovulatory period is always fraught with some risks. If it were possible to anticipate and determine the precise time of ovulation, the method would still be inaccurate because of the variability in life-span of spermatozoa. The only reasonable way of calculating the pre-ovulatory infertile period is to say that it finishes five days before the earliest temperature rise as recorded during previous cycles. The taking of a basal temperature is not within the capabilities of many individuals because they have trouble reading a thermometer, plotting an accurate graph and ensuring that the temperature is taken accurately and that it is genuinely a basal temperature.

Even accepting accuracy in the taking and recording of a basal temperature chart, there can be difficulty in its interpretation. This is because the post-ovulatory temperature rise can be slow or step wise. If these readings are used to calculate the day of ovulation, and this calculation then used to work out the safe period according to the calendar, inaccuracies can arise.

Post-ovulatory Infertile Period

The length of the post-ovulatory infertile period varies between one woman and another and there is also a variation between cycles in the same individual. In the majority of cycles the post-ovulatory period is 12–16 days before the onset of the next menstrual period and so the post-ovulatory infertile period is a few days less than this. The exact relationship between the post-ovulatory temperature rise and ovulation itself is somewhat variable. This rise may be due to the effect of progesterone or its metabolites on the hypothalamic temperature regulating centre. Significant production of progesterone by the corpus luteum starts at a time which varies from woman to woman, sometimes occurring within 24 hours, and sometimes up to 48 hours after ovulation. After the temperature has been raised for three consecutive days fertilisation is very unlikely.

There is no direct evidence as to how long after ovulation it is that an ovum can be fertilised, but it is probable that the maximum time is 48 hours. Conception is much more likely during the day or two preceding the temperature rise, which is probably the time of ovulation.

Another method of recognising ovulation is the onset of mild, mid cycle lower abdominal pain (mittelschmerz) but this occurs in a recognisable manner in only a minority of women.

Cervical Mucus

Observation of cervical mucus was originally described as an adjunct to the calendar or temperature methods. It involves the recognition of the profuse, clear, watery discharge of cervical mucus which occurs at the time of ovulation. It is recommended that the woman uses a tissue to wipe the inside of her vagina to assess the quantity and characteristic of the mucus. There is no conclusive evidence that the time relationship between peak mucus production and ovulation is sufficiently constant for accurate prediction of the latter, or that the alteration in mucus flow is sufficiently great to be noticeable in most women.

Cycle Regulation

For theological reasons some patients request that they might take a hormonal preparation to regulate their menstrual cycles so that they can use a rhythm method of contraception. Some physicians may prefer to prescribe a combined oral contraceptive, tongue in cheek. Others may give a progestagen like dydrogesterone cyclically; this is reputed not to stop ovulation. Others may not be prepared to compromise with the intellectual dishonesty involved, but they should remember that they have their patient's psyche to consider as well as their own consciences.

Few physicians would consider it justifiable to regulate ovulation with clomiphene and related drugs for this purpose. Even with short-term use there are the possible hazards of ovarian cyst formation and haemorrhage therein, and the potential hazards of use of clomiphene over many years are unknown. Gonadotrophin-releasing factors are being taken to regulate ovulation and thereby facilitate the rhythm method in some South American centres.

Use-effectiveness of Rhythm Methods

To measure the effectiveness of these methods as contraceptive techniques several factors, which are difficult to separate, must be considered. These are the precise technique used to predict ovulation and the problems of assessing method failures as distinct from patient failures. The population studied to measure use-effectiveness have varied so much that it is not possible to compare them closely, and the rates given may have little validity for other users.

The calendar method is not at all effective, with failure rates of up to 30 per 100 woman-years. For the reasons already stated, and the fact that many studies are retrospective, it is extremely difficult to disentangle patient and method failures.

The temperature method is most reliable if intercourse is restricted to the post-ovulatory infertile period, commencing three days after the ovulatory temperature rise and continuing up to the beginning of menstruation. The World Health Organisation in 1967 reported on contraceptive efficiency. They felt that the definition of the post-ovulatory infertile period by temperature-charting was reliable. Their figure for the use-effectiveness of this period, based on four European studies, was 0.8–1.4 pregnancies per 100 woman-years. Three of these studies were retrospective and no allowance was made for following up patients who did not reply to the questionnaire. Despite the fact that the failure rate among drop-outs was considerably higher, the results are still surprisingly low. The second study, reported by Marshall (1968a) involved 502 couples of whom only 16 were not followed up. The failure rate in this study, again of the post-ovulatory infertile period, was 6.6 pregnancies per 100 woman-years, of which 4.2 pregnancies per 100 woman-years were due to patient failure — that is, the couple had had intercourse outside the strictly defined time.

It seems that if the couple restrict themselves to the post-ovulatory infertile period rigidly, contraception is quite effective. The problems occur in regular temperature taking and the restriction of intercourse to less than half of the menstrual cycle. Once intercourse takes place outside the strictly defined post-ovulatory infertile period and is allowed during the pre-ovulatory period then the method is much less effective. Reputed failure rates for intercourse during both pre- and post-ovulatory periods range from 0.7 per 100 woman-years (Rötzer, 1968) to 19.5 per 100 woman-years (Bartzen, 1967). This illustrates again the difficulty in drawing valid conclusions from any one study, but the general impression is that pregnancy rates of over 10 per 100 woman-years must be expected.

The cervical mucus method is ineffective, with pregnancy rates as high as 25.4 per 100 woman-years (Marshall, 1972).

The reasons for the relative ineffectiveness of these methods are the difficulties in timing ovulation from the temperature chart, the varying survival times of sperm and ovum, and finally the possibility that ovulation may occur at other times of the cycle. The mechanism of rupture of the follicle and expulsion of the ovum is still obscure. It is known that there are smooth muscle fibres within the ovary and it may be that stimulation of these or the release of some chemical mediator by intercourse can lead to rupture of the follicle and ovulation.

Advantages of Rhythm Methods

These are the only methods available to strict Roman Catholics, and they involve no expense except for a thermometer. A potential advantage that has been suggested is that by timing coitus the couple may be able to have some control over the sex of the ensuing offspring (*see* Rinehart, 1975 for review). Some evidence suggests that the Y-bearing sperm has less nuclear material, can swim faster but loses fertilising capacity more rapidly. A male child is then more likely at the time of ovulation, when cervical mucus is most easily penetrated (Kleegman, 1954); if insemination takes place before ovulation a female child is more likely. These studies are based on artificial insemination. Other theories have been propounded with the opposite relationship of fetal sex to the timing of intercourse and the ovulatory rise in basal body temperature. Guerrero (1974) found that the longer before or after the time of basal temperature rise that natural intercourse took place, the greater the likelihood of a male child.

There are so many factors involved in whether conception does or does not take place, apart from the type of spermatozoa, that accurate analysis of this type of data is virtually impossible. Coital timing to produce a male child may well be a more effective contraceptive than a sex determinant.

Disadvantages of Rhythm Methods

These include the necessity of frequent basal temperature-taking, the relatively high failure rate, and the increased risks of abnormal pregnancy and offspring should the method fail, and of psychological stresses within the marriage.

The main problem is the evidence that conception occurring other than at mid cycle can lead to abnormal handling of the conceptus by the female genital tract. It may be that attempted rhythm contraception, with conception late in the cycle, is responsible for many tubal pregnancies (Iffy, 1961, 1963a). It is also possible that late implantation of the blastocyst can encourage both spontaneous abortion and, if the pregnancy continues, placenta praevia (Iffy, 1963b). Additional evidence comes from Guerrero (1973) who found that insemination nine days before the ovulatory temperature rise, thereby involving aged spermatozoa, lead to a 14.3% chance of spontaneous abortion. Insemination three days after ovulation involving ageing ova led to a 30% incidence of spontaneous abortion.

There is some evidence that ageing of sperm within the female genital tract of animals can lead to chromosomal abnormalities, which if they are not too gross to permit fetal development may result in congenital abnormalities (Thibault, 1970). In man no relationship between the age of sperm and the incidence of congenital abnormalities has been demonstrated (Marshall, 1968b), but further confirmatory evidence would be desirable before drawing definite conclusions.

The fertilisation of ageing ova has a definite teratogenic effect in animals (Blandau and Young, 1936; Thibault, 1970) and probably in humans. It is possible that the increased incidence of congenital abnormalities occurring in babies born to older women is because the ova are older and have undergone degenerative changes before ovulation. Some evidence to this effect has been available for years but has attracted little notice. Hertig and Shea (1967) studied 34 early embryos which had been removed before the first missed menstrual period at the time of hysterectomy from women with regular cycles. Examination of these embryos revealed that if ovulation took place on Day 14 of the cycle, 12 out of 13 embryos were normal. If ovulation took place on Day 15 or later, then only 9 out of 21 embryos were normal and the other 12 would probably have aborted. Thus any factor that delays conception for a day or two after mid cycle tends to increase the rate of abortion or, if the pregnancy continues, of congenital abnormality. Further evidence that ageing of the ova causes abnormalities has been produced by Cross (1961) who suggested to 16 women who had had between one and seven previously abnormal pregnancies that they had intercourse at mid cycle only. Fifteen of them subsequently delivered themselves of normal offspring. These results are not conclusive but are suggestive of the role of ageing ova in the aetiology of congenital abnormalities. More research is necessary in this field, but our present knowledge indicates that an increased risk of congenitally abnormal babies is a potential hazard of the rhythm methods. Perhaps the scant attention given to the problem is justified, as the guilt that could be generated in parents who have had an abnormal baby after a failure of rhythm contraception could be considerable. Liberalisation of theological views on contraception could lead to more objective evaluation of the risks of periodic abstinence.

The incidence of psychological stress induced by the necessary periods of abstinence will vary greatly with the libido of the couple. It is probable, with the greater use of conventional contraceptive techniques among Roman Catholics, that those couples with a strong sex drive will employ them, while those with less interest in sex will be content with the rhythm methods.

ABSTINENCE

Abstinence from intercourse is undoubtedly the most effective method of preventing pregnancy! At times of financial hardship or stress such as economic depression and war, the birth rate drops and it is probable that abstinence plays some part in this. It is interesting to note that animals deprived of food and in a state of hardship tend to be more fertile. Are the high birth rates among the different peoples of the world a similar phenomenon or are they due to increased sexual drive prompted by a need to preserve the species? The falling birth rate of Western society is due to the increasing knowledge and availability of contraception and abortion and the desire to improve the financial status of the family. Affluence and preoccupation with the material things of life may also lead to a reduction in sexual drive. This relative abstinence may be a small contributory factor in the current reduced birth rate in developed countries.

Among young single people in Western society at the present time abstinence from sexual intercourse is rapidly decreasing. This is reflected by a rising incidence of gonorrhoea and abortion. There is today less and less mystique and romance about sex, and its physical pleasure and purely biological role is increasingly emphasised. The change in attitude has been brought about by the influence on young people of advertising, films, television, books, magazines, and by pressure from their own peer group.

There is no evidence that abstinence from heterosexual intercourse is physiologically or psychologically harmful in any way. Culturally enforced abstinence conditioned by late marriage in some communities, and celibacy of the clergy or prisoners have had no harmful physical effects on the individuals concerned. It is possible that homosexual *practices* may be more prevalent in such groups, but unlikely that homosexual *tendencies* are more common than might be expected to result from selection of an appropriate community by deviant individuals.

REFERENCES

BARTZEN, P.J. (1967). Effectiveness of the temperature rhythm system of contraception. *Fert. Steril.,* **18**, 694—706

BLANDAU, R.J. and YOUNG, W.C. (1936). Ovum age and pregnancy in the guinea pig. Data from 462 artificially inseminated females. *Anat. Rec.,* **67**, supplement 1, 33

CARTWRIGHT, A. (1970a and b). In *Parents and family planning services.* pp. 37 and 149 respectively. Routledge and Kegan Paul, London

CROSS, R.G. (1961). Prevention of anencephaly and foetal abnormalities by a preconceptional regimen. *Lancet,* ii, 1124

GUERRERO, R. (1973). Possible effects of the periodic abstinence method. *Proceedings of a Research Conference on Natural Family Planning,* 96—105. Ed. Uricchio, W.A. and Williams, M.K. Human Life Foundation, Washington

GUERRERO, R. (1974). Association of the type and time of insemination within the menstrual cycle with the human sex ratio at birth. *New Engl. J. Med.,* **291**, 1056–1059

HERTIG, A.T. and SHEA, S.M. (1967). Human trophoblast: normal and abnormal. *Am. J. clin. Path.,* **47**, 249–268

HOLLINGSWORTH, T.H. (1965). A demographic study of the British ducal families. In *Population in History*, 354–378. Ed. Glass, D.V. and Eversley, D.E.C. Arnold, London

IFFY, L. (1961). Contribution to the aetiology of ectopic pregnancy. *J. Obstet. Gynaec. Br. Commonw.,* **68**, 441–450

IFFY, L. (1963a). The role of premenstrual post-mid-cycle conception in the aetiology of ectopic gestation. *J. Obstet. Gynaec. Br. Commonw.,* **70**, 996–1000

IFFY, L. (1963b). The time of conception in pathological gestations (The scope of the reflux theory). *Proc. R. Soc. Med.,* **56**, 1098–1100

KLEEGMAN, S.J. (1954). Therapeutic donor insemination. *Fert. Steril.,* **5**, 7–31

MARSHALL, J. (1968a). A field trial of the basal-body temperature method of regulating births. *Lancet,* **ii**, 8–10

MARSHALL, J. (1968b). Congenital defects and the age of spermatozoa. *Int. J. Fert.,* **13**, 110–120

MARSHALL, J. (1972). Ovulation method of family planning. *Lancet,* **ii**, 1027–1028

MURAMATSU, M. (1967). In *Japan's experience in family planning – past and present*, 58–59. Family Planning Federation of Japan, Tokyo

PEEL, J. (1970). The Hull family survey. I. The survey couples, 1966. *J. biosoc. Sci.,* **2**, 45–70

PEEL, J. (1972). The Hull family survey. II. Family planning in the first 5 years of marriage. *J. biosoc. Sci.,* **4**, 333–346

PELLER, S. (1965). Births and deaths among Europe's ruling families since 1500. In *Population in History*, pp. 87–100. Ed. Glass, D.V. and Eversley, D.E.C. Arnold, London

POTTS, D.M. (1973). Coitus interruptus. *Aust. & N.Z. J. Obstet. Gynaecol.,* **13**, supplement, 241–250

RINEHART, W. (1975). Sex preselection – not yet practical. *Population Reports,* **I**, number 2, 21–32

RÖTZER, J. (1968). Supplemental basal body temperature and regulation of conception. *Arch. Gynaek.,* **206**, 195–214

ROYAL COMMISSION ON POPULATION (1949). *Family Limitation and its Influence on Human Fertility During the Past Fifty Years*, volume I, 67. Her Majesty's Stationery Office, London

STYCOS, J.M. (1968). In *Human fertility in Latin America. Sociological Perspectives*, p. 318. Cornell University Press, Ithaca, New York

TAYLOR, H.C. (1954). Pelvic pain based on a vascular and autonomic nervous system disorder. *Am. J. Obstet. Gynec.,* **67**, 1177–1196

THIBAULT, C. (1970). Normal and abnormal fertilisation in animals. *Adv. Biosci.,* **6**, 63–85

WORLD HEALTH ORGANIZATION (1967). Biology of fertility control by periodic abstinence. *Techn. Rep. Ser. Wld Hlth Org.,* **360**, 20

WYON, J.B. and GORDON, J.E. (1971). *The Khanna Study. Population Problems in the Rural Punjab.* Harvard University Press, Cambridge, Massachusetts

Part III
Intra-uterine Contraception

9 Intra-uterine Devices

Consideration of the history of intra-uterine devices is of some significance. The problems which their use presented in the past were much the same as those met with today. Changes in standards of acceptability to patients and physicians over the years have been greater than any improvements in effectiveness or reductions in the untoward consequences of the procedure.

The use of devices inserted into the uterine cavity to prevent conception was developed in Germany in the 1920s. Initially, loops of silkworm gut, a suture material extracted as a single thread from a silkworm killed at the inception of its cocoon-spinning stage, were employed. They commonly had a strand lying through the cervix with a button or silver wire to facilitate removal. Gräfenberg, in Berlin, noting the severe ascending sepsis sometimes associated with the intracervical wishbone and stem pessaries which had been used for years, introduced the concept of an entirely intra-uterine device. At first he used silkworm gut tied in the form of stars, but these tended to be expelled. He then developed the spiral rings made of coiled silver, gold or German silver — an alloy of copper, zinc and nickel — which bear his name (Gräfenberg, 1931; Tietze, 1962; Tatum, 1972). Gräfenberg rings, often made of silver—copper alloys (Tatum, 1972), were widely used in the 1930s. Apart from the need to remove some of the rings for pain or bleeding there were reports of expulsions, pregnancies, abortions and perforations of the uterus. Severe infections occurred in many patients and a number of deaths were reported. In consequence, the American Medical Association Committee on Contraceptive Practices in 1937 indicated its complete disapproval of intra-uterine methods of contraception.

During the next two-decades intra-uterine devices were widely condemned in Western countries. Their use continued in Japan and in 1959 Ishihama reported on some 20 000 cases; in the same year Oppenheimer reviewed 28 years' experience in Israel. In 1969 Hill reported on 1070 patients studied in Australia over a 32 year period. Limited use continued in England (Jackson, 1962; Hawkins, 1973) and in the United States of America (Hall and Stone, 1962). Pregnancy rates were low and although there were many patients with pain and bleeding very few major catastrophes were recorded. On the other hand, it is clear from the report of Wren (1962) of 12 cases of serious complications of Gräfenberg rings admitted to a single hospital in Western Australia during the years 1954 to 1961 that infections and perforations with intestinal obstruction were still occurring.

Against the background of a pressing need for world population control, widespread interest in intra-uterine devices revived with the introduction of inexpensive plastic devices in the early 1960s. The Lippes loop, the Margulies spiral and the Birnberg bow were publicised by the first and second International Conferences on Intra-uterine Contraception, held in New York in 1962 (Tietze and Lewit, 1962) and 1964 (Segal *et al.*, 1965) respectively. Since then large-scale programmes have developed which have resulted in wide publicity such that 15 000 000 women in the world now employ intra-uterine devices for contraception. Numerous research and development projects have resulted in over 200 new types and modifications of device being tested clinically. Large-scale statistically controlled evaluation programmes involving hundreds of thousands of women have been conducted. The numbers of publications in medical and lay literature dealing with intra-uterine devices run into thousands.

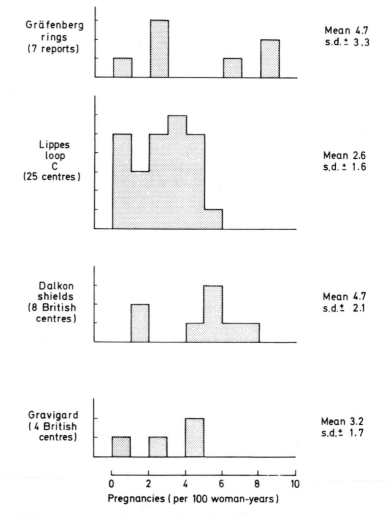

Figure 9.1 Pregnancy rates with intra-uterine devices. Histograms showing centre to centre variation (Data from Tietze, 1962; Pathfinder Fund, 1969; Williams and Snowden, 1974).

It is a sobering thought that there has been little change in the pregnancy rate (*Figure 9.1*), the major complications and the minor side-effects associated with the devices since the days of Gräfenberg.

MODE OF ACTION

A number of hypotheses have been formulated as to the mode of action of intra-uterine devices in preventing pregnancy. It is clear that in the human there are no relevant systemic effects. The normal endocrinological functions are not disturbed and ovulation takes place normally in the presence of a device.

In rodents and in sheep the presence of a foreign body in the uterine cavity causes the uterus to release prostaglandin $F_{2\alpha}$ which accelerates degeneration of the corpus luteum (Poyser *et al.*, 1970, 1971; Blatchley *et al.*, 1972). In the guinea-pig the prostaglandin synthetase inhibitor indomethacin inhibits the luteolytic effect of the foreign body in the uterus, confirming that the effect is mediated by release of prostaglandin (Donovan, 1975). It seems unlikely that these mechanisms are operative in humans since plasma progesterone levels are normal in the luteal phase in patients with intra-uterine devices (Brenner and Mishell, 1975).

Tubal Transport of Ova

It has been suggested that the presence of a device in the uterus causes an increase in motility of the fallopian tubes, expediting the progress of the ovum through the tube and reducing the opportunity for fertilisation and for early divisions of the fertilised ovum which usually take place there. Mastroianni and Rosseau (1965) showed in monkeys that an intra-uterine device accelerates the tubal transport of ova to the uterus, without affecting migration of spermatozoa. Kymographic studies in female patients by Makhlouf and Abdel-Salam (1970) demonstrated that a device causes an increased basal tonus and increased rate and magnitude of pressure oscillations in the fallopian tubes, presumably reflecting increased tubal peristalsis. Erb and Obelensky (1972) showed that tubes excised from women wearing devices had increased motility. Tietze and Lewit (1970) found that the incidence of ectopic pregnancy with a device *in situ* was only 0.1 per 100 woman-years, one-tenth of the rate for unprotected intercourse. This suggests an influence on the tube either preventing fertilisation or encouraging the transport of fertilised ova to the uterus. On the other hand, Tietze's (1966) calculation of an ectopic pregnancy rate of 0.8–1.2 ectopic pregnancies per 100 woman-years in the absence of contraception is theoretical and assumes ovulation 13 times a year, fertilisation of 20–30% of ova produced, and an ectopic rate of 0.3 per 100 fertilised ova. These assumptions may be incorrect and there is some evidence that tubal transport of ova, fertilised or unfertilised, is not affected by a device (Noyes *et al.*, 1966; World Health Organisation, 1968). Whilst occasional fertilised ova have been recovered from the fallopian tubes of women with devices, it is possible that the chance of fertilisation is reduced, either because of a reduction in the number of spermatozoa reaching the tubes or because their ability to effect fertilisation has been impaired. On the whole it seems unlikely that the fallopian tubes themselves play any major role in the mode of action of intra-uterine contraceptive devices.

Cervical Mucus

Changes in cervical mucus may affect the ability of spermatozoa to fertilise the ovum. The cervix of the parous woman with an intra-uterine device, particularly if it has a 'tail' or nylon threads lying in the canal, is often patulous, with an excessive secretion of watery mucus. It is not uncommon to find some degree of ectropion, either persisting post-partum or developing after insertion of the device. Abnormalities in the secretion could possibly affect the reputed power of cervical mucus to enhance the ability of spermatozoa to fertilise, though it is not clear that 'capacitation' of spermatozoa by the mucus is essential for fertilisation in humans. In the presence of a Lippes loop, spermatozoal penetration of the cervical mucus is actually increased (Ansbacher and Campbell, 1971).

The Intra-uterine Environment

The composition of uterine luminal fluid in women with and without intra-uterine devices was examined by Kar *et al.* (1968). The only changes they found in the presence of a device were an accumulation of metabolically inert protein and of non-protein nitrogenous material. They did not test whether or not the fluid was toxic to spermatozoa. Bacterial contamination of the uterine cavity is unlikely to be important with respect to the mode of action of the device as there is evidence that the cavity is sterile one month after insertion (Mishell *et al.*, 1966). Ishihama *et al.* (1970) reported finding corynaebacteria, anaerobes or *Gaffkya tetragena* in the endometrial fluid of 12 out of 180 device users, but this incidence was not significantly greater than the two positives found in 60 non-users, using the same methodology.

Of considerable interest is work suggesting that in the presence of Lippes loop endometrial aspirates contain large numbers of neutrophil leucocytes and macrophages which phagocytose spermatozoa (Sağiroğlu and Sağiroğlu, 1970; Sağiroğlu, 1971). These authors concluded that most of the spermatozoa present in the uterine cavity were phagocytosed or destroyed within 16 hours of intercourse, though Morgenstern *et al.* (1966) found that some still penetrate to the tubes in the chronic presence of a device. This view of the mode of action is consistent with Tietze and Lewit's (1970) computation that the number of tubal pregnancies is reduced by the presence of a device. If the device is the stimulus to phagocytosis, then it is also consistent with the demonstration by Davis and Lesinsky (1970) and Huber *et al.* (1975) that efficacy of the devices varies directly with their surface area (*Table 9.1*). It has been suggested that the

Table 9.1 PREGNANCY RATES AT TWO YEARS RELATED TO THE SURFACE AREA OF DIFFERENT TYPES OF INTRA-UTERINE DEVICES (DAVIS AND LESINSKI, 1970)

Type of device	Surface area (sq. mm)	Pregnancy rate (%)
Small bow	390	16.1
Small loop	527	9.3
Large bow	730	7.1
Small coil	960	4.5
Large loop	960	4.1
Large coil	1200	2.2

leucocytes concerned have increased lysosome hydrolase activity with a high potential for phagocytosis and intracellular digestion (Baron and Esterly, 1972). The phagocytic response has been thought to be particularly related to the points of contact with the endometrium, but devices which have angles in proximity to the tubo-uterine junctions seem to be no more effective than other devices not so shaped.

Mechanical Effects

Although the larger devices seem to convey increased protection against pregnancy (*Table 9.1*), it seems unlikely that reduction of area of endometrium available for implantation is a primary factor, since small loops of silkworm gut, covering only a small area of the endometrium, exert a contraceptive effect. The possibility of a shearing action of the device on the endometrium, dislodging a fertilised ovum, must be considered — some evidence for this will be found in *Table 9.2*. The proportion of posterior fornix pool cytological smears containing

Table 9.2 VAGINAL CYTOLOGY (POSTERIOR FORNIX) IN PATIENTS WEARING LIPPES LOOP AND METAL SPRING (M–213) INTRA-UTERINE DEVICES (BENSTER AND HAWKINS, UNPUBLISHED RESULTS)

	Lippes loop	*M–213*
Cases	124	87
Endometrial cells		
In clusters	2%	6%
Single cells	7%	13%

endometrial cells is greater with the M–213 device (Silberman *et al.*, 1969), which has sharp edges, than with the smoothly contoured Lippes loop (Benster and Hawkins, unpublished observations). On the other hand, the M device is no more effective than the Lippes loop in preventing pregnancy (Bernard, 1972). Mann (1962) showed that the Lippes loop is compressed like an accordion when the uterus contracts and this might have a shearing action. It has also been suggested (Rozin *et al.*, 1969) that plastic and other rigid devices distort and distend the cavity of the uterus, converting the potential cavity into a fluid-filled space in which the blastocyst lacks contact with the endometrium.

Myometrial Activity

It would be expected that the presence of a foreign body in the uterus would stimulate myometrial contractions, and it is conceivable that such activity would tend to prevent implantation. Bengtsson and Moawad (1967) and Moawad and Bengtsson (1970) recorded intra-uterine pressures in women with Lippes loops *in situ*. They found that there was little effect on small, spontaneous uterine contractions until the fourth or fifth post-ovulatory day. After that the device caused a precocious development of the less frequent contractions of high amplitude which normally precede menstruation. Thus uterine contractions of a magnitude over 100 mmHg (13 kPa), normally only seen on the day before menstruation, occurred as early as Day 22 of the cycle if a device were present. Such myometrial contractions might well interfere with the implantation of the blastocyst.

The observations on the four sizes of Lippes loop in *Table 9.3* are relevant in this respect: the larger the loop, the smaller the pregnancy rate and the greater the expulsion rate. This is consistent with the idea that increased myometrial activity in response to the device is linked with contraceptive efficacy. Coutinho (1971) found that intraluminal pressures at menstruation are increased in the uterus which contains a device. It is possible that such activity could result in expulsion of an early embryo — use has been made of stimulation of uterine contractions with prostaglandins at the time of menstruation to interfere with

Table 9.3 LIPPES LOOPS. NET CUMULATIVE EVENT RATES FOR ONE YEAR OF USE PER 100 USERS (SNOWDEN, 1975a)

	Pregnancies	*Expulsions*	*Removals (bleeding or pain)*
Loop A (smallest)	4.4	15.6	4.7
Loop B	3.6	12.2	5.9
Loop C	2.8	10.4	7.1
Loop D (largest)	2.4	5.9	8.1

nidation. It has been suggested that prostaglandins released locally in response to the presence of an intra-uterine device may be involved in the consequent increased motility. It is unlikely that the luteolytic effect of these agents has much effect during the secretory phase of the cycle, as plasma progesterone levels and the endometrial responses appear normal. The luteal phase is shortened by an average of two days (Nygren and Johansson, 1973) but this seems to be due to a tendency for 'breakthrough' bleeding from the endometrium, not to changes in hormone levels (Brenner and Mishell, 1975). If luteal function is inadequate at the end of a cycle when fertilisation has occurred, deficient progesterone influence might then not only enhance uterine motility but also affect nidation adversely. Chaudhuri (1971) suggested that prostaglandins may stimulate uterine motility directly and that this could be important in contraceptive efficacy. He was unable to demonstrate that indomethacin, which inhibits prostaglandin synthetase and hence prostaglandin release, impaired the contraceptive effect of intra-uterine devices in rats (Chaudhuri, 1973). In fact, indomethacin itself has a contraceptive action in rodents (Marley and Smith, 1974). This is more in line with the concept suggested by previous workers that the primary effect of prostaglandins during the cycle in which fertilisation takes place is to aid conception (Hawkins and Labrum, 1961; Hawkins, 1968; Bygdeman *et al.*, 1970) though it does not conflict with an abortifacient effect when prostaglandins are given two or three weeks after conception. It is possible that prostaglandins released from the uterus containing an intra-uterine device and from leucocytes adherent to the device (Myatt *et al.*, 1977) expedite expulsion of the endometrium at the end of a menstrual cycle and that this may discourage nidation.

Effects on the Endometrium

Minor gross morphological, maturational, inflammatory and biochemical changes in the endometrium have been reviewed by Eckstein (1970), who considers that the value of the available information is somewhat less than its bulk, as well as by Tatum (1972) and Johannisson (1973).

The endometrium of both anterior and posterior surfaces of the uterine cavity shows the imprint of the device; under the rim or loops of the device the endometrium is compressed, between loops it is oedematous and sometimes hyperaemic or haemorrhagic (Israel and Davis, 1966).

It has repeatedly been suggested, on the basis of endometrial biopsies, that the menstrual changes in the endometrium are altered by an intra-uterine device so that it is no longer in phase with the time of ovulation. On the other hand, as Eckstein (1970) has pointed out, when complete hysterectomy specimens are examined, endometrial 'dating' appears essentially normal and in phase with the ovarian cycle. It may be that in some women an intra-uterine foreign body has a luteolytic effect, mediated by prostaglandin release, with impairment of endometrial development as occurs in rodents and cows. This is not the case in the great majority of women using devices who have normal plasma progesterone levels in the second half of the cycle, and normal endometrium in which the ultrastructural changes of the secretory phase tend to occur a day or two prematurely (Wynn, 1968).

Numerous experimental and clinical reports testify to leucocytic proliferation of varying degree in the endometrium when a device is *in situ*. In some reports it appears that the response is generalised; others emphasise its relation to points of contact with the device. The cells infiltrating the endometrium are mainly polymorphonuclear leucocytes, but macrophages, mononuclear cells and plasma cells are often prominent. It is quite clear that the inflammatory response is not to bacterial invasion of the endometrial cavity (Mishell *et al.*, 1966). No bacterial contamination of the endometrial cavity was found in hysterectomy specimens removed more than 30 days after insertion of a device, though many showed the histological changes of 'chronic endometritis'. There is evidence that the changes are related to the presence of phagocytic leucocytes which engulf spermatozoa in the endometrial cavity (Sağiroğlu, 1971; Tatum, 1972). It is possible that such a response could also render the endometrium hostile to implantation, but the exact mechanism is obscure.

A marked increase in acid phosphatase activity in the endometrium at mid cycle in the uterus containing an inert device has been demonstrated, whilst there was no such change in the normal uterus (Joshi and Sujan-Tejuja, 1969). Whether or not these findings bear any relation to contraceptive activity is unknown. Other observations were that the increases in total protein and RNA which normally occur at mid cycle were produced about a week earlier in endometrium with a device present. This may well be a reflection of asynchronous change in areas of the endometrium in close contact with the device, rather than a generalised endometrial reaction.

Action of Inert Devices

It therefore appears that the most likely modes of action of the inert devices are:

(1) Reduction of the number of spermatozoa reaching the tubes or impairment of their capacity to fertilise;

(2) A direct mechanical effect in prevention of implantation;
(3) Production of a change in the endometrium rendering it hostile to implantation and early development of the blastocyst;
(4) A stimulant effect on myometrial activity resulting in very early abortion.

PHARMACOLOGICALLY ACTIVE INTRA-UTERINE DEVICES

In the past, Gräfenberg rings were made of various alloys and often contained copper and sometimes zinc or nickel. Ions passing into solution may have had a toxic effect on spermatozoa or influenced endometrial reaction. We found that 6 out of 24 women using Gräfenberg rings made of 92.5% silver and 7.5% copper and zinc had chronic endometritis with infiltration of the endometrium by histiocytes, lymphocytes and plasma cells (Hawkins and Nixon, unpublished observations).

What is not widely known is that medical grades of stainless steel vary in their composition and this may influence endometrial reaction. The Majzlin spring was found by Ober *et al.* (1970) to produce focal and diffuse acute inflammatory changes in the endometrium, and, when the spring had been *in situ* for some months, chronic endometritis with diffuse infiltration of the endometrium by lymphocytes, plasma cells and scattered eosinophils. There was a good correlation between complaints of abnormal bleeding, pain and discharge and the presence of endometritis. The spring is made of type 303 stainless steel containing a maximum of 0.15% carbon, 2.0% manganese, 0.045% phosphorus, 0.03% sulphur, 1.0% silicon, 18% chromium and 9% nickel. The M–213 device is made of a type 316 stainless steel, containing 0.08% carbon, 2.0% manganese, 0.045% phosphorus, 0.03% sulphur, 1.0% silicon, 17% chromium, 12% nickel and 2.5% molybdenum (Bernard, personal communication). The M–213 does not appear to give rise to the inflammatory effects described by Ober *et al.* (1970), and endometrium from women using it does not differ from that of women using plastic Lippes loops (Thomlinson, J., personal communication). Perhaps the molybdenum in the M–213 protects the endometrium from the effects of the other metals, either because the type 316 steel is harder and more resistant to corrosion or by pharmacological antagonism of the effects of other metallic ions.

Devices Containing Copper

In 1969, Zipper, Medel and Prager in Chile, demonstrated that a small piece of copper or zinc wire inserted within the uterus of a rabbit greatly reduced the number of implantation sites in that horn compared with the control horn. Zipper, Tatum *et al.* (1969) proceeded to show that the addition of 30 sq. mm of exposed copper in the form of copper wire wound round a T shaped device which previously had an unacceptably high pregnancy rate (18 per 100 woman-years) reduced this to approximately 5 per 100 woman-years. There is a direct relationship between the area of exposed copper on the device, and contraceptive efficacy (Orlans, 1973). Subsequent work (Orlans, 1973; Williams and Snowden, 1974) has demonstrated pregnancy rates which do not differ markedly from those with some inert devices. It appears that the addition of metallic copper to a relatively inefficient device may improve contraceptive efficacy but conveys little improvement in performance in comparison with a good inert device.

A copper ion concentration as high as 1.8×10^{-3} M ($115 \mu g/ml$) can appear after 18 hours incubation of metallic copper, surface area 400 sq.mm, in a mixture of human uterine secretion and saline (Oster, 1972). A 200 sq.mm copper surface releases about $50 \mu g$ of copper per day, causing about a sixfold increase in the concentration of copper in the uterine fluid (Hagenfeldt, 1972a). These levels are maintained for at least a year after insertion, but eventually decrease as the available copper is dissolved. Laufe *et al.* (1974) found with Copper-7 devices that after three to six months the dose of copper in the uterus is of the order of $40 \mu g/day$ whilst after ten months it is about $18 \mu g/day$. There are increased copper concentrations in the endometrium and cervical mucus (Hagenfeldt, 1972b). The amounts of copper in the uterine secretion are sufficient to inhibit growth of human amniotic fluid cells and fetal fibroblasts and epithelioid cells (Jones, Gregson and Elstein, 1973) and human cervical cells (Hounsell and Hawkins, 1974) in tissue culture. Systemic absorption of the dissolved intra-uterine copper has been demonstrated in rats (Okereke *et al.*, 1972) but in humans the copper absorbed is insufficient to cause a measurable change in serum copper (Hagenfeldt, 1972b; Laufe *et al.*, 1974).

Available information on the mode of action of copper in preventing pregnancy was reviewed by Tatum (1973), Johannisson (1973), Orlans (1973), Hagenfeldt (1973), Oster and Salgo (1975) and Hsu *et al.* (1976). The presence of copper in the uterus does not affect ovulation or fertilisation *per se*. Copper causes small globules to form in the cervical mucus channels (Daunter, 1976) and may well affect penetration of spermatozoa. It tends to depress spermatozoal activity (Chattopadhyay *et al.*, 1976) and is spermicidal in higher concentrations of the order of 0.1–0.2 mM (White, 1955; Loewit, 1971), but the amounts released by a copper device into human uterine fluid take several hours to produce any reduction of spermatozoal motility (Jecht and Bernstein, 1973).

The principal relevant effects seem to be on the endometrium. Hsu *et al.* (1976) found that Copper T devices eroded the endometrium causing focal superficial chronic endometritis, with infiltration of the endometrium by polymorphonuclear leucocytes, mononuclear and plasma cells in relation to the site of the device. Copper depresses oestrogen binding in the endometrium and it also depresses uptake of thymidine into DNA in the endometrial cells, suggesting that it interferes with metabolism and growth processes in these cells. It impairs glycogen storage in the endometrium. In addition copper can compete with zinc, a co-factor in the carbonic anhydrase reaction, which is needed to deal with carbon dioxide produced by the implanting blastocyst. In fact, levels of the trace elements zinc and manganese in the endometrium are decreased after months of exposure to a copper device. Lactate dehydrogenase isoenzymes containing the M subunit are inhibited (Wilson, 1977). Acid phosphatase activity in the endometrium is increased in the proliferative phase and both β-glucuronidase and alkaline phosphatase are depressed in the secretory phase. Copper is potent in producing a leucocytic reaction, particularly in the uterine cavity.

Forder (1974) suggested that copper ions tend to alter prostaglandin synthesis from production of prostaglandin E_2 to prostaglandin $F_{2\alpha}$. If uterine production of these substances has any relevance to the contraceptive effect of intra-uterine devices in humans then the latter compound might be expected to have a greater effect in impairing corpus luteum function and in enhancing uterine motility.

It should be noted that low concentrations of copper ions ($10^{-3.5}-10^{-5}$ M) facilitate the colonisation by viruses of cells in tissue culture (Wyler and Wiesendanger, 1975). The possibility that viruses play a role in the chronic endometritis associated with intra-uterine devices has not been excluded, though we have so far been unable to grow the usual pathogenic viruses from the cervix of patients with devices (Hawkins and Murdoch, unpublished observations).

Some or all of the effects on the endometrium prevent implantation of the blastocyst. HCG is detectable in the serum of patients with copper devices in 12–19% of luteal phases, suggesting that fertilisation has occurred but the blastocyst has then degenerated (Landesman *et al.*, 1976). Insertion of a copper device up to five days post-coitum can prevent pregnancy, presumably by preventing nidation (Tatum and Lippes, 1975). All the effects of the copper are readily reversible on removal of its source. Copper does not disturb the growth of blastocysts which are already implanted and there is no evidence that the presence of a device containing copper causes any fetal abnormality or interferes with fetal growth or with the pregnancy and confinement (Snowden, 1976). This argues against any specific toxic effect on early development of the embryo.

Recently, it has been suggested that a silicone rubber device which releases both metallic copper and zinc acts as a cation exchanger and lowers the intra-uterine pH (Anderson, 1974). It is claimed that this renders the intra-uterine environment hostile to spermatozoa.

Devices Containing Progesterone

T-shaped intra-uterine devices which release progesterone, 100–150 µg per day for months, are more effective in preventing pregnancy than inert devices of the same shape. Scommegna *et al.* (1974) found that the progesterone does not interfere with plasma hormone levels, ovulation or cervical mucus and concluded that the contraceptive efficacy was due to a local decidual stromal reaction in the endometrium, rendering it hostile to implantation.

The pregnancy rates with progesterone-releasing devices (Scommegna *et al.*, 1974; Place and Pharriss, 1974) are no lower than those cited in early reports of the performance of comparable copper-wound devices. Preference might be given to use of the hormone on the grounds that it is endogenous to the endometrium and is metabolised there, but copper is also a normal constituent of endometrium. The number of patients requiring removal of progesterone devices for bleeding problems in the early months is considerable, and it is tempting to conclude that the devices combine the disadvantages of intra-uterine contraceptives with those of low-dose progestagen oral contraception!

The Progestasert is a relatively flexible T-shaped device containing 38 mg of progesterone crystals intended to be released at about 65 µg per day (which may be compared with the systemic production of 25 mg per day by a mature corpus luteum). The device is intended to be replaced annually.

It has recently been suggested that use of the Progestasert is associated with an unduly high incidence of ectopic gestation (Tatum and Schmidt, 1977; Snowden, 1977), and it has been withdrawn in Great Britain, pending further assessment.

Conclusion

We are at the present time left with the concept that all intra-uterine devices lead to changes in the intra-uterine environment which tend to impair the ability of spermatozoa to effect fertilisation and to prevent implantation of the blasto-cyst. The nature of the changes specifically responsible is not clear, but factors likely to be involved are impairment of the endometrial surface, increased uterine motility, a phagocytic leucocyte response and inflammatory and bio-chemical changes in the endometrium. These changes may be enhanced by incorporation of substances such as copper or progesterone in the devices.

EVALUATION OF INTRA-UTERINE DEVICES

Clinical reports in the general medical literature must be regarded as providing only preliminary information as to the performance of a given intra-uterine device. Such reports are particularly susceptible to local environmental influences on both the motivation and reaction of the patients and on the physician's value judgements and policies of management. On the whole, preg-nancy rates are more influenced by these factors than removal or complication rates, but even in well regulated trials pregnancies with a Lippes loop size C appear to vary from 0.0 in Bombay to 5.8 per 100 woman-years in Beer-Sheba (Pathfinder Fund, 1969) and with standard size Dalkon shields from 1.4 in Dublin (Miller *et al.*, 1975) to 8.6 in Boston (Perlmutter, 1974). An additional problem is the 'lost to follow-up' patient, who should be regarded as at risk for pregnancy or complications until such time as the device is known to have been formally removed. These patients are often either left out of an assessment or the assumption is made that they will have the same complication rates as patients still under study. In fact the incidence of complications tends to be higher in the segment of the population least accessible to follow-up (Sims, 1973). Patients with an intra-uterine device catastrophe do not in general return to the clinic where the device was fitted but have recourse to a hospital with an acute gynaecological unit, and resist contact for follow-up purposes. This is not just a matter of resentment — patients are loyal and do not like to upset the doctor who fitted the device by reporting a failure (Hawkins, 1969).

It is not always easy to demonstrate the relationship of event rates to 'lost to follow-up' rates, as the data are often confounded by other variables (Snowden and Williams, 1972). On the other hand the data collected by the Pathfinder Fund (1969) on 25 trials of Lippes loop C with at least 90% follow-up, from centres around the world, show a positive correlation between pregnancy rates and follow-up rates (*Figure 9.2*). The better the follow-up, even within the range 90–100%, the higher the pregnancy rate found. It follows that pregnancy rates based on series with only 90% follow-up are likely to be underestimates and to be sure of the data a 99% follow-up is required.

It is well established that the demographic characteristics of the population influence pregnancy rates. Many studies have shown that the older the patients the lower the pregnancy rate. Since in general the effect of parity is confounded with that of age, it may sometimes appear that more parous patients, who are older, have lower pregnancy rates. Tietze and Lewit (1970) have found that, within the separate age groups 15 to 24 years and 35 to 49 years, pregnancy rates actually increase with parity. It could be that in both these groups high parity is associated with women who ovulate consistently. The relation may be partly due to the effect of repeated pregnancy in enlarging the uterine cavity. In more parous women the surface area of the endometrium is proportionately larger, compared with the surface area of the device.

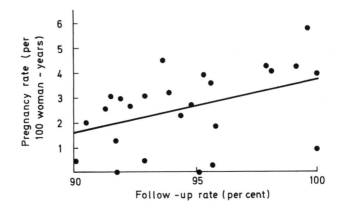

Figure 9.2 Relationship between reported pregnancy rates with Lippes loop C and follow-up rate. All studies had loss to follow-up less than 10% (Pathfinder Fund, 1969). The regression is significant (P<0.05).

Cultural and economic pressures in the community also affect failure rates. At first sight it would seem that intra-uterine devices should be independent of such effects, but in practice factors bearing primarily on patient motivation may affect the number of pregnancies. This reflects the ability of the patients not only to detect whether or not spontaneous expulsion of the device has occurred but also then to take alternative precautions and see a physician for advice. The attitude of the physician is important. Careful instruction of patients on verifying that the device is *in situ* and ready access of patients to their doctor if expulsion is suspected improve results.

Failures may be more common in women who have intercourse frequently. This may be involved in the higher pregnancy rates in younger women. Conversely, in communities where religious and cultural factors or adverse publicity lead to lack of trust in the efficacy of devices, infrequent intercourse may give better results. The custom of prolonged lactation and breast feeding in some countries contributes to low pregnancy rates in patients having a device fitted after a confinement. Of course any community where fertility is low – for example where pelvic inflammatory disease is common – will have low pregnancy rates.

Short of the performance of double-blind comparative trials of efficacy, which are difficult to arrange except when closely similar devices are being assessed, it is necessary to document and evaluate centre to centre variation in performance, rather than to control this variable. The difficulty is illustrated by Snowden (1972) and Snowden *et al.* (1973), who describe the extent of variation to be found between clinics in the same county. In one study the clinics in two towns a few miles apart were conducted by the same doctor who used the same device. The groups of patients had the same age and parity structure and the studies were concurrent. The pregnancy rate in one town was consistently three times that in the other. Even assessment of sexual habits and incidence of gonorrhoea is unlikely to provide a complete explanation of such a difference. In such circumstances more useful information may be obtained by regarding the difference as an expression of centre to centre variation (*Figure 9.1*) than by attempting to analyse it further.

Reported rates of complications in patients using devices are very much more susceptible to such influences than are pregnancy rates. Certainly spontaneous expulsions are commoner with some devices than with others, but they are also influenced by racial factors, age and parity structure of the population and incidence of spontaneous and therapeutic abortion (Bernard, 1970), all of which affect the size, configuration and physiological activity of the uterus and the competence of the cervix. Bernard (1970) also suggests that skill at insertion influences liability to expulsion. Expulsion undetected by the patient is common and reported rates are much influenced by whether or not patients verify the presence of the device by self-examination, by their observation of menstrual loss and by attendance at clinics for follow-up examinations.

Reported rates of removal of devices because of medical complications such as excessive bleeding, pain or discharge are influenced by all the above factors but are very susceptible indeed to the effect of patient motivation, and more particularly to the experience, beliefs, attitudes and skills of the physician. It has been shown (Hawkins, 1973) that modern plastic devices have the same list of major and minor complications as the Gräfenberg ring 40 years ago, and the same wide range in the reporting of these complications. Data presented at the Second International Conference on Intra-uterine Contraception (Segal *et al.*, 1965) held in New York in 1964, before it became fashionable to show a low complication rate, gave incidences of intermenstrual bleeding from 2 to 78%, of menorrhagia from 3 to 40%, of lower abdominal pain from 2 to 58% and of vaginal discharge from 3 to 40%. These side-effects still occur but in general patients have been trained to accept them. Strongly motivated patients from communities where family limitation is at a premium tolerate severe side-effects without even mentioning them to their doctors. Where the devices are unpopular for religious, political or economic reasons, or where there has been adverse publicity, medical complication rates are high. Even more important are the attitudes of physicians (Snowden, 1972, 1973a; Hawkins, 1973; Moignard, 1973). Enthusiasm for intra-uterine contraception has sometimes led to loss of perspective and in many instances a situation where success of an IUD programme has become the primary objective of the physician, overshadowing the primary purpose of provision of effective contraception by the best means appropriate to the patient. Moignard (1973) concludes by quoting Bernard to the effect that 'mental preparation of both doctor and patient', rather than medical skill, is a challenge 'on whose mastery may well depend the future of the IUD method of contraception'. Specialist gynaecologists, who could have added balance and perspective to the provision of contraceptive services but who have tended over the years to delegate the task to enthusiasts, must accept a major share of the responsibility for the development of such restricted outlooks. Regrettably, personal, financial, political and even racial attitudes of physicians are sometimes concerned in their attitude to medical complications of intra-uterine contraception and are reflected in the complication and removal rates they report.

'Continuation rate' — that is, the proportion of patients continuing to use a device after a given time — is a meaningless statistic from a medical point of view. It is inversely related to the pregnancy, expulsion and removal and is thus affected by all the variables influencing these rates, and is in addition dependent on the desire of the patient for additional children, and removals for this purpose. For these reasons continuation rates are mainly of interest to politicians and economists engaged in the assessment of population control programmes.

Even in large-scale studies, reporting of rare but major complications is likely to be defective. For example, few realise that intra-uterine devices have been directly responsible for a death rate of about 20 per million users per year (Meeker, 1969) equivalent to that from pulmonary embolism and cerebral thrombosis in women using full oestrogen dose oral contraceptives (Inman and Vessey, 1968).

A very large number of cases is required to establish the occurrence of a low-incidence complication as due to more than chance. Physicians are reluctant to report a relatively rare complication and create alarm on a basis which has dubious statistical validity. Low-incidence major complications are particularly likely to be located in the 'lost to follow-up' group, the consequences having been dealt with in circumstances far removed from the clinic where the device was fitted, with delay and often failure in determining what has happened to the patient. These factors have sometimes resulted in complications being observed by clinicians before they are made known by large-scale monitoring programmes. For example, the high proportion of ectopic gestations amongst women who do become pregnant with an intra-uterine device *in situ* was reported from a clinical source (Ramkissoon-Chen and Kong Ta-Ko, 1966) before it was revealed by the Cooperative Statistical Program for the Evaluation of Intra-Uterine Devices (Tietze, 1966).

National and International Sources of Data

It was appreciated early in the 1960s that the standard procedures for reporting results of clinical research by means of publications in the literature from individual centres were inadequate for full evaluation of intra-uterine contraceptive devices. Adequate assessment involves not only data from a number of environments, preferably international, but also analysis of factors influencing centre to centre variation in results. The Cooperative Statistical Program for the Evaluation of Intra-Uterine Devices was initiated in the United States of America by the National Committee on Maternal Health, at the request of the Population Council (Tietze, 1966). It was largely responsible for the introduction of actuarial methods of computing results and has produced a series of valuable reports.

A consistent attempt was made in the reports of the Pathfinder Fund (for example, *see* Bernard, 1969a) to incorporate only data from centres where high follow-up rates are obtained. Double-blind studies to control for variation in patient and medical environments have been encouraged (Bernard, 1969b). Recently, the Family Planning Research Unit at the University of Exeter has been producing useful reports analysing data from a number of centres which are representative of Great Britain. Other organisations have concentrated on the assembly and presentation of representative reports on contraception; the

Studies on Family Planning and the *Country Profiles* of the Population Council and the *Population Reports* from the George Washington University Medical Center are particularly useful.

It is of primary importance for physicians to understand that individual reports on a device, whether from medical or commercial sources, are of little significance until the results they quote have been confirmed by a large-scale multicentre programme. At the same time it must be appreciated that such programmes are manned by individuals who, from the highest motives, are concerned with techniques for population control on a widespread basis rather than the individual patient, and are financed from sources with political and economic bias. The physician must retain responsibility for interpreting findings with regard to the welfare of the individual patient.

Analysis of 'Use-Effectiveness'

The first consistent procedure for evaluating contraceptive efficacy was Pearl's Index (Pearl, 1932). To calculate this, total accidental pregnancies are divided by total months of contraceptive exposure and multiplied by 1200 to give the number of pregnancies per 100 years of contraceptive exposure. The index is somewhat susceptible to bias (Potter, 1966). If the population under study contains a large number of poorly motivated individuals who are careless in their application of contraceptive methods or in reporting suspected expulsion when they are using intra-uterine devices, this results in an artificially high pregnancy rate in a short-term study. As successive months of exposure elapse, the accident-prone are selectively removed from the study and the bulk of the data is accumulated from the most strongly motivated group, giving an artificially low pregnancy rate in a long-term study. The latter effect is also automatically ensured if the population contains a proportion of women who were infertile from the start — the longer the study proceeds, the greater the influence of the infertile group and the lower the apparent pregnancy rate. Finally, the Pearl Index is said to give a favourable view if a large number of 'spacers' — women who have just given birth and wish to postpone the next pregnancy for a few months or perhaps a year — are included in a study of short duration. These are a relatively infertile group, many of which have not resumed ovulation and who leave the study before the real risk of pregnancy arises.

The use of actuarial procedures — the 'life-table method' developed by Potter (1966) and Tietze (1967) — was widely applied by the Cooperative Statistical Program and has now become a common form for reporting results. The status of participants in the study is assessed after each successive month of exposure and in this way the occurrence of pregnancy or other mishaps is expressed sequentially, month by month, in relation to the number of women actually exposed for that period of time. A cumulative pregnancy rate can be computed — the usual figure quoted is the gross cumulative one year failure rate. This is the proportion of women who would be expected to conceive during one year of use of the device if there were no discontinuation for reasons other than accidental pregnancy.

Life-table methods have several advantages. They minimise the effect of the main source of bias such as the short-term spacer and the long-term subfertile group to which the Pearl Index is so susceptible, and at the least permit evaluation of such effects by study of the successive monthly failure rates. The approach has facilitated acquisition of data which can be used for comparison of contraceptive efficacy in a short period of time. On the other hand it is widely believed that life-table procedures eliminate the sources of bias completely. This is not the case and values obtained in this way are still influenced by inclusion, for example, of a large number of postpartum women who use the method for a short time (Hawkins and Benster, 1977). Discontinuation rates can readily be broken down according to cause: pregnancy, expulsion or removal for various reasons. The calculations are not too complex to perform by hand (Tietze and Lewit, 1973), but are fairly readily programmed for a computer. Finally, an expression of the error of a given calculated rate can be derived. A pregnancy rate obtained by a life-table method is usually presented in the form 'per 100 woman-years ± standard error'. It should be understood that this is not a sampling standard error with a given number of degrees of freedom, like that usually presented with the means of a series of numerical observations. It is an approximation to the standard error in a large population. An exact computation is given by Potter (1969). Tietze and Lewit (1973) describe a much simpler procedure which yields a reasonable approximation to the standard error, provided the number of couples at risk does not fall below about 100. They also give a procedure for estimating 95% confidence limits for the rates.

Large samples are required before a valid mathematical deduction can be made as to the significance of a difference between two rates. A common assumption is that if the standard errors quoted for the rates overlap, then the difference between the rates has not been demonstrated to be of importance. This is a reasonable interpretation, provided it is realised that if the standard errors do not overlap no real difference necessarily exists. If, as sample sizes increase to large numbers, the gap between the two values plus or minus their standard errors remains constant or increases, the difference can be regarded as important.

Evaluations of contraceptive efficacy have generated appropriate jargon. *Events* include the occurrence of pregnancies, expulsions and removals for medical or personal reasons or for a planned pregnancy — 'use-related terminations'. *Non-related events* include 'loss to follow-up', removal at the investigator's choice and a category of *release from follow-up*. The last represents patients using a device satisfactorily who move out of the area or out of the country for personal reasons; sometimes the qualification that they are formally transferred to the care of another doctor is required. *Closures* include pregnancies, expulsions and removals where the device is not replaced, and release from follow-up. *Event rates* are either *net* or *gross*. *Net rates* are useful for assessing the overall performance of a device, being designed to measure the incidence of each type of event in the presence of all other types of event. They are estimated using a *multiple decrement table* (Potter *et al.*, 1969). Net cumulative event rates have the useful property that they are additive. For example, the sum of the net rates for closures for different reasons gives a total closure rate, and this subtracted from 100 gives the net continuation rate. *Gross rates* are designed to measure the incidence of each type of event separately, independent of that of other events. They are calculated using a *single decrement table* (Potter, 1966). They are always higher than *net rates* and cannot be added to give a cumulative total event rate. Gross rates are most useful for comparison of a single type of event among several different devices or several different groups of users.

In most studies a 'cut-off date' is employed. All the information that can be obtained is completed to this date, using retrospective follow-up of defaulters where necessary, and submitted to analysis. Patients about whom no recent facts up to the last appointment before the cut-off date are available are classified as 'lost to follow-up'.

The Cooperative Statistical Program employed an analysis which assumes that event rates in the 'lost to follow-up' group are the same as those in patients kept under study — an assumption that may not be justified. Other analyses can be devised which regard 'loss to follow-ups' as a separate category of event. Some computer programmes incorporate a feature particularly applicable to intra-uterine device studies — when a previously 'lost to follow-up' patient is located, all the relevant information becomes available and the patient is automatically reinstated in the study.

Jain and Sivin (1977) have drawn attention to minor differences in definitions of 'months of use', categories of termination and treatment of incomplete observations between different procedures described for life-table computations. The results for a single year of study are little affected, but quite marked discrepancies in rates derived can arise in studies lasting several years. It is important to specify the exact computation employed. As is so often the case in clinical trials, a comparison between a new device or procedure and one that is well established, with the same doctors employing the same procedures in a single environment, and analysing the results the same way, is of much greater value than any attempt to define arbitrary average rates which might have general applicability. The pooled results of multicentre trials of a single device provide mean rates of more theoretical than practical interest. The value of multicentre studies lies in the range of centre to centre variation in rates which they indicate.

Monitoring of low-incidence major complications such as perforation of the uterus by a device has not so far been well conducted in large-scale programmes. One reason for this is the assumption that the events are rare and can easily be appraised; another is that the rare catastrophes tend to occur in patients recorded as 'lost to follow-up'. The only answer to this problem is a serious attempt to obtain 100% follow-up and application of sequential 'control chart' statistical approaches, where a single event cumulating to a deviation from the expected normal variation is promptly noted.

TYPES OF DEVICE

Gräfenberg rings are now seldom used. They are relatively easy to insert, and with experience can be removed easily using Gräfenberg's hook. They are associated with the same risk of pregnancy as the newer devices (*Figure 9.1*) and the same side-effects (Hawkins, 1973). The reasons for their loss of popularity are that they are expensive and they are 'closed ring' devices, which if they do perforate the uterus have been known to strangulate bowel (Wren, 1962). Similar considerations apply to the Hall ring. The Ota rings, made in metal or plastic, resembled Gräfenberg rings but had central spokes which prevented bowel entanglement if they perforated. They were widely used in

Japan with moderate success (Ishihama, 1959) but dilatation of the cervix under anaesthesia was often necessary to ensure that they were correctly placed in the uterus.

The plastic devices introduced in the years 1960 to 1964 had the advantages that they could be made inexpensively, that they could be readily introduced without anaesthesia, and that their presence could be verified by a 'tail' protruding through the cervix.

The device which has been most extensively used since its introduction (Lippes, 1962) is the Lippes loop — it is probably still the most widely used intra-uterine device in the world today. Enormous experience has been gained and published with the loops, and the physician who uses them routinely can have the confidence that their properties and all the complications that can arise have been fully documented in the last decade. When all factors are evaluated it is difficult to prove that any of the, literally, hundreds of devices which have been developed since have any overall advantage over the loops for routine use.

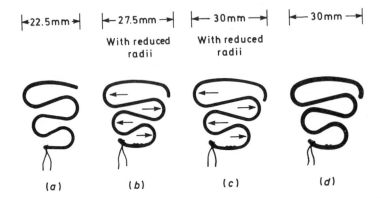

Figure 9.3 Lippes loops: (a) Blue thread, weight 290 mg; (b) Black thread, weight 526 mg; (c) Yellow thread, weight 615 mg; (d) White thread, weight 709 mg. (Courtesy of Ortho Pharmaceuticals Ltd.).

Lippes loops (*Figure 9.3*) are polythene double S's which are introduced through a plastic cylinder inserted through the cervix and unfold *in situ*. Two threads attached to the tail protrude through the cervix for verification of the presence of the device and to facilitate removal. There have been minor changes in the devices over the years. The plastic is now radio-opaque and gum silicone is incorporated in the blend. The threads are ultrasonically welded in place. Originally, the devices were sold in bulk, sterilised in 0.1–1.0% benzalkonium chloride solution and loaded in an inserter immediately before use. More recently they have become available in individual sterile packs, pre-loaded in disposable inserters. It is perhaps worth noting that the change in presentation was associated with a very considerable increase in price (Drug and Therapeutics Bulletin, 1973).

Particularly with older Lippes loops, manufacturing faults eventually come to light. Sometimes when a device is removed the plastic is found to have 'lost its memory' — the shape the unrestricted device assumes is distorted. Occasionally the loop has fragmented *in utero* — one particular batch manufactured in the Far

East became notorious for this defect. Devices removed after several years in the uterus may be pitted. They sometimes have calcium carbonate deposits (Howard, 1971) which also contain magnesium, iron, phosphate, uric acid and protein (Engineer *et al.,* 1970; Dasgupta *et al.,* 1971), and there is often adherent mucoid and collagenous material which contains white cells which have migrated from the endometrium (Potts and Pearson, 1967). On the other hand many loops removed after five to ten years are in remarkably good condition.

The loops are made in sizes A to D (*Figure 9.3*). Size C is the first choice for the average parous female. Size D has the same overall dimensions but the plastic is thicker, rendering the device less easily compressed and expelled. It is tolerated well by many women who have had two or three children, and is particularly indicated for those who have expelled a size C loop. The B loop is narrower than the C, and is suitable for some nulliparous women and some patients who have had discomfort wearing a C loop. The A loop is narrower still and the curves have wider radii than B or C loops. In practice it is not often used, but may be appropriate for the young nullipara with a noticeably small uterus on examination.

The effect of size of the loops, pregnancy rates and expulsion rates being less with the larger sizes, is shown in *Table 9.3*. Removals for complaints of bleeding or pain are not consistently related to the size of loop (Tietze and Lewit, 1970) being influenced primarily by the attitudes of patients and physicians, though Snowden (1975a) found that on average the larger loops gave more trouble of this sort. There is the usual variation in pregnancy rates in studies from different environments. In 25 trials of the C loops, the Pathfinder Fund (1969) study recorded between nil and 5.8 pregnancies per 100 woman-years during the first year of use (*see Figures 9.1* and *9.2*, pp. 164, 174). As with all inert devices the annual pregnancy rate steadily decreases with each successive year of use. With the D loop, Tietze and Lewit (1970) found a decrease from 2.7 pregnancies per 100 woman-years in the first year of use, to 0.9 in the sixth year of use.

The Margulies spiral proved to be associated with relatively high rates of bleeding and expulsion (Tietze and Lewit, 1970). This may have been associated with the rigid plastic tail. The Birnberg bow required some skill at insertion, undergoing an acute angulation on release in the uterus before resuming its shape. This may have been responsible for some of the uterine perforations reported (Nakamoto and Buchman, 1966). The bow has two closed rings and if it perforates has been known to cause bowel strangulation.

The double spiral Saf-T-Coil was found in the Cooperative Statistical Program (Tietze and Lewit, 1970) to have a high expulsion rate and high removal rate for bleeding and pain. This may have been partly due to misplacements — if the device is allowed to expand low in the uterine cavity instead of at the fundus it can cause severe symptoms. The Saf-T-Coil and its modifications are widely used in Great Britain and the United States of America and pregnancy rates seem to be relatively low (Tattersall, 1971; Huber *et al.,* 1975; Snowden *et al.,* 1977).

Efforts to deal with the problem of spontaneous expulsion led to the introduction of two steel spring devices — the Majzlin spring (Solish and Majzlin, 1968) and the M device (Silberman *et al.,* 1969). These were intended to be 'fundus-seeking', lateral compression due to uterine contractions tending to drive the device upwards. The Majzlin spring tended to create deep grooves in the endometrium, though apparently not into the myometrium, and many difficulties were encountered in removal (Solish and Majzlin, 1969). The M device was also difficult to remove, general anaesthesia often being required. In the United Kingdom a perforation rate of 0.23% of insertions was recorded (Hawkins, 1970). This may have been partly due to problems at insertion, and partly due to the fundus-seeking property — a number of perforations have been recorded with Dalkon shields, which are inserted by a different technique but share the fundus-seeking property. Although the Majzlin spring and the M device resulted in a marked reduction in spontaneous expulsions (Solish and Majzlin, 1969; Bernard, 1972) this is of little value if it results in an increase in perforations. The latter complication is of course rare but its consequences can be lethal (Scott, 1968) and the metal spring devices have lost favour.

As information has accumulated on the properties needed for an effective device — easy insertion, large surface area, resistance to expulsion, innocuousness if perforation occurs and easy removal — large numbers of new devices have been introduced. Some idea of the great variety available can be obtained from reviews (Bluett, 1973; Drugs and Therapeutics Bulletin, 1973; Huber *et al.*, 1975; Monks, 1976). Unfortunately the ingenuity of the inventors has not been matched by significant improvement in performance characteristics. The pattern is consistent; initial enthusiasm, one or two reports of excellent results and then independent evaluation under practical working conditions with the conclusion that the new device conveys little or no advantage over existing models.

The Dalkon shield, introduced by Davis (1970), was designed to have a large surface area and was shown to provoke an endometrial leucocyte and plasma cell response (Davis and Lesinski, 1970). It had lateral fins which tended to orientate it within the uterine cavity and caused the device to be fundus-seeking in response to lateral compression by uterine contractions. The small amount of copper the device contained was shown in a controlled trial to be insufficient to affect the performance of the device (Snowden and Williams, 1974b). Initial results (Davis and Lesinski, 1970) were encouraging, with pregnancy and expulsion rates of only 1.1 and 2.3, respectively, per 100 woman-years. Subsequent independent multicentre trials demonstrated pregnancy rates within the same range as other intra-uterine devices (Snowden and Williams, 1973; Jones, Parker and Elstein, 1973; Templeton, 1973; Snowden and Williams, 1975a). Expulsion rates were quite low. Several uterine perforations were reported (Snowden and Williams, 1972, 1973; Sprague and Jenkins, 1973; Snowden, 1974a). The shield can be quite difficult to remove and general anaesthesia may be required.

The Dalkon shield possessed properties in common with many of the other new devices. It was shown to be effective in the patient who had previously expelled another device or had to have another device removed (Bluett and Hawkins, 1974) and for insertion at the time of therapeutic abortion (Rumpus, 1973; Newton *et al.*, 1974). Lippes loops sizes C and D (Andolšek, 1967; 1972; Goldsmith *et al.*, 1972), Saf-T-Coils (Cabrera, 1968), DANA devices (Koukar and Němec, 1970; Poradovský *et al.*, 1972; Huber *et al.*, 1975) and Gravigards (Newton *et al.*, 1974) have also been used after abortions, but the use of the Dalkon shield was of interest in that it is a relatively small device which lay freely within the bulky post-abortion uterine cavity. The strings often disappeared but at follow-up when the uterus had involuted it was found to be correctly placed with the strings protruding through the cervical os.

Dalkon shields were withdrawn from the market following reports from the United States of America of four fatal cases of sepsis in patients who became pregnant with the standard size device *in situ* (Christian, 1974). Although the plaited strings of the device were shown to be capable of carrying bacteria upwards by capillary action (Tatum *et al.*, 1975), the case was never proved since the smaller size shields, which had the same tails, did not convey the same risk of sepsis (Cates *et al.*, 1976). Out of 50 abortions occurring with the device *in situ* in British studies only two became septic (Snowden, 1974a).

The Wing Antigon device (Lebech *et al.*, 1971; Snowden and Williams, 1975b; Wiese, 1976) seems to share some of the properties of the Dalkon shield and is suitable for use immediately after therapeutic abortion and in patients who have previously expelled another device, though some models have the disadvantage that they are closed rings. We have also found the Combined Multiload CU-250 (Snowden, 1975b) useful if there has been a previous expulsion, though care must be taken not to tear the cervix when this device is removed.

The use of the Gravigard, or 'Copper 7', was first reported on in 1972 (*see* Orlans, 1973; Williams and Snowden, 1974). The simple form of this device facilitates use in the nullipara. As with the Copper T device (Zipper *et al.*, 1969), from the point of view of contraceptive efficacy geometrical simplicity is compensated by a winding of copper wire which exposes 200 sq. mm of metallic copper. The Gravigard has been independently evaluated in a multi-centre trial; pregnancy rates varied from 0.9 to 4.4 per 100 woman-years (*Figure 9.1*). Expulsion and complication rates recorded so far differ little from those with other devices.

It is a matter of some concern to the authors to note that several of the newer devices seem to depend for retention on what might be described as 'prongs' which are likely to embed in the uterine wall. Timonen *et al.* (1972) found the arms of 13 out of 15 T devices had embedded and of 39 T devices examined *in situ* by hysterosalpingography by Kemal *et al.* (1973), 32 were found to be lying within the uterine cavity in positions suggesting that one or both arms of the 'T' were embedded in the myometrium. It is not uncommon to find that when a Gravigard has been inserted in a nulliparous uterus, its lower extremity extends further down the cervical canal than would be so if it were lying correctly. This implies that the angle of the '7' is unduly extended and the two upper extremities are pressed against the uterine wall in a way that would encourage embedding. The Petal (Copper Lem) device depends on four shaped prongs for retention. The long-term effects of embedding of the prongs of devices of this sort in the uterine wall have yet to be ascertained.

We are similarly concerned at the possibility of damage to the uterus in the region of the internal os when some of the newer devices are removed. The M device, the Majzlin spring, the Dalkon shield, the Copper Omega and the Combined Multiload CU-250 are often difficult to remove, and it is sometimes obvious that the junction of uterine cavity and cervical canal is torn internally during the process. Again, long-term effects are as yet unknown.

It is therefore of some interest to consider two devices which are flexible. Brief preliminary reports on the 'Latex Leaf', designed by Anderson were made by Snowden (1973b) and Anderson (1974). The Leaf is a small flat leaf-shaped device made of flexible silicone rubber and impregnated with powdered copper and zinc. It was intended to be replaced every six months. Samples evaluated had minor defects — for example the strings were readily torn off. On the other hand there was a minimum of complaints of cramps or bleeding and a modified device of this type might well be acceptable to patients. Similar comments apply to the fluid-filled device described by Futoran and Kitrilakis (1974). This is a soft pliable silicon pouch which is easily inserted into the uterine cavity and subsequently filled with saline, the filling tube then being tied off. Most of the endometrial surface is then contacted by the device without mechanical insult to the tissues. Side-effects were minimal in the first trials but a subsequent report (Andolšek and Thomas, 1976) is not encouraging.

SELECTION OF PATIENTS

The intra-uterine device is not the most effective contraceptive, nor is it free from minor and occasional major complications. On the other hand, for a proportion of women it is the best available contraceptive when all factors have been considered. The selection of a contraceptive procedure requires value judgements to be made by the patient; the role of the physician should be to provide the information and such advice as is desired to enable the patient to make those judgements.

Age and Parity

With nulliparous women under the age of 20, significant problems are associated with the use of intra-uterine contraception (Snowden *et al.*, 1977). These can all be related to the small size of the uterus and its cavity, but doubtless anxiety, social circumstances and sometimes lack of motivation are also involved. Insertion may be difficult and painful; sometimes general anaesthesia may be indicated. Post-insertion pain may be considerable. Expulsion rates are very high — between 20 and 50% of young nulliparous women are likely to expel an orthodox device within a year; if it is replaced it is likely to be expelled again. Painful and heavy menstruation, intermenstrual bleeding and dyspareunia are common. Pregnancy rates are also higher than in older and parous women. This may be partly due to unnoticed expulsion, and partly to frequent intercourse and high fecundity. The risk of perforation of the uterus, either at insertion or later on, is likely to be increased.

All these problems can be somewhat reduced by selection of appropriate devices such as the Lippes loop A or B, the nulliparous Saf-T-Coil, the Gyne T (copper T) and the Gravigard device (Snowden *et al.*, 1977). The last is relatively easy to insert, but tends to lie in a narrow uterine cavity in an unduly angulated position. In general it is wise to consider alternative methods of contraception for the young nullipara, particularly if she has a small and narrow uterus, with a tight cervical canal.

As age and parity increase all the difficulties and complications steadily diminish (Tietze and Lewit, 1970; Bernard, 1970; Snowden *et al.*, 1977), and it seems likely that this is due to the greater capacity of the uterus to accommodate the device. With reduced expulsions, diminished frequency of intercourse and diminished liability to conceive, failure rates are lower in older women.

Bernard (1970) has observed in Israel that in the highly parous women, expulsion is more likely if she has a history of multiple abortions. Similarly, in a Yugoslav population, older women who have had many abortions are likely to expel a device. These relationships are probably due to incompetence of the cervix.

Finally, it should be noted that as age increases so does the proportion of collagen relative to smooth muscle in the uterus, the uterus becoming more rigid. This increases the theoretical risk of perforation in the woman over 40.

Environment

It was thought initially that intra-uterine devices would be more successful in underdeveloped than in sophisticated communities since the patients would be less worried by minor side-effects. In some environments this has proved to be the case. In others, lack of contact with physicians makes follow-up impossible, and unreported expulsions and complications such as perforation of the uterus can be hazardous. The devices have on the whole been unsuccessful in countries where cultural factors make life difficult for women who suffer from intermenstrual bleeding or menorrhagia, which are common side-effects in the first few months of use.

Contra-indications

Acute or purulent cervicitis conveys a risk of introducing bacterial infection into the uterine cavity and this may spread to involve the rest of the pelvis and peritoneal cavity; minor trauma to the uterus during insertion may facilitate spread of infection by the bloodstream. If the cause is gonorrhoea, even when it has been treated successfully, consideration should be given to the fact that an intra-uterine device conveys no protection against reinfection, whilst barrier methods of contraception may provide some defence. Trichomonal cervicitis is easily treated and of itself gives rise to no particular risk, but it may facilitate bacterial invasion from the vagina and is in some communities commonly associated with gonorrhoea. Patients with candidiasis should have the infection treated before insertion of a device, though the risk of systemic dissemination of the infection is minute provided the patient is not suffering from a chronic debilitating illness, diabetes or bronchiectasis. The presence of a device need not interfere with diagnosis of underlying conditions in patients with recurrent candidiasis. Occasionally patients are encountered in whom no underlying cause can be found, who suffer from recurrent infections until the device is removed permanently.

Virus infections of the cervix as with herpesvirus hominis type 2, cytomegalovirus, or the organism of non-specific urethritis are not known to cause endometritis but they might facilitate bacterial invasion and if these conditions are present in the cervix it would seem wise on general principles to defer insertion. A cervical smear examined cytologically can only detect a limited proportion of cases of virus cervicitis, and diagnostic culture for viruses is necessary if these conditions are suspected.

'Chronic cervicitis' with erosions, Nabothian follicles, chronic discharge and sometimes cervical and parametrial tenderness is probably best treated by cautery or cryosurgery and allowed to heal before a device is inserted. Though chronic cervicitis is usually regarded as a non-infective condition, there is little doubt that sometimes it provides a portal of entry for low-grade infection, and insertion of a device may exacerbate symptoms. Congenital or postpartum ectropions are not a firm contra-indication to insertion, though epithelialisation may be delayed with a device *in situ*; if they later become symptomatic the device may either be blamed by the patient or may have to be removed to permit treatment and healing. Some authorities (Sobrero and Goldsmith, 1973) advocate cauterisation of a simple ectropion at the time of insertion.

Active pelvic inflammatory disease is an obvious contra-indication to insertion of an intra-uterine device. What is in doubt is whether or not insertion should be undertaken at all in a woman with a history of pelvic inflammatory disease. If this is done there is certainly some risk of exacerbation, even if anti-biotic cover such as tetracycline, ampicillin or trimethoprim with cotrimoxazole and metronidazole, is given for two weeks. There is a small risk to the patient's future fertility. Four of the ten deaths associated with intra-uterine devices reported by Scott (1968) were due to post-insertion pelvic sepsis proceeding to overwhelming infection. On the other hand many thousands of women with known or unsuspected quiescent pelvic inflammatory disease have been fitted without ill consequences. The decision must be made in the light of the known history of the patient, the extent and severity of the disease, and the physical findings on examination, together with an appraisal of the patient's desire to have a device, the alternatives available to her, her life-style and her reaction to knowledge of potential complications.

The glib statement that carcinoma of the cervix or corpus of the uterus are absolute contra-indications to insertion of a device is usually pronounced. In fact, diagnosis and treatment preclude the need for contraception. The comment is presumably intended to draw attention to the need for vigilance in suspecting the presence of cancer of the uterus in women presenting for contraceptive advice. Routine cervical smears should be taken before insertion and any abnormal bleeding or physical signs require appropriate investigation and treatment. Sobrero and Goldsmith (1973) comment that it might be excusable to insert a device to prevent conception whilst suspected malignancy is investigated. This seems unreasonable and could conceivably lead to dissemination of a cancer or perforation of the uterus. Barrier methods should be advised until a diagnosis is made. There is no evidence that intra-uterine devices ever caused endometrial cancer or carcinoma *in situ* of the cervix, but we have some reservations about using potentially irritant foreign bodies in women with endometrial hyperplasia or who have had a cone biopsy for carcinoma *in situ*.

Irregular uterine bleeding and benign lesions of the cervix such as polyps merely require diagnosis and treatment before insertion of a device. On the other hand, menorrhagia of dysfunctional origin being treated medically after organic pathology has been excluded, is a reasonable contra-indication. Intra-uterine devices have a tendency to exacerbate pre-existing menorrhagia.

Caesarean section and other scars in the uterus are not contra-indications, but it must be accepted that there is a small risk of perforation of a weak scar, either at insertion or later on. The uterus of the woman who has had a Caesarean section followed by one or more vaginal deliveries is at particular risk. It follows that such patients should be advised of the risk, special care should be taken over placement using general anaesthesia if necessary, and careful follow-up instituted, the patient palpating the strings weekly and attending for examination at three-to six-monthly intervals. Fibromyomata distorting the uterine cavity not only predispose to perforation at insertion, to expulsion of the device and to menor-rhagia but also impair contraceptive efficacy. Congenital abnormalities of the uterus do not necessarily contra-indicate, provided the anatomy of the situation is known and placement is careful, but efficacy may be reduced in an arcuate uterus with a bulky cavity. Insertion of a device in one horn of a bicornuate uterus is said to exert a contraceptive effect but is unlikely to have a high degree of efficacy.

Medical Complications

It is important that patients with cardiac, renal or pulmonary disease, in whom infection might have serious consequences, be carefully appraised. Factors to be considered include the relative risks of alternative methods of contraception and of pregnancy or, in the event of an unwanted pregnancy, therapeutic abortion. The prognosis of the patient's condition for the remainder of her reproductive life must be taken into account in relation to her views on planning her future family. The situation often calls for a frank and accurate statement of a progno-sis from knowledge of which she has hitherto been protected by her medical attendants. In such circumstances consultation with her other medical atten-dants is essential in order to avoid confusion. At the same time the potential for rapid progress of medical science in some fields must be recognised and due allowance made. Ten years ago the suggestion that a single girl with a successful kidney transplant might consider marriage and parenthood would have seemed quite unreasonable and sterilisation might well have been advised. It is now well established that such patients can undertake a successful pregnancy and that their expectation of life, with the possibility of further transplants or haemo-dialysis, is indefinite. In these circumstances it is now reasonable practice to temporise with an intra-uterine device until marriage and a desire for a child ensue. The cumulative increase in the risk of pregnancy with an intra-uterine device as the years go by must also be considered, even though the annual risk diminishes each year. A 5% risk of pregnancy in the first year may be acceptable for the woman who wishes to temporise. A 15—20% risk over five years may not be acceptable for a teenage girl, especially as risks of complications cumulate concurrently.

The one general medical condition which it is reasonable to regard as an absolute contra-indication to the use of an intra-uterine device for contraception is valvular heart disease. Patients with congenital or rheumatic heart disease who are at risk for bacterial endocarditis should not be provided with an additional portal of entry for infection. There is some risk that blood-borne infection may be introduced at the time of insertion. Even if this procedure is covered by antibiotics, subsequent development of a low-grade endometritis which might be harmless to the average patient, could have serious results in those with anatomical lesions in the heart.

In general the days when *ex cathedra* advice from physicians was enough are gone. Consultation with a patient who is as fully informed as her understanding will permit is now necessary to arrive at advice which is really given 'in good faith', over such a personal matter as family planning in circumstances where health and perhaps life are involved.

Similar considerations apply to patients who have a blood dyscrasia or who are on anticoagulant therapy. There is some risk of uterine bleeding with a device, which can only really be determined by a therapeutic trial. The decision to use an intra-uterine device must be an appropriately balanced judgement made with patient involvement.

Patients with backache should not receive short-wave or microwave diathermy to the abdomen or lower back areas whilst wearing a device containing metal, or heat injury to the surrounding tissues may result. Copper devices are of course contra-indicated in patients with copper allergy or Wilson's disease.

Patients with psychiatric problems may give rise to difficulties with follow-up and the early reporting of complications. Collaboration with home-visiting medical social workers may be necessary to ensure adequate supervision. Occasionally psychiatric patients react adversely to the thought of a foreign body in their uterus. Some women are motivated, for diverse and often obscure reasons, to remove the device themselves and conceal the fact. Each case must be judged on its merits.

The best person to advise on the suitability of an intra-uterine device for a patient with a relevant medical disorder is a gynaecologist who is not a committed enthusiast for the use of the device, but who has a balanced approach to the use of all contraceptive methods.

Social and Personal Factors

It was thought at one time that the devices would solve the problem of the poorly motivated patient, in that their effectiveness would be independent of the patient's attitudes. It appeared that the all too frequent and bitterly regretted 'wilful exposure to unwanted pregnancy' (Lehfeldt, 1959) problem had been solved. In fact this has not proved to be the case. In the years 1956 to 1961, study of a series of 16 psychiatric patients with Gräfenberg rings showed that within two years all had contrived to have them removed, mainly on the basis of minor and perhaps exaggerated side-effects (Hawkins and Nixon, unpublished observations). Well balanced women commonly express an underlying desire for pregnancy, however inconvenient this may be, as intolerance in the form of discomfort, irregular or heavy bleeding, vaginal discharge, dyspareunia and anxiety about possible ill consequences, including cancer. These reactions often start at or shortly after insertion, but sometimes occur later on with the realisation that the device is proving effective. Not uncommonly, such women attend a doctor other than the physician who inserted the device, either requesting removal or presenting symptoms of a severity which justify removal. Another expression of poor motivation is concealment of expulsion — either the patient is not sure whether or not the device has been expelled or it is inconvenient for her to be seen at once, and she becomes pregnant in the interim. The power of these mechanisms is such that the physician must not necessarily anticipate being any more successful with intra-uterine devices than with other contraceptive procedures when dealing with poorly motivated patients. He may encounter reflections of the husband's lack of family planning motivation. Patients often return for removal with the comment that 'their husband does not approve' or complaints that he finds the strings irritant during intercourse. Some account of the husband's feelings about the matter should be obtained before a device is fitted.

An intra-uterine device may not be the ideal contraceptive method for the patient whose sexual activity is unconventional. It conveys no protection against gonorrhoea, and it is quite likely that the risk of pregnancy is greater with frequent intercourse.

Ethical and Legal Considerations

Intra-uterine devices are not the only contraceptive method and in general the choice should be that best suited to the needs of the patient since it is commonly conditioned by personal rather than medical circumstances. It is important that patients for whom insertion is considered should appreciate the possibilities of other contraceptive procedures. This understanding is best achieved in a clinic where advice on other techniques is freely available. If a clinic is solely devoted to the use of intra-uterine devices, then preliminary counselling on choice of method should be conducted before the patient's appointment is booked.

Intra-uterine contraception places the physician in a position of greater personal responsibility than other methods of family planning. With barrier procedures, after appropriate instruction the onus of performance is on the patient. Even with oral contraceptives, it is up to the patient to take the pills as directed. In contrast, an intra-uterine device is inserted by a physician, and usually stays in place regardless of the patient's feelings and activities, until it is removed by a physician. It therefore behoves the doctor to pay considerable attention to ethical and legal considerations and the adequacy of consent procedures for intra-uterine contraceptives. Insertion of an intra-uterine device should be regarded as a minor operative procedure, requiring the informed consent of the patient. It is desirable that this be given in writing, signed and witnessed, and should include a statement that the purpose of the procedure and its possible complications have been understood. In this litigious age, it is best to include a statement that the patient understands that, as with other contraceptive procedures, there is a small risk of failure and that, rarely, pregnancy can occur with a device *in situ*. In countries with abortion laws such as those in Great Britain, it is important to make it clear that contraceptive failure *per se* does not constitute grounds for therapeutic abortion. Even in environments where abortion is available on demand, the physician may feel it necessary to establish that he personally would be under no obligation to terminate an unwanted pregnancy.

The discussion of these matters with the patient is far more important than a signature on a consent form. The latter has little legal weight unless the meaning has been fully explained to the patient and her understanding ascertained.

It is commonly stated that consent of the patient's consort should also be obtained. This requirement is often unrealistic. Many husbands are reluctant to spare the time to attend a clinic with their wife for a full discussion and those who will not come may represent the group of couples where the wife is most in need of contraception. The physician would do well to ascertain the legal position in his own country. In Great Britain a woman can consent to insertion of a device in her own right, but she still takes the risk of marital disharmony if her husband does not agree, and the matter could possibly be used against her in divorce proceedings. The fact that he has acted 'in good faith' in his patient's interest provides adequate defence for the physician inserting the device. The most practical solution is then to secure from the patient the statement that either she has discussed the problem with her consort and he agrees to the insertion or that she understands the possible marital consequences of having a device without his consent. At the other extreme, there are still countries where a wife may be the property of her husband, culturally and legally. In such an environment the husband's direct consent to insertion of a device should always be obtained, however the physician personally feels about the morality of the situation.

It is generally accepted that minors — the age limit in a community is usually defined — are not competent to give consent to operative procedures on themselves except in emergency situations. In Great Britain, it is unwise to insert a device in a girl under 16 years of age without the consent of both parents and the patient, especially as pain, menstrual disturbance and expulsion are quite likely to occur in this group of patients. Some practitioners feel that it is ethical to give contraceptive advice to young teenagers without their parent's knowledge, but they would be ill-advised to use an operative procedure with known complications. Even with the parent's knowledge and consent there is still the question of encouraging illegal intercourse under 16 years of age, but in Great Britain the police usually decline to prosecute in such cases if the girl has reached the age of 14. The physician must sometimes make his own ethical decision, giving priority to the interests of his patient.

It is obviously unethical to insert a device without the patient's previous consent, given with the understanding that the device will prevent conception. Sometimes it may seem to be in the interests of the patient or her environment to provide effective contraception without their understanding of the procedure. Nonetheless, it is unethical to put a device in a mentally incompetent person or one who is incapable of understanding its significance because of cultural background or lack of education.

It is now generally accepted that closed-ring devices convey some additional hazard of bowel strangulation in the rare event of their perforating the uterus. If such a device is employed, it would seem reasonable to inform the patients of the reason why, and of the slight additional risk.

When a device is inserted the patient's permission to inform her family medical practitioner should be obtained, and he should be told the nature of the device used. Sometimes the patient prefers that her own doctor should not be informed. If it is agreed to take on a patient on those terms, then the responsibility to provide 24 hour a day cover in the event of complications must also be accepted. This is easier to do in hospital practice than in an isolated clinic.

The most important specific functions of follow-up visits are to check that the device has not been expelled unnoticed, to verify that it has not perforated the uterus, and to determine that the patient has not developed pelvic inflammatory disease. The extent of responsibility for patients who default from their follow-up appointments is ill-defined. The assumption that failure to attend is always the patient's fault is not always valid — failure to emphasise the importance of periodical review or administrative errors may well be responsible. Patients who do not attend should therefore be sent a reminder. If they do not reply it should suffice to notify their family practitioner that they are wearing a device but no longer attending the clinic.

Some of the pregnancies which occur are due to unnoticed expulsion, or occasionally perforation of the uterus by the device. Should conception occur with a device *in situ*, abortion occurs spontaneously in 40–60% (Lewit, 1970; Alvior, 1973; Snowden, 1974b; Vessey *et al.*, 1974). In the remainder the pregnancy continues normally and there is no evidence of increased fetal abnormality or perinatal mortality. With Lippes loops then extraction of the device during the first trimester is compatible with continuation of the pregnancy (Alvior, 1973). With some other devices it is clear that a general policy of removal during pregnancy increases the abortion rate. The differences are probably due to some devices tending to be pushed down into the lower part of the cavity, whence they are easily recoverable without disturbing the conceptus, whilst 'fundal-seeking' and 'tail-less' devices tend to stay high in the uterus and become entangled in the conceptus. Abortion at the time a device is removed during pregnancy, or within a day or two, is not uncommon and the patient may then interpret the procedure as termination of pregnancy unless the reason why the physician advises removal is fully explained in advance.

Finally, we have encountered patients who have had occasion to resent the fact that they were not informed that intra-uterine devices do not prevent the acquisition of venereal disease. Women suspected to have unconventional sexual proclivities should be advised that the devices convey no protection against infection. In communities where venereal disease is rife, all patients should be so warned.

REFERENCES

ALVIOR, G.T. (1973). Pregnancy outcome with removal of intrauterine device. *Obstet. Gynec., N.Y.*, **41**, 894–896

AMERICAN MEDICAL ASSOCIATION COMMITTEE ON CONTRACEPTIVE PRACTICES (1937). Dangers of Gomco intra-uterine silver ring. *J. Am. med. Ass.*, **108**, 413

ANDERSON, I. (1974). The leaf IUD. In *Intrauterine Devices. Development, Evaluation and Program Implementation*, pp. 199–202. Ed. Wheeler, R.G., Duncan, G.W. and Speidel, J.J. Academic Press, New York, San Francisco, London

ANDOLŠEK, L. (1967). Insertion of IUDs after abortion – preliminary report. *Proceedings of the Eighth International Conference of the International Planned Parenthood Federation, Santiago, Chile, 9–15 April 1967*, pp. 285–289. Ed. Hankinson, R.K.B., Kleineman, R.L. and Eckstein, P. Austin, Hertford

ANDOLŠEK, L. (1972). Experience with immediate post-abortion insertions of the IUD. *Family Planning Research Conference: a Multidisciplinary Approach; held at the University of Exeter, Exeter England. September 27–28, 1971. Excerpta Medica International Congress Series No. 260*, pp. 55–58. Ed. Goldsmith, A. and Snowden, R. Excerpta Medica, Amsterdam

ANDOLŠEK, L. and THOMAS, M. (1976). Use of the fluid-filled Tecna device in Ljubljana, Yugoslavia. *Contraception*, **14**, 435–445

ANSBACHER, R. and CAMPBELL, C. (1971). Cervical mucus sperm penetration in women on oral contraception or with an IUD *in situ*. *Contraception, 3*, 209–217

BARON, D.A. and ESTERLY, J.R. (1972). Lysosomal hydrolases in exudates stimulated by an intrauterine device. *J. reprod. Med., 9*, 27–31

BENGTSSON, L.P. and MOAWAD, A.H. (1967). The effect of the Lippes loop on human myometrial activity. *Am. J. Obstet. Gynec., 98*, 957–965

BERNARD, R.P. (1969a). *IUD Performance Patterns. January 1969. Tables and Charts Prepared for Investigators*. Pathfinder Fund, Boston

BERNARD, R.P. (1969b). *IUD Performance Patterns. Geographic Series No. 1, October 1969. Tables and Charts and Comments Prepared for Investigators. The Yugoslavia Multi-Clinic IUD Trial*. Pathfinder Fund, Boston

BERNARD, R.P. (1970). IUD Performance patterns – a 1970 world view. *J. Int. Fed. Gynecol. Obstet., 8*, 926–940

BERNARD, R.P. (1972). The 'M'–IUD: an international clinical trial. *Am. J. publ. Hlth, 62*, 828–845

BLATCHLEY, F.R., DONOVAN, B.T., HORTON, E.W. and POYSER, N.L. (1972). The release of prostaglandins and progestin into the utero-ovarian venous blood of guinea-pigs during the oestrous cycle and following oestrogen treatment. *J. Physiol., Lond., 223*, 69–88

BLUETT, D. (1973). Clinical experiences with the Dalkon shield including the insertion of the Dalkon shield in chronic expellers of other devices. In *Dalkon Shield Symposium, London, October 11th 1972*, pp. 21–26. Ed. Templeton, J.S. A.H. Robins, Horsham, Sussex

BLUETT, D.G. and HAWKINS, D.F. (1974). The use of the Dalkon shield among users with previous unsuccessful experience with other IUDs. *See* Snowden, R. and Williams, M. (1974). *Family Planning Research Unit Report No. 12*, pp. 11–19. University of Exeter

BRENNER, P.F. and MISHELL, D.R., Jr. (1975). Progesterone and oestradiol patterns in women using an intrauterine contraceptive device. *Obstet. Gynec., N.Y., 46*, 456–459

BYGDEMAN, M., FREDRICSSON, B., SVANBORG, K. and SAMUELSSON, B. (1970). The relation between fertility and prostaglandin content of seminal fluid in man. *Fert. Steril., 21*, 622–629

CABRERA, R. (1968). Aplicacion postaborto del D.I.U. Saf-T-Coil 33s. *Rev. Chil. Obstet. Ginec., 33*, 215–220

CATES, W., Jr., ORY, H.W., ROCHAT, R.W. and TYLER, C.W., Jr. (1976). The intra-uterine device and deaths from spontaneous abortion. *New Engl. J. Med., 295*, 1155–1159

CHATTOPADHYAY, S.K., AHUJA, J.M. and KHANNA, S.D. (1976). Effect of copper ionisation of the cervix on sperm migration. *Contraception, 14*, 331–341

CHAUDHURI, G. (1971). Intrauterine device: possible role of prostaglandins. *Lancet, i*, 480

CHAUDHURI, G. (1973). Release of prostaglandins by the I.U.C.D. *Prostaglandins, 3*, 773–784

CHRISTIAN, C.D. (1974). Maternal deaths associated with an intrauterine device. *Am. J. Obstet. Gynec., 119*, 441–444

COUTINHO, E.M. (1971). Intrauterine devices and their mechanism of action. Discussion. *Nobel Symposium 15. Control of Fertility*, pp. 194–195. Ed.

Diczfalusy, E. and Borell, U. Wiley, New York, London Sydney: Almqvist and Wiksell, Stockholm

DASGUPTA, P.R., KAR, A.B. and ENGINEER, A.D. (1971). Uric acid in the uterine fluid of women fitted with Lippes loop and in deposits found on used devices. *Am. J. Obstet. Gynec.,* **110**, 593–594

DAUNTER, B. (1976). The scanning electronmicroscopy of human cervical mucus in the non-pregnant and pregnant states. *Br. J. Obstet. Gynec.,* **83**, 738–743

DAVIS, H.J. (1970). The shield intrauterine device. A superior modern contraceptive. *Am. J. Obstet. Gynec.,* **106**, 455–456

DAVIS, H.J. and LESINSKI, J. (1970). Mechanism of action of intrauterine contraceptives in women. *Obstet. Gynec., N.Y.,* **36**, 350–358

DONOVAN, B.T. (1975). Indomethacin, ketoprofen and corpus luteum regression in the guinea-pig. *Br. J. Pharmac.,* **53**, 225–227

DRUG AND THERAPEUTICS BULLETIN (1973). Intrauterine contraceptive devices. Volume 11, number 17, pp. 65–68.

ECKSTEIN, P. (1970). Mechanisms of action of intrauterine contraceptive devices in women and other mammals. *Br. med. Bull.,* **26**, 52–59

ENGINEER, A.D., DASGUPTA, P.R. and KAR, A.B. (1970). Chemical composition of the deposit formed on the Lippes loop after prolonged use. *Am. J. Obstet. Gynec.,* **106**, 315–316

ERB, H. and OBOLENSKY, W. (1972). Effect of intrauterine devices on the tube motility of women. *Acta europaea fertil.,* **3**, 109–117

FORDER, J.V.H. (1974). Intrauterine device, prostaglandins and copper. *Lancet,* **ii**, 1009

FUTORAN, J.M. and KITRILAKIS, S. (1974). Experience with a fluid-filled intra-uterine device. *Obstet. Gynec., N.Y.,* **43**, 81

GOLDSMITH, A., GOLDBERG, R., EYZAGUIRRE, H., LUCERO, S. and LIZANA, L. (1972). IUD insertion in the immediate postabortal period. *Proceedings of the Family Planning Research Conference, a Multidisciplinary Approach, Exeter, England, September 27–28, 1971. Excerpta Medica International Congress Series No. 260,* pp. 59–67. Ed. Goldsmith, A. and Snowden, R. Excerpta Medica, Amsterdam

GRÄFENBERG, E. (1931). An intrauterine contraceptive method. *The Practice of Contraception. An International Symposium and Survey,* pp. 33–56. Ed. Sanger, M. and Stone, H.M. Williams and Wilkins, Baltimore

HAGENFELDT, K. (1972a). Intrauterine contraception with the copper-T device. 4. Influence on protein and copper concentrations and enzyme activities in uterine washings. *Contraception,* **6**, 219–230

HAGENFELDT, K. (1972b). Intrauterine contraception with the copper-T device. 1. Effects on trace elements in the endometrium, cervical mucus and plasma. *Contraception,* **6**, 37–54

HAGENFELDT, K. (1973). *Bibliography on Copper IUDs.* Reproduction Research Information Service, Cambridge

HALL, H.H. and STONE, M.L. (1962). Observations on the use of intrauterine pessary, with special reference to the Gräfenberg rings. *Am. J. Obstet. Gynec.,* **83**, 683–688

HAWKINS, D.F. (1968). Relevance of prostaglandins to problems of human subfertility. *Prostaglandin Symposium of the Worcester Foundation for*

Experimental Biology, October 16–17, 1967, pp. 1–7. Ed. Ramwell, P.W. and Shaw, J.E. Interscience, New York

HAWKINS, D.F. (1969). Complications with IUDs. *Br. med. J.,* **ii**, 381

HAWKINS, D.F. (1970). *Perforation of the uterus by M-213 devices in Great Britain. Report to the Medical Advisory Committee.* Pathfinder Fund, Boston

HAWKINS, D.F. (1973). On-going studies with the Dalkon shield in special situations. *Dalkon Shield Symposium. London, October 11th 1972*, pp. 14–16. Ed. Templeton, J.S. A.H. Robins, Horsham, Sussex

HAWKINS, D.F. and BENSTER, B. (1977). A comparative study of three progestagens (chlormadinone acetate, 0.5 mg; megestrol acetate 0.5 mg in oil; norethisterone, 0.35 mg) used as oral contraceptives. *Br. J. Obstet. Gynaec.,* **84**, 708–713

HAWKINS, D.F. and LABRUM, A.H. (1961). Semen prostaglandin levels in fifty patients attending a fertility clinic. *J. Reprod. Fert.,* **2**, 1–10

HILL, A.M. (1969). Contraception with the Gräfenberg ring. A review of 33 years' experience. *Am. J. Obstet. Gynec.,* **103**, 200–212

HOUNSELL, P.G. and HAWKINS, D.F. (1974). Effect of copper on growth of human cervical epithelial cells in tissue culture. *J. Obstet. Gynaec. Br. Commonw.,* **81**, 712–718

HOWARD, G. (1971). The significance of calcium deposits occurring on intrauterine devices. *J. Obstet. Gynaec. Br. Commonw.,* **78**, 861–862

HSU, C., FERENCZY, A., RICHART, R.M. and DARABI, K. (1976). Endometrial morphology with copper-bearing intrauterine devices. *Contraception,* **14**, 243–260

HUBER, S.C., PIOTROW, P.T., ORLANS, B. and KOMMER, G. (1975). IUDs reassessed – a decade of experience. *Population Reports,* series B, number 2, 21–48

INMAN, W.H.W. and VESSEY, M.P. (1968). Investigation of deaths from pulmonary, coronary and cerebral thrombosis and embolism in women of child-bearing age. *Br. med. J.,* **ii**, 193–199

ISHIHAMA, A. (1959). Clinical studies on intrauterine rings, especially the present state of contraception in Japan and the experiences in the use of intrauterine rings. *Yokohama med. Bull.,* **10**, 89–105

ISHIHAMA, A., NISHIJIMA, M. and WADA, H. (1970). Bacteriological study on the users of intrauterine contraceptive devices. *Acta obstet. gynaec. jap.,* **17**, 77–80

ISRAEL, R. and DAVIS, H.J. (1966). Effect of intrauterine contraceptive devices on the endometrium. *J. Am. med. Ass.,* **195**, 764–768

JACKSON, M.C.N. (1962). The Gräfenberg silver ring in a series of patients who had failed with other methods. *Intrauterine Contraceptive Devices. Proceedings of the Conference April 30–May 1, 1962, New York City. Excerpta Medica International Congress Series No. 54*, pp. 37–40. Ed. Tietze, C. and Lewit, S. Excerpta Medica, Amsterdam

JAIN, A.K. and SIVIN, I. (1977). Life-table analysis of IUDs: problems and recommendations. *Stud. Fam. Plann.,* **8**, 25–47

JECHT, E.W. and BERNSTEIN, G.S. (1973). The influence of copper on the motility of human spermatozoa. *Contraception,* **7**, 381–401

JOHANNSSON, E. (1973). Recent developments with intrauterine devices. *Contraception,* **8**, 99–112

JONES, R.W., GREGSON, N.M. and ELSTEIN, M. (1973). Effect of copper-containing intrauterine contraceptive devices on human cells in culture. *Br. med. J.,* **ii**, 520–523

JONES, R.W., PARKER, A. and ELSTEIN, M. (1973). Clinical experience with the Dalkon shield intrauterine device. *Br. med. J.,* **iii**, 143–145

JOSHI, S.G. and SUJAN-TEJUJA, S. (1969). Biochemistry of the human endometrium in users of the intrauterine contraceptive device. *Fert. Steril.,* **20**, 98–110

KAR, A.B., ENGINEER, A.D., GOEL, R., KAMBOJ, V.P., DASGUPTA, P.R. and CHOWDHURY, S.R. (1968). Effect of an intrauterine contraceptive device on biochemical composition of uterine fluid. *Am. J. Obstet. Gynec.,* **101**, 966–970

KEMAL, I., GHONEIM, M., TALAAT, M. and MALLAWANI, A. (1973). The anchoring mechanisms of retention of the copper-T device. *Fert. Steril.,* **24**, 165–169

KOUKAR, J. and NĚMEC, M. (1970). Insertion of IUD after termination of pregnancy. *Čslká Gynek.,* **35**, 465–467

LANDESMAN, R., COUTINHO, E.M. and SAXENA, B.B. (1976). Detection of human chorionic gonadotropin in blood of regularly bleeding women using copper intrauterine contraceptive devices. *Fert. Steril.,* **27**, 1062–1066

LAUFE, L.E., GIBAR, Y., McCLANAHAN, B.J. and WHEELER, R.F. (1974). Volume and copper concentration of menstrual discharge from women employing Copper-7 and other types of contraceptives. *Adv. planned Parenthood,* **9**, 38–42

LEBECH, P.E., ANDERSON, E.S., BERGGREEN, K. and NEUMANN, E. (1971). Intrauterine contraception with a new Antigon model, and investigation of the mechanism of action of intrauterine devices. *Dan. med. Bull.,* **18**, 146–151

LEHFELDT, H. (1959). Wilful exposure to unwanted pregnancy (WEUP). Psychological explanation for patient failures in contraception. *Am. J. Obstet. Gynec.,* **78**, 661–665

LEWIT, S. (1970). Outcome of pregnancy with intrauterine devices. *Contraception,* **2**, 47–57

LIPPES, J. (1962). A study of intrauterine contraception: development of a plastic loop. *Intrauterine Contraceptive Devices. Proceedings of the Conference, April 30–May 1, 1962, New York City. Excerpta Medica International Congress Series No. 54,* pp. 69–75. Ed. Tietze, C. and Lewit, S. Excerpta Medica, Amsterdam

LOEWIT, K. (1971). Immobilization of human spermatozoa with iron. Basis for a new contraceptive? *Contraception,* **3**, 219–224

MAKHLOUF, A.M. and ABDEL-SALAM, A.F. (1970). Kymographic studies of the fallopian tubes after insertion of intrauterine contraceptive devices using the Lippes loop and the nylon ring. *Am. J. Obstet. Gynec.,* **106**, 759–764

MANN, E.C. (1962). Cineradiographic observations on intra-uterine contraceptive devices. *Intra-uterine Contraceptive Devices. Proceedings of the Conference, April 30–May 1, 1962, New York City. Excerpta Medica International Congress Series No. 54,* pp. 91–103. Ed. Tietze, C. and Lewit, S. Excerpta Medica, Amsterdam

MARLEY, P.B. and SMITH, C.C. (1974). The source and a possible function in fertility of seminal prostaglandin-like material, in the mouse. *Br. J. Pharmac.,* **52**, 114P

MASTROIANNI, L. and ROSSEAU, C.H. (1965). Influence of the intrauterine coil on ovum transport and sperm distribution in the monkey. *Am. J. Obstet. Gynec.*, **93**, 416–420

MEEKER, C.I. (1969). Use of drugs and intrauterine devices for birth control. *New Engl. J. Med.*, **280**, 1058–1060

MILLER, J.F., SNOWDEN, R., LOUGHRAN, J.T. and ELSTEIN, M. (1975). Comparison of use of the Dalkon shield in Dublin and Southampton. *Br. med. J.*, **ii**, 599–601

MISHELL, D.R., BELL, J.H., GOOD, R.G. and MOYER, D.L. (1966). The intrauterine device: a bacteriological study of the endometrial cavity. *Am. J. Obstet. Gynec.*, **96**, 119–126

MOAWAD, A.H. and BENGTSSON, L.P. (1970). The long-term effect of Lippes loop on the *in vivo* motility patterns of the non-pregnant human uterus. *Acta obstet. gynec. scand.*, **49**, supplement 6, 31–34

MOIGNARD, J. (1973). The importance of high continuation rates and of good physician/patient rapport in IUD practice. *Dalkon Shield Symposium, London, October 11th, 1972*, pp. 4–7. Ed. Templeton, J.S. A.H. Robins, Horsham, Sussex

MONKS, I. (1976). The current state of IUCDs. *J. mat. Child Hlth*, August, 10–15

MORGENSTERN, L.L., ORGEBIN-CRIST, M.-C., CLEWE, T.H., BONNEY, W.A. and NOYES, R.W. (1966). Observations on spermatozoa in the human uterus and oviducts in the chronic presence of intrauterine devices. *Am. J. Obstet. Gynec.*, **96**, 114–118

MYATT, L., CHAUDHURI, G., GORDON, D. and ELDER, M.G. (1977). Prostaglandin production by leucocytes attached to intrauterine devices. *Contraception*, **15**, 589–599

NAKAMOTO, M. and BUCHMAN, M.I. (1966). Complications of intrauterine contraceptive devices. Report of 5 cases of ectopic placement of the bow. *Am. J. Obstet. Gynec.*, **94**, 1073–1078

NEWTON, J., ELIAS, J. and JOHNSON, A. (1974). Immediate post-termination insertion of Copper 7 and Dalkon shield intrauterine contraceptive devices. *J. Obstet. Gynaec. Br. Commonw.*, **81**, 389–392

NYGREN, K.-G. and JOHANSSON, E.D.B. (1973). Premature onset of menstrual bleeding during ovulatory cycles in women with an intrauterine contraceptive device. *Am. J. Obstet. Gynec.*, **117**, 971–975

NOYES, R.W., CLEWE, T.H., BONNEY, W.A., BURRUS, S.B., DE FEO, V.J. and MORGENSTERN, L.L. (1966). Searches for ova in the human uterus and tubes. I. Review, clinical methodology and summary of findings. *Am. J. Obstet. Gynec.*, **96**, 157–167

OBER, W.B., SOBRERO, A.J. and CHABON, A.B. (1970). Endometrial findings after insertion of stainless steel spring IUD. *Obstet. Gynec., N.Y.*, **36**, 62–68

OKEREKE, T., STERNLIEB, I., MORELL, A.G. and SCHEINBERG, I.H. (1972). Systemic absorption of intrauterine copper. *Science, N.Y.*, **177**, 358–360

OPPENHEIMER, W. (1959). Prevention of pregnancy by the Gräfenberg ring method. A re-evaluation after 28 years' experience. *Am. J. Obstet. Gynec.*, **78**, 446–454

ORLANS, F.B. (1973). Intrauterine devices. Copper IUDs; performance to date. *Population Reports*, series B, number 1, 1–20

OSTER, G.K. (1972). Chemical reactions of the copper intrauterine device. *Fert. Steril.*, **23**, 18–23

OSTER, G.K. and SALGO, M.P. (1975). The copper intrauterine device and its mode of action. *New Engl. J. Med.*, **293**, 432–438

PATHFINDER FUND (1969). *International IUD Program. 1-year baseline. January 1969*. Pathfinder Fund, Boston

PEARL, R. (1932). Contraception and fertility in 2000 women. *Hum. Biol.*, **4**, 363–407

PERLMUTTER, J.F. (1974). Experience with the Dalkon shield as a contraceptive device. *Obstet. Gynec., N.Y.*, **43**, 443–446

PLACE, V.A. and PHARRISS, B.B. (1974). Progress in the development of the Progestasert TM 65 progesterone therapeutic system for contraception. *J. reprod. Med.*, **13**, 66–68

PORADOVSKÝ, K., MÉSZÁROSOVÁ, A. and HOLLER, J. (1972). Experience with intra-uterine contraceptive devices, type DANA, inserted immediately following termination of pregnancy. *Čslká Gynek.*, **37**, 497–499

POTTER, R.G., Jr. (1966). Application of life table techniques to measurement of contraceptive effectiveness. *Demography*, **3**, 297–304

POTTER, R.G. (1969). Use-effectiveness of intrauterine contraception as a problem in competing risks. In *Family Planning in Taiwan. An Experiment in Social Change*, pp. 458–484. Ed. Freedman, R. and Takeshita, J.Y. Princeton University Press, Princeton, New Jersey

POTTER, R.G., Jr., CHOW, L.P., JAIN, A.H. and LEE, C.H. (1969). Effectiveness of intrauterine contraception: termination levels and correlates. *Ibid*, Chapter 10, pp. 241–279

POTTS, M. and PEARSON, R.M. (1967). A light and electron microscope study of cells in contact with intrauterine contraceptive devices. *J. Obstet. Gynaec. Br. Commonw.*, **74**, 129–136

POYSER, N.L., HORTON, E.W., THOMPSON, C.J. and LOS, M. (1970). Identification of prostaglandin $F_{2\alpha}$ released by distension of the guinea-pig uterus, *in vitro*. *J. Endocr.*, **48**, xliii

POYSER, N.L., HORTON, E.W., THOMPSON, C.J. and LOS, M. (1971). Identification of prostaglandin $F_{2\alpha}$ released by distension of the guinea-pig uterus, *in vitro*. *Nature, Lond.*, **230**, 526–528

RAMKISSOON-CHEN, R. and KONG TA-KO. (1966). Extrauterine pregnancy and intrauterine devices. *Br. med. J.*, **i**, 1297

ROZIN, S., SCHWARTZ, A. and SCHENKER, J.G. (1969). The mode of action of an intrauterine contraceptive device. *Int. J. Fert.*, **14**, 174–179

RUMPUS, M.F. (1973). The insertion of the Dalkon shield at pregnancy termination. *Dalkon Shield Symposium. London, October 11th 1972*, pp. 16–18. Ed. Templeton, J.S. A.H. Robins, Horsham, Sussex

SAĞIROĞLU, N. (1971). Phagocytosis of spermatozoa in the uterine cavity of women using intrauterine devices. *Int. J. Fert.*, **16**, 1–14

SAĞIROĞLU, N. and SAĞIROĞLU, E. (1970). Biological mode of action of the Lippes loop in intrauterine contraception. *Am. J. Obstet. Gynec.*, **106**, 506–515

SCOMMEGNA, A., AVILA, T., LUNA, M., RAO, R. and DMOWSKI, W.P. (1974). Fertility control by intrauterine release of progesterone. *Obstet. Gynec., N.Y.*, **43**, 769–779

SCOTT, R.B. (1968). Critical illnesses and deaths associated with intrauterine devices. *Obstet. Gynec., N.Y.*, **31**, 322–327

SEGAL, S.J., SOUTHAM, A.L. and SHAFER, K.D. (1965). Editors, *Intrauterine*

Contraception. Proceedings of the Second International Conference October 2–3, 1964, New York City. Excerpta Medica International Congress Series No. 86. Excerpta Medica, Amsterdam

SILBERMAN, E., STONE, M.L. and CONNELL, E.B. (1969). The "M", a new intra-uterine contraceptive device. *Am. J. Obstet. Gynec.,* **105**, 279–281

SIMS, A.C.P. (1973). Importance of a high tracing-rate in long-term medical follow-up studies. *Lancet,* **ii**, 433–435

SNOWDEN, R. (1972). Social and personal factors involved in the use effective-ness of the IUD. *Proceedings of the Family Planning Research Conference, a Multidisciplinary Approach. Exeter, England, September 27–28, 1971. International Congress Series No. 260,* pp. 74–81. Ed. Goldsmith, A. and Snowden, R. Excerpta Medica, Amsterdam

SNOWDEN, R. (1973a). Social factors in the use-effectiveness of the Dalkon shield and other intra-uterine devices. *Dalkon Shield Symposium. London, October 11th 1972,* pp. 7–10. Ed. Templeton, J.S. A.H. Robins, Horsham, Sussex

SNOWDEN, R. (1973b). Preliminary assessment of the Latex Leaf. *Family Planning Research Unit Reports, No. 5.* University of Exeter

SNOWDEN, R. (1974a). Pelvic inflammation, perforation and pregnancy out-come associated with the use of IUDs. *Family Planning Research Unit Report No. 15.* University of Exeter

SNOWDEN, R. (1974b). An enquiry into ectopic pregnancy and the intrauterine device. *Family Planning Research Unit Report No. 11,* pp. 1–14. University of Exeter

SNOWDEN, R. (1975a). Recent studies in intrauterine devices: a reappraisal. *J. biosoc. Sci.,* **7**, 367–375

SNOWDEN, R. (1975b). Preliminary assessment of the Combined Multiload CU-250 intrauterine device. *Family Planning Research Unit Report No. 18* University of Exeter

SNOWDEN, R. (1976). IUD and congenital malformations. *Br. med. J.,* **i**, 770

SNOWDEN, R. (1977). The Progestasert and ectopic pregnancy. *Br. med. J.,* **ii**, 1600–1601

SNOWDEN, R., ECKSTEIN, P. and HAWKINS, D. (1973). Social and medical factors in the use and effectiveness of IUDs. *J. biosoc. Sci.,* **5**, 31–49

SNOWDEN, R. and WILLIAMS, M. (1972). The Dalkon shield. *Family Planning Research Unit Report No. 2.* University of Exeter

SNOWDEN, R. and WILLIAMS, M. (1973). The use-effectiveness of the Dalkon shield in the United Kingdom. *Contraception,* **7**, 91–104

SNOWDEN, R. and WILLIAMS, M. (1974a). The United Kingdom field trial of the Dalkon shield (second report). *Family Planning Research Unit Report No. 7* University of Exeter

SNOWDEN, R. and WILLIAMS, M. (1974b). Two Dalkon shield studies. Copper versus non-copper. Previous IUD expulsion or removal. *Family Planning Research Unit Report No. 12,* pp. 2–10. University of Exeter

SNOWDEN, R. and WILLIAMS, M. (1975a). The United Kingdom Dalkon shield trial: two years of observations. *Contraception,* **11**, 1–13

SNOWDEN, R. and WILLIAMS, M. (1975b). The United Kingdom field and clinical trials of the Antigon device. *Family Planning Research Unit Report No. 17,* pp. 1–38. University of Exeter

SNOWDEN, R., WILLIAMS, M. and HAWKINS, D. (1977). *The IUD. A Practical Guide.* Croom Helm, London

SOBRERO, A.J. and GOLDSMITH, A. (1973). *Intrauterine devices. A Manual for Clinical Practice*, Ed. Cosby, M.L. Pathfinder Fund, Boston

SOLISH, G.I. and MAJZLIN, G. (1968). New stainless steel spring for intrauterine contraception. *Obstet. Gynec., N.Y.*, **32**, 116–119

SOLISH, G.I. and MAJZLIN, G. (1969). The Majzlin spring-study of over 1500 insertions. *Advances in Planned Parenthood – V. Proceedings of the Seventh Annual Meeting of the American Association of Planned Parenthood Physicians. Excerpta Medica International Congress Series No. 207*, pp. 117–122. Ed. Sobrero, A.J. and Lewit, S. Excerpta Medica, Amsterdam

SPRAGUE, A.D. and JENKINS, VAN R. II (1973). Perforation of the uterus with a shield intrauterine device. *Obstet. Gynec., N.Y.*, **41**, 80–82

TATTERSALL, J.M. (1971). A comparison of the Lippes loop C and the Saf-T-Coil over four years in an FPA clinic. *FPA Medical Newsletter*, number 39, September

TATUM, H.J. (1972). Intrauterine contraception. *Am. J. Obstet. Gynec.*, **112**, 1000–1023

TATUM, H.J. (1973). Metallic copper as an intrauterine contraceptive agent. *Am. J. Obstet. Gynec.*, **117**, 602–618

TATUM, H.J. and LIPPES, J. (1975). In "Fellows succeed in IUD work". *ACOG Newsletter*, **19**, number 11, p. 6

TATUM, H.J. and SCHMIDT, F.H. (1977). Contraceptive and sterilization practices and extrauterine pregnancy: a realistic perspective. *Fert. Steril.*, **28**, 407–421

TATUM, H.J., SCHMIDT, F.H., PHILLIPS, D., McCARTY, M. and O'LEARY, W.M. (1975). The Dalkon shield controversy. Structural and bacteriological studies of IUD tails. *J. Am. med. Ass.*, **231**, 711–717

TEMPLETON, J.S. (1973). Editor. *Dalkon Shield Symposium. London, October 11th 1972.* A.H. Robins, Horsham, Sussex

TIETZE, C. (1962). Intrauterine contraceptive rings: history and statistical appraisal. *Intrauterine Contraceptive Devices. Proceedings of the Conference, April 30–May 1, 1962, New York City. Excerpta Medica International Congress Series No. 54*, pp. 9–20. Ed. Tietze, C. and Lewit, A. Excerpta Medica, Amsterdam

TIETZE, C. (1966). Contraception with intrauterine devices, 1959–1966. *Am. J. Obstet. Gynec.*, **96**, 1043–1054

TIETZE, C. (1967). Intrauterine contraception: recommended procedures for data analysis. *Stud. Fam. Plann.*, **18**, supplement, 1–6

TIETZE, C. and LEWIT, S. (1962). Editors. *Intrauterine Contraceptive Devices. Proceedings of the Conference, April 30–May 1, 1962, New York City. Excerpta Medica International Congress Series No. 54.* Excerpta Medica, Amsterdam

TIETZE, C. and LEWIT, S. (1970). Evaluation of intrauterine devices: ninth progress report of the Cooperative Statistical Program. *Stud. Fam. Plann.*, **55**, 1–40

TIETZE, C. and LEWIT, S. (1973). Recommended procedures for the statistical evaluation of intrauterine contraception. *Stud. Fam. Plann.*, **4**, 35–41. *See also Clin. Obstet. Gynec.*, **17**, 121–138

TIMONEN, H., LUUKKAINEN, T., RAINIO, J. and TATUM, H.J. (1972). Hysterographic studies with the copper T (TCu 200) *in situ. Contraception*, **6**, 513–521

VESSEY, M.P., JOHNSON, B., DOLL, R. and PETO, R. (1974). Outcome of pregnancy in women using an intrauterine device. *Lancet*, **i**, 495–497

WHITE, I.G. (1955). The toxicity of heavy metals to mammalian spermatozoa. *Aust. J. exp. Biol.,* 33, 359–366

WIESE, J. (1976). A study of four antigon models and factors in the use-effectiveness of the IUD. *Contraception,* 14, 687–701

WILLIAMS, M. and SNOWDEN, R. (1974). The United Kingdom field trial of the Gravigard device. *Family Planning Research Unit Report No. 8.* University of Exeter

WILSON, E.W. (1977). The effect of copper on lactic dehydrogenase isoenzymes in human endometrium. *Contraception,* 16, 367–374

WORLD HEALTH ORGANIZATION (1968). Intra-uterine devices: physiological and clinical aspects. Report of a WHO scientific group. *Tech. Rep. Ser. Wld Hlth Org.,* No. 397, p. 32

WREN, B.G. (1962). Complications associated with the use of the Gräfenberg ring. *Aust. & N.Z. J. Obstet. Gynaecol.,* 2, 7–9

WYLER, R. and WIESENDANGER, W. (1975). The enhancing effect of copper, nickel and cobalt ions on plaque formation by Semliki Forest Virus (SFV) in chicken embryo fibroblasts. *Archs Virol.,* 47, 57–69

WYNN, R.M. (1968). Fine structural effects of intrauterine contraceptives on the human endometrium. *Fert. Steril.,* 19, 867–882

ZIPPER, J. A., MEDEL, M. and PRAGER, R. (1969). Suppression of fertility by intra-uterine copper and zinc in rabbits: a new approach to intrauterine contraception. *Am. J. Obstet. Gynec.,* 105, 529–534

ZIPPER, J.A., TATUM, H.J., PASTENE, L., MEDEL, M. and RIVERA, M. (1969). Metallic copper as an intrauterine contraceptive adjunct to the 'T' device. *Am. J. Obstet. Gynec.,* 105, 1274–1278

10 Procedures for Intra-uterine Contraception

INSERTION PROCEDURES

Time of Insertion

In the woman who has not had a recent pregnancy the most propitious time for insertion of an intra-uterine device is the first half of the menstrual cycle, preferably between Days 10 and 14. The diameter of the cervical canal is greater at this time than during the secretory phase (Johnstone *et al.*, 1974). The uterus is relaxed and myometrial contractions, which might tend to cause expulsion, are at a minimum. In addition, the risk that the patient is already pregnant is low at this time. Some authorities have advocated insertion during menstruation (Sobrero, 1971; Monks, 1976), arguing that the cervix is even more lax at that time, but this seems unwise as a routine procedure. There is a chance that infection may be introduced directly into the open venous sinusoids and post-insertion bleeding may be quite heavy. In addition, some patients resent gynaecological assaults during menstruation and the logistics of arranging appointments to coincide with menstruation are troublesome for both patient and doctor.

With postpartum women the problem is much simpler, insertion being easy four to six weeks after delivery. It has been suggested that at this time motivation is high (American College of Obstetricians and Gynecologists, 1968) but this is only relatively true, the sample being biased by the absence of women who failed to attend for a postnatal examination. Attempts have been made to overcome this problem by inserting devices a few days after delivery, before the patient has left hospital. Results have not been encouraging, expulsion rates with Lippes loops size D, Petal devices and Saf-T-Coils being very high (Emens, 1973a; Shervington, 1974). Emens (1973a) found that only 10% of Dalkon shield devices so inserted had been expelled within the following month, an improvement on the results of Diamond and Freeman (1973) who found that 48% were expelled. Emens (1973b) observed that in most cases the device becomes correctly orientated and the strings are present six weeks postpartum. Bluett (1973a) considers that the shield should be put into the puerperal uterus at the level of the internal os. If this is done the device can sometimes end up embedded in the lower segment and cervical canal as the uterus involutes. There is probably an increased risk of perforation and infection associated with early postpartum insertion, but these risks vary widely with the population studied and the skill of the doctors concerned. In general, early postpartum insertion is unwise. It may be true that some poorly motivated patients could be provided in this way with contraception which they really need, but this is the very group of women who are liable to neglect the problems arising and are thereby more prone to serious consequences.

If one waits much more than six weeks after delivery to insert the device, a small proportion of patients will have already become pregnant before they can attend, and clinical diagnosis of the pregnancy can be difficult. In addition, insertion becomes progressively more uncomfortable for the patient as the cervical canal continues to shrink.

Insertion at the time of therapeutic abortion in the first trimester seems to be safer and more effective than insertion soon after delivery. The patients are more strongly motivated and the uterus is firmer and smaller than in the postpartum woman. The risks of perforation and sepsis are less as the opportunity is available to perform the procedure under general anaesthesia in the best conditions in an operating theatre. Andolšek (1972) and Goldsmith *et al.* (1972) had few problems with this approach. Larger and less easily expelled devices are preferable – Andolšek (1972) recorded only 2.8 expulsions per 100 users within a year with Lippes loops size D but the corresponding figure for size C was 9.8%.

Insertion of a device when an apparently spontaneous abortion occurs and retained products of conception are evacuated under general anaesthesia is unwise. Even if the abortion was in fact spontaneous there has usually been bleeding. The uterus is soft and boggy and to empty it without damage and secure haemostasis is the primary consideration. A device may easily perforate the uterus or cause further bleeding. In practice, if immediate contraceptive precautions are requested there is a considerable risk that the abortion was caused by interference. There is an implied risk of intra-uterine infection and it would then be rash to insert a device.

Facilities

The lithotomy position is highly desirable for insertion, and an examination couch with lithotomy poles and good light should be available. Apart from the usual equipment for a general medical and gynaecological examination a vulsellum or a single tooth tenaculum and a uterine sound should be on the sterile trolley. The equipment for Papanicolaou smears, microscopy of wet preparations of vaginal secretion and bacteriological culture is desirable.

A couch or bed where a patient with discomfort after insertion can rest for several hours if necessary should be available, and hospital admission for observation may be needed if there is bleeding or suspicion of perforation of the uterus.

Preparation of Devices

Some guidance on choice of device for different age and parity groups is given by Snowden *et al.* (1977).

Many devices are now available in a pre-packed form, already sterilised and loaded into an inserter.

If purchased unsterilised, plastic devices and inserters should not be boiled or autoclaved, and are best washed carefully in water containing 0.1% benzalkonium chloride and then left to soak in a similar solution for 24 hours before use. Alternatively, 1% benzalkonium chloride may be used for six hours and the devices rinsed in a more dilute solution before use. They can also be sterilised with iodine, which has the advantage that it is rapidly bactericidal and virucidal (Chang, 1958; Ten Have and Stuht, 1964). Insertion into diluted tincture of iodine or an iodine-iodide mixture containing 0.04% of elemental iodine for five minutes before use suffices, rinsing in sterile water before insertion. Plastic devices should not be left in contact with iodine for long periods but should be washed and stored dry. Iodine cannot be used with plastic devices containing copper, zinc or other metals. These devices must be sterilised in benzalkonium chloride.

Devices made entirely of metal may be autoclaved or boiled. Otherwise they can be sterilised in aqueous benzalkonium chloride. They should not be exposed to iodine.

After sterilisation a device may be loaded into an inserter using sterile gloves and instruments.

Procedure

A medical, obstetric and gynaecological history should be taken and a general physical examination including urine analysis should be carried out, unless the patient is well known to the physician and has recently been examined. The insertion procedure should be explained, and, unless there is a specific reason to the contrary, the patient should be shown the device. She may have many questions about intra-uterine devices which need to be answered (Snowden *et al.*, 1977).

Insertion is best conducted in the lithotomy position, though it can be achieved in a left lateral position or in the dorsal position, supporting the buttocks with a cushion if necessary. The cervix should be inspected carefully and a Papanicolaou smear taken if no recent result is available. In appropriate cases, and in some areas in all cases, swabs from the cervix should be taken for microscopy of a wet preparation and culture for gonorrhoea. A small clean ectropion of congenital, postpartum or hormonal contraceptive origin is no bar to insertion, and electrocautery (Sobrero, 1971) or the cryoprobe may be used to treat the cervix immediately before insertion. If there is acute cervicitis, or a purulent discharge, or any condition which can be labelled 'chronic cervicitis' or 'endocervicitis' it is wise to defer insertion until a bacteriological culture is available and the condition has been treated. A viral cervicitis may be suspected if there is a history of urethral irritation in the consort or if a Papanicolaou smear shows inclusion bodies in desquamated squamous cells, and may be sometimes be confirmed by virus culture. If Papanicolaou smears are not readily available, either painting the cervix with Schiller's iodine (iodine 0.3%, potassium iodide 1.2%, in water) or the use of a colposcope may indicate the need for punch biopsy of a suspicious lesion. It is our experience that scrupulous attention to the state of the cervix before insertion reduces the incidence of subsequent sepsis and other complications to a very low figure.

The uterus is examined bimanually, with special attention to its position, size, regularity, consistency, mobility and sensitivity to palpation. Any adnexal tenderness requires careful evaluation and adnexal swellings need investigation. Pelvic inflammatory disease contra-indicates insertion.

Mucus and debris are removed from the cervix, which is then mopped with an antiseptic (aqueous iodine, 0.04%, merthiolate, 0.1%, chlorhexidine 0.1%, or benzalkonium chloride, 1%, are suitable). It is after this that opinions on technique differ. Some gynaecologists feel that a vulsellum should always be applied to the cervix which is then drawn down to straighten the canal and align the cavity in the same plane, and that a sound should be passed to measure the cavity and confirm its direction. Application of a vulsellum is usually felt and is often quite painful. The uterine sound may cause considerable discomfort as it passes the internal os and again when it reaches the fundus. Sobrero (1971) has made the point that attempts to measure the uterine lumen with a sound are unnecessary with simple devices. In study programmes using a single size of device rates of spontaneous expulsion or removal for pain or bleeding are no lower than in those which try to individualise the size of the device to be inserted. Others believe that the use of vulsellum and sound cause unnecessary discomfort, in general add no information and predispose to perforation of the uterus by the device. The best compromise is to adjust the technique to the patient. If the uterus can be defined bimanually with ease, its axis is relatively near to the axis of the vagina, and the canal is fairly lax, then insertion can often be accomplished easily and safely without vulsellum or sound. If the uterus is difficult to define, or markedly anteflexed or retroflexed, then a vulsellum may draw it into a position where its axis can be readily confirmed by gentle sounding. Application of a single tooth tenaculum is less painful than that of a vulsellum, but the tooth may tear the cervix if firm traction is needed. If the impression is gained that the canal may be tight, a 3 or 4 mm diameter Hegar dilator is a better and less uncomfortable instrument for exploration than a sound.

Inserters are of four main types. Those used with linear devices such as the Lippes loop are inserted to occupy only the cervical canal with or without gentle traction on the cervix. Pressing the plunger then expels the device into the uterine cavity where it assumes its unrestrained shape, and the inserter is withdrawn leaving the strings in the canal. Some leave the strings 5 cm long but they can then irritate the husband and it is probably better to cut them 1–2 cm below the external os. Another alternative is to leave them at 5 cm and trim them to 2 cm at the first follow-up visit when the device can be assumed to have settled into its most natural position in the uterus.

The second type of inserter is used for more complex devices which are folded up within it, and are intended to pass into the uterine cavity. The sleeve is then withdrawn, keeping the plunger stationary, thus allowing the device to expand within the cavity.

With the Gravigard device, Newton *et al.* (1974) recommend measuring the length of the uterine cavity with a sound first. The cervical stop on the inserter is then set to this distance and the inserter introduced into the uterus. The outer sheath is withdrawn 2.5 cm to free the transverse arm, and then held steady. The inserter rod is gently pushed to ensure that the device is at the fundus. The withdrawal of the sheath is then completed and the rod and then the sheath removed.

The third type consists of a hooked carrying rod to which the device, generally partly folded, is attached. This type was employed with Dalkon shields, which are thrust into the uterine cavity with the rod. The latter is then rotated to disengage it from the device and withdrawn.

The fourth type of inserter, used with the Antigon device, remains at the external os of the cervix, the folded device being extruded through the cervical canal, to expand in the uterine cavity.

It is essential that the instructions for the device employed be read carefully and followed strictly if perforation of the uterus is to be avoided. For example, to pass an inserter of the second type into the uterus and then press the plunger instead of withdrawing the sleeve, simply forces the device into the uterine wall.

The device should be inserted in the plane of the uterine lumen. This mini-mises the risk of perforation or embedding in the uterine wall. In addition, it reduces the pain which many patients feel as the more rigid models are inserted, the device expanding naturally to lie in the cavity without tension on the walls. If the uterus is markedly anteflexed or retroflexed, traction on the cervix tends to draw it into an axial position, enabling insertion to be accomplished.

Truthful explanation and gentle but secure handling are the keys to successful insertion. Accurate pelvic examination and careful asepsis prevent complications.

Difficulties with Insertion

The patient who cannot relax sufficiently to permit adequate determination of the size and position of the uterus, exposure of the cervix and introduction of the inserter, should be taken seriously. Apart from the discomfort and embarras-sment occasioned to patient, physician and sometimes others in the clinic by attempting to wrestle with the problem, the situation may predispose to perfo-ration of the uterus (Hawkins, 1970).

Sometimes the aetiology is obvious – misunderstanding of the procedure or the nature of the device. If this is the case it is possible that reassurance and explanation will enable the patient to relax, but once the problem has arisen, it is likely to recur at a further attempt at the same or at a subsequent clinic session. The difficulty can sometimes be resolved by changing circumstances such as the position for examination, the physician or the venue (for example, operating room instead of clinic) sufficiently to permit the patient to blame her nervousness at the first attempt on such factors. Intelligent anticipation that the difficulty may arise is the best preventive measure. Preliminary explanation tailored to the needs of the individual patient, persuasion of the patient to relax completely in the lithotomy position, and avoidance of clumsiness in the examination are particularly important. Sometimes the nervous nullipara who finds a dorsal or lithotomy position difficult will relax completely in a left lateral or Sims' position, provided the move is made immediately there are indications of trouble. Nursing assistance is necessary to manipulate buttocks, speculum and lighting in these positions.

Commonly the roots of the problem lie deeper. They may be associated with poor motivation for contraception or conflict between environmental pressures for family planning and a strong desire to have another baby. Otherwise they may reflect marital and sexual difficulties or any of the factors which lead some women to dislike or resent gynaecological procedures.

Some authorities try again after premedication with a sedative. It is our view that if the simplest manoeuvres to overcome the problem fail, it is better to admit the patient to hospital for a few hours and insert the device under a brief general anaesthetic. It is the patient who has had an unpleasant experience with insertion who resents the device, is intolerant of minor side-effects, is unco-operative with follow-up procedures and who fails to report if something goes wrong. The risks which such patients run counterbalance the very small risk of general anaesthesia for insertion.

Other conditions which call for general anaesthesia for insertion are difficulty in determining the size and position of the uterus and any gynaecological history or physical findings which could be interpreted as providing an indication for curettage.

A tight cervical canal is best dealt with by asking the patient to return on the third or fourth day of menstruation, but may require passage of a sound and one or more dilators to permit introduction of the inserter. This process is commonly painful. It used to be said that dilatation of the cervix without premedication or general anaesthesia could lead to 'cervical shock', presumably vagal in nature, which could be fatal. With the degree of dilatation required to introduce a device syncope is not uncommon. Atropine sulphate, 0.6 mg, should be given intra-venously at once (Menzies, 1978); inhalation of aromatic spirits of ammonia and rest in a horizontal position are said to help. No fatal cases of cervical shock associated with insertion of a device have yet been reported, though hundreds of thousands of women must have had some dilatation performed for this purpose without anaesthesia. On the other hand Conrad *et al.* (1973) found that six women in a series of 7140 in Atlanta, Georgia, had acute neurovascular sequelae, including convulsions and syncope, following insertion or removal of a device. Such patients should be investigated for neurological or cardiovascular abnor-mality, and if further intra-uterine manipulation is attempted, it should be under general anaesthesia after premedication including atropine (Hawkins, 1977).

Jackson (1973) uses inhalation of an ampoule of amyl nitrite to facilitate dilatation of the cervix and insertion of a device, though the patient may get an unpleasant headache after this. A paracervical block may be used injecting 5 ml of 1% lignocaine into the cardinal and uterosacral ligaments on each side. Intra-cervical block, using three injections of 4 ml of 1% lignocaine at 12, 4 and 8 o'clock, has also been employed, though the patient who has just undergone an unsuccessful attempt to negotiate her cervical canal is not the most tolerant of the manipulations involved in inserting the block. In cases of real difficulty, admission for examination under general anaesthesia, dilatation and insertion is the best answer.

Pain, in the form of uterine cramps immediately after insertion, is quite common. It is usually comparable in severity to dysmenorrhoea and resolves with a few minutes' rest or simple analgesics, preferably prostaglandin synthe-tase inhibitors such as aspirin, indomethacin or flufenamic acid, perhaps con-tinued for 24 hours. Occasionally syncope with measurable hypotension results and several hours rest and observation may be indicated. The anxious nullipara can hyperventilate and become hysterical in response to post-insertion pain. In a few women the reaction to the pain is sufficiently severe that the physician may feel prompt removal of the device to be the only answer.

Bleeding after insertion can also be troublesome. If it is at all heavy and does not resolve fairly soon, the presence of either an unsuspected pregnancy or intra-uterine pathology may be responsible. The need for hospital admission, examination under anaesthesia and, if the device is correctly *in situ*, removal and curettage, should be assessed.

Most perforations of the uterus either occur or are initiated by embedding of the device in the uterine wall at the time of insertion. Perforation should be suspected when the device is felt to slide in a direction incompatible with the axis of the uterus, when pain or bleeding are severe or persistent, or when the strings or tail of the device disappear upwards into the uterus. In any of these circumstances, hospital admission, cross-matching of blood and subsequent removal of the device should be considered. If the strings of the device are readily accessible, this manoeuvre can be safely achieved in the ward, but the access and asepsis provided in an operating theatre is an advantage even though anaesthesia may not be required. If perforation of the uterus is confirmed but the device can be removed *per vaginam* it is rare that laparotomy is needed. Usually two to three days' observation, with a five-day course of broad-range antibiotics, suffices for any bleeding or pelvic tenderness to resolve and to confirm that pelvic infection is unlikely. If the device has disappeared through the uterine wall then investigation and operative removal may be necessary.

Advice after Insertion

After a successful insertion the patient should be instructed how to examine herself to detect the presence of the threads in the cervical canal. She should perform this examination at least monthly, preferably after each menstrual period, as this is the most likely time for unnoticed expulsion of the device. If she cannot feel the threads she should regard herself as unprotected against pregnancy and seek medical advice. If the threads have really disappeared, other possibilities are perforation or the occurrence of pregnancy with the device *in situ*. With post-menstrual self-examination the patient might also detect downward displacement of the device into the cervical canal.

Should the patient require greater security against pregnancy than is provided by the device alone, some authorities prescribe the additional use of chemical contraceptives. Snowden and Williams (1975) noted that with the Dalkon shield, the clinic with the lowest pregnancy rate was one where half the patients were advised to use an additional procedure, generally a spermicide. On the other hand, in a large-scale multicentre trial of the M-213 device, our 400 patients were supplied with and advised to employ a vaginal foam containing 12.9% of the spermicide nonoxynol-9 to provide additional security. The pregnancy rate over the first year was 5.4 per 100 woman-years (Murdoch and Hawkins, unpublished results) whilst rates from other centres in Great Britain varied between nil and 6.2. We therefore feel that any effect of such advice on pregnancy rate is trivial compared with between-clinic variation. We have met several poorly motivated patients who have been given supplies of spermicide when a device was fitted, subsequently expelled the device, and attended the clinic several months later with an early pregnancy and the comment that they 'thought it would be all right if they just used the spermicide'. We consider that if increased protection is required the patient should be advised to use either condoms or a diaphragm with the usual contraceptive cream, at mid cycle. Others advise a low-dose progestagen oral contraceptive to supplement the effect of the device, provided the patients tolerate such preparations without menstrual disturbance.

The patient should be advised that she may notice uterine cramps or other mild pelvic discomfort, some irregular bleeding or spotting, and a slight vaginal discharge for a few weeks. The next menstrual period may well be more uncomfortable and heavier than usual. The patient should be reassured along the lines that these problems usually resolve after a month or two. If she develops worsening or severe pain or bleeding, or symptoms of pyrexia, she should seek medical advice promptly.

In the United States of America, the Department of Health, Education and Welfare's Food and Drug Administration (1977) has published a document intended to be given to patients having intra-uterine devices fitted. Apart from providing far too much information for the average patient the document contains extensive lists of adverse reactions and side-effects which can only create inappropriate anxiety in both patient and doctor. It also states that if pregnancy occurs with a device *in situ* and the tails are visible the doctor should remove the device, and suggests that termination of the pregnancy should be considered. In our opinion, and in that of many American doctors, this document represents an unethical intrusion on the doctor—patient relationship.

Follow-up Visits

Apart from the desirability of periodic review of general welfare and gynaecological health, an annual Papanicolaou smear, and marital, sexual and family planning counselling follow-up visits serve three purposes. Review and management of minor side-effects of the device are important; verification at intervals that neither expulsion nor perforation has occurred and ascertaining that chronic pelvic inflammatory disease has not developed should be incumbent on the physician who inserted the device.

These purposes can in general be accomplished with routine visits one month and six months after insertion, followed by six-monthly or annual visits if all is well. An interval of one year may be too long if silent perforation of the uterus is to be detected in patients whose palpation of the strings is unreliable.

The patient must also appreciate that she can attend at any time if she has problems. If a full-time service cannot be provided, as in clinics not attached to hospitals, then patients should be given an appropriate port of call in emergency, their family practitioners being fully acquainted with the circumstances.

Follow-up visits involve full discussion, examination and documentation (Snowden *et al.,* 1977). Devices wound with copper wire are said to need replacement after an appropriate interval, usually one to two years, as the release of copper steadily decreases until it reaches an ineffective level. The reduction in copper release can be accentuated by calcium deposits on the device (Gosden *et al.,* 1977) and this may leave the patient protected only by a relatively inefficient inert device. At the present time it is probably wise to follow the manufacturer's recommendations though these may be biased by commercial considerations. Liability to pregnancy decreases year by year with continued use of inert devices. It may be that this mechanism will maintain apparent efficacy after the first year or two, although the amount of copper release has declined.

Sound data to enumerate the risks of leaving a copper device *in situ* for several years will be of interest.

Replacement of plastic devices after a year or two has been recommended, in view of their tendency to accumulate calcareous deposits, but there is no evidence that these are harmful. We have removed Lippes loops that have remained efficient and caused no problems over eight to ten years. The Family Planning Research Unit (1977) concluded that there is little relation between the occasional occurrence of disintegration, distortion, calcification or embedding of Lippes loops and the time for which they have been worn. Hata *et al.* (1969) carried out endometrial biopsies on 518 women who had worn intra-uterine devices (Yusei or Ota rings) for up to 15 years. Minor inflammatory changes were more common in the endometrium than in women who did not use devices, but there was no correlation between duration of use and the histological appearances and there was no malignancy. Even so, in our present state of ignorance of the very long-term effects, it is probably a wise precaution to change any device after five years and perform endometrial biopsy or take uterine washings as described by Wachtel *et al.* (1973) for cytological examination at that time.

There is little agreement as to when an intra-uterine device which is still *in situ* at the time of the menopause should be removed (Family Planning Research Unit, 1977). Some workers feel that it should be removed promptly or the uterine wall, protected only by atrophic endometrium, may become eroded.

Vaginal Cytology

It has been reported that cervical and posterior fornix smears from patients with Lippes loops have a low karyopryknotic index, with marked attenuation in the normal mid cycle increase in cornification of the desquamated epithelial cells (Sammour *et al.*, 1967). There was an incidence of 35% of smears showing heavy infiltration with leucocytes and bacteria during the first three cycles after insertion, but this had decreased to 5% in smears taken one year or more later.

These findings should be borne in mind in interpreting smears from patients with devices.

Documentation

Insertion of an intra-uterine device is a procedure for which the physician should accept responsibility for maintenance of supervision. In order to arrange for this it is necessary to maintain not only full documentation but also a mechanism for tracing and visiting those who default from clinic attendance.

REMOVAL

A proportion of women, depending on the population studied, eventually have the device removed because they want another baby. Tietze and Lewit (1970) list other common non-medical reasons for requesting removal as including fear of injury, lack of confidence, religious reasons, unspecified objections by the husband or by a doctor not concerned in fitting the device, separation, divorce or widowhood, and elective sterilisation.

Procedure

Most simple devices can be removed in the out-patient clinic without difficulty. The lithotomy position is desirable but not essential. The position of the uterus should first be ascertained; if it is acutely anteflexed or retroflexed, a tenaculum is attached to the cervix and gentle traction applied to align the uterine cavity towards the axis of the vagina. Aseptic and antiseptic precautions are employed. A sponge-holding forceps or similar instrument is used to grasp both strings of devices that have two. Steady and equal traction on the strings in the axis of the cervical canal and uterine cavity usually results in removal without much difficulty.

Metal spring devices such as the M device or the Majzlin spring can be quite difficult to remove; success depends on equal traction on the two sides in the axis of the uterus. Removal of Dalkon shields can be uncomfortable for the patient; Bluett (1973b) feels that application of firm and continuous traction until initial resistance is overcome is needed to avoid spasm of the cervix. He also recommends use of general anaesthesia for removal from nulliparous patients in whom difficulty is anticipated.

Closed-ring devices without tails can usually be removed from parous women with Gräfenberg's (1931) hook or a similar instrument under out-patient conditions. If the strings of a device have disappeared, its presence low in the uterus can usually be confirmed with a uterine sound. Sobrero and Goldsmith (1973) describe the out-patient removal of devices whose tail has disappeared using uterine forceps without anaesthesia.

When the strings are absent it is our feeling that, unless the cervix is patulous and the end of the device can be grasped easily with Spencer Wells or polyp forceps, removal should be conducted under general anaesthesia. Similar considerations apply when the strings are torn off the device during an attempted removal. Under anaesthesia the cervix is dilated to Hegar 6 or more, the cavity explored using some traction on the cervix, and the device removed with forceps. A Gräfenberg hook may be useful. If the device is embedded in the myometrial wall or if there is difficulty at the internal os, the uterus may be damaged internally, but major degrees of laceration are rare and bleeding is not usually heavy or persistent. Nonetheless, if a tear is suspected, observation for a day or two and perhaps a course of antibiotics are indicated.

Fertility after Removal

Fertility does not seem to be impaired after removal of a device, provided there has been no episode of inflammatory disease whilst the device was *in situ*. Sixty per cent of women who have a device removed in order to conceive do so within three months; 85–90% within a year (American College of Obstetricians and Gynecologists, 1968; World Health Organisation, 1968; Tietze, 1968; Tietze and Lewit, 1970). Hata *et al.* (1969) found lower figures but it is not clear that all their patients were trying to conceive. They observed that the ability to conceive was not related to the time for which the device had been used, but Tietze (1968) showed that conception rates in patients who had worn a device for more than 20 months were consistently lower than those with a shorter duration of use.

POSTCOITAL CONTRACEPTION

Tatum and Lippes (1975) have found that insertion of a copper intra-uterine device can act as an effective postcoital contraceptive. There were no pregnancies among the 150 women studied who had had the device inserted within three to five days of unprotected intercourse. This procedure seems preferable to the use of large doses of oestrogen for rape victims, in view of the side-effects and potential dangers of the drugs.

REFERENCES

AMERICAN COLLEGE OF OBSTETRICIANS AND GYNECOLOGISTS (1968). Intra-uterine devices. *ACOG Technical Bulletin,* **10**, 2

ANDOLŠEK, L. (1972). Experience with immediate post-abortion insertions of the IUD. *Family Planning Research Conference. A Multidisciplinary Approach, Exeter, England, September 27–28 1971. Excerpta Medica International Congress Series, No. 260*, pp. 55–58. Ed. Goldsmith, A. and Snowden, R. Excerpta Medica, Amsterdam

BLUETT, D. (1973a and b). *Dalkon Shield Symposium. London, October 11th 1972*, pp. 26–27 and 29, respectively. Ed. Templeton, J.S., A.H. Robins, Horsham, Sussex

CHANG, S.L. (1958). The use of active iodine as a water disinfectant. *J. Am. pharm. Ass. Sci. Edn*, **47**, 417–423

CONRAD, C.C., GHAZI, M. and KITAY, D.Z. (1973). Acute neurovascular sequelae to intrauterine device insertion or removal. *J. reprod. Med.,* **11**, 211–212

DIAMOND, R.A. and FREEMAN, D.W. (1973). Insertion of intrauterine devices in the early postpartum period. *Minn. Med.,* **56**, 49–50

EMENS, M. (1973a and b). The insertion of the Dalkon shield post-partum. *Dalkon Shield Symposium, London, October 11th 1972*, pp. 18–21 and 29, respectively. Ed. Templeton, J.S. A.H. Robins, Horsham, Sussex

FAMILY PLANNING RESEARCH UNIT (1977). Long term use of the Lippes loop intrauterine device. *Memorandum 2/77, October 1977.* University of Exeter

FOOD AND DRUG ADMINISTRATION. DEPARTMENT OF HEALTH, EDUCATION AND WELFARE (1977). Intrauterine contraceptive devices: professional and patient labelling. *Federal Register,* **42**, 23772–23783

GOLDSMITH, A., GOLDBERG, R., EYZAGUIRRE, H., LUCERO, S. and LIZANA, L. (1972). IUD insertion in the immediate postabortal period. *Proceedings of the Family Planning Research Conference, a Multidisciplinary Approach, Exeter, England, September 27–28, 1971. Excerpta Medica International Congress Series No. 260*, pp. 59–67. Ed. Goldsmith, A. and Snowden, R. Excerpta Medica, Amsterdam

GOSDEN, C., ROSS, A. and LOUDON, N.B. (1977). Intrauterine deposition of calcium on copper-bearing intrauterine contraceptive devices. *Br. med. J.,* **i**, 202–206

GRÄFENBERG, E. (1931). An intrauterine contraceptive method. *The Practice of Contraception. An International Symposium and Survey*, pp. 33–56. Ed. Sanger, M. and Stone, H.M. Williams and Wilkins, Baltimore

HATA, Y., ISHIHAMA, A., KUDO, N., NAKAMURA, Y., MIYAI, T., MAKINO, T. and KAGABU, T. (1969). The effect of long-term use of IUD. *Acta obstet. gynaec. Jap.*, **16**, 73–78

HAWKINS, D.F. (1970). *Perforation of the uterus by M-213 devices in Great Britain. Report to the Medical Advisory Committee.* Pathfinder Fund, Boston

HAWKINS, D.F. (1977). Cervical shock. *Practitioner*, **218**, 181–182

JACKSON, M. (1973). *Dalkon Shield Symposium. London, October 11th 1972,* p. 28. Ed. Templeton, J.S. A.H. Robins, Horsham, Sussex

JOHNSTONE, F.D., BOYD, I.E., McARTHY, T.G. and BROWNE, J.C. McC. (1974). The diameter of the uterine isthmus during the menstrual cycle, pregnancy and the puerperium. *J. Obstet. Gynaec. Br. Commonw.*, **81**, 558–562

MENZIES, D.N. (1978). Vasovagal shock after insertion of intrauterine device. *Br. med. J.*, **i**, 305

MONKS, I. (1976). The current state of IUCDs. *J. mat. Child Hlth*, August, 10–15

NEWTON, J., ELIAS, J., McEWAN, J. and MANN, G. (1974). Intrauterine contraception with the Copper-7: evaluation after two years. *Br. med. J.*, **iii**, 447–450

SAMMOUR, M.B., ISKANDER, S.G. and RIFAI, S.F. (1967). Combined histologic and cytologic study of intrauterine contraception. *Am. J. Obstet. Gynec.*, **98**, 946–956

SHERVINGTON, P. (1974). Cited by Elder, M.G. *Obstetric Therapeutics*, p. 548. Ed. Hawkins, D.F. Baillière Tindall, London

SNOWDEN, R. and WILLIAMS, M. (1975). The United Kingdom Dalkon Shield trial: two years of observation. *Contraception*, **11**, 1–13

SNOWDEN, R., WILLIAMS, M. and HAWKINS, D. (1977). *The IUD. A Practical Guide*, Croom Helm, London

SOBRERO, A.J. (1971). Intrauterine devices in clinical practice. *Fam. Plann. Perspect.*, **3**, number 1, 16–24

SOBRERO, A.J. and GOLDSMITH, A. (1973). *Intrauterine devices. A Manual for Clinical Practice.* Ed. Cosby, M.L. Pathfinder Fund, Boston

TATUM, H.J. and LIPPES, J. (1975). Fellows succeed in IUD work. *ACOG Newsletter*, **19**, number 11, p. 6

TEN HAVE, R. and STUHT, J. (1964). The use of an itinerant physician to introduce the intra-uterine contraceptive device in medically disadvantaged areas. *Intra-uterine Contraception. Proceedings of the Second International Conference, October 1964, New York City. Excerpta Medica International Congress Series No. 86*, pp. 52–59. Ed. Segal, S.J., Southam, A.L. and Shafer, K.D. Excerpta Medica, Amsterdam

TIETZE, C. (1968). Fertility after discontinuation of intrauterine and oral contraception. *Int. J. Fert.*, **13**, 385–389

TIETZE, C. and LEWIT, S. (1970). Evaluation of intrauterine devices: ninth progress report of the Cooperative Statistical Program. *Stud. Fam. Plann.*, **55**, 1–40

WACHTEL, E., GORDON, H. and WYCHERLEY, J. (1973). The cytological diagnosis of endometrial pathology using a uterine aspiration technique. *J. Obstet. Gynaec. Br. Commonw.*, **80**, 164–168

WORLD HEALTH ORGANIZATION (1968). Intra-uterine devices: physiological and clinical aspects. Report of a WHO scientific group. *Tech. Rep. Ser. Wld Hlth Org.*, **397**, 23

11 Complications of Intra-uterine Contraception

PREGNANCY

Pregnancy rates of the order of 2—3 per 100 woman-years are usually quoted for reasonably effective forms of intra-uterine device. Tietze and Lewit (1970) concluded from six years of study by the Co-operative Statistical Program that no single type of device has consistently lower or higher pregnancy rates than the others. They found no consistent difference between devices with plastic tails or springs and those without such as Gräfenberg rings or Birnberg bows. The only important difference between devices was that larger sizes of loops and spirals tended to have a lower pregnancy rate than smaller sizes of the same device. Snowden (1975), reporting on the multicentre studies of the Family Planning Unit of the University of Exeter, found mean pregnancy rates between 2.4 and 4.4 per 100 users in the first year of use for the different devices they have tested in Great Britain.

We have already given reasons for believing that if complete follow-up can be achieved true mean rates may be as high as 5 per 100 woman-years. The exact figure is unimportant. It should be recognised that the major source of variation is environmental rather than the nature of the device employed. If the extent of 'between-centre' variation in the Exeter studies (Snowden, 1975) is examined, it will be found that pregnancy rates with a single device can vary between 1.5 and 7.0 per 100 woman-years, according to locality within Great Britain. Some of this variation is attributable to the time for which a centre has been using a device, to differences between single-doctor and multi-doctor clinics, to religious and ethnic differences in the patients, to varying frequencies of follow-up and to the use of supplementary methods of contraception.

The likelihood of unwanted pregnancy in women employing intra-uterine devices is reduced in older women, but increased parity conveys an increased risk of pregnancy when women of the same age groups are compared (Tietze and Lewit, 1970; Snowden et al., 1977).

With all inert devices the pregnancy risk decreases with each year of use. Tietze and Lewit's (1970) figures for the Lippes loop D are shown in *Table 11.1* and it will be seen that in the third and fourth years the pregnancy risk has fallen to less than half of that in the first year. The mechanism of this is not entirely clear. It is not primarily due to progressive damage to the uterus since Hata et al. (1969) showed that fertility after removal of a device is unrelated to the number of years for which it has been used. Women at the highest risk are

Table 11.1 LIPPES LOOP D, EVENT RATES (TIETZE AND LEWIT, 1970)

	Net annual rates per 100 woman-years					
	1st year	*2nd year*	*3rd year*	*4th year*	*5th year*	*6th year*
Pregnancies	2.7	2.0	1.2	1.4	0.6	0.9
Expulsions	9.5	2.5	1.6	0.8	0.2	0.0
Removals for bleeding and pain	11.7	7.6	7.5	5.6	2.7	2.5

progressively eliminated from the studies due to the occurrence of pregnancy. Removal from the studies for other reasons may well leave a low-risk group continuing — we have found that women who expel devices have an increased chance of conceiving with a device *in situ* (Bluett and Hawkins, unpublished observations).

It must not be forgotten that although *annual* risk of pregnancy decreases year by year, the *cumulative* risk of failure steadily increases. Even on Tietze and Lewit's figures (*Table 11.1*), which we regard as optimistic, the woman who uses a Lippes loop D for six years stands a 1 in 10 chance of acquiring an unwanted pregnancy during that time. The woman who needs very effective contraception for a period of years should be advised that an intra-uterine contraceptive device used alone is not her best choice. The woman who has used a device successfully for five years and wishes advice poses a problem in subjective probability. She is in the same position as the gambler who has made five tosses of a coin and obtained tails each time. The practical prognosis may be somewhere between the 0.9% chance of conception as a sixth year user and the primary prediction of a 9.3% chance of conception within six years, depending on how much of the success was due to factors determining her 'low-risk' category and how much to good luck! The 0.9% figure may be particularly optimistic, as failures after several years of use are notoriously hard to trace.

Copper-wound devices were originally designed with a view to providing effective contraception over a period of four years. In practice the rate of release of the copper decreases to one-sixth of the initial rate over the first 21 months of use (Orlans, 1973). Nonetheless the copper T and 7 devices tend to show some decrease in pregnancy rate in the second and third years of use (Zipper *et al.*, 1973; Newton *et al.*, 1974; Sivin, 1976). The efficacy of devices containing progestagen is of course reduced after the progestagen has been released, but retention of the inert container would be expected to convey some protection against pregnancy.

Devices inserted during the weeks following delivery appear to be more effective initially, particularly as some women are breast-feeding and have lactation amenorrhoea.

When a pregnancy occurs and examination reveals that the tails of the device are no longer palpable in the cervix, or the device has no tail, then expulsion or silent perforation of the uterus must always be considered as possible causes. In either case, no immediate action is indicated. If there are indications for terminating the pregnancy then a postero-anterior x-ray of the abdomen and pelvis will confirm the presence or absence of the device. Should the device obviously be lying outside the uterus, then recovery may be effected by laparotomy, laparoscopy or colpotomy at the time of the abortion. A similar course of action should be followed if the device is apparently in the uterus but cannot be found when the products of conception are evacuated. A pregnancy which is a consequence of unnoticed expulsion should be normal. In the absence of symptoms, an inert device that has perforated the uterus is usually best left alone and recovered after the confinement, but copper-loaded devices which have perforated the uterus should be removed as they cause peritoneal reaction and adhesions (Tatum, 1973; Newton *et al.*, 1974).

Many pregnancies occurring with a device in the uterus terminate in apparently spontaneous abortion in the first or second trimester. Lewit (1970) found that abortions occurred in 54% of pregnancies with devices that had a plastic tail or strings protruding through the cervix, compared with 43% abortions where a wholly intra-uterine tailless device was *in situ*. Vessey *et al.* (1974) found an abortion rate of 52% in women using Lippes loops or Saf-T-Coils. Snowden (1974a) observed an abortion rate of 58% amongst women becoming pregnant with a device *in situ*, and Steven and Fraser (1974) recorded a similar figure. It is difficult to be certain that some of these abortions were not caused by interference. Should the pregnancy continue with an inert or a copper device in place it is established that there is no increase in the incidence of congenital abnormality of the fetus (Tietze, 1968; Steven and Fraser, 1974; Snowden, 1976). It is very important to convey to the patient that if she does not miscarry, she may expect a normal baby. Pregnancy is usually uncomplicated, but we have noted an increased incidence of uterine bleeding, both before and after 28 weeks' maturity, without any particular ill-effects to mother or fetus.

Management

Opinions differ as to the advisability of trying to remove the device when pregnancy occurs. Alvior (1973) removed Lippes loops provided that the maturity of the pregnancy was less than three months, the threads were still visible at the cervical os and there was no undue resistance when traction was put on the strings. These are the cases where the loop is situated in the lower part of the uterus, well below the conceptus. Subsequent abortion occurred in only 30% of cases and this provides evidence that no particular harm results from removal under these specified conditions. The difference between this figure and the 40–60% abortion rate reported in practice is accounted for by exclusion of cases of threatened abortion, incomplete abortion, known interference and those where the thread was not visible. It does not provide evidence that removal tends to conserve the pregnancy, nor does the figure of 48% abortions which Alvior cites for cases where the device was left alone, since the selection of these cases differed and the potential for interference remained. Lewit (1970) found that with devices with tails or strings showing it made little difference to the outcome whether or not the device was removed. With tailless devices such as Gräfenberg rings or Birnberg bows, soundings, attempts at removal or successful removal increased the abortion rate to 82%. With the Dalkon shield, reputed to be a 'fundus-seeking' device, the abortion rate was increased from 52 to 86% by removal (Snowden, 1974a).

Following Christian's (1974) report of fatal cases of uterine sepsis occurring in pregnancies with Dalkon shields *in situ*, Templeton (1974) suggested that when a patient with one of these devices is found to be pregnant, it should promptly be removed by traction on the strings. Apart from the fact that this is likely to cause abortion — a rash procedure to conduct in a family planning clinic — it seems more likely to cause bleeding and sepsis than to prevent them (Hawkins, 1974). It has been confirmed in the United States of America that although very small, the risk of fatal septic abortion is increased if a device, particularly a Dalkon shield, is left *in situ* during pregnancy (Kahn and Tyler, 1975, 1976; Cates *et al.*, 1976). No confirmation of these observations has been obtained in Great Britain. Of 368 pregnant women with devices present, studied by Snowden (1974a), only two developed septic abortions; one was due to gonorrhoea and interference was suspected in the other. If the device is embedded in the softened uterus or has silently perforated the lower part of the uterus leaving the strings in the cervix, attempted removal may result in a serious laceration of the uterus. If an undiagnosed ectopic gestation is present, heavy bleeding may result from manipulation.

It seems therefore that during the first 12 weeks of pregnancy, no harm results from removing a Lippes loop by gentle traction on the strings, though if abortion subsequently occurs the patient may well think this was the cause. In other circumstances and particularly with tailless devices and Dalkon shields the pregnancy is most likely to continue normally if the device is left alone. If it is decided to continue with the pregnancy a high vaginal swab should be sent for culture and the patient instructed to report promptly if she develops symptoms of pyrexia or general malaise.

If the device is not identified at the confinement, ultrasonography, exploration of the uterus or hysterosalpingography during the puerperium may be necessary to verify that it is still in the uterus.

EXPULSION

Disappearance of the Transcervical Appendage

This is a common problem and may indicate expulsion unnoticed by the patient. The disappearance should always be confirmed by bimanual examination because the tails are sometimes palpable when they are not visible. In addition, careful exploration of the canal with a pair of artery forceps will sometimes reveal them. If this is the case and the patient is not pregnant, it is wise to replace the device, leaving the tails 5 cm long. The possibility that pregnancy has occurred, drawing the device up into the uterus, should be considered and if there is any doubt, further investigations should be postponed until a negative pregnancy test has been obtained. With careful aseptic precautions, passage of a sound may reveal the presence of the device in the uterine cavity, but this may not exclude partial perforation of the uterus. A single antero-posterior x-ray can confirm absence of the device from the pelvis and abdomen. If the device is seen, it is often difficult to determine whether or not it is in the uterus, even with the aid of a lateral film. Hysterosalpingography may be necessary to confirm that the device is intra-uterine by radiological means. Where ultrasonography is available, this is the best procedure for localising the device; if pregnancy has occurred then it will not be disturbed by ultrasonography.

Downward displacement of the device into the cervical canal may occur without complete expulsion. Even if the cause is pregnancy, it is then reasonable to remove the device, though the patient should be observed for a while after-wards and warned of the possibility of bleeding from the cervix.

Spontaneous Expulsion

The majority of spontaneous expulsions of the device take place within a few months of insertion, the expulsion rate steadily decreasing with increasing years of use (*Table 11.1*, p. 214), Expulsion is much commoner if the device has been inserted within four weeks of delivery; subsequently it is commoner at the time of menstruation. Large devices are less easily expelled. With Lippes loops the gross expulsion rates during the first two years found by Tietze and Lewit (1970) ranged from 26 to 13 per 100 users for sizes A to D respectively. Snowden's (1975) findings in Great Britain are similar (*Table 9.3*, p. 168). More rigid devices such as the Birnberg bow are less easily expelled but convey an increased risk of perforation of the uterus, though this is a much rarer event. Similar considerations apply to the 'fundus-seeking' devices such as the M device and the Dalkon shield. Expulsion rates are lower but perforations of the uterus are more common.

A number of factors have been found to be associated with spontaneous expulsion. The device is less likely to be expelled from older and more parous women. This may be related to the increased collagen content and decreased elasticity and contractility of the uterus. At the same time the uterine cavity is generally larger and able to accommodate the device more readily.

Bernard (1971) has investigated the rather complex interrelations between a history of therapeutic abortions, age, parity and the risk of expulsion. He was able to show that amongst women of low parity in Yugoslavia, the expulsion rate was least in those who had had two or three therapeutic abortions and greatest in those who had had either none or one, or who had had four or more abortions. His hypothesis to explain this finding was that up to three early pregnancies and abortions may make the uterus more tolerant of an internal foreign body; beyond that the damage caused by repeated surgical assaults on the cervix may affect its competence, permitting easier expulsion. Racial factors affect the situation — for example, expulsion rates are higher in Africans than in non-Africans living in the same area — and there are wide variations depending on geographic regions.

Management

According to Mishell (1974), after expulsion of a Lippes loop D, the patient has a 68% chance of retaining it if it is re-inserted, and after two expulsions she has a 34% chance of retaining the third device. Sobrero and Goldsmith (1973) state that the chances of repeated expulsion are two to three times higher than the chance of expulsion after a first insertion. Replacement with a larger device improves the chances of retention. We have examined the results of inserting Dalkon shields in women who have previously expelled another device (Bluett and Hawkins, 1974) and obtained greater success, but the shields are no longer available and the best device currently available for replacement after an expul-sion is probably a Wing Antigon (Monks, 1976). In our study there was no relation between the number of previous expulsions and whether or not the replacement shield was expelled, which led us to question the meaning of the concept of 'chronic expulsion'. It may be not so much that these women have a hyperactive uterus or lax cervix but that the shape of their uterine cavities is such that a device which fits well would have been retained in the first place. Although the rate of repeated expulsion was low, we did note a slightly higher pregnancy rate in these women who had expelled more than one device before.

BLEEDING

Following insertion, many patients experience slight bleeding for a few days. If a moderate loss persists for a week or if bleeding is heavy, they should be seen for review. Apart from checking the haemoglobin level and the extent of the blood loss, the possibilities of perforation of the uterus, of abortion of an unsuspected early pregnancy, of pelvic inflammatory disease or of intra-uterine pathology should be suspected. If bleeding is slight, the patient is not anaemic, and there are no pelvic findings suggesting pathology, an expectant policy may be pursued, with frequent review. Otherwise it may be desirable either to remove the device and await events or to admit the patient for examination under anaesthesia and curettage.

Menorrhagia

Intra-uterine devices tend to shorten the luteal phase of the menstrual cycle (Nygren and Johannsson, 1973). Brenner and Mishell (1975) have confirmed that in the presence of a device the onset of the menses can occur when plasma

Table 11.2 INFLUENCE OF INTRA-UTERINE DEVICES ON AVERAGE MENSTRUAL BLOOD LOSS (ml PER CYCLE) IN THREE ENVIRONMENTS (HEFNAWI *et al.*, 1974; ISRAEL *et al.*, 1974; LAUFE *et al.*, 1974)

	Cairo	California	Pennsylvania
Controls	37	–	21
Lippes loop	78	75	–
Copper 7	50	–	30
Copper T		54	–
Dalkon shield	–	60	62
Saf-T-Coil	–	–	45
Oral contraception	20	–	5

oestradiol and progesterone levels are higher than in control cycles. On average the menstrual loss is increased by between 50 and 200% (*Table 11.2*) and menstruation prolonged by two to four days (Ostergard and Broen, 1972). These figures give little idea of the proportion of women who suffer a blood loss which is sufficient to render continued use of a device unacceptable. The proportion of women who discontinue use of a device because of bleeding problems depends on the attitude of their physicians, the attitude of the patients and on the environment, and removal rates vary between nil and 15% during the first year of use. The proportion of women in whom an excessive loss is due to underlying uterine pathology is unknown.

We feel that there are dangers to the patient in the adoption of either the single-minded attitude of the physician with great enthusiasm for intra-uterine contraception or the *laissez-faire* attitude of some physicians who have wide experience of the use of devices. There is no doubt that chronically increased menstrual loss due to an intra-uterine device can cause anaemia (Zadeh *et al.*, 1967). This can be debilitating and can have particularly serious consequences among women who have poor diets or who live in areas with a high incidence of parasite infections. Undiagnosed pelvic inflammatory disease can prejudice the patient's future fertility. However rare, undiagnosed endometrial carcinoma can lead to a patient's death. On the other hand we appreciate that a formal curettage performed on every patient with an increased menstrual loss in association with a device would not be feasible, though there are those who would advocate the use of out-patient endometrial cytological examinations using endometrial brushes (Ayre, 1955), vacuum (Vabra) curettage (Jensen, 1970; Holt, 1970), endometrial lavage (Wachtel *et al.*, 1973) or endometrial cell sampling (Isaacs and Wilhoite, 1974) where these procedures are available.

In general, patients who report an increased but tolerable menstrual loss should have haemoglobin estimations in addition to a pelvic examination and vaginal cytology carried out at their follow-up visits. It is unusual for increased menstrual loss due to a device to return to normal whilst the device remains *in situ*. Those who are anaemic, who report a loss which they consider inconvenient or who describe a loss in terms of passage of clots, 'flooding' or use of towels, and which the physician considers to be a cause for concern, should have the device removed. A judgement must then be made on the basis of the patient's age, medical and gynaecological history and physical findings as to whether or not to recommend a diagnostic examination under anaesthesia and curettage. With younger patients who have only used the device for a few months and who have negative clinical and laboratory findings it may be reasonable to pursue an expectant policy, otherwise the device may be removed, alternative contraception advised as an interim measure, and, if the patient so wishes, a device less likely to cause menorrhagia (*Table 11.2*, p. 218) inserted at a later date. When a patient who has used a device satisfactorily for months develops a progressive or abrupt increase in menstrual loss, pathology should be suspected. When incomplete abortion, perforation of the uterus, pelvic inflammatory disease, ectopic gestation or malignancy are possible, or there is heavy bleeding, it is advisable to admit the patient to hospital with the device *in situ* and proceed accordingly.

It has been shown that functional menorrhagia caused by a device is associated with increased local fibrinolytic activity (Bonnar and Allington, 1974). In a number of studies it has been demonstrated that aminocaproic acid, 3 g four times a day by mouth during menstruation, will markedly reduce the blood loss. We have reservations about the use of aminocaproic acid in this context. There is a risk of masking intra-uterine pathology unless this has been excluded by curettage. The side-effects of aminocaproic acid are considerable — Kasonde and Bonnar (1975) found that 78% of patients experienced mild to moderate symptoms such as nausea, headache and dizziness. The mechanism of these effects, and the possible effects on renal function of long-term administration of an inhibitor of fibrinolysis are unknown. It seems quite unreasonable to administer an agent with symptomatic effects to treat a localised iatrogenic problem due to a device which is not essential to life or health, when the problem can be promptly cured by removal of the device and alternative contraceptive advice.

The best advice to the patient who continues to have menorrhagia following removal, curettage, exclusion of pathology and replacement with another device is to use a different contraceptive procedure. Nonetheless there are some women who have strong personal reasons for wishing to continue to use a device. It is sometimes possible to maintain their haemoglobin with a daily iron tablet, and it may be worth trying Clemetson and Blair's (1962) regime of iron, ascorbic acid and a vitamin P preparation such as hesperidin, rutin or hydroxyethylrutosides (Paroven). An alternative is the use of the oral prostaglandin synthetase inhibitor, mefenamic acid (Ponstan), 500 mg eight hourly, during menstruation (Guillebaud *et al.*, 1978). If the patient has, or develops, dyspepsia, mefenamic acid is contra-indicated.

Intermenstrual Bleeding

The patient whose only symptom is intermenstrual spotting or brown discharge during the first few months of use of a device should be examined to determine if there is vulvitis, vaginitis or cervicitis. A Papanicolaou smear and a cervical swab for bacteriological culture are taken and a saline preparation of vaginal secretion examined for trichomonads. If a bimanual examination reveals only a simple cervical erosion or a slightly bulky and tender uterus compatible with the presence of an intra-uterine device and no adnexal pathology, and the investigations are negative, then it is reasonable to reassure the patient and review the situation in three months.

Intermenstrual loss of fresh blood for more than a day or two, or prolongation of menstruation for much more than a week, require examination and investigation along lines similar to those employed in managing menorrhagia. Small episodes of bleeding, spotting or brown discharge are extremely common with an intra-uterine device, particularly during the first few months of use. Spotting or discharge may well be harmless. Development of intermenstrual bleeding in a previously asymptomatic patient should indicate the need for a careful review.

It has been shown that oral aminocaproic acid will reduce intermenstrual spotting after insertion of a device (Kullander, 1970) but we have the same reservations about its use in this way as we have with respect to menorrhagia.

PELVIC PAIN

The majority of patients experience some lower abdominal pain and backache resembling dysmenorrhoea after insertion of a device. If this does not wear off in an hour or two it is usually relieved by simple analgesics such as aspirin or paracetamol. If the pain does not respond or is preventing normal activities 24 hours after insertion, undiagnosed pelvic inflammatory disease, misplacement or partial expulsion of the device or perforation of the uterus should be suspected. If these can be excluded, the pain may be due to an unduly large device in a small uterus or one with high myometrial tonus or simply to anxiety and low pain threshold on the part of the patient. In any of these events it may be necessary to remove the device and advise alternative contraception or perform reinsertion at a later date, perhaps with a different device.

Some patients experience continuing low-grade pelvic discomfort and excessive dysmenorrhoea when a device is *in situ*. In the reports at the Second International Conference (Segal *et al.,* 1965), the incidence of complaints of pelvic pain varied from 4% to 58%. A decision must be made on management which should depend on the patient's values and not those of the physician! The patient may be sufficiently enamoured of the virtue of the device that she will tolerate a trivial discomfort. Otherwise, replacement with another type of device or alternative contraception should be considered.

If a patient who presents, either within a few days of insertion or at any time thereafter, with pelvic pain which has developed acutely or is of increasing severity, the cause may be partial or complete expulsion of the device, obvious on inspection with a vaginal speculum. If this is not the case and there is any chance of ectopic gestation, extensive pelvic examination should be deferred until the patient has been admitted to hospital and blood cross-matched. The differential diagnosis of pelvic inflammatory disease, ectopic gestation and perforation of the uterus should be considered. In some cases none of these will be considered likely and after 24 hours of observation the only physical findings will be uterine tenderness and vague adnexal tenderness but no adnexal swellings. The device should then be removed and the symptoms and signs may resolve completely within a day or two. Nonetheless, the possibility of missing an early ectopic gestation should not be ignored and the patient kept under observation as an out-patient until the risk is considered to be over.

With some patients presenting with the development of pelvic pain, the physician may be sufficiently confident of the absence of serious pathology that examination under anaesthesia, curettage and removal of the device after an interval of days or weeks may be reasonable.

VAGINAL DISCHARGE

Most patients with an intra-uterine device have a slight watery or mucoid leucorrhoea, often in association with a cervical erosion which is unlikely to heal whilst the strings remain in the cervix. Cervical erosions are particularly common in the presence of copper-containing devices (Rubinstein, 1974). The likely cause is the effect of copper on the growth of cervical epithelial cells, because concentrations of the ion comparable to those achieved in uterine secretion inhibits the growth of these cells in monolayer culture (Hounsell and Hawkins, 1974). If the increased secretion is a nuisance and no other cause can be found, the device should be removed, the erosion or 'endocervicitis' treated with the cryoprobe or by electrocautery, barrier contraception used as an interim measure, and the device replaced after a month or two, when the cervix has healed.

If vaginal discharge is noted, either by the patient or by the physician at a follow-up visit, it should always be investigated. Examination when the device was inserted should have excluded vaginitis and cervicitis at that time but a device presents no barrier to subsequent infection. Investigation should include examination of a saline suspension of secretion for trichomonads, vaginal and cervical cytological smears, culture of high vaginal swab for *Candida albicans* and other pathogens including anaerobic organisms, and examination of Gram-stained urethral and cervical smears for *Neisseria gonorrhoea*. History of an irregular liaison or presence of ulcerative lesions may indicate the need for a Wassermann or similar test for syphilis. If there are ulcerative or vesicular lesions of the cervix or vulva or an irritant vaginal discharge for which no other cause can be found, virus culture and serum agglutinations for *Herpesvirus hominis* type 2 infection may be needed. It is possible that copper-containing devices might predispose to virus infection – the copper ion facilitates entry of viruses into cells in tissue culture (Wyler and Wiesendanger, 1975). A history of non-specific urethritis in the consort may suggest virus infection in the female genital tract. Failure to account for vulval, vaginal or cervical lesions with these tests calls for a detailed gynaecological investigation for all the less common causes of disease of the lower genital tract.

Most of the causes of vaginitis mentioned can be treated with the device *in situ*, provided that there is no evidence of inflammatory disease of the uterus and adnexa. This may be difficult to ascertain in the presence of a severe trichomonal, candidal or herpetic infection. If symptoms are strictly local, there is no abdominal tenderness, and distinct adnexal tenderness cannot be felt at a bimanual one-finger vaginal or rectal pelvic examination then it is reasonable to treat the vaginitis first, and re-examine the pelvic organs when local tenderness has subsided. Gonorrhoea must be presumed to have involved the pelvic reproductive organs, and in our view, treatment should be initiated, the device removed after 24 or 48 hours, and then antibiotic treatment completed.

From time to time patients will be seen who are susceptible to recurrent or trichomonal infections. Having exhausted the diagnostic and therapeutic armamentarium on both the patient and her consort, one may be driven to the reluctant conclusion that a combination of the device and chronic cervicitis are contributing to the recurrences, perhaps by harbouring organisms in the cervix. It is then reasonable, as a last resort, to remove the device, treat the cervix, and advise barrier contraception, preferably together with an antiseptic spermicide.

PELVIC INFLAMMATORY DISEASE

It is likely that, in common with the other side-effects of intra-uterine devices, the occurrence of this problem has changed little since the time of Gräfenberg (Hawkins, 1973). What has changed is the ability to treat the infections consequent on insertion of a foreign body into the uterus. The availability of antibiotics was a major reason for the resurgence of interest in intra-uterine contraception which occurred in the 1960s.

The incidence of acute episodes of pelvic inflammatory disease following insertion of a device can vary between 1 and 2% in selected high-income patients and between 8 and 10% in indigent and other populations where the incidence of pre-existing chronic pelvic inflammatory disease is high, when other variables are comparable (Willson *et al.*, 1967). The majority of these infections are probably exacerbations of quiescent chronic pelvic inflammatory disease, often previously undiagnosed. This seems clear as the incidence of pelvic infection is less well related to method of contraception employed than it is to the characteristics of the population studied. A few infections are due to careless aseptic and anti-septic technique at insertion or to insertion through an infected cervix. The vaginal cavity and cervix are impossible to sterilise completely and a few infections must result from the inevitable carriage of vaginal saprophytes into the uterus. In general, bacteria from the endocervix introduced into the endometrial cavity with insertion are soon eliminated, the uterine cavity becoming sterile again within 30 days (Mishell *et al.,* 1966). The migration of white cells into the cavity which takes place in response to the device (Moyer *et al.,* 1970) doubtless plays a part in eliminating bacteria, and an increased serum immunoglobulin response has also been found (Holub *et al.,* 1971; Gump *et al.,* 1973). Fortunately, pelvic infections with *Clostridia* do not seem to occur after insertion of a device, though these organisms are not uncommon in the vagina; serious post-insertion infections with *β-haemolytic streptococcus,* Group A and particularly Group B, or *bacteroides sp.* are seen from time to time.

In some populations it is clear that pelvic infection arising *de novo* two months or more after insertion of a device may often be due to gonorrhoea or is otherwise related to intercourse. In other areas, where the causes of pelvic inflammatory disease are less well defined, there is little evidence that the presence of a device affects the patterns of infection predisposed to by debility, chronic ill health or other factors. Burnhill (1973) believes that a progressive endometritis leading to serious pelvic infection can arise from the presence of a device.

Management is that of pelvic inflammatory disease. A high vaginal swab is taken for culture, and in severe cases blood cultures performed. Full-dose antibiotic therapy is instituted promptly without waiting for the bacteriological results, and modified only if the patient fails to respond or if an unusual organism is isolated. The manifestations of severe and spreading infection are treated appropriately.

In our opinion the device should be removed at once in mild and moderate infections, or after 24 hours of antibiotic therapy in severe infections. It has been claimed by a number of workers that pelvic infection can be treated effectively with the device in place. We feel that this contradicts the basic principle of extracting a readily removable and dispensable foreign body from an inflammatory situation. Patients who elect to use intra-uterine devices are expecting to have a pregnancy at some future date, and they should not be exposed to management that might delay resolution of the infection, with subsequent chronic inflammatory disease and impaired fertility.

Severe and Unusual Infections

One-third of hospital admissions for intra-uterine device complications are for infection (Huber *et al.,* 1975). Pelvic infection associated with intra-uterine devices can proceed to tubo-ovarian abscess, appendicitis, pelvic peritonitis, pelvic abscess, general peritonitis or septicaemia. In the 1967 American College of Obstetricians and Gynecologists' survey, two-thirds of the cases of critical illness associated with devices were due to pelvic inflammatory disease and seven of the ten deaths involved pelvic infection (Scott, 1968).

Schiffer *et al.* (1975) in New York have reported ten cases of actinomycosis of the female genital tract associated with use of devices.

PERFORATION OF THE UTERUS

The glib statement that 'all perforations occur at insertion' is often made. When cases are produced where a device has been demonstrated to lie in the uterus and is subsequently found in the abdomen, it is then said that 'perforations either occur or are initiated at insertion'. When it is known that 80% of some devices are embedded in the myometrium at insertion but overall only about 0.1% perforate, the amended comment loses its significance, as embedding at insertion clearly does not necessarily predispose to perforation.

The majority of perforations do occur at insertion; some of these are incomplete, the device later migrating or being expelled through the uterine wall. Some devices damage the wall of the uterine cavity at insertion, and some of these become partly embedded in the uterine wall. These are sometimes detected by hysterosalpingography; more commonly by difficulty in removal. Some devices which lie under tension within a uterine cavity to whose contours they are not well adapted probably erode the endometrium and become embedded later. In a small proportion of cases subsequent migration through the wall, perhaps aided by myometrial contractions associated with menstruation, leads to perforation. It is possible that the occurrence of a pregnancy with a device *in situ* may assist migration, though in most cases of 'pregnancy perforation' the perforation has preceded the pregnancy.

Incidence

In the Co-operative Statistical Program (Tietze and Lewit, 1970) this varied from nil with spirals and Saf-T-Coils to 0.1% with Lippes loops and 1.2% with bows. In 29 of the 49 patients concerned the discovery of the perforation was associated with a pregnancy. The high figure for bows, in conjunction with the fact that the bow is a closed loop and thus capable of strangulating bowel if it does perforate, was largely responsible for the decline in its popularity.

There is a tendency for perforations to be underreported. This is partly because patients fitted with a device in a family planning clinic are commonly dealt with in an acute hospital unit elsewhere; other perforations are asymptomatic and may not be identified. Perforation rates as high as 0.7–0.9% for Lippes loops were found in Singapore (Kanagaratnam, 1968; Ratnam and Yin, 1968).

At times the data has suggested that 'fundus-seeking' devices such as the M device and the Dalkon shield had particularly high perforation rates, contrasting with reduced rates of spontaneous expulsion. The M device was withdrawn from the Pathfinder Fund programme because of a perforation rate of 0.23% in Great Britain (Hawkins, 1970). On the other hand, in the more recent Exeter studies (Snowden, 1974a), the perforation rates found were: Lippes loops 0.11%, Dalkon shields 0.08%, Copper 7's 0.05%. Both the M device and the Dalkon shield were associated with new methods of insertion; withdrawal of a guard tube in the first case and thrusting the device through cervix on a supporting rod in the second. It is likely that some of the perforations recorded with these devices were due to inadequate training in insertion techniques.

In summary it seems that the perforation rate for intra-uterine devices in the hands of trained physicians should not be higher than 0.3% (Snowden *et al.*, 1977).

Factors Predisposing to Perforation

We consider that nulliparous patients with a history of severe spasmodic dysmenorrhoea, patients who have recently had several pregnancies in rapid succession, grande multiparae, patients over 40 years of age, those with a history of either expulsion or pregnancy with a previous device, those with a retroverted uterus, those with a uterine scar from a Caesarean section or a plastic repair of the uterus and those with a soft bulky uterus after an abortion or confinement constitute groups where the small risk of perforation is somewhat increased; insertion should be conducted with caution by an experienced physician. Scrupulous follow-up procedures should be applied to these patients. Patients with uterine fibromyomata or with a history of pelvic inflammatory disease are high risk groups; in both of these situations alternative contraception should be seriously considered because of the associated hazards of intra-uterine devices.

As a matter of general principle, particular care should also be taken where there is difficulty in defining the uterus bimanually, where the patient does not relax well and where there is difficulty in negotiating the cervix. In these three circumstances the alternative of insertion under general anaesthesia should be considered. Whether or not the use of a uterine sound or of a vulsellum on the cervix prevent or predispose to perforation is a point on which opinions differ widely. What is clear is that the experience of the physician and the care and diligence with which he applied the training he has received and the insertion instructions for the device he is using are of great importance in reducing the risk of perforation.

Diagnosis. Observations suggesting the possibility of perforation include difficulty, sudden pain or bleeding at insertion; subsequent episodes of pain, bleeding or pelvic sepsis; or the occurrence of pregnancy; all associated with disappearance of the strings. Many perforations are silent, the only sign being asymptomatic disappearance of the strings. On the other hand, perforation of the lower part of the uterus can occasionally occur, leaving the tail of the device *in situ* in the uterus.

If perforation is suspected, and there is nothing to suggest pregnancy, probing the uterine cavity with a sterile sound may reveal the device to be normally situated. There is a slight risk of introducing infection if the probing is extensive, and the patient should be reviewed a few days later to check that all is well; if the strings are absent, replacement of the device may be desirable, leaving the strings of the new device fairly long for a few weeks.

In most cases of suspected perforation the most valuable investigation is an ultrasound B-scan. This enables exact location of the device in relation to the uterus. If diagnostic ultrasound is not available, a straight x-ray of the abdomen will in general only indicate whether or not the device has been expelled or has left the pelvis to lie in mid or upper abdomen. If the device is still in the pelvis it can be very difficult to decide if it is intra- or extra-uterine, even with the aid of lateral or oblique views. Hysterography with a radio-opaque medium instilled into the uterine cavity is then required for localisation

If the patient is pregnant, ultrasound is again the best diagnostic manoeuvre.

If it is not available, antero-posterior and lateral x-rays convey no proven risk to the fetus and may enable localisation. Sometimes the device will be visualised in the pelvis without it being possible to determine its exact location. If the patient is asymptomatic and it is intended that the pregnancy continue, most obstetricians will adopt a conservative approach, seeing the patient fairly frequently and requesting her to report promptly if any untoward symptoms develop. There are small risks of sepsis, haemorrhage and amniotic fluid infusion with this approach, but unless removal of the device before delivery is determined upon, further diagnostic procedures might as well be left until after the confinement.

Management

There is little doubt that a closed-ring device which has perforated the uterus should be removed promptly because of the risk of bowel strangulation. Similarly, a copper device should be removed because of the severe peritoneal reaction it can cause (Tatum, 1973; Newton *et al.,* 1974). It is our view that all devices which perforate the uterus should be removed surgically. The urgency of the situation will be dictated by the symptomatology and any complications of the perforation. Some gynaecologists feel that an asymptomatic perforation should be managed expectantly. We cannot support this view. Many of the cases of peritonitis associated with intra-uterine devices have been due to previously asymptomatic perforation. One of the ten fatal cases reported by Scott (1968) was associated with perforation followed sometime later by peritonitis; two others with perforation, subsequent pregnancy, and amniotic fluid infusion at the confinement.

If a device which has perforated is palpable *per vaginam*, it may often be removed by anterior or posterior colpotomy. Sometimes the device will move out of reach if a formal colpotomy is conducted. If the device can be felt immediately deep to the vaginal skin where a small incision can be made directly onto it at any point not involving bladder or rectum, this should be done and the device firmly grasped at once with forceps before it moves away. The least traumatic route for extracting it can then be decided at leisure. If the device can be felt in the pouch of Douglas but readily moves upwards, an abdominal approach may give less trouble.

The laparoscope is a most valuable instrument for visualising a device and assisting with its removal from the abdominal cavity. Having localised the device, it is simple to make a tiny secondary flank incision, introduce a large pair of forceps and remove the device by that route under direct laparoscopic vision. Attempts at removal along the laparoscope cannula can be traumatic and sometimes unsuccessful.

If resort has to be made to laparotomy for removal it is helpful to obtain an accurate localisation with an ultrasound scan shortly before. Failing this, antero-posterior and lateral localising x-rays can be taken with the patient on the operating table. It is a distressing experience to venture on laparotomy to recover a device and then to have to close the abdomen without having found it!

ECTOPIC GESTATION

The incidence of ectopic gestation in patients who become pregnant with an intra-uterine device *in situ* has been reported as 1 in 23 by the Co-operative

Statistical Program, based on 23 917 patients, mainly in the United States of America, of whom 783 became pregnant with a device in the uterus (Tietze and Lewit, 1970). The comparable figure based on 16 180 insertions in Great Britain is 1 in 27 (Snowden, 1974b), corresponding to about 0.06 ectopic pregnancies per 100 woman-years in the first year of use (Snowden, personal communication, 1977). About one-ninth of the ectopic gestations are ovarian pregnancies (Lehfeldt *et al.*, 1970).

Ectopic gestation is a potentially lethal condition which was responsible for 12 maternal deaths per year in England and Wales, 1970–1972, accounting for 10% of the total maternal deaths directly due to pregnancy (Arthure *et al.*, 1975). It is therefore of the utmost importance that the symptoms and signs of ectopic gestation be borne in mind at all times by physicians supervising intra-uterine device patients and by gynaecologists who see these patients when complications arise.

At the present time there is no evidence that intra-uterine devices *cause* ectopic gestation. The devices prevent intra-uterine implantation but cannot be expected to prevent ectopic gestation effectively, and this accounts for the high relative incidence of tubal pregnancy if patients wearing a device conceive. The high relative incidence of ovarian pregnancy amongst those who do have an ectopic gestation suggests that the devices do have some effect in preventing tubal pregnancy but none in preventing ovarian pregnancy (Lehfeldt *et al.*, 1970).

It has recently been contended that intra-uterine devices can cause ectopic gestation. In England and Wales, over the last few years, the ectopic gestation incidence in the general population lay between 0.28 and 0.38 per 1000 women of reproductive age per year (Beral, 1975). It is a reasonable assumption that only half these women are exposed to sexual activity and that at least half of these are using either barrier or oral contraception which preclude the opportunity to achieve an ectopic gestation. The ectopic gestation incidence in the 'at risk' group, the great majority of which are not users of devices, is of the order of 1.1–1.5 per 1000 per year. In known users of intra-uterine devices the ectopic gestation rate is 0.5–2.0 per 1000 per year (assuming a pregnancy rate of 2 to 4 per 100 woman-years). There is thus no evidence that in Great Britain devices have any more effect than to prevent intra-uterine pregnancy. The increased incidence of ectopic gestation which has been observed since 1970 (Beral, 1975) is likely to be due to the aftermath of the Abortion Act, 1967, the chronic inflammatory sequelae of therapeutic abortion.

The overall incidence of ectopic gestation is much increased in large urban communities with high proportions of non-white and low socio-economic status inhabitants (Erhardt and Jacobzmer, 1956; Lehfeldt *et al.*, 1970). This is presumably partly due to pelvic inflammatory disease. The incidence of ectopic gestation in users of intra-uterine devices must be expected to be correspondingly increased in such populations.

Diagnosis and Management

Diagnosis calls for an increased index of suspicion engendered by the knowledge that the patient has an intra-uterine device and readiness to advise hospital admission, laparoscopy or laparotomy when indicated. Management is that of the ectopic gestation. It is rash to attempt removal of the device before the diagnosis is made laparoscopically, as heavy bleeding can be initiated.

DISCOMFORT TO HUSBAND

Occasionally husbands complain of penile discomfort during intercourse, attributing this to the device. Tietze and Lewit (1970) quote a removal rate of 0.1 per 100 woman-years for this reason with Lippes loops and Saf-T-Coils. With Margulies spirals, which had a rigid plastic stem lying in the cervical canal, the removal rate for husband discomfort was much higher, 2.4 per 100 woman-years. Actual abrasions or lacerations of the penis have been reported but they are very rare.

Sometimes when the patient's husband has complained it will be found that there has been some downward displacement of the device and its stem is palpable in the cervical canal. Removal and replacement with another device such as a smaller Lippes loop or a device such as an Antigon which has no downward stem will solve this problem. If only the strings are palpable they can sometimes be shortened with symptomatic relief.

It must be borne in mind when this complaint is made that the husband sometimes has another reason for avoiding intercourse or wishing for the device to be removed which he has not shared with his consort.

CANCER

There is no evidence that intra-uterine devices cause carcinoma *in situ* or invasive carcinoma of the cervix or that they cause carcinoma of the endometrium.

In Israel, Oppenheimer (1959) conducted a study in which women continued the use of a Gräfenberg ring for 10 to 20 years without finding any case of cancer. In Japan, Hata *et al.* (1969) reported a study of over 10 000 women screened for uterine cancer. Of these 1333 had intra-uterine devices and about half of these had used the device for at least five years. There was no increased incidence of carcinoma *in situ* or invasive cancer in the women with devices and no case of endometrial cancer was detected. With women who had dysplasia of the cervix, Richart and Barron (1967) showed that wearing a device did not increase the chance that the disorder would progress to carcinoma *in situ*.

Patients with devices are susceptible to regular cancer-screening in relation to their follow-up visits. In nearly 24 000 patients recorded by the Cooperative Statistical Program during six years, 71 cases of carcinoma were reported, of which 46 were known to be carcinoma *in situ* and five invasive cancer. In the first *month* of use, the detection rate was 2.02 per 100 woman-years – the result of the screening examination conducted at the time of insertion. Over the next six years the detection rate remained steadily at about 0.08 per 100 woman-years, an average figure for patients in the reproductive age group after primary screening.

MORTALITY ASSOCIATED WITH INTRA-UTERINE DEVICES

The commonest causes of fatality associated with intra-uterine devices have not changed in character since the days of stem pessaries and Gräfenberg rings, though with better patient supervision, antibiotics and intensive care a fatal outcome should now be very rare. All the deaths reviewed by the American Medical Association Committee on Contraceptive Practices in 1937 were due to peritonitis or septicaemia; some were secondary to perforations. The majority were due to stem pessaries, rather than rings. Of the ten deaths reported by Scott in 1968, four were due to sepsis occurring within a few days of insertion, three to sepsis of later onset, one of these following a perforation. The remaining three deaths were associated with pregnancy, one with a septic abortion, the other two with perforation and amniotic fluid infusion at the time of the confinement. Of the 39 deaths identified by the United States Food and Drug Administration (Jennings, 1974), 35 were due to sepsis, 18 of these being septic abortions.

Cates *et al.* (1976) noted that all of 50 deaths from septic abortion associated with intra-uterine devices occurred after the 11th week of gestation. Most of the women who died with a device in place complained of fever as the initial symptom. The onset of the illness with septicaemia contrasts with that in the customary form of septic abortion, which tends to start with uterine pain and bleeding. The number of cases where the sepsis was a result of interference is quite unknown.

Meeker (1969) estimated an overall mortality from intra-uterine contraception of 20 per million users per year, based on the American College of Obstetricians and Gynecologists' survey (Scott, 1968). The United States Department of Health, Education and Welfare (1974) was more optimistic, estimating between one and ten deaths per million users per year. The risk is probably about the same as that associated with currently available combined oral contraceptives and about a tenth of that arising from the consequences of unprotected intercourse.

REFERENCES

ALVIOR, G.T. (1973). Pregnancy outcome with removal of intrauterine device. *Obstet. Gynec., N.Y.,* **41**, 894–896

AMERICAN MEDICAL ASSOCIATION COMMITTEE ON CONTRACEPTIVE PRACTICES (1937). Dangers of Gomco intra-uterine silver ring. *J. Am. med. Ass.,* **108**, 413

ARTHURE, H., TOMKINSON, J., ORGANE, Sir G., LEWIS, E.M., ADELSTEIN, A.M. and WEATHERALL, J.A.C. (1975). Report on confidential enquiries into maternal deaths in England and Wales 1970–1972. *D.H.S.S. Rep. Hlth soc. Subj.,* No. 11. Her Majesty's Stationery Office, London

AYRE, J.E. (1955). Rotating endometrial brush: new technic for the diagnosis of fundal carcinoma. *Obstet. Gynec., N.Y.,* **5**, 137–141

BERAL, V. (1975). An epidemiological study of recent trends in ectopic pregnancy. *Br. J. Obstet. Gynaec.,* **82**, 775–782

BERNARD, R.R. (1971). Factors governing IUD performance. *Am. J. publ. Hlth,* **61**, 559–567

BLUETT, D.G. and HAWKINS, D.F. (1974). The use of the Dalkon shield among users with previous unsuccessful experience with other IUDs. *See* Snowden, R. and Williams, M. (1974). *Family Planning Research Unit Report No. 12,* pp. 11–19. University of Exeter

BONNAR, J. and ALLINGTON, M. (1974). Cited by Kasonde, J.M. and Bonnar, J. (1975). *Br. med. J.*, **iv**, 17–19

BRENNER, P.F. and MISHELL, D.R. Jr. (1975). Progesterone and oestradiol patterns in women using an intrauterine contraceptive device. *Obstet. Gynec., N.Y.*, **46**, 456–459

BURNHILL, M.S. (1973). Syndrome of progressive endometritis associated with intrauterine contraceptive devices. *Adv. planned Parenthood*, **8**, 144–150

CATES, W. Jr., ORY, H.W., ROCHAT, R.W. and TYLER, C.W. Jr. (1976). The intrauterine device and deaths from spontaneous abortion. *New Engl. J. Med.*, **295**, 1155–1159

CHRISTIAN, C.D. (1974). Maternal deaths associated with an intrauterine device. *Am. J. Obstet. Gynec.*, **119**, 441–444

CLEMETSON, C.A.B. and BLAIR, L.M. (1962). Capillary strength of women with menorrhagia. *Am. J. Obstet. Gynec.*, **83**, 1269–1279

ERHARDT, C.L. and JACOBZINER, H. (1956). Ectopic pregnancies and spontaneous abortions in New York City — incidence and characteristics. *Am. J. publ. Hlth*, **46**, 828–835

GUILLEBAUD, J., ANDERSON, A.B.M. and TURNBULL, A.C. (1978). Reduction by mefenamic acid of increased menstrual blood loss associated with intrauterine contraception. *Br. J. Obstet. Gynaec.*, **85**, 53–62

GUMP, D.W., MEAD, P.B., HORTON, E.L., LAMBORN, K.R. and FORSYTH, B.R. (1973). Intrauterine contraceptive device and increased serum immunoglobulin levels. *Obstet. Gynec., N.Y.*, **41**, 259–264

HATA, Y., ISHIHAMA, A., KUDO, N., NAKAMURA, Y., MIYAI, T., MAKINO, T. and KAGABU, T. (1969). The effect of long-term use of IUD. *Acta obstet. gynec. jap.*, **16**, 73–78

HAWKINS, D.F. (1970). *Perforation of the uterus by M-213 devices in Great Britain. Report to the Medical Advisory Committee*, Pathfinder Fund, Boston

HAWKINS, D.F. (1973). On-going studies with the Dalkon shield in special situations. *Dalkon Shield Symposium. London, October 11th, 1972*, pp. 14–16. Ed. Templeton, J.S. A.H. Robins, Horsham, Sussex

HAWKINS, D.F. (1974). Septic abortion and the Dalkon shield. *Br. med. J.*, **iii**, 113–114

HEFNAWI, F., ASKALAMI, H. and ZAKI, K. (1974). Menstrual blood loss with copper intrauterine devices. *Contraception*, **9**, 133–139

HOLT, E.M. (1970). Out-patient diagnostic curettage. *J. Obstet. Gynaec. Br. Commonw.*, **77**, 1043–1046

HOLUB, W.R., REYNER, F.C. and FORMAN, G.H. (1971). Increased levels of serum immunoglobulins G and M in women using intrauterine contraceptive devices. *Am. J. Obstet. Gynec.*, **110**, 362–365

HOUNSELL, P.G. and HAWKINS, D.F. (1974). Effect of copper on growth of human cervical epithelial cells in tissue culture. *J. Obstet. Gynaec. Br. Commonw.*, **81**, 712–718

HUBER, S.C., PIOTROW, P.T., ORLANS, B. and KOMMER, G. (1975). IUDs reassessed — a decade of experience. *Population Reports*, series B, number 2, 21–48

ISAACS, J.H. and WILHOITE, R.W. (1974). Aspiration cytology of the endometrium: office and hospital sampling procedures. *Am. J. Obstet. Gynec.*, **118**, 679–687

ISRAEL, R., SHAW, S.T. Jr. and MARTIN, M.A. (1974). Comparative quantitation of menstrual blood loss with the Lippes loop, Dalkon shield and Copper T intrauterine devices. *Contraception*, **10**, 63–71

JENNINGS, J. (1974). Report of safety and efficacy of the Dalkon shield and other IUDs. Cited by Huber, S.C., Piotrow, P.T., Orlans, F.B. and Kommer, G. (1975). *Population Reports*, series B, number 2, p. 36

JENSEN, J.G. (1970). Vacuum curettage. Out-patient curettage without anaesthesia. *Dan. med. Bull.*, **17**, 199–202

KAHN, H.S. and TYLER, C.W. Jr. (1975). Mortality associated with the use of IUDs. *J. Am. med. Ass.*, **234**, 57–59

KAHN, H.S. and TYLER, C.W. Jr. (1976). An association between the Dalkon shield and complicated pregnancies among women hospitalized for intrauterine contraceptive device-related disorders. *Am. J. Obstet. Gynec.*, **125**, 83–86

KANAGARATNAM, K. (1968). Singapore: the national family planning program. *Stud. Fam. Plann.*, number 28, 1–11

KASONDE, J.M. and BONNAR, J. (1975). Aminocaproic acid and menstrual loss in women using intrauterine devices. *Br. med. J.*, **iv**, 17–19

KULLANDER, S. (1970). Experiences with an IUCD (Margulie's coil). *Fert. Steril.*, **21**, 482–489

LAUFE, L.E., GIBAR, Y., McCLANAHAN, B.J. and WHEELER, R.F. (1974). Volume and copper concentration of menstrual discharge from women employing Copper-7 and other types of contraceptive. *Adv. planned Parenthood*, **9**, 38–42

LEHFELDT, H., TIETZE, C. and GORSTEIN, F. (1970). Ovarian pregnancy and the intrauterine device. *Am. J. Obstet. Gynec.*, **108**, 1005–1009

LEWIT, S. (1970). Outcome of pregnancy with intrauterine devices. *Contraception*, **2**, 47–57

MEEKER, C.I. (1969). Use of drugs and intrauterine devices for birth control. *New Engl. J. Med.*, **280**, 1058–1060

MISHELL, D.R. Jr. (1974). Current status of contraceptive steroids and the intrauterine device. *Clin. Obstet. Gynec.*, **17**, 35–51

MISHELL, D.R. Jr., BELL, J.H., GOOD, R.G. and MOYER, D.L. (1966). The intrauterine device: a bacteriological study of the endometrial cavity. *Am. J. Obstet. Gynec.*, **96**, 119–126

MONKS, I. (1976). The current state of IUCDs. *J. mat. Child Hlth*, August, 10–15

MOYER, D.L., MISHELL, D.R. and BELL, J. (1970). Reactions of human endometrium to the intrauterine device. 1. Correlation of the endometrial histology with the bacterial environment of the uterus following short-term insertion of the IUD. *Am. J. Obstet. Gynec.*, **106**, 799–809

NEWTON, J. ELIAS, J., McEWAN, J. and MANN, G. (1974). Intrauterine contraception with the Copper-7: evaluation after two years. *Br. med. J.*, **iii**, 447–450

NYGREN, K. G. and JOHANSSON, E.D.B. (1973). Premature onset of menstrual bleeding during ovulatory cycles in women with an intrauterine contraceptive device. *Am. J. Obstet. Gynec.*, **117**, 971–975

OPPENHEIMER, W. (1959). Prevention of pregnancy by the Gräfenberg ring method. A re-evaluation after 28 years' experience. *Am. J. Obstet. Gynec.*, **78**, 446–454

ORLANS, F.B. (1973). Intrauterine devices. Copper IUDs: performance to date. *Population Reports*, series B, number 1, 1–20

OSTERGARD, D.R. and BROEN, E.M. (1972). Clinical experience with the Dalkon shield. *Advances in Planned Parenthood, Vol. 7. Proceedings of the 9th Annual Meeting of the American Association of Planned Parenthood*

Physicians, Kansas City, Missouri, April 5–6, 1971, pp. 81–83. Ed. Sobrero, A.J. and Harvey, R.M. Excerpta Medica, Amsterdam

RATNAM, S.S. and YIN, J.C.K. (1968). Translocation of Lippes loop (the missing loop). *Br. med. J.*, i, 612–614

RICHART, R.M. and BARRON, B.A. (1967). The intrauterine device and cervical neoplasia. *J. Am. med. Ass.*, **199**, 817–819

RUBINSTEIN, E. (1974). The copper-7 device in chronic and IUD-induced acute cervicitis treated with oral estriol. *Contraception*, **10**, 673–681

SCHIFFER, M.A., ELGUEZABAL, A., SULTANA, M. and ALLEN, A.C. (1975). Actinomycosis infections associated with intrauterine contraceptive devices. *Obstet. Gynec., N.Y.*, **45**, 67–72

SCOTT, R.B. (1968). Critical illnesses and deaths associated with intrauterine devices. *Obstet. Gynec., N.Y.*, **31**, 322–327

SEGAL, S.J., SOUTHAM, A.J. and SHAFER, K.D. (1965). Editors, *Intra-uterine Contraception. Proceedings of the Second International Conference October 2–3, 1964, New York City. Excerpta Medica International Congress Series No. 86.* Excerpta Medica, Amsterdam

SIVIN, I. (1976). A comparison of the Copper T-200 and the Lippes loop in four countries. *Stud. Fam. Plann.*, **7**, 115–123

SNOWDEN, R. (1974a). Pelvic inflammation, perforation and pregnancy outcome associated with the use of IUDs. *Family Planning Research Unit Report No. 15*, pp. 1–6. University of Exeter

SNOWDEN, R. (1974b). An enquiry into ectopic pregnancy and the intrauterine device. *Family Planning Research Unit Report No. 11*, pp. 1–14. University of Exeter

SNOWDEN, R. (1975). Recent studies in intrauterine devices: a reappraisal. *J. biosoc. Sci.* **7**, 367–375

SNOWDEN, R. (1976). IUD and congenital malformation. *Br. med. J.*, i, 770

SNOWDEN, R., WILLIAMS, M. and HAWKINS, D. (1977). *The IUD. A Practical Guide.* Croom Helm, London

SOBRERO, A.J. and GOLDSMITH, A. (1973). *Intrauterine Devices. A Manual for Clinical Practice*, Ed. Cosby, M.L., p. 4. Pathfinder Fund, Boston

STEVEN, J.D. and FRASER, I.S. (1974). The outcome of pregnancy after failure of an intrauterine device. *J. Obstet. Gynaec. Br. Commonw.*, **81**, 282–284

TATUM, H.J. (1973). Metallic copper as an intrauterine contraceptive agent. *Am. J. Obstet. Gynec.*, **117**, 602–618

TEMPLETON, R.S. (1974). Septic abortion and the Dalkon shield. *Br. med. J.*, ii, 612

TIETZE, C. (1968). Fertility after discontinuation of intrauterine and oral contraception. *Int. J. Fert.*, **13**, 385–389

TIETZE, C. and LEWIT, S. (1970). Evaluation of intrauterine devices: ninth progress report of the Cooperative Statistical Program. *Stud. Fam. Plann.*, **55**, 1–40

UNITED STATES DEPARTMENT OF HEALTH, EDUCATION AND WELFARE, CENTER FOR DISEASE CONTROL (1974). IUD safety: report of a nationwide physician survey. *Morbidity and Mortality*, **23**, 226–231

VESSEY, M.P., JOHNSON, B., DOLL, R. and PETO, R. (1974). Outcome of pregnancy in women using an intrauterine device. *Lancet*, i, 495–498

WACHTEL, E., GORDON, H. and WYCHERLEY, J. (1973). The cytological diagnosis of endometrial pathology using a uterine aspiration technique. *J. Obstet. Gynaec. Br. Commonw.*, **80**, 164–168

WILLSON, J.R., LEDGER, W.J. and LOVELL, J. (1967). Intrauterine contraceptive devices: a comparison between their use in indigent and private patients. *Obstet. Gynec., N.Y.,* **29**, 59–66

WYLER, R. and WIESENDANGER, W. (1975). The enhancing effect of copper, nickel and cobalt ions on plaque formation by Semliki Forest Virus (SFV) in chicken embryo fibroblasts. *Archs Virol.,* **47**, 57–69

ZADEH, J.A., KARABUS, C.D. and FIELDING, J. (1967). Haemoglobin concentration and other values in women using an intrauterine device or taking corticosteroid contraceptive pills. *Br. med. J.,* **iv**, 708–711

ZIPPER, J., MEDEL, M. PASTENE, L. and RIVERA, M. (1973). Factors that limit the efficacy of copper-carrying IUDs. In *Intrauterine Devices. Development, Evaluation and Program Implementation,* pp. 235–241. Ed. Wheeler, R.G., Duncan, G.W. and Speidel, J.J. Academic Press, New York

Part IV
Legal Abortion

12 Abortion Counselling

The need for abortion seems to be a product of current civilisation which has to be accepted. The majority of countries have recognised this by liberalising their abortion laws to some degree during the last decade.

There is ample evidence that this need is generated by the pressures of society in developed countries. The fact that there is no demand for abortion in communities in the West Indies and some southern states in the United States of America, where illegitimacy carries no stigma, proves this point. Free abortion has a much more dramatic effect on birth rates than contraceptive advice programmes (Potts, 1967; Tietze, 1969; Potts, 1970; Jurukovski and Sukarov, 1971; Kotasek, 1971; Gordon, 1972; Tietze and Murstein, 1975) and countries with a population problem have found it politically expedient, at least tacitly, to support increased facilities for abortion.

The idea that the increasing responsibility of women is expressed by liberalising the availability of abortion was pilloried years ago by Dr Elizabeth Tylden, who said, 'How can you expect a woman who has just displayed her complete irresponsibility by acquiring an unwanted pregnancy to be treated as a wholly responsible individual?' This is only one reason why the legal responsibility for making decisions about abortion has devolved on to the medical profession. The main reason is that members of the public at large are aware that abortion is either wrong or at least a medically and psychologically unsatisfactory solution to social problems and yet they want to have the process available as an expedient. The traditional recipients of the problems that such conflicts create are the Church, the State and the medical profession. The Church is faced with the difficulty that it cannot enforce its views without losing its adherents; most politicians who are the executives of the State are similarly reluctant to accept the label of 'abortionist' in relation to the next election. It has therefore fallen to the medical profession to bear the public conscience by accepting the responsibility for decisions as to whether or not an abortion shall be carried out.

This responsibility has been accepted by the profession as the least of several evils. If abortion is to be available it is best that it be conducted by doctors in the safest environment. The very marked decrease in morbidity and mortality resulting from illegal abortion since the Abortion Act became law in Great Britain in 1967 is good evidence for this. If abortion is to be conducted by doctors within a legal framework, it is reasonable that those who perform the operation should have the responsibility of assessing whether or not the individual case is justified by the law and whether or not the operation is in the best

237

interests of the patient. If the legal framework permitting the abortion is phrased, as is the case in Great Britain, in a form requiring medical judgements, then it is implicit that doctors must be involved in making the decisions. Abortions have their sequelae, medical and psychological as well as social, and it is desirable that those who have to repair the damage should be involved at an earlier stage.

Few doctors are happy with those aspects of society which produce the need for abortion; fewer still are satisfied with an environment which generates defects in motivation to employ effective contraceptive measures. Be that as it may, whatever long-term moves we may support to rectify these situations, the current problem of the individual patient has to be faced and dealt with within the available legal framework in such a way as to benefit that patient.

The reaction of the obstetricians and gynaecologists who have to work with liberalised abortion statutes varies according to their personal ethics and values. In Great Britain only 6% of consultant obstetricians and gynaecologists have a conscientious objection to abortion in all circumstances (Royal College of Obstetricians and Gynaecologists, 1970). It is our opinion that a specialist who has these reservations should make that fact known to patients seeking his advice, and make clear to them their right to obtain an opinion elsewhere. At the other extreme, only 4% of specialists favoured 'abortion on demand', where the decision is based solely on the fact that the patient requested abortion. Ninety per cent of obstetricians and gynaecologists in Great Britain are therefore faced with making a separate decision on each case, and it is inevitable that the patient's views and values will be a factor. This decision-making process involving doctor and patient is currently dignified by the term 'abortion counselling'.

In environments where permissive abortion laws lead to a situation of abortion on request', much the same techniques of abortion counselling have been applied to women who have made such a request. The object of the exercise is then to assist the patient to rationalise and accept her own decision to have an abortion and to attenuate the emotional trauma of the procedure itself. The possibility of group counselling should be considered for younger patients. Most women prefer individual counselling but younger patients react better to the abortion after group counselling than they do after individual counselling (Bracken *et al.*, 1973). Older women react better after individual counselling. Abortion counselling is not an emergency, and it is our view that a child under the age of 16 should be accompanied by a parent or guardian when she comes to indicate unequivocal parental consent to the counselling and examination of the child.

THE LEGAL BACKGROUND

The situation with respect to abortion varies from country to country. In the United States of America, although legislation differs from one state to another, Supreme Court rulings made in 1973 indicate that the decision whether or not to have an abortion is protected by the constitutional right of privacy, and the implementation of the decision is a matter only for the pregnant woman with her physician. Abortion may not be prohibited by State law during the first six months of pregnancy or before viability, and if there is prohibition thereafter, this must give way when the woman's life or health are at stake (Mears, 1975).

Geographical differences between countries have been reviewed by Tietze and Murstein (1975), Lee (1973), Mears (1975) and Zimmerman (1976), amongst others.

In Great Britain, the Abortion Act (1967) is an example of a law which provides for legal abortion on broad grounds. Those who drafted the Act have stated that it was not intended to provide abortion on demand; privately some of those associated with it have said that their objective was to get as near to abortion on demand as Parliament would tolerate. In fact the law permits a registered medical practitioner to carry out an abortion provided that two registered medical practitioners are of the opinion, formed in good faith:

(1) that the continuance of the pregnancy would involve *risk to the life* of the pregnant woman, or of *injury to the physical or mental health* of the pregnant woman or *any existing children of her family*, greater than if the pregnancy were terminated, or
(2) that there is a *substantial risk* that if the child were born it would suffer from such physical or mental abnormalities as to be *seriously handicapped*.

In determining whether the continuance of a pregnancy would involve such risk of injury to health as in (1), *account may be taken of the pregnant woman's actual or reasonably foreseeable environment*.

When a registered medical practitioner is of the opinion, formed in good faith, that urgent termination of a pregnancy is necessary to save the life or to prevent grave permanent injury to the physical or mental health of the pregnant woman, he may proceed without consultation with a second practitioner.

Risk to the Life of the Pregnant Woman

It has been contended that now the mortality of legal abortion (9.2 and 3.6 per 100 000, in 1972 and 1973, respectively; Registrar General, 1972, 1973) may be less than the maternal mortality (between 10.2 and 12.2 per 100 000 maternities in 1972 to 1976; Department of Health and Social Security, 1972–1977) in England and Wales, abortion on demand could be legal in Great Britain. This argument is invalid when applied to the individual patient, since with abortion it is the healthy young woman who may be at risk, whilst mortality in relation to a confinement occurs largely in older women with major medical or obstetric complications.

There are very few circumstances in which the continuation of a well managed pregnancy can be held to be a direct risk to life, in the sense that an obstetrician would advise termination of a wanted pregnancy. In carcinoma of the cervix diagnosed in early pregnancy, the conceptus succumbs to the treatment whether it be radiotherapy or surgery. In very severe heart conditions such as Eisenmenger's syndrome, in which a confinement is commonly followed by reversal of the cardiac shunt and maternal death, there is doubt if the risk following abortion is much less. With established renal disease in pregnancy, culminating in renal failure, there is no real evidence that terminating the pregnancy adds anything to the situation except complications to the management of the renal failure. Similar considerations apply to liver failure and to most major medical disorders; in the past, many pregnancies have been terminated in life-threatening situations on an empirical basis rather than because there was any good evidence that the prognosis would be improved. A life actually saved by therapeutic abortion is very rare — we recall a single case of status epilepticus coming on in early pregnancy which repeatedly failed to respond to therapeutic measures short of general anaesthesia, and resolved after a therapeutic abortion. The 'risk to life' cited in some 6% of notifications of legal abortion in England and Wales between 1968 and 1971 (Committee on the Working of the Abortion Act, 1974a) must be regarded as remote, with social and psychological factors being the prime indications. In fact, the proportion of notifications under the 'risk to life' heading decreased steadily from 13% in 1968 to 3% in 1971.

The threat to commit suicide if the pregnancy continues, whilst it may indicate severe emotional disturbance, cannot be considered a major risk to life. Patients occasionally make hysterical suicide attempts to draw attention to the severity of their problems but very rarely make use of methods and circumstances where their attempt is likely to be successful. Sim (1963) found that during a seven year period in Birmingham, 119 women under 50 committed suicide but not one was pregnant. Similar conclusions have been reached in Brisbane (Whitlock and Edwards, 1968) and the United States of America (Bolter, 1962). In Sweden, of 13 500 women who were refused abortion between 1938 and 1958, only three committed suicide. Suicide is undoubtedly rare in pregnant women; when it does occur, the primary reason is not usually the pregnancy *per se* (*see* Gardner, 1971b, for review).

We have noted that in recent years, since abortion on broad indications has been made legal, very few patients threaten suicide if the pregnancy continues. This manoeuvre is no longer necessary to justify a legal abortion.

Injury to the Physical Health of the Woman

The British Medical Association Committee on Therapeutic Abortion (1968) gave an exhaustive list of medical conditions which might be considered to constitute a risk to health in pregnancy. The great majority of these conditions can be treated in pregnancy just as well as in the non-pregnant woman. In 1968 there were very few conditions in which it was seriously believed that pregnancy actively contributed to the progress of the disease, and it is now difficult to name a disease where there is good evidence that pregnancy actually causes irreversible deterioration. On the other hand the term 'health' is a generalisation synonymous with 'well-being', and there are many medical disorders such as diabetes mellitus and major degrees of heart disease where management in pregnancy is troublesome, involving much hospitalisation, and others such as musculo-skeletal and neurological disorders in which pregnancy can provide an additional physical burden which may honestly be said to affect physical health. In the appraisal of these conditions it should be remembered that if the same patient presented with a much wanted pregnancy, the obstetrician would be expected to accept responsibility for management of the pregnancy and confinement. It follows that, once the patient has been presented with an honest prognosis for the pregnancy, the assessment to be made is of her values and of the social and psychological factors contributing to the request for abortion, not her medical status.

There are a few physical disorders in which the prognosis for a successful pregnancy in the future, as well as that for the medical problem, is improved if the current pregnancy is terminated, and treatment undertaken before another pregnancy is initiated. A clear example is congenital heart disease such as a Fallot's tetralogy, if open heart surgery is indicated. A less dramatic indication is found in conditions of the renal pelvis and ureter when operative repair, best undertaken in the non-pregnant state, may reduce the chances of urinary tract infections in a subsequent pregnancy.

Injury to the Mental Health of the Woman

This group comprises by far the largest proportion of women having legal abortions in Great Britain. Mental health means the same as mental well-being and the interpretation of this is the prerogative of the individual physician, varying from 'transient distress caused by inconvenience' to 'major breakdown necessitating mental hospitalisation which can be expected to be permanent unless the pregnancy is terminated'. Patients falling in the latter category are rare, in fact it is uncommon to find a case where a psychiatrist will certify that *mental illness* or *psychiatric* harm will result if a pregnancy continues. These specialists usually find it more honest to talk in terms of damage to *psychological* well-being, or of 'inability to cope'. Many physicians equate the prospect of weeks or months of distress and unhappiness with 'injury to mental health'.

We can only make a few points in this context. The judgement will be conditioned by the ethics, beliefs and training of the physician.

Arén and Åmark (1961) followed up 142 patients who had been granted a legal abortion on socio-psychiatric grounds in Sweden, but who had been persuaded to change their minds or in whom the pregnancy was too advanced for the abortion to be performed. In this very extensive assessment, only 8% of the patients were subsequently unequivocally worse off from a social, mental and physical point of view because the abortion had not been performed. In our opinion it is more important that appropriate management be provided for the 8% who would be worse off without an abortion, than to make an accurate decision based on an arbitrary criterion in the remaining applicants, who are distressed enough to request an abortion and are convinced that this is what they want.

Paradoxically, it is the normally well balanced patient with an acute reactive depression or anxiety state who benefits symptomatically by her 'mental health' being restored after a legal abortion, rather than the chronic psychiatric patient, whose psychiatric status is often unchanged or even worsened by the operation.

We feel that whilst it is unimportant whether or not a specialist psychiatrist is consulted before a decision is made with respect to most patients, it is important a psychiatrist be involved in the assessment, management and follow-up of any patient with a history of psychiatric disorder or who displays the symptoms and signs of a current psychiatric disorder. There are two reasons for this — to prevent or treat any unwanted psychiatric reactions and because the reaction to an unwanted pregnancy or to an abortion sometimes provides an entrée into the patient's psyche which can be of great value in psychiatric management.

There are two classes of patient in which we have subsequently had occasion to question the wisdom of an apparently sound decision to terminate a pregnancy under this clause. The first class comprises patients with 'inadequate personalities' whose aberrant life-style is perpetuated by society's repetitively solving their problems each time they occur and then leaving them to generate the next one. The second consists of patients with unrecognised psychopathic personalities. Both of these classes of patient are drawn to one's attention by their return with an identical set of problems a few months after the abortion has been performed.

Injury to the Physical or Mental Health of any Existing Children

This, taken in conjunction with the provision that account may be taken of the current or foreseeable environment, is the so-called 'social' clause. Applied strictly, it is rarely applicable. If 'health' is interpreted as 'well-being' it may be taken to encompass any parous woman who has an unwanted pregnancy and who is subject to the social and financial pressures which are currently widespread. In practice, decisions made under this clause involve value judgements on the part of the physician and of the patient. The risks of mortality or serious morbidity after abortion are small, but they should be taken into account as their consequences in a family already under stress could be disastrous.

Substantial Risk of a Seriously Handicapped Child

With respect to familial and genetic disorders, patients, and sometimes their doctors, may be under illusions as to the magnitude of the risk involved and it is necessary to obtain expert genetic counselling before the facts are considered. This should be done before any diagnostic procedure such as amniocentesis, which carries a risk to a normal pregnancy, is conducted. It must not be assumed that because there is a substantial risk of transmission of serious abnormality to the fetus that the patient will wish to have an abortion. Some patients prefer to continue the pregnancy, even if the presence of a condition such as sickle cell disease (haemoglobin S/S) is demonstrated and it is pointless to endanger the pregnancy by amniocentesis if the result will not affect management.

If a patient has an abortion because of the risk of transmission of a hereditary disorder which is not detectable in the fetus antenatally, then it is logical to suggest sterilisation of husband or wife. If this is not acceptable, then the real reason for requesting abortion is unlikely to be the chance of an abnormal baby.

Patients who are undergoing or are about to undergo radiotherapy for malignant disease of the pelvis or systemic cytotoxic therapy with drugs known to cause fetal abnormality such as methotrexate and some alkylating agents, may be taken to incur a substantial risk to the fetus. On the other hand, many patients taking azathioprine, some taking mercaptopurine, and a few on chlorambucil or busulphan are known to have completed successful pregnancies. The risk of fetal abnormality with the use in pregnancy of anti-epileptic drugs without folic acid is probably about 6% (Smithells, 1976); whether or not a 17 to 1 chance that a baby will be completely normal can be considered to contain a 'substantial risk' is a value judgement. Treatment with steroids, chloroquine or other agents where a very small or unproved association with fetal abnormality has been suggested cannot be taken as incurring a substantial risk. Serologically proven rubella during the first trimester of pregnancy is known to engender a substantial risk; with other virus infections in pregnancy the risk is small or unproved.

Patients who present requesting termination because they are aged over 40 years, because they have become pregnant whilst taking an oral contraceptive, because they have been given an oral pregnancy test, because they have been taking drugs with a tenuous and unproven association with fetal abnormality, or because they have had an x-ray in early pregnancy, do not in our opinion have a *substantial* risk of the fetus being affected. They should be reassured and informed of the chances that their baby will be normal. If they persist in requesting an abortion then the real reason for the request should be ascertained and assessed.

Immediate Termination to Preserve Life or Prevent Serious Disability

We know of few examples where use of this clause is appropriate. The need can arise when immediate surgery is necessary for life-threatening pelvic disease or trauma.

ABORTION COUNSELLING IN PRACTICE

The pattern of interview is necessarily individual to the doctor and must be appropriate to the patient. We shall indicate guide lines that we have found useful.

Confirmation of the pregnancy should be obtained before counselling begins, and the maturity of the pregnancy should be confirmed on examination before the interview is concluded. In our opinion the objectives of abortion counselling should be:

(1) to ascertain whether or not the situation conforms to the requirements for legal abortion;
(2) to detect equivocation on the part of the patient;
(3) to detect and predict any possible harm that might come to the patient if an abortion is performed;
(4) to determine whether or not a psychiatric or other medical opinion or a social report should be obtained before arriving at a decision;
(5) to inform the patient fully about the procedures involved in abortion and their possible consequences and
(6) to provide for continuing emotional and practical support for the patient, whichever decision is made.

Circumstances of the Conception

Having documented demographic, medical, gynaecological and obstetric histories, it is desirable to enquire into the causation of the unwanted pregnancy.

Facetious answers at this stage suggest either lack of concern or hysteria. Belligerent replies suggest emotional disturbance. Details should be sought of the putative father, his circumstances, whether or not he knows about the pregnancy, and his reaction to it if he does.

Use of Contraception

Enquiry into what precautions were taken against conception usually produces revealing replies. Stories of contraceptive failure may be viewed with scepticism but there is no real need to indicate this to the patient. Contraceptive failure does not provide any legal grounds for abortion. The point behind the questions is that they lead to some understanding of the patient's motivation.

In the study by Bracken *et al.* (1973) only one half of the women seeking abortion had used a contraceptive within the preceding year and only one fifth claimed to be practising contraception at the time they conceived. Anderson *et al.* (1977) reported from New York State that 57% were not using contraception when they conceived an unwanted pregnancy. In our own work (Morgan, I. and Hawkins, D.F., unpublished observations) very few women requesting abortion in North West London had not had the knowledge or means to prevent pregnancy available to them. Richardson and Dixon (1976) found that despite good contraceptive advice, 91 out of 211 women who had become pregnant again after a legal abortion did so within one year. Much more work is needed to obtain knowledge of the factors which lead women wilfully to expose themselves to unwanted pregnancy.

Consequences of Pregnancy and Confinement

Enquiry into the potential consequences of continuing the pregnancy usually reveals the nature of the problem. If the patient is unable to specify the untoward consequences of continuing pregnancy it is likely that she is still in a state of emotional disturbance which precludes rational assessment of values, and it is unwise to arrive at decisions without allowing her as long as necessary to rationalise her situation. We feel that this may be more important from the point of view of the patient's subsequent psychological status than the slight increase in risks of physical complications of abortion attendant on a week or two's delay in operating.

In the case of an unmarried woman, enquiries as to whether or not the parents or other relatives are aware of the situation and their reaction to the pregnancy often provide revealing answers with respect to the patient's background. Fifteen years ago the suggestion of the continuation of the pregnancy, social support, care in a mother and baby home during the final months and adoption of the baby was often acceptable to an unmarried mother as an alternative to abortion. These patients seemed to do very well. They were distressed when they gave up the baby but accepted this as a cold decision made in the best interests of the baby. Today the situation in Great Britain has changed radically. The social support that can be provided is inadequate and the social workers who should assist often merely encourage the patient to request a legal abortion. Mother and baby accommodation is unobtainable in many areas. Women are much less ready to have a baby resulting from an unplanned or unwanted pregnancy adopted; adoption procedures are more exacting. The legislation entitling an adopted child to information about its real parents will act as a major deterrent to adoption in Great Britain. The predictions of the social scientists that the baby is best off with its unmarried mother have not been justified — many of these children end up in a succession of foster homes and many develop social or psychiatric problems.

In this social climate, little positive encouragement can be given to the patient to solve her problems by continuing with an unwanted pregnancy as an alternative to abortion. What support is available is usually allocated to those who are equivocal about abortion or who are strong-minded enough to want to accept the responsibility of a pregnancy and confinement.

Environmental Pressures

Many patients who do not really want an abortion are subjected to pressure from parents, consorts and sometimes well-meaning social workers, local authority employees and even doctors. Whenever such pressures are suspected — as in the case of teenage girls, or patients referred by or in the care of the social services — it is important to see the patient alone and ascertain her personal views in depth before hearing those who are applying the pressure. In a sense, the need for abortion is dependent on environmental pressure in very nearly all cases, but it is important to delineate exogenous threats from other individuals which the patient recognises as such, from factors which she accepts as part of the normal environment. It is all too easy to be led into operating on a patient to relieve the anxiety of another individual such as the patient's mother or husband. This can result in the exact opposite of the patient's expectations, a state of permanent resentment being generated. In the marital situation, it is our opinion that an abortion, or for that matter, having a baby, never either strengthened a marriage or caused one to break up. The expense to a local authority of maintaining a mother and baby is a matter which is totally irrelevant to the terms of the Abortion Act.

Equivocation

The detection of any equivocation on the part of the patient is a red light indicating a potential psychiatric breakdown if abortion is proceeded with, however good the case may appear. It is our practice to refer these cases to a psychiatrist who has a balanced viewpoint and who will provide appropriate support if the patient eventually does commit herself to an abortion. Regrettably, our failure to detect equivocation is sometimes only demonstrated by the patient's not attending for operation, or even discharging herself from hospital before the abortion is performed.

Depression

If questions about appetite and sleep are included in a routine systematic enquiry the patient may answer these without appreciating that they relate to this diagnosis. Sometimes patients with severe depression are quite unaware that this is obvious, even to someone who has never met them before, and these patients should be treated with great circumspection. Some women will consciously produce a demonstration of weeping and other indications of depression for the benefit of the physician. What they do not realise is that it is very difficult for a well-balanced individual to simulate depression effectively, and that if they can perform in this way they are probably far more emotionally disturbed by the pregnancy than they themselves appreciate.

Examination

Unless the size of the uterus and the state of the pelvis has been previously assessed, we find it desirable to examine the patient at this point, before proceeding to matters which involve knowledge of the maturity of the pregnancy.

Type of Operation

With middle trimester pregnancies it is important that the patient understands that currently accepted procedures take many hours and involve spontaneous passage of the conceptus and often evacuation of retained products of conception under general anaesthesia. She should also accept the small chance that the procedure could fail, and that she might require hysterotomy to terminate the pregnancy. If this chance is not acceptable, then the grounds for termination of the pregnancy cannot be strong.

The Aftermath of Abortion

The news media and the advocates of abortion on request have presented the public with an image of abortion as a very simple procedure with no complications. It is only fair that the patient should be informed of the facts. It is reasonable to state that mortality is extremely low and that acute complications can nearly always be dealt with readily and effectively. On the other hand it is not reasonable to conceal from the patient the fact that legal abortion conducted in the best circumstances still conveys some risk to her future fertility. There is a real chance of either infertility due to pelvic inflammatory disease or of spontaneous abortion or premature labour occurring in pregnancies subsequent to legal abortion; the exact magnitude of the risk is currently unknown. Nonetheless, it is of particular importance that nulliparous patients should be made aware of these hazards.

The magnitude of the risk of psychiatric sequelae to legal abortion is equally unknown. Patients who develop such problems seldom return to report them to the doctor who performed the abortion, and the social respectability which has been conferred on abortion encourages the patient to feel ashamed if she develops such sequelae and to conceal them from doctors. The risks to patients with a psychiatric history and to those who equivocate have already been mentioned. We have also found that there is cause for concern in patients who have conceptualised the uterine contents as a fetus or miniature baby, rather than just an 'unwanted pregnancy', by the time they come for counselling (Goldie, L., personal communication). It is also worth discussing the patient's religious convictions should they be relevant. Frank discussion of any conflict may well avert a subsequent guilt reaction.

Contraception and Sterilisation

These topics should be discussed and appropriate plans for preventing recurrence of the situation agreed. It is of little value to recommend subsequent attendance at a family planning clinic. The contraceptive measure — starting on an oral contraceptive, an injected long-acting contraceptive or insertion of an intra-uterine device — should be conducted before the patient leaves hospital. Some patients will claim that an intention of abstinence will be adequate protection; this should be countered along the lines that bitter experience has repeatedly shown that such a resolve confers inadequate protection. For similar reasons, if female sterilisation has been definitely desired by both husband and wife before the unwanted pregnancy, then it is our view that it should be combined with the abortion procedure. On the other hand if either the patient or her husband has any doubt at all about the desire for sterilisation, or it transpires that this is the first occasion on which they have considered the possibility of sterilisation, then contraceptive measures should be instituted at the time of the abortion and the possibility of sterilisation discussed at a later date when the pressures have lessened and the emotional reaction to abortion has settled down. The sterilisation procedure can then be conducted with the patient's rational understanding and complete agreement.

Rejection of Requests for Legal Abortion

When the physician considers that there are no legal grounds for abortion, his opinion may sometimes be reinforced by showing the patient a printed list of the legal indications for abortion. It is our custom when these circumstances occur to inform the patient that at best we can only give an opinion formed in good faith, that we will inform her family practitioner in detail about the reasons for that opinion, and that we will state that if he wishes to refer her elsewhere for another opinion we will have no objection. When we telephone or write to the family practitioner we also offer to supervise and support the patient through the course of the pregnancy and we say that should her condition deteriorate we would be prepared to see her at any time and reassess the grounds for abortion.

Special Cases

Teenage Girls

It is of course essential to obtain the consent of a parent or guardian of a girl under sixteen years of age to a legal abortion except in the very rare case in which a pregnancy has to be terminated in the course of emergency treatment of a medical situation where the patient's life is at risk or serious disability may result from delay. We meet three particular problems in counselling girls under the age of 16 years. The first is to ascertain the feeling and wishes of the patient herself, as distinct from those of her mother or family. The second is that these patients often conceal the pregnancy, presenting at a stage when the physical risks of abortion can confidently be stated to outweigh all but the strongest grounds for termination. In fact, the psychiatric hazards to such girls from going through a pregnancy are small, provided that they can be protected from social and family pressures and adequate arrangements can be made for care of the baby and for continuation of the patient's education. The third difficulty which sometimes occurs is that of convincing the patient's mother that her daughter will be in need of contraceptive advice after an abortion. In the Aberdeen study nearly a quarter of the 14 and 15 year old girls were pregnant again within a year after a legal abortion (Aitken-Swan, 1973). It is seldom difficult to convince the patient herself and to come to an arrangement with her and her family practitioner which ensures that contraceptive measures are instituted. In Great Britain, the Medical Defence Union (1974) advises that a doctor who provides contraception for a girl under the age of 16 is not acting unlawfully if he does so in good faith to protect the girl against the potentially harmful effects of intercourse. If a patient under 16 refuses permission for her parents to be consulted about the provision to her of contraceptive advice or her parents refuse permission for her to be so advised, the physician is in a difficult position. If he performs a vaginal examination or inserts an intra-uterine device this may be, in law, a technical assault (Committee on the Working of the Abortion Act, 1974b). It is unlikely that a physician who prescribes an oral contraceptive for a girl under 16 without her parent's consent is at any serious medico-legal risk if he is of the opinion that his actions are in his patient's best interests.

The Married Woman

It is always desirable to obtain the consent of the husband or consort to performing legal abortion.

If the indication for termination of pregnancy is risk to the life or physical or mental health of the patient it is not necessary in law in Great Britain to obtain the husband's consent (Medical Defence Union, 1974). Nonetheless, the patient should be advised that she is risking the stability of her marriage should she either conceal the facts from him or have the operation in the face of his objections. The patient should be warned that whilst every effort can be made to conceal the nature of her operation from her husband if she so desires, no guarantee can be given in an ordinary hospital that he could not find a way of discovering what has happened. It is always possible that the husband might attempt to make use of this knowledge in the course of divorce proceedings.

If the indication is risk to the physical or mental health of existing children an interview with the husband present should normally form part of abortion counselling and assessment of the grounds for legal abortion.

If an abortion for risks to existing children or for risk of fetal abnormality is performed in the face of the husband's objections, it is always possible that he might sue the surgeon for depriving him of his child. In Great Britain, such a legal action would be unlikely to succeed if the surgeon acted in good faith in what he considered to be the best interests of his patient (Medical Defence Union, 1974). In the United States of America, even in States where laws have been passed requiring husband's consent to abortion, when cases have been brought to court they have not succeeded, the laws being declared unconstitutional.

Late Abortions

The risks of complications to the operative procedure of abortion steadily increase with increasing maturity of the pregnancy. After 16 weeks' maturity only clear medical or psychiatric grounds or evidence of an abnormal fetus are likely to outweigh the physical risks of the operation. After 20 weeks' maturity it is unwise to perform abortion except for the strongest medical reasons. After 28 weeks' maturity the fetus is legally viable and the question does not arise. In the United States of America the definition of fetal viability varies, being 20 weeks' maturity in Massachusetts, and less well defined in some other States.

The doctor who undertakes a late abortion may rarely encounter the problem of a fetus which shows some of the signs of life, even if intra-uterine injections are employed to procure the abortion. In New York State and in the Commonwealth of Massachusetts it is the legal duty of a physician to support life in a fetus born alive, whether it is born naturally or aborted, and regardless of whether or not it has been judged viable. When undertaking the abortion of a patient whose pregnancy exceeds 20 weeks' maturity, a doctor should carefully consider his ethical, legal and personal position should the fetus be delivered alive.

Mentally Incompetent Patients

It is our opinion that it is unethical to perform an abortion on a patient who is incapable of understanding the significance of the operation and giving her informed consent, except as an essential part of management of a life-threatening situation or one which could cause serious disability. We feel that pressures from relatives or social or medical agencies in this respect should be resisted, however socially desirable the operation may seem. The proper role of these individuals and agencies is to provide the mentally incompetent patient with an environment where pregnancy does not occur in the first place, not to approve abortion in a patient whose own health will not benefit from the operation.

USE FOR MEDICAL RESEARCH OF PRODUCTS OF CONCEPTION OBTAINED AT ABORTION

Objections to the use of fetal material are in general emotional rather than rational, but in order to protect those engaged in research it has proved necessary to evolve guidelines to define a reasonable approach to the problem.

It is, in the opinion of the Department of Health and Social Security (1972), unethical for a medical practitioner to administer drugs or carry out procedures on the mother with the deliberate intent of ascertaining the harm that these might do to the fetus, notwithstanding that arrangements have been made to terminate the pregnancy and even if the mother is willing to give her assent to such an experiment. If the fetus proved to be alive on termination of the pregnancy and survived but was handicapped the investigator would be liable to civil action for compensation in Great Britain. If the fetus was born alive and was handicapped or subsequently died as a result of the experiments, those concerned would be liable to prosecution.

The Department's recommendations with respect to the use of pre-viable fetuses for research are as follows. Dissection or experiments should not take place in the operating theatre or place of delivery. Only fetuses weighing less than 300 g should be used. The responsibility for deciding that the fetus may be used is that of the medical attendants and not of the research worker. There should be no monetary exchange for fetuses or fetal material. The research should be carried out in departments directly related to a hospital and with the direct sanction of the ethical committee of that hospital. The ethical committee should satisfy itself on the validity of the research, that the information cannot be secured in any other way and that the investigators have the necessary facilities and skill. Full records should be maintained by the institution.

There is little official guidance on the need for consent of the patient to the use of fetal material from an abortion for research, though the Department expresses the view that the patient must be offered the opportunity to declare any special directions about the disposal of the fetus. Examination of the products of conception by a pathologist is desirable in any event, to determine their completeness and normality. Some ethical committees require informed consent of the patient to the use of any fetal tissue; others require informed consent with material from middle trimester abortions. In our opinion this is absurd. It is excessively cruel to present a woman who is already in a state of emotional crisis with such a requirement. There may even be a risk of causing serious psychiatric harm if the nature of the research involves conceptualisation of the products as a fetus by a woman who until that time has simply regarded it as an unwanted pregnancy (Goldie, L., personal communication).

The Viable Fetus

In Great Britain, the Department of Health and Social Security (1972) recommends that the minimum limit of viability for human fetuses should be taken as '20 weeks' gestational age' — a somewhat confusing term which, taken literally means 22 weeks maturity of the pregnancy, measured in the usual way from the first day of the last menstrual period. This is said to correspond to a weight of 400–500 g. The Department also considers that when a fetus is viable in these terms and is born alive, then it is unethical to carry out any experiments with it which are inconsistent with treatment necessary to promote its life.

When a viable fetus is dead on separation from the mother there are no statutory restrictions in Great Britain on the use of part or whole of the fetus for research. As it is of less than 28 weeks' maturity there is no legal necessity to register its disposal but it is advisable to keep records of the use of such material. The Department recommends that dissection or experiments do not take place in the operating theatre, that no monetary exchanges are involved in the use of the material and that the mother should have had an opportunity to declare any views she may have had about disposal of the products. When a viable fetus is born alive and then dies in consequence of removal from the mother it should be registered as a live birth and a neonatal death. The permission of the mother is then required for autopsy or use of fetal materials for research.

It will be noted that there are no specific recommendations in Great Britain with respect to fetuses over 300 g in weight but less than 22 weeks' maturity which show some sign of life. Medical practitioners would be well advised to avoid experimental use of such material except in exceptional circumstances and with the strongest ethical and legal backing. In the United States of America a physician was successfully prosecuted in the Commonwealth of Massachusetts for employing a live fetus from a second trimester abortion for experimental work and this has left the legal position unsettled. It was held that whilst the destruction of the fetus within the mother is a legal procedure, should the fetus be extracted alive, then a new individual has been born and a procedure which causes its death is manslaughter (Mears, 1975).

Use of placenta, membranes, amniotic fluid and fragments of fetuses removed during abortions is subject to no legal restriction, but the approval of the hospital ethical committee is desirable.

MORTALITY OF LEGAL ABORTION

In England and Wales, the mortality directly attributable to legal abortion fell from 20 to 4 per 100 000 from 1969 to 1973 (*Table 12.1*). Over the same period the number of legal abortions performed on residents increased from 50 000 to

Table 12.1 MORTALITY FROM LEGAL ABORTION IN RESIDENTS OF ENGLAND AND WALES (REGISTRAR-GENERAL, 1969–1973)

	Legal abortions	*Deaths*	*Mortality per 100 000*
1969	49 829	10	20.1
1970	75 962	10	13.2
1971	94 570	12	12.7
1972	108 565	10	9.2
1973	110 568	4	3.6

111 000 per year. The improvement in the mortality rate may be due to improved techniques, to greater experience of the surgeons, and to a greater proportion of the operations being performed at an earlier stage of pregnancy. It may be partly due to a decreasing proportion of the operations being performed on medical grounds, a correspondingly greater proportion being concerned with previously healthy women.

Data from 2 820 920 legal abortions in the United States of America are shown in *Table 12.2*. The overall mortality is of the order of 4 per 100 000 operations. Before 11 weeks' maturity the risk is less than half this figure; from 13 to 15 weeks it is double. Past 16 weeks the mortality is increased tenfold.

In other developed countries, abortion mortality has been between 1 and 7 per 100 000 operations in recent years (Tietze and Murstein, 1975).

The mortality associated with legal abortion is small, but it is best mentioned to the patient, if only to put it in perspective. When a gynaecologist conducts a

Table 12.2 MORTALITY OF LEGAL ABORTION BY TYPE OF PROCEDURE AND WEEKS OF GESTATION. DEATH RATES PER 100 000 ABORTIONS, UNITED STATES OF AMERICA, 1972–1975 (FROM CATES *et al.*, 1977)

	Weeks' gestation						
	≤8	9–10	11–12	13–15	16–20	≥21	Total
Surgical evacuation*	0.5	1.8	5.0	9.1	9.4	–	1.9
Intra-amniotic hypertonic saline instillation	–†	–	–	–	29.3	30.1	22.9
Prostaglandin instillation	–	–	–	–	11.9	–	17.8
Hysterotomy or hysterectomy	–	–	–	–	–	–	45.0
All methods	0.6	2.0	4.9	11.5	23.4	37.3	3.7

*Surgical – dilatation and curettage, vacuum evacuation of products.
†Dash indicates too few cases to derive a meaningful rate.

procedure which results in the deaths of several women a year in Great Britain and about 25 women a year in the United States of America, it is important that he has clear views about the grounds which justify the operation.

SEQUELAE OF LEGAL ABORTION

It is now ten years since the Abortion Act was passed in Great Britain. In that time more than one million legal abortions have been fully documented, performed and notified to the Chief Medical Officer of the Department of Health and Social Security. It is astonishing that with such an unrivalled opportunity for determining facts, the number of publications giving serious information on the long-term consequences of legal abortion coming from Great Britain in that time can be counted on the fingers of one hand. The report of the Committee on the Working of the Abortion Act (1974c) devotes eight pages to an inconclusive review of the literature on the late and latent ill consequences of abortion, compared to hundreds of pages on the problems of women in securing abortions.

It seems likely that the public at large, the Government and the medical profession who perform the abortions have no wish to ascertain the facts of long-term sequelae. This ostrich-like attitude is regrettable. If abortion counselling is to be on a rational basis, it is important that doctor and patient should be aware of the magnitude of the long-term hazards involved.

Two aspects of the sequelae of legal abortion frequently present themselves to the practising obstetrician and gynaecologist. Currently, infertility clinics are populated by many women who have had one or more legal abortions in the past, and then find difficulty in conceiving when they want to, the cause being chronic pelvic inflammatory disease involving the fallopian tubes. Also, the number of women who need a Shirodkar suture to prevent subsequent abortion or premature labour has been markedly increased by patients with a history of legal abortion. Patients are also seen with ectopic gestations due to chronic pelvic inflammatory disease, or in whom caesarean section is indicated in labour because of doubts about the integrity of a hysterotomy scar.

Information on the long-term psychiatric and social sequelae of legal abortion is very limited; what there is is partly anecdotal in character.

Infertility

The principal cause of failure to conceive years after a legal abortion seems to be chronic pelvic inflammatory disease, often otherwise asymptomatic. On general principles it must be presumed that the causes are intra-uterine manipulation and retained products of conception providing a nidus for the low-grade infection so introduced.

The incidence of post-abortion sterility is really unknown. Gardner (1971a) has pointed out that some figures from Eastern Europe or Japan may have been 'politically adjusted', to use Sir Norman Jeffcoate's phrase. Some of the figures are low due to defective follow-up. Kotasek's (1971) report from Czechoslovakia is of interest in that the patients had their abortions performed by vacuum curettage during the course of a three to five day hospital admission. He found that 20–30% of the patients subsequently had pelvic inflammatory disease, were sterile or had had an ectopic gestation, though it is not clear how the diagnosis of sterility was made. The best estimate of the incidence of sterility is probably somewhere near the middle of the range of 1–6% found in the European literature by Lindahl (1959) and Wynn and Wynn (1972) – a significant risk for a nulliparous patient who may want a family in the future. In our experience the commonest mechanisms of infertility after legal abortion are adhesions and inflammatory damage in relation to the fallopian tubes, but the work of Momose (1966) may indicate another cause. Hysterographic observations by this author showed an incidence of intra-uterine adhesions which increased from 3% after one previous curettage to 5% after two instrumentations, to 7% after three and to 23% after four or more curettages. This incidence is significantly reduced by the use of vacuum aspiration of the uterine contents.

Ectopic Gestation

It is known that there is an association between a history of illegal abortion and subsequent ectopic pregnancy (Panayotau *et al.*, 1972). There have been reports (Novak, 1963; Kotasek, 1971) suggesting that the incidence of subsequent ectopic gestation is also increased in patients who have had a legal abortion, presumably due to pelvic inflammatory disease. On the other hand, in controlled studies in Japan (Sawazaki and Tanaku, 1966) and Yugoslavia (Hren *et al.*, 1974) no association was detected. Berić and Kupresanin (1971) found no evidence of an increase in ectopic gestations after vacuum aspiration compared with classical techniques.

In Great Britain the incidence of ectopic gestation steadily increased after the Abortion Act was passed in 1967. According to Beral (1975) there were 2673 ectopic gestations in 1966 (28.4 per 100 000 women; 3.2 per 1000 conceptions), whilst in 1972 there were 3447 (36.6 per 100 000 women; 4.3 per 1000 conceptions). Beral considers it unlikely that the increase in ectopic pregnancies is related to the increase in legal abortions, pointing out that the time trends in the age groups do not correspond. It is difficult to accept this argument; there is

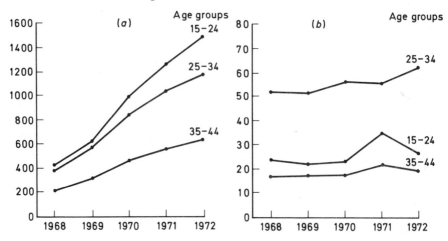

Figure 12.1 England and Wales. (a) Legal abortions per 100 000 women, by age groups (Registrar General, 1968–1972) and (b) ectopic pregnancies per 100 000 women, by age groups (Beral, 1975). The increase in legal abortion started in 1968 to 1969; that in ectopic gestation began in 1971.

in fact a time lag between the increase in abortions and the increase in ectopic gestations (*Figure 12.1*), which is explicable if silent pelvic inflammatory disease takes a year or two to cause damage and many patients avoid pregnancy scrupulously for a year or two after a legal abortion. Beral (1975) also presents data showing a correlation between the legal abortion rate and the incidence of ectopic gestations in different towns in Great Britain (*Table 12.3*). Even though, as she suggests, intra-uterine contraceptive devices and low-dose progestagen oral contraceptives may have played a part in causing the increase in ectopic

Table 12.3 RELATION BETWEEN ANNUAL LEGAL ABORTION RATES (WOMEN AGED 15 TO 49) AND ANNUAL ECTOPIC PREGNANCY RATES (WOMEN AGED 15 TO 44) IN ENGLAND, 1971/1972. CORRELATION COEFFICIENT = +0.54, EXCLUDING LONDON (BERAL, 1975)

Region	Legal abortions per 1000 women	Ectopic pregnancies per 100 000 women
Leeds	6.53	26.1
Sheffield	6.88	29.2
Liverpool	7.02	23.8
Wessex	7.18	30.7
Manchester	7.38	34.5
Oxford	7.55	35.6
Newcastle	7.56	29.1
East Anglia	7.85	21.7
South Western	8.11	34.7
Birmingham	8.90	37.8
London:		
North East*	9.90	41.2
South East*	10.63	36.5
South West*	13.67	39.9
North West*	15.00	37.4

*Excluding teaching hospitals

gestations, it is difficult to escape the conclusion that legal abortion is primarily responsible.

In the Lane Report (Committee on the Working of the Abortion Act, 1974d) the point is made that broad use of legal abortion reduces the number of term pregnancies but not the number of ectopic pregnancies, and therefore the proportion of ectopic gestations will appear to be increased. This factor cannot explain the increase in the absolute number of ectopic gestations, and it is not consistent with the time lag shown in *Figure 12.1*.

In Japan there have been a number of cases of cervical ectopic pregnancy reported since 1953. Shinagawa and Nagayama (1969) found that 13 out of 19 such patients had previously had an induced abortion performed by dilatation and curettage. In each instance, hysterectomy was required to control haemorrhage.

Cervical Incompetence and Spontaneous Abortion

It seems clear that legal abortion can result in incompetence of the cervix. Kotasek (1971) says that the incidence after vacuum curettage performed during the first trimester is high and Stallworthy *et al.* (1971) found demonstrable cervical lacerations in 4.8% of cases. Tietze and Lewit (1972) give an incidence of cervical damage of only 0.9% after termination of pregnancy by dilatation and curettage or vacuum curettage; Richardson and Dixon's (1976) estimate was 5.2%. Damage to the cervix which is not obvious until the patient conceives again may be more common. It is sometimes assumed that the incompetence is caused by forceful dilatation of the cervix and that the increased risk of incompetence after a middle trimester abortion (Wright *et al.*, 1972; Richardson and Dixon, 1976) is due to the greater degree of cervical dilatation necessary to effect abortion. Johnstone *et al.* (1976) found that dilatation beyond 12 mm at termination of pregnancy is associated with increased cervical diameters subsequently. The thesis that use of a small flexible catheter (*see* Karman and Potts, 1972) with a paracervical block leads to less cervical damage (Potts, 1973) may merely replace the problem with chronic pelvic inflammatory disease arising from retained products of conception (Berić *et al.*, 1972). There is also a risk of cervical incompetence when prostaglandins are used to procure a middle trimester abortion (Wright *et al.*, 1972) though Mackenzie and Hillier (1977) did not find this a problem. Kajanoja *et al.* (1974) have reported the occurrence of cervico-vaginal fistula and it must be concluded that forceful uterine contractions can damage the cervix without any instrumentation.

The extent of the problem is such that it has become our practice to insert a Shirodkar suture promptly in the cervix with any symptom or sign suggesting incompetence, in a patient giving a history of legal abortion. We also suture the cervix in patients with this history who are admitted with a threatened abortion, if the bleeding stops and the pregnancy continues.

The incidence of spontaneous abortion in a subsequent pregnancy may be increased (Richardson and Dixon, 1976; Mackenzie and Hillier, 1977) though Roht and Aoyama (1974) obtained no evidence of this in their surveys in Japan. This risk of abortion in a subsequent pregnancy may be higher after a previous middle trimester abortion. Wright *et al.* (1972) found that spontaneous middle trimester abortion occurred in eight out of 91 patients with a history of a previous legal abortion but in only 1% of age-matched controls with a previous spontaneous abortion. Of the eight patients who miscarried, only one had had the previous legal abortion before ten weeks' maturity. Richardson and Dixon (1976) found that of 11 cases in which the cervix had been lacerated during dilatation only one of the subsequent pregnancies continued beyond the 36th week and only five babies survived.

It is not entirely clear whether or not all the abortions and premature labours in subsequent pregnancies are due to cervical incompetence or if some are due to other uterine damage such as over-enthusiastic curettage causing subsequent difficulties with implantation and development of the placenta. We would also question data on the actual incidence of spontaneous abortion in patients with a history of a previous legal abortion. Controlled comparisons (Wright *et al.,* 1972; Richardson and Dixon, 1976; Mackenzie and Hillier, 1977) confirm that there is an excess of miscarriages in this group but the figures for abortions in the control groups, 5.5%, 2.8% and 6.4% respectively, are surprisingly low. The overall incidence of spontaneous abortion in any pregnancy is 10–15% and one must conclude that a number of early abortions in both 'control' and 'previous legal abortion' groups occur before the patients ever reach a specialist clinic, and considerable bias could arise.

Premature Labour

Again, it seems likely that the incidence of premature labour is somewhat increased in women who have previously had a legal abortion; the magnitude of any such effect is in doubt. Richardson and Dixon (1976) found an incidence of 13.7% of premature deliveries in a series of 211 patients who had had a legal abortion compared with 5.2% in a matched control series who had had a previous spontaneous abortion.

The figures from Yugoslavia between the years 1960 to 1970 cited by Berić and Kupresanin (1971) are not helpful as the number of legal abortions did not increase dramatically over that period. Potts (1967) concluded that in Hungary legal abortion had contributed to a doubling of the perinatal mortality rate in subsequent pregnancies. He considered that the high prematurity rate in towns (15% compared with an overall rate of 11–12%) was also attributable. The Hungarian data given by Klinger (1970) is of particular interest not so much because it shows an increase in prematurity rate as the numbers of legal abortions have increased, but because it establishes a clear association between the number of legal abortions which a patient has had and the subsequent risk of a premature baby (*Table 12.4*). Data from the Hungarian Central Statistical Office cited by Tietze and Dawson (1973) shows that only the magnitude of the effect is modified by cross-classification according to parity. The Lane Report (Committee on the Working of the Abortion Act, 1974c) suggests other factors such as classification differences which could possibly account for the changes in reported prematurity rates in Hungary between 1960 and 1968 but the consistency of the prematurity rate for women with no previous abortions (*Table 12.5*) speaks against this and these changes do not affect the relationship with the number of previous abortions. The report also points out that in Aberdeen the prematurity rate varied from 3% in social class 1 to 15% in social class 5 and that the Hungarian figures may be biased by underprivileged patients

Table 12.4 PREMATURE LIVE BIRTHS (UNDER 2500 g) BY NUMBER OF PREVIOUS INDUCED ABORTIONS IN HUNGARY (KLINGER, 1970)

Number of previous induced abortions	Premature live births (%)		
	October 1960	April 1964	1968
0	8.0	9.6	9.3
1	11.1	13.7	13.0
2	12.2	15.2	16.6
3+	13.9	20.1	20.6
Total	8.3	10.5	10.5

who used abortion for family planning rather than contraception. Whilst such a group might bias the magnitude of the effect, it seems unlikely that it could account for a clear quantitative relationship such as that in Klinger's data for 1968 (*Table 12.4*), from a prematurity rate of 9.3% with no previous abortions to 20.6% after three or more previous abortions.

On the other hand Roht and Aoyama (1974) conducted two surveys in the Kochi prefecture in Japan, one based on a mailed questionnaire, the other on interviews conducted by Public Health Nurses. They were unable to detect any increase in prematurity rate in subsequent pregnancies in women who had had abortions.

In practice, in Great Britain there has been no relevant change in the proportion of low birth weight babies born in the decade since the Abortion Act was passed in 1967 (*Table 12.5*), although the legal abortions in residents have increased from 22 000 in 1968 to 101 000 in 1976. The latter figure, for 1976, is equivalent to one-fifth of the live birth rate. It must be concluded either that the

Table 12.5 BABIES OF LOW BIRTH WEIGHT (2500 g OR LESS) BORN ALIVE IN ENGLAND AND WALES, 1957 to 1976, AS PERCENTAGES OF TOTAL LIVE BIRTHS. (DEPARTMENT OF HEALTH AND SOCIAL SECURITY, 1972–1977)

	'Premature' live births	Percentage of total live births
1957	50 168	6.9
1958	50 742	6.9
1959	50 130	6.7
1960	52 633	6.7
1961	54 632	6.7
1962	55 999	6.7
1963	56 172	6.6
1964	55 852	6.4
1965	54 743	6.3
1966	55 205	6.5
1967	53 804	6.5
1968	54 180	6.6
1969	53 406	6.7
1970	53 514 (50 766)*	6.8 (6.8)*
1971	49 886 (47 202)*	6.4 (6.3)*
1972	(45 366)*	(6.6)*
1973	(40 628)*	(6.4)*
1974	(38 889)*	(6.4)*
1975	(36 493)*	(6.4)*
1976	(35 440)*	(6.4)*

*Figures in parentheses are for England only.

ready availability of legal abortion has had no effect on the incidence of pre-mature labour or that any such effect has been compensated by improvements in obstetric care.

It might be considered that prophylactic use of Shirodkar sutures in women who have previously had therapeutic abortions would have prevented adverse effects on the premature live birth in Great Britain. Mackenzie and Hillier (1977) found that previous prostaglandin abortions did not significantly affect duration of gestation, if cervical sutures were only inserted when there was positive clinical indication.

Perinatal Mortality

A factor which increases the risk of premature labour is likely to result in an increase in perinatal mortality. It has been suggested that the perinatal mortality rate might be increased by about 16 per 1000 among women who have previously had a legal abortion (Ogborn, 1973).

Valid evidence about this is lacking. It was suggested by Jurukovski and Sukarov (1971) from Yugoslavia that perinatal mortality rates in that country doubled after the liberalisation of abortion laws. In contrast a detailed analysis from the Hungarian Central Statistical Office, cited in the Lane Report (Committee on the Working of the Abortion Act, 1974c) showed no evidence of consistent change in the national perinatal mortality rate since abortion was made legal in 1958. In Great Britain a number of factors have contributed to reductions in the perinatal mortality rate during the last decade and it would not be possible to isolate any effect of legal abortion on national statistics of this type. Such perinatal mortality surveys as are available have failed to separate data for patients who have had legal abortions from those who have had spontaneous abortions. Well controlled prospective follow-up studies will be required before any conclusions can be drawn.

Hysterotomy Scars

The risk of rupture of the hysterotomy scar in a subsequent pregnancy can be reduced by using low transverse uterine incisions for hysterotomy (Chapter 13, p. 300), and that of endometriosis in the scars by careful packing to avoid spilling decidua in the wound. The risk of uterine scar rupture cannot be completely eliminated — we have seen dehiscence of a low transverse hysterotomy scar in labour, and caesarean sections will still be conducted for *suspected* scar rupture. It is sad that it is sometimes the young teenager who has concealed her condition until mid-pregnancy who ends up with a hysterotomy scar which prejudices her obstetric future.

Psychiatric Sequelae

It is our view that the psychiatric sequelae of legal abortion are neither so rare as the protagonists of abortion on demand would have us believe nor so common or serious as the anti-abortion lobby consider.

Few reports give any hard evidence on this matter. They must be viewed in relation to Arén and Åmark's (1961) finding that the socio-psychiatric status of 8% of women who had been granted legal abortion, but in whom it was not carried out, deteriorated meaningfully.

Pare and Raven (1970) were not impressed by the psychiatric sequelae of legal abortion, though many patients had feelings of guilt or remorse and in 13% these persisted for more than three months. These authors felt that failure to terminate the pregnancy often led to regrets and sometimes resentment against the baby. McCance *et al.* (1973), in the Aberdeen study, could find no greater incidence of depression in women who had a legal abortion 15 months previously than in women who had gone through with the unwanted pregnancy. Berić *et al.* (1973) in Yugoslavia found depression after legal abortion to be associated with ambivalence towards the procedure, often persisting after the operation, but soon resolving and leaving no lasting sequelae. The predominant reaction in most of their cases was one of relief that the situation had been resolved.

Mackenzie and Hillier (1975) found that of 266 personal reports from patients, four reported depressive illnesses, but that of their 41 patients who did not reply, enquiries made to their family practitioners disclosed that six had had depressive illnesses. This illustrates well the problems involved in interpreting such data. Patients with depression may conceal that fact in their replies, they may not be aware that they have a depressive illness or they may not reply to enquiries and come into a 'lost to follow-up' category.

We consider that with patients who have either medical or social — as distinct from psychiatric — grounds for termination of pregnancy, the stronger the patient understands those grounds to be, the less likely is she to have an un-toward psychiatric reaction. With psychiatric grounds for abortion, the normally well-balanced patient with an acute anxiety state or depressive reaction has a good prognosis in this respect, provided she has a week or two to get over any initial acute stress reaction and readjust her values between discovering she is pregnant and the operation. This often involves a temporary replacement of moral values by expediency, but subsequent guilt reactions are relatively rare. The postoperative prognosis in psychiatric patients is not nearly so good and psychiatric support for these women is desirable.

Other Sequelae

In a somewhat emotionally-charged review, Wynn and Wynn (1972) suggested that legal abortion can cause disorders of menstruation, and in a subsequent pregnancy, antepartum haemorrhage, retained placenta, postpartum haemor-rhage, and the birth of a dysmature baby or one that is physically or mentally abnormal. Whilst we have some sympathy with the objectives of the Wynn report — the sequelae of abortion have certainly been under-publicised — we do not feel that evidence adequate to substantiate any of these associations has been presented.

Potts (1967) found an association of previous abortion with abruptio placentae, placenta praevia and prolonged labour in the Czechoslovakian data, and Mackenzie and Hillier (1977) have suggested that placenta praevia and prolonged labour in multigravidae might be associated with previous legal abortion. The numbers of actual cases involved in these studies were small and these results must be considered inconclusive.

Conclusion

The reasonably well established long-term sequelae of legal abortion are rhesus isoimmunisation, which should be completely preventable (Chapter 13, p. 263); pelvic inflammatory disease leading to infertility in a small proportion of patients, and to a slight risk of ectopic gestation; and cervical incompetence with some chance of spontaneous abortion or premature labour which can be reduced by early diagnosis and treatment.

REFERENCES

AITKEN-SWAN, J. (1973). Epidemiological background. In *Experience with Abortion. A Case Study of North-East Scotland*, pp. 12—46. Ed. Horobin, G. Cambridge University Press

ANDERSON, J.E., MORRIS, L. and GESCHE, M. (1977). Contraceptive use at time of conception for pregnancies resulting in unwanted births. *Contraception,* **15**, 705—710

ARÉN, P. and AMARK, C. (1961). The prognosis in cases in which legal abortion has been granted but not carried out. *Acta psychiat. neurol. scand.,* **36**, 203—278

BERAL, V. (1975). An epidemiological study of recent trends in ectopic pregnancy. *Br. J. Obstet. Gynaec.,* **82**, 775—782

BERIĆ, B.M. and KUPRESANIN, M. (1971). Vacuum aspiration using para-cervical block, for legal abortion as an out-patient procedure up to the 12th week of pregnancy. *Lancet,* **ii**, 619—621

BERIĆ, B.M., KUPRESANIN, M. and HULKA, J.F. (1972). The Karman catheter: a preliminary evaluation as an instrument for termination of pregnancies up to twelve weeks of gestation. *Am. J. Obstet. Gynec.,* **114**, 273—275

BERIĆ, B., KUPRESANIN, M. and KAPOR-STANULOVIC, N. (1973). Accidents and sequelae of medical abortions. *Am. J. Obstet. Gynec.,* **116**, 813—821

BOLTER, S. (1962). The psychiatrist's role in therapeutic abortion: the unwitting accomplice. *Am. J. Psychiat.,* **119**, 312—316

BRACKEN, M.B., GROSSMAN, G., HACHAMOVITCH, M., SUSSMAN, D. and SCHRIER, D. (1973). Abortion counselling: an experimental study of three techniques. *Am. J. Obstet. Gynec.,* **117**, 10—20

BRITISH MEDICAL ASSOCIATION COMMITTEE ON THERAPEUTIC ABORTION (1968). Indications for termination of pregnancy. *Br. med. J.,* **i**, 171—175

CATES, W. Jr., GRIMES, D.A., SMITH, J.C. and TYLER, C.W. Jr. (1977). The risk of dying from legal abortion in the United States, 1972—1975. *Int. J. Gynaecol. Obstet.,* **15**, 172—176

COMMITTEE ON THE WORKING OF THE ABORTION ACT (1974a, b, c and d). *Report*, volume I, pp. 14, 77—78, 246—253 and 250, respectively. Her Majesty's Stationery Office, London

DEPARTMENT OF HEALTH AND SOCIAL SECURITY. Scottish Home and Health Department. Welsh Office. (1972). *The Use of Fetuses and Fetal Material for Research. Report of the Advisory Group.* Her Majesty's Stationery Office, London

DEPARTMENT OF HEALTH AND SOCIAL SECURITY (1972—1977). *On the State of Public Health. The Annual Reports of the Chief Medical Officer of the Department of Health and Social Security for the years 1971 to 1977.* Her Majesty's Stationery Office, London

GARDNER, R.F.R. (1971a, b). *Abortion. The Personal Dilemma,* pp. 217, 224—225 respectively. Paternoster Press, Exeter

GORDON, H. (1972). Contraception or abortion? (b) Is abortion a form of contraception? *R. Soc. Hlth J.,* **92**, 194—199

HREN, M., TOMAŽEVIČ, T. and SEIGAL, D. (1974). Ectopic pregnancy. In *The Ljubljana Abortion Study, 1971–1973,* pp. 34—38. Ed. Andolšek, L. National Institutes of Health Center for Population Research, Bethesda, Maryland

JEFFCOATE, T.N.S. (1970). In *Morals and Medicine,* p. 32. British Broadcasting Corporation, London

JOHNSTONE, F.D., BEARD, R.J., BOYD, I.E. and McCARTHY, T.G. (1976). Cervical diameter after suction termination of pregnancy. *Br. med. J.,* **i**, 68—69

JURUKOVSKI, J. and SUKAROV, L. (1971). A critical review of legal abortion. *Int. J. Gynaecol. Obstet.,* **9**, 111—117

KAJANOJA, P., JUNGNER, G., WIDHOLM, O., KARJALAINEN, O. and SEPÄLÄ, M. (1974). Rupture of the cervix in prostaglandin abortions. *J. Obstet. Gynaec. Br. Commonw.,* **81**, 242—244

KARMAN, H. and POTTS, M. (1972). Very early abortion using syringe as vacuum source. *Lancet,* **i**, 1051—1052

KLINGER, A. (1970). Demographic consequences of the legalization of induced abortion in Eastern Europe. *Int. J. Obstet. Gynaecol.,* **8**, 680—691

KOTASEK, A. (1971). Artificial termination of pregnancy in Czechoslovakia. *Int. J. Gynaecol. Obstet.,* **9**, 118—119

LEE, L.T. (1973). Five largest countries allow legal abortion on broad grounds. *Population Reports,* series F, number 1, 1—8

LINDAHL, J. (1959). In *Somatic Complications following Legal Abortion,* pp. 144—151. Heinemann, London, Melbourne, Toronto

MACKENZIE, I.Z. and HILLIER, K. (1975). Delayed morbidity following prostaglandin-induced abortion. *Int. J. Gynaecol. Obstet.,* **13**, 209—214

MACKENZIE, I.Z. and HILLIER, K. (1977). Prostaglandin-induced abortion and outcome of subsequent pregnancies: a prospective controlled study. *Br. med. J.,* **ii**, 1114—1117

McCANCE, C., OLLEY, P.C. and EDWARD, V. (1973). Long-term psychiatric follow-up. In *Experience with Abortion. A Case Study of North-East Scotland,* pp. 245—300. Ed. Horobin, G. Cambridge University Press

MEARS, J. (1975). *The Abortion Controversy – a Doctor's Guide to the Law.* American Civil Liberties Union Foundation, New York

MEDICAL DEFENCE UNION (1974). In *Consent to Treatment,* p. 24. The Medical Defence Union, London

MOMOSE, K. (1966). Intrauterine adhesions as seen with hysterosalpingography in relation to the intrauterine instrumentation with pregnancy. In *Harmful Effects of Induced Abortion,* pp. 44—48. Ed. Koya, Y. Family Planning Federation of Japan, Tokyo

NOVAK, F. (1963). Effects of legal abortion on the health of mothers in Yugoslavia. In *Changing Patterns in Fertility,* pp. 223—224. Excerpta Medica Foundation, New York and Singapore

OGBORN, A. (1973). Latent morbidity after abortion. *Br. med. J.,* **ii**, 114—115

PANAYOTOU, P.P., KASKARELIS, D.B., MIETTINEN, O.S., TRICHOPOULOS, D.B. and

KALANDIDI, A.D. (1972). Induced abortion and ectopic pregnancy. *Am. J. Obstet. Gynec.*, **114**, 507–510

PARE, C.M.B. and RAVEN, H. (1970). Follow-up of patients referred for termination of pregnancy. *Lancet*, **i**, 635–638

POTTS, M. (1967). Legal abortion in eastern Europe. *Eugen. Rev.*, **59**, 232–250

POTTS, M. (1970). Postconceptive control of fertility. *Int. J. Gynaecol. Obstet.*, **8**, 957–970

POTTS, M. (1973). Latent morbidity after abortion. *Br. med. J.*, **i**, 739–740

REGISTRAR-GENERAL, THE. *Statistical Review of England and Wales for the Years 1969, 1970, 1971, 1972 and 1973, respectively. Supplements on Abortion.* Her Majesty's Stationery Office, London

RICHARDSON, J.A. and DIXON, G. (1976). Effects of legal termination on subsequent pregnancy. *Br. med. J.*, **i**, 1303–1304

ROHT, L.H. and AOYAMA, H. (1974). Induced abortion and its sequelae: prematurity and spontaneous abortion. *Am. J. Obstet. Gynec.*, **120**, 868–874

ROYAL COLLEGE OF OBSTETRICIANS AND GYNAECOLOGISTS (1970). The Abortion Act, (1967). Findings of an inquiry into the first year's working of the Act conducted by the Royal College of Obstetricians and Gynaecologists. *Br. med. J.*, **ii**, 529–535

SAWAZAKI, C. and TANAKA, S. (1966). The relationship between artificial abortion and extrauterine pregnancy. In *Harmful Effects of Induced Abortion*, pp. 49–63. Ed. Koya, Y. Family Planning Federation of Japan, Tokyo

SHINAGAWA, S. and NAGAYAMA, M. (1969). Cervical pregnancy as a possible sequelae of induced abortion: report of 19 cases. *Am. J. Obstet. Gynec.*, **105**, 282–284

SIM, M. (1963). Abortion and the psychiatrist. *Br. med. J.*, **ii**, 145–148

SMITHELLS, R.W. (1976). Environmental teratogens of man. *Br. med. Bull.*, **32**, 27–33

STALLWORTHY, J.A., MOOLGAOKER, A.S. and WALSH, J.J. (1971). Legal abortion: a critical assessment of its risks. *Lancet*, **ii**, 1245–1249

TIETZE, C. (1969). Abortion laws and abortion practices in Europe. In *Advances in Planned Parenthood – V. Proceedings of the Seventh Annual Meeting of the American Association of Planned Parenthood Physicians, San Francisco, April 1969. Excerpta Medica International Congress Series No. 207*, pp. 194–212. Excerpta Medica, Amsterdam

TIETZE, C. and DAWSON, D.A. (1973). Induced abortion: a factbook. *Reports on Population/Family Planning*, number 14, 1–56

TIETZE, C. and LEWIT, S. (1972). Joint program for the study of abortion (JPSA): early medical complications of legal abortion. *Stud. Fam. Plann.*, **3**, 97–122

TIETZE, C. and MURSTEIN, M.C. (1975). Induced abortion: 1975 factbook. *Reports on Population/Family Planning*, number 14, 2nd edition, 1–76

WHITLOCK, F.A. and EDWARDS, J.E. (1968). Pregnancy and attempted suicide. *Compr. Psychiat.*, **9**, 1–12

WRIGHT, C.S.W., CAMPBELL, S. and BEAZLEY, J. (1972). Second-trimester abortion after vaginal termination of pregnancy. *Lancet*, **i**, 1278–1279

WYNN, M. and WYNN, A. (1972). *Some Consequences of Induced Abortion to Children Born Subsequently*, p. 30. Foundation for Education and Research in Child-bearing, London

ZIMMERMAN, M. (1976). Abortion law and practice – a status report. *Population Reports*, series E, number 3, 25–40

13 Techniques

The pioneers in the field of 'lunch-hour' abortions, conducted with local anaesthesia and a plastic catheter, have demonstrated that the risk of immediate medical complications is acceptable (Lewis *et al.*, 1971). Most subsequent reports suffer from defective follow-up, making it difficult to assess the post-operative complications, but Andolšek *et al.* (1977) have reported a controlled study with a nearly complete follow-up at four weeks. They were able to show that the use of local instead of general anaesthesia and discharge on the day of operation instead of an overnight stay in hospital made no difference to the rates for physical complications.

We have reservations about out-patient abortion under local anaesthesia because of the distress caused to a proportion of patients, and the unknown incidence of chronic pelvic inflammatory disease due to incomplete evacuation of the uterus and subsequent infertility. A number of patients complain of anxiety before the operation, of the indignity of the procedure, of severe pain during the abortion and of emotional disturbance subsequently. Our personal knowledge of this problem is limited to a North London environment, but the pain involved and the high proportion of psychiatric reactions are well documented (Lewis *et al.*, 1971; Stringer *et al.*, 1975). In many instances the patients do not return to the gynaecologist performing the operation, preferring to go elsewhere with their complaints, and this may have led to lack of appreciation of the problem. Even when the out-patient vacuum aspiration is supplemented by curettage, the uterus is often incompletely emptied, and from general principles the sequelae of chronic inflammatory disease and subsequent infertility are likely to be appreciable. The views of those who wish therapeutic abortion to be regarded as a freely available and trivial procedure, of those whose primary concern is financial economy or of those whose objective is population control should not be considered in preference to the welfare of individual patients.

We not infrequently admit young, healthy and emotionally stable patients early on the morning of the operation for termination of pregnancy under general anaesthesia, and offer them discharge from hospital the same evening if all is well. They usually prefer a night's rest and observation in hospital afterwards.

Rhesus Isoimmunisation

It is now well recognised that all methods of therapeutic abortion after six weeks from the last menstrual period convey a risk of isoimmunisation from a rhesus positive fetus. Transplacental bleeding from fetus to mother occurs in 25% of induced abortions (Matthews and Matthews, 1969). All rhesus negative women having a therapeutic abortion should receive anti-D(Rh$_0$) immunoglobin intra-muscularly, within 48 hours after the abortion. The usual dose is 50 μg for pregnancies of up to 20 weeks' maturity and 100 μg thereafter. Some practitioners check the proportion of fetal cells in the patient's blood by the Kleihauer method after the operation and give an increased dose if feto-maternal transfusion has been excessive.

SURGICAL PROCEDURES IN THE FIRST TRIMESTER

Before the end of the 12th week of pregnancy, as measured from the first day of the last normal menstrual period, the size of the uterus and its contents are such that abortion can be carried out surgically *per vaginam* with reasonable safety. Before the advent of suction techniques the conventional surgical approach was dilation of the cervix and removal of the uterine contents with sponge forceps and a blunt curette. This procedure is now relatively uncommon in Great Britain since it is said to carry a higher incidence of trauma to the uterus, including perforation, and a greater blood loss than the use of suction.

Before 8 weeks' maturity termination can be performed by insertion of a suction tube into the uterine cavity, without dilation of the cervix, and aspiration of the contents. Between 8 and 12 weeks, cervical dilation is essential if complete evacuation of fetus and placenta is to be ensured; the uterine cavity can be emptied by means of a larger bore suction curette.

The Karman Catheter

In 1970, Karman first described the use of a flexible plastic catheter (Karman and Potts, 1972) for the vacuum aspiration of first trimester pregnancies. This catheter is 6 mm in diameter with two triangular openings just below the blunt tip. A negative pressure of 600 mmHg (80 kPa) is applied, rotating the catheter and moving its tip up and down from internal os to fundus until the uterus seems to be empty. The negative pressure is greater than that needed for wide bore cannulae.

The advantages of the Karman cannula are that its small bore and flexibility allow easy introduction through an undilated or minimally dilated cervix, that it rarely perforates the uterus and that it does not cause cervical laceration and subsequent cervical incompetence. In an early study of the technique, Berić *et al.* (1972) found that a significant proportion of patients had residual products of conception as determined by curettage after vacuum aspiration; at 6 weeks' maturity the proportion of patients having retained products was 12%, but by 8 weeks it was 85% and after 9 weeks evacuation of the uterus was inadequate in all patients. With increasing maturity of the pregnancy the size of fetal parts are such that they will not pass through the aspiratory openings or the evacuatory opening in the catheter, the areas of these being only 35 mm^2 and 28 mm^2 respectively. Despite the narrow bore of the catheter, in 4.6% of patients (Berić *et al.*, 1972) its passage through the cervix requires cervical dilatation after the insertion of a paracervical block. The flexibility of the catheter can make it difficult to traverse a relatively tight cervix. Berić *et al.* (1972) overcame this problem by inserting a uterine sound into the catheter to stiffen it during its passage through the cervix. This increases the risk of uterine perforation.

A varying range of sizes of Karman catheter has been introduced, to avoid the problem of a high incidence of incomplete abortion after 8 to 9 weeks' gestation. Using the original 6 mm cannula for pregnancies up to 8 weeks, an 8 mm cannula for 9 to 10 weeks, and a 10 mm cannula for 11 to 13 weeks' gestation Liu and Hudson (1974) found that complete emptying of the uterus was possible if suction was followed by curettage with a small curette. Only 0.1% of their patients needed a repeat curettage for recurrent bleeding. General anaesthesia was used and cervical dilatation was required in most patients, though in the multiparous patient with a 6 to 8 week sized uterus the small cannula would pass through the cervix. The immediate complication rate among 2045 patients was 4.4%. The complications included cervical lacerations, uterine perforations and infections of the chest, urinary tract and genital tract.

Despite the general impression that the Karman catheter of 6 mm diameter is inadequate for terminating pregnancies of more than 6 to 8 weeks, some authors have reported good results with its use up to 10 weeks. Goldsmith and Margolis (1971) used it in 72 patients, most of whom were 9 or 10 weeks pregnant. In only 5 was cervical dilatation necessary and in only 5 was uterine evacuation incomplete, when the cavity was explored with a small curette.

'Menstrual Regulation'

This term is used to describe evacuation of the uterine cavity when a menstrual period is up to about three weeks overdue, with the intention of procuring abortion should the patient be pregnant. In environments such as Spain and most South American and Moslem countries, where statutes require proof of pregnancy before an abortion can be considered criminal, the procedure is legal without further ado. In Great Britain and France, and in most of their ex-colonies, it is the *intent* to procure abortion that can be illegal, and full documentation under the Abortion Act of 1967 is required before performing the aspiration (Lee and Paxman, 1975).

Following encouraging reports (Van der Vlugt and Piotrow, 1973a, 1974) of the use of the Karman catheter for 'menstrual regulation', Stringer *et al.* (1975) made a study of its use on 424 women outpatients in London teaching hospitals. Ninety per cent of the women were no more than 14 days overdue for menstruation and 67% of these had histological evidence of pregnancy. The 4 mm catheter was inserted without dilatation of the cervix in most patients. A few required dilatation, larger cannulae or repeated insertion. Without anaesthesia 59% of the pregnant patients described the pain they experienced as moderate, severe or unacceptable. When intracervical block with 12 ml of 1% lignocaine (lidocaine) was used, 35% of pregnant patients still had severe pain. An even greater proportion of those eventually proved not to have been pregnant experienced severe pain. About one-fifth of the patients suffered nausea, vomiting and faintness. Subsequently, 3.4% of patients were pyrexial, 2.8% needing evacuation of retained products of conception. Of the 260 patients who were proved to have been pregnant, 12 still had a positive pregnancy test at the follow-up visit 6 weeks later. It is surprising that the authors proceeded to build up a series of this size with a procedure which caused so much pain and could not even be guaranteed to cause abortion. Atienza *et al.* (1975) in Baltimore had even worse results – of 76 women in their series who were pregnant, abortion was incomplete in 5 and pregnancy continued in 6. Goldthorp (1977) found personal interest, experience and ability of the surgeon to be of great importance; pregnancy continued in only 2 of his 75 pregnant patients.

Vacuum Curettage

This has, during recent years, become the standard method of terminating first trimester pregnancies. A metal (Bierer) or rigid plastic (Berkeley) cannula with two or more holes for suction (*see* Van der Vlugt and Piotrow, 1973b) is inserted into the uterus. The negative pressure exerted is 600 mmHg (80 kPa). The rigid tube allows for easy curettage of the uterine contents from the wall, and the diameter of the tube allows for easy aspiration of the products of conception. It is necessary to increase the diameter used as maturity of the pregnancy increases so that at 12 weeks it is necessary to use a cannula of 10 mm diameter. The procedure, unlike the Karman catheter technique, requires cervical dilatation and this has to be done either under general anaesthesia or paracervical block. Vacuum curettage can be either an in-patient or out-patient procedure.

Technique

As a rule we use general anaesthesia. We do not normally catheterise the bladder. If the maturity of the pregnancy is at least 10 weeks the cervix is dilated to Hegar 11. Ergometrine (ergonovine), 0.5 mg, is then given intravenously. An appropriate size vacuum curette (a 10 mm curette is suitable at 10 weeks' maturity) is introduced into the uterus and suction applied. It is best if the pressure rises quickly. The curette is moved up and down, traversing all the walls of the uterine cavity in turn. The pressure is released from time to time, and always when it reaches 600 mmHg (80 kPa). When the uterus feels empty, the walls gripping the curette, the latter is removed and the uterine cavity scraped with a blunt spoon uterine curette. If bleeding continues further ergometrine or oxytocin is given, and, if necessary, the uterine cavity re-explored.

Some gynaecologists use local anaesthesia for vacuum curettage (Kerslake and Casey, 1967; Berić and Kupresanin, 1971) while many employ general anaesthesia. The chief advantages of local anaesthesia (paracervical block) are that cervical dilatation becomes easy and the gynaecologist feels more confident in discharging the patient home the same day (Strausz and Schulman, 1971). These authors found that the use of 4 paracervical injections of 5–6 ml of 1% lignocaine gave good or excellent anaesthesia in 96% of 500 patients. Alternative techniques are detailed by Van der Vlugt and Piotrow (1973b). The overall incidence of reactions to the local anaesthetic may be high, varying from 0.6 to 12%, but convulsive reactions are rare (0.3 per 1000). In a well-controlled trial, Andolšek *et al.* (1977) could detect no objective difference in physical complications between patients having local anaesthesia and those having general anaesthesia.

General anaesthesia is used in many centres to carry out vaginal terminations of pregnancy. Gaseous anaesthesia is probably conducive to more uterine bleeding due to myometrial relaxation and for this reason the use of ether or halothane is undesirable. The extent of uterine bleeding associated with the use of other gaseous anaesthetics depends in part on the depth of anaesthesia and the amount and route of administration (intramuscular or intravenous) of the oxytocic drug employed.

An alternative to conventional general anaesthesia is the use of intravenous diazepam, 10 mg, pentazocine, 30 mg, methohexitone, 100 mg and ergometrine, 0.5 mg. This technique provides good cervical relaxation for dilatation and reduces the blood loss (Loung *et al.*, 1971).

Complications of Vacuum Curettage

All patients undergoing termination of pregnancy by vacuum curettage should have a routine haemoglobin estimation, and blood should be sent to the laboratory for ABO and Rhesus grouping and the serum saved. Negro patients should have a test for sickle-cell trait performed at the same time. If the maturity of the pregnancy is greater than 10 weeks or the patient is anaemic it is desirable to cross-match at least one unit of blood, in case of emergency.

Short-term complications include haemorrhage, perforation of the uterus, cervical laceration, vault and vaginal haematomata, infection and secondary bleeding. The incidence of complications is directly related to the period of gestation, but the incidence of death due to these complications is very low.

Complications are a little more common in patients in their first pregnancy and in those who had an induced or spontaneous abortion in a previous pregnancy. Otherwise, there is no particular relation to age, marital status or parity (Cheng *et al.*, 1977).

Haemorrhage at the time of operation increases with gestation. The average blood loss at 6–7 weeks' maturity has been reported to be only 40–65 ml; at 12 weeks it is 160–200 ml, according to Berić and Kupresanin (1971). No indication was given as to how blood loss was measured. Loung *et al.* (1971), in their series of 1000 cases of pregnancies terminated using intravenous diazepam, methohexitone, pentazocine and ergometrine instead of formal general anaesthesia, found that 70% of patients lost less than 200 ml. Sixty-one patients lost more than 500 ml of blood, 16 of these requiring blood transfusion. Our own experience, using the same method of anaesthesia, has shown a lower incidence of significant blood loss, with only one patient among 400 needing a blood transfusion (Stone *et al.*, 1977). Haemorrhage at operation is treated by intravenous ergometrine, 0.5 mg, repeated if necessary, and intravenous oxytocin, 5 units. If bleeding does not cease promptly, blood transfusion may be necessary, and cautious re-exploration of the uterus performed with ovum forceps and a blunt spoon curette to detect unsuspected perforation. If the uterus is intact, retained products may be removed. With a bulky atonic uterus and severe bleeding bimanual compression or even dilatation of the cervix with large Hegar dilators to permit exploration with one or two fingers may rarely be necessary. Some gynaecologists still flush the uterus with 0.9% saline at 40 °C through a blunt flushing curette if bleeding persists. This procedure has the disadvantage that debris may be washed into the tubes and the open venous sinusoids and perhaps predispose to infection and also that the uterus tends to relax and start bleeding again half an hour later. Packing the uterine cavity is in general an unsatisfactory manoeuvre. It can conceal true causes of the haemorrhage such as perforation or retained products and predispose to infection. The very bulky and truly atonic uterus is not only susceptible to perforation during the packing procedure, but also difficult to pack effectively, as it continues to relax. Unsuspected haemorrhage into a large pack may be very considerable. In patients properly prepared in hospital, the need for hysterectomy or ligation of the hypogastric or internal iliac arteries to control haemorrhage due to such conditions as a massive laceration, undetected and lacerated uterine fibroids or a bleeding diathesis is extremely rare.

Estimates of abnormal bleeding in the weeks following the abortion are difficult to obtain as follow-up procedures are in general defective. Andolšek *et al.* (1977) have conducted a study where they achieved nearly 100% follow-up at 4 weeks after the operation. The incidence of prolonged bleeding (greater than normal menstruation and lasting for more than 7 days) or heavy bleeding (soaking several pads in 2 or 3 hours) was 8.5% in Ljubljana and 2.5% in Singapore.

Perforation of the uterus can occur during uterine sounding or cervical dilatation and is only rarely caused by the suction curette (Andolšek, 1974). For this reason it is advisable not to sound the uterus but to assess its size and position by a careful bimanual examination.

In large units handling numerous cases of termination of pregnancy the incidence of recorded uterine perforation at vacuum curettage is low though of course that of unrecognised perforation may be considerable. These accidents occur more commonly during the early stages of an operator's training. Figures varying between 0.04% (Berić and Kupresanin, 1971) and 1.7% (Stallworthy *et al.,* 1971) have been reported. In our recent experience of 400 cases of vacuum curettage no perforations were observed. It is likely that the risk of perforation of the uterus increases with gestation.

If the uterus is perforated and the gestation sac unruptured, the safest approach is to terminate the pregnancy by abdominal hysterotomy, either immediately if the patient has previously consented to additional procedures, or the following day if consent is needed. The question of whether or not the indication for termination of the pregnancy was strong does not enter into the decision. If termination was justified in the first place, then whatever procedure is necessary to accomplish it with safety is justified. An alternative approach is to wait two weeks, and then terminate the pregnancy with a prostaglandin, preferably used intravenously to avoid further intrauterine manipulation. The disadvantage of waiting is that a large rupture of the uterus or bowel damage may be revealed in that time by the complications of intra-abdominal haemorrhage or peritonitis respectively, when they could have been dealt with effectively by immediate laparotomy. The advantage of waiting is that laparotomy is avoided in the great majority of cases.

If the gestation sac has been ruptured by the time a perforation is discovered but there is not much bleeding then it is probably best to leave well alone, give a course of antibiotics and ergometrine and observe the patient in hospital for a week. It is unlikely that vaginal or abdominal exploration of the uterus will be necessary within that time, but subsequent irregular bleeding and discharge may well call for a cautious curettage.

When the uterus is perforated with a sound or dilators early in the proceedings and there is no heavy bleeding it is generally advised that the patient be returned to the ward and observed. It is tempting for the experienced surgeon to modify this rather inconclusive approach. Should he be confident that the perforation is small and fundal, and, after bimanual examination, sure of the contour and position of the uterus, dilatation of the cervix and cautious exploration of the uterine cavity with large ovum forceps or even a large suction curette could be entertained. Having ascertained that the perforation is not large enough to permit passage of the instrument chosen, equally cautious evacuation of at least some of its contents, using the ovum forceps or a reduced vacuum pressure, could be performed. The risks are of enlarging the perforation and causing haemorrhage and of penetrating the wall of the uterus and damaging the abdominal viscera. Subsequently, there is a risk of intra-abdominal haemorrhage and infection.

When perforation of the uterus is appreciated at a time when the evacuation of the products is nearly complete it is a mistake to resort to laparotomy unless bleeding is heavy. In general, observation of vaginal loss, temperature and bowel function in hospital for 3 to 4 days will reveal no serious consequences.

If perforation of the uterus is associated with heavy and uncontrollable bleeding, either external or into the abdomen, then laparotomy and repair of the damage or, very rarely, hysterectomy or ligation of one or both internal iliac arteries, are the only options.

Laceration of the cervix is a fairly common complication of vacuum curettage. Strausz and Schulman (1971) recorded an initial incidence of 7.1%. These lacerations nearly always occur at the side of the cervix, and Strausz and Schulman found that their occurrence could be much reduced if the tenacula were applied to the cervix laterally, to 'protect' it during dilatation. Prostaglandins given by vaginal or intrauterine routes several hours preoperatively have been used to obtain some degree of cervical dilatation before vacuum aspiration (Toppozada *et al.*, 1973; and *see* Bygdeman and Bergström, 1976). Although the gastrointestinal side-effects can be uncomfortable for the patients the manoeuvre is usually successful.

If laceration is detected it should be explored and repaired accurately, using heavy (No. 2) chromic catgut or even a non-absorbable suture, if it is to heal adequately. If the tear appears to run up into the vault, then traction with vulsella on the lower extremities may reveal the apex within the cervical canal. Very rarely, a lateral laceration extends up into the corpus of the uterus, and there is a risk of damage to the uterine artery or even the ureter. Laparotomy is then required to repair the damage.

Haematomata of the vagina or its vault can be caused by adherence of the vacuum curette as it is inserted or withdrawn, and can assume a large size. They can extend up into the broad ligament or retroperitoneally. In general haematomata should not be explored or drained, even if blood transfusion is necessary. Direct surgical attack on the source of bleeding is extremely difficult, working through oedematous tissue saturated with extravasated blood, and all that may eventually be achieved by laparotomy is ligation of the internal iliac arteries. Drainage merely predisposes to infection.

Retained products of conception are the commonest cause of haemorrhage during the first few postoperative days. The incidence of significant quantities of retained products following suction curettage has been estimated at between

0.4% (Hodgson and Portman, 1974), 1.3% (Pakter *et al.*, 1971) and 2.9% (Loung *et al.*, 1971). These are almost certainly underestimates. When we adopted the approach that any episode of increased bleeding or lower abdominal pain during the first two postoperative weeks was likely to be due to retained products and required curettage, we found that 2.7% of patients had retained products; a further 0.7% had a negative curettage (Stone *et al.*, 1977). When the uterus is examined by ultrasonic B-scanning (Stone and Elder, 1974) the incidence of significant amounts of retained products of conception after vacuum curettage is found to be much higher than suspected. These cases are usually associated with increased vaginal bleeding and lower abdominal pain. Our experience has been that between 6 and 8 weeks' maturity, 7% of patients have retained products justifying re-evacuation of the uterus, whilst at 10 to 12 weeks, the corresponding figure is 11%. This is in keeping with the overall increase in complications with gestation shown by Pakter *et al.* (1971) who found a four-fold increase after 12 weeks' maturity.

Retained products of conception can and often will, lead to acute post-operative intrauterine infection. Many authors do not quote figures for immediate postoperative pyrexia, but a rate of 1.2% has been given by two groups (Loung *et al.*, 1971; Pakter *et al.*, 1971). Our own experience has been that the rate is much higher − 4.2% (Stone *et al.*, 1977).

Postoperative pyrexia is not always specifically due to retained products of conception, and can often be treated medically (Hodgson and Portman, 1974).

Acute pelvic infection after vacuum termination occurs in about 5% of patients (Kotasek, 1971). The causes are probably organisms which are sapro-phytic in the vagina and cervix, infection introduced by amateur attempts at interference with the pregnancy, and deficiencies of aseptic technique. After intracervical swabs have been taken for culture, our first resource is amoxy-cillin for a low grade infection or intramuscular pencillin and streptomycin if pyrexia is high or pelvic findings indicate severe infection. The majority of patients respond satisfactorily. The indication for changing the antibiotics is either failure of clinical response after 48 hours or culture of an unusual organism. The amendments are then guided by the laboratory reports, but metronidazole is commonly included in the regimen, as *bacteroides* and other Gram-negative pathogens are sometimes undetected by routine culture. If there is clinical suspicion of retained products re-evacuation of the uterus may be indicated after the infection is controlled, and very occasionally, when it fails to respond.

Andolšek *et al.* (1977) found clinical evidence of pelvic inflammatory disease in 1.9−2.4% of patients examined 4 weeks after vacuum termination of pregnancy.

Chronic pelvic inflammatory disease, proceeding silently but leading to sub-fertility, infertility or ectopic gestation has been estimated by Kotasek (1971) to occur in 25% of women after vacuum termination of pregnancy. He based his findings on patients whose pregnancies were terminated by vacuum curettage under general anaesthesia and who were kept in hospital for 3−5 days after the operation. This must be compared with the data of Kolstad (1957) who used dilatation and curettage up to 12 weeks and abdominal hysterotomy after. He was able to show that only 4 out of 119 women who later wanted to have children were found to be sterile.

It is our clinical experience that the incidence of chronic pelvic inflammatory disease after termination of pregnancy is often underestimated. It may not be manifested by the signs of postoperative haemorrhage, pyrexia or pelvic pain, and may only be found at subsequent laparoscopy or laparotomy carried out for the investigation of infertility. On the basis that asymptomatic chronic pelvic infection may be caused by retained products of conception, we advocate ultrasonic B-scanning whenever there is any doubt about complete evacuation of the uterus, or even routinely, 2 days after the abortion and repetition of the operative procedure if there is any suspicion of retained products in the sonar scan.

Incompetence of the cervix leading to subsequent spontaneous abortion or premature labour is a further long-term complication of vacuum termination of pregnancy. It has been shown that vaginal termination is likely to be followed by a subsequent spontaneous abortion or premature labour due to cervical incompetence (Horksý, 1971; Kotasek, 1971; Wright *et al.*, 1972).

Mortality

The mortality associated with vacuum termination of pregnancy in England and Wales during the years 1969 to 1972 was 7.5 per 100 000 abortions (Registrar General, 1969 to 1972); more recently (1972 to 1975), in the United States of America, it had fallen to 1.9 per 100 000 abortions (Center for Disease Control, 1977). This last figure may be compared with a mortality rate of 2.6 per 100 000 abortions for termination of pregnancy by dilatation and curettage.

The causes of death are perforation, uterine rupture, haemorrhage, infection, anaesthetic hazards and associated medical disorders.

Dilatation and Curettage

The conventional technique for terminating an early pregnancy using ovum forceps and a blunt curette has been largely superseded in Great Britain by vacuum curettage. As vacuum aspiration became popular throughout the world during the nineteen sixties, so the use of simple curettage has declined. Reporting in 1971 from New York City, Pakter *et al.* recorded an incidence of termination of pregnancy of 38.8% by dilatation and curettage and 39.0% by suction curettage, but in the United States of America as a whole in 1972 to 1975 the proportion was 13.6% and 75.9% respectively (Center for Disease Control, 1977).

Dilatation and curettage has been abandoned in favour of suction curettage because the risk of operative and immediate postoperative complications is reduced. Uterine perforation occurs in 0.09% to 6.0% of terminations of pregnancy by dilatation and curettage according to Kerslake and Casey (1967), whilst the same authors did not find reports of any perforations in 14 000 cases of vacuum aspiration. However Pakter *et al.* (1971) reported very similar perforation rates for dilatation and curettage and for vacuum aspiration, these being 0.28% and 0.25% respectively. Obviously much depends on the skill of the operator, but the need to insert metal instruments into the uterus many times is likely to increase the risk, especially in relatively inexperienced hands. Damage to the uterine wall is also said to be less with vacuum aspiration than with dilatation and curettage by Kerslake and Casey (1967), though one source they cite reported finding muscle fibres in the aspirations from 20% of patients.

Because the fetus is removed in relatively large fragments especially when the gestation is 10 to 12 weeks, greater dilatation of the cervix is usually necessary than when the suction curette is inserted. This may render the cervix incompetent and predispose to subsequent abortions or premature labour.

Blood loss is greater with dilatation and curettage, being 18–57% higher than with suction curettage (Kerslake and Casey, 1967; Pakter *et al.*, 1971). This appears to be because the abortion procedure takes a much longer time, during which partially removed pieces of placental tissue within the uterine cavity cause bleeding. Finally, the risk of retained products of conception, with the possible sequelae of secondary haemorrhage and subsequent infection is greater with curettage.

In our units there have been no terminations of pregnancy performed by dilatation and curettage in recent years. It is our opinion that the procedure is no longer appropriate for the termination of first trimester pregnancy.

INTRAVENOUS PROSTAGLANDINS

The First Trimester

Irrespective of the trimester of pregnancy intravenous administration of prostaglandin E_2 (Prostin E2, dinoprostone) is appreciably more effective in causing abortion than the use of prostaglandin $F_{2\alpha}$ (Prostin F2 alpha, dinoprost) even when given in lower doses. The incidence of gastro-intestinal side-effects such as nausea, vomiting and diarrhoea is high, especially in the first trimester when higher doses are needed than in later weeks.

Using intravenous prostaglandin E_2 at infusion rates of 2–5 μg/min, Embrey (1970, 1971a and b) reported success rates of 75–80% without gastro-intestinal side-effects. In a larger series of 62 patients Karim and Filshie (1972) found that 58 aborted but in half of these the abortion was incomplete, so that evacuation of the uterus under general anaesthesia was required. The infusions were at the rate of 5–20 μg/min and lasted up to 48 hours. They resulted in a number of side-effects including nausea, vomiting, diarrhoea, pyrexia, headache and local phlebitis. The overall success rates of eight studies involving 90 patients was 70% (Sparks and Lee, 1973).

Anderson *et al.* (1972b) described three successful first trimester abortions in ten cases using infusion rates of prostaglandin $F_{2\alpha}$ varying from 25 to 200 μg/min. There was a high incidence of side-effects. The overall success rate of ten small studies combined was 55%, with infusion rates of $F_{2\alpha}$ varying from 13 to 300 μg/min (Sparks and Lee, 1973).

The success rate of these methods in the first trimester is not in general high enough to justify the incidence of side-effects, and so the attention of investigators has turned to other modes of administering prostaglandins at this stage of pregnancy.

The Middle Trimester

The use of intravenous prostaglandin E_2 in inducing abortion in the middle trimester has been studied quite extensively. With an infusion rate of 5–20

μg/min of E_2 for up to 48 hours Karim and Filshie (1972) reported 62 abortions from 67 patients, but in 7 the abortion was incomplete. Significant side-effects have been reported with these doses of E_2 (Karim and Filshie, 1972; Hillier and Embrey, 1972). The unwanted effects included tachycardia, vomiting, diarrhoea, pyrexia, headache and phlebitis at the intravenous infusion site.

Using prostaglandin $F_{2\alpha}$, Wiqvist *et al.* (1971) reported a 27% incidence of abortion with an infusion rate of 50 μg/min. When this was increased to 100 μg/min the incidence of abortion rose to 75%. Brenner (1972) feels that increasing the prostaglandin $F_{2\alpha}$ dose does not increase the abortifacient efficacy. Numerous authors have now published series on the efficacy of intravenous prostaglandin $F_{2\alpha}$ (Sparks and Lee, 1973). Infusion rates of 50–300 μg/min are needed for up to 2 days. Some of the best results have been achieved by resting the patients overnight and resuming the infusion on the next day. If this regime is used sensibly, then abortion occurs in 30–100% of patients. Unwanted effects, particularly diarrhoea, nausea, vomiting and dizziness, are common, and the larger the doses of prostaglandin employed the more common they are.

The intravenous route of administration of prostaglandins has certain disadvantages which limit its use as a method of inducing abortion. Plasma concentrations of prostaglandins required to cause abortion are five to ten times those required to induce labour (Karim and Filshie, 1970; Embrey, 1970). Unwanted gastro-intestinal effects are quite common, with both E_2 and $F_{2\alpha}$. Other side-effects include headache, fever, bronchoconstriction and peripheral vasodilatation, as well as a local inflammatory reaction at the needle site. Localised tissue reactions are more common with E_2, while the infusion of $F_{2\alpha}$ more often leads to gastro-intestinal side-effects. E_2 may have some protective value in patients prone to thrombosis, causing a rise in plasma antithrombin and euglobulin lysis activities (Howie *et al.*, 1973). Another problem is that with pregnancies of greater than 16 weeks' maturity the fetus sometimes shows the signs of life for a short while after the abortion.

Intravenous Prostaglandin with Oxytocin

A reduction in the dose of prostaglandin can be compensated for by the use of intravenous oxytocin and by the fact that the action of this on the myometrium is enhanced by prostaglandins (Hall and Pickles, 1963). This would seem to be a better approach as the incidence of side-effects is diminished.

In the first and middle trimester the uterus is relatively insensitive to the administration of oxytocin (Caldeyro-Barcia and Sereno, 1961; Bengtsson and Csapo, 1962). Burnhill *et al.* (1962) tried using large doses of intravenous oxytocin for the termination of mid-trimester pregnancies, with success in only 5 out of 10 cases. They employed large doses of oxytocin, up to 3 400 mu/min. The induction abortion intervals were between 24 and 54 hours whilst side-effects included headache, dizziness, nausea, flushing and phlebitis at the infusion site.

The potentiating effect of prostaglandins on the myometrial sensitivity to oxytocin makes this a combination that deserves further study, despite the relatively high incidence of vomiting. The concurrent use of intravenous oxytocin and prostaglandin E_2 has been tried successfully, all 19 patients in a small series having a successful abortion (Coltart and Coe, 1975). The longest induction-delivery interval was 24.5 hours, involving a total amount of prostaglandin E_2 of 9.5 mg and of 173 units of oxytocin. Most patients vomited, but in only 2 cases out of 19 was this distressing. Considerable caution should be used with respect to the dose of oxytocin. There is a real risk of cervical laceration or rupture if uterine activity is stimulated too much.

INTRAMUSCULAR PROSTAGLANDINS

The 15-methyl analogues of prostaglandins, and particularly those of prostaglandin E_2, have a greater duration of action and have been used by the intramuscular route for the termination of mid trimester pregnancies. Recent studies have suggested that intermittent divided doses of 15(S)15-methyl-prostaglandin E_2 methyl ester (the prefix '15(S)' indicates the pharmacologically active stereo-isomer) given intramuscularly, are effective as an abortifacient. Bienarz *et al.* (1974) gave 3 μg/100 lb (0.07 μg/kg) per hour intramuscularly and achieved a 100% abortion rate in 30 women with a mean injection abortion time of 13 hours. There was a high incidence of vomiting (73%) with an average of almost 3 episodes of vomiting per patient. Brenner *et al.* (1974) used 5 μg of the 15-methyl derivative intramuscularly every 4 hours. This regimen led to a much longer injection abortion interval, only 65% of patients aborting within 24 hours and 85% within 48 hours. The mean injection abortion interval was 21 hours. Diarrhoea and vomiting each occurred in 35% of patients whilst shivering and fever were the commonest side-effects, occurring in 65% and 60% of patients respectively.

15(S)15-Methyl-prostaglandin $F_{2\alpha}$ also conveys an unpleasant incidence of severe gastro-intestinal toxic effects when used in larger doses (125–250 μg 3-hourly) by the intramuscular route to procure a middle trimester abortion (Greer *et al.*, 1975; Ballard and Slaughter, 1976). Four patients in these studies developed acute respiratory distress with bronchospasm. Lauersen and Wilson (1975) obtained similar results using 250–750 μg 2 hourly. Of their 35 patients, 32 vomited, 25 had diarrhoea and 8 became pyrexial during the treatment.

INTRA-AMNIOTIC PROSTAGLANDINS

An advantage of the intra-amniotic injection of a prostaglandin compared with either oral or intravenous administration is a lower incidence of systemic side-effects and in particular a reduction in untoward gastro-intestinal responses. The advantage of a single intra-amniotic injection over a series of smaller doses infused through an intra-amniotic catheter is a reduced risk of infection. A single injection is also easier to administer and supervise than a continuous extra-amniotic infusion. With late abortions (after 16 weeks) the fetus is sometimes aborted alive and dies after a short while.

Intra-amniotic prostaglandin $F_{2\alpha}$ has been used to induce mid trimester abortions with varying degrees of success (Toppozada *et al.*, 1971; Brenner *et al.*, 1972a; Brenner *et al.*, 1973; Wiqvist *et al.*, 1973; Fraser and Brash, 1974; Elder, 1974). There is somewhat less information on the use of intra-amniotic prostaglandin E_2 (Karim and Sharma, 1971a; Craft, 1973). Although abortion occurs in most patients given either drug, the use of intra-amniotic prostaglandin $F_{2\alpha}$ has been much more extensive because approval of the use of prostaglandin E_2 was delayed by the Federal Drug Administration in the United States of America. This was because the original preparations of E_2 were unstable on keeping – a pharmaceutical problem that has now been solved. The synthetic derivatives 15-methyl-prostaglandin E_2 and 15-methyl-prostaglandin $F_{2\alpha}$ methyl ester have been employed in the same way (Karim *et al.*, 1972; Amy *et al.*, 1973; Wiqvist *et al.*, 1973).

Apart from the uterine contractions caused by prostaglandins the drugs may cause uteroplacental ischaemia, with a reduction in the production of 17β-oestradiol, progesterone and placental lactogen from the feto-placental unit. The drop in plasma progesterone may be at least partially responsible for the progressive uterine contractions seen throughout the abortion process (Csapo *et al.*, 1972b). The later the gestation the less was the drop in plasma progesterone level. This may account for the increase in injection-abortion interval found with increasing maturity from 13 to 20 weeks (Dillon *et al.*, 1974). On the other hand, Karim and Filshie (1972) did not find marked falls in plasma hormone levels until after abortion had occurred.

Increased uterine tone can lead to early rupture of the membranes, and loss of the prostaglandin reservoir injected into the amniotic fluid, with consequent diminution of uterine activity. If the regimen is one of frequent injections of small doses of prostaglandin through an intra-amniotic catheter, uterine action may be maintained, but a single injection can fail to produce abortion unless an intravenous infusion of oxytocin is used to maintain uterine contractions. The mid trimester uterus is normally relatively insensitive to oxytocin but in these circumstances usually responds, perhaps due to placental damage and reduction of progesterone influence, perhaps due to the prostaglandins causing enhancement of oxytocin action. Quite small doses of oxytocin starting with 10 or 20 drops/min of 5 u/l (3–6 mu/min) sometimes suffice but the dose may be increased at intervals if necessary. The enhanced response to oxytocin is sometimes marked, and it is important not to start with too large a dose if a precipitate abortion with damage to the cervix is to be avoided.

If there is little progress after 24 hours, it is reasonable to repeat the intra-amniotic injection of prostaglandin. In the few cases where the cervix has not dilated much 48 hours after the first injection, we tend to use extra-amniotic infusion of prostaglandins with antibiotic cover.

One alternative procedure when the membranes rupture and uterine contractions cease is to give 0.5 mg ergometrine (ergonovine) maleate with 5 u of oxytocin 6 hourly by intramuscular injection. Another is to use an intravenous infusion of prostaglandin.

Contra-indications

Only relative contra-indications to the use if intra-amniotic prostaglandins for mid trimester abortion can be defined. Patients who might be psychologically intolerant of an abortion process lasting many hours and culminating in expulsion of the products of conception are best dealt with operatively under general anaesthesia. Similar considerations apply to patients with a history of drug addiction, who might well require tranquillisers or narcotics during a prostaglandin abortion.

For patients in whom complications might be expected from transabdominal insertion of a needle into the uterus, an alternative procedure should be selected. Examples are women with a history of extensive abdominal wall or lower abdominal surgery, of extensive abdominal inflammatory conditions such as severe peritonitis, or Crohn's disease, or of treated or untreated malignant disease. Local uterine conditions such as fundal fibroids may preclude successful injection. If active pelvic inflammatory disease is present it should be under effective antibiotic control.

The principal side-effects of prostaglandins are vomiting and diarrhoea and even local intra-uterine administration is best avoided in a patient with a gastric ulcer or ulcerative colitis. The drugs have a hypotensive action in large doses and some gynaecologists may wish to avoid their use in women with major cardiovascular disorders. It is stated by the manufacturers that prostaglandins should be used with caution in patients with glaucoma or raised intra-ocular pressure.

There are reports of bronchospasm occurring during prostaglandin administration, and some confusion in the literature as to the pharmacological effects of these agents on the bronchi in humans. All prostaglandins are irritant when inhaled as aerosols. When given parenterally in large enough doses, prostaglandin $F_{2\alpha}$ and its metabolites have a bronchoconstrictor effect in humans; prostaglandin E_2 is a bronchodilator. It follows that prostaglandin $F_{2\alpha}$ should not be used to terminate pregnancy in an asthmatic patient (or one with history of an allergic diathesis), but it is reasonable to use prostaglandin E_2 in asthmatics well controlled by drugs. There are also rare reports of convulsions occurring during prostaglandin administration, but the risk is very small in well-controlled epileptics taking anticonvulsant drugs. Nevertheless many gynaecologists prefer to perform therapeutic abortion in an epileptic surgically, under general anaesthesia.

Prostaglandin E_2

Intra-amniotic prostaglandin E_2 has in general given more favourable results than prostaglandin $F_{2\alpha}$ (Mackenzie *et al.*, 1974). Administration has been by a single injection and the mode of action is probably similar to that of prostaglandin $F_{2\alpha}$. The pattern of uterine contractions induced seems to resemble that induced by prostaglandin $F_{2\alpha}$ but to be more effective in inducing abortion (Roberts *et al.*, 1972).

The doses used have been three injections of 1 mg each (Roberts *et al.*, 1972); 2.5 mg (Karim and Sharma, 1971a; Craft, 1973); 10 mg (Craft, 1973; Fraser and Brash, 1974); two doses of 10 mg (Mackenzie *et al.*, 1974) and 20 mg (Craft, 1973). The dose regimen using 3 mg led to a high success rate, 11 patients out of 13 aborting, but the injection-abortion interval varied between 8 and 70 hours (Roberts *et al.*, 1972). Using 5 mg, 10 mg or 10 mg repeated, abortion rates of over 95% have been reported (Craft, 1973; Mackenzie *et al.*, 1974), with an injection-abortion interval ranging from 4 to 19 hours (Karim and Sharma, 1971a; Fraser and Brash, 1974; Mackenzie *et al.*, 1974). The efficacy of intra-amniotic E_2 seems to be greater than that of $F_{2\alpha}$, without increase in the incidence of unwanted side-effects. The number of cases studied has so far been small, because prostaglandin E_2 is more difficult to handle from the manufacturing point of view and it is only recently that stable preparations have become available for clinical use in Great Britain. Mackenzie *et al.* (1974) compared an average induction-abortion time of 12 hours with intra-amniotic E_2 (10 mg plus 10 mg) to a time of 32 hours using $F_{2\alpha}$ (25 mg), and Fraser and Brash (1974) had similar results.

Prostaglandin $F_{2\alpha}$

A single intra-amniotic injection of $F_{2\alpha}$ has been used in doses of 15 mg (Brenner *et al.*, 1972a); 25 mg (Brenner *et al.*, 1973; Wiqvist *et al.*, 1973); 40 mg (Anderson *et al.*, 1972a; Fraser and Brash, 1974; Elder, 1974) and 100 mg (Craft, 1973).

The large bolus of injected prostaglandin $F_{2\alpha}$ diffuses slowly across the membranes, and acts on the myometrium for some hours. Increased uterine tone of up to intra-amniotic pressures of 30–40 mmHg (4–5 kPa) occurs rapidly – usually within 20 minutes of the intra-amniotic injection. This is followed within 1 hour by the onset of uterine contractions, at a frequency of 1.5 to 2 per minute, tending to diminish to 1 per minute. The basal tone remains at about 30 mmHg (4 kPa), whilst the amplitude of the contractions varies between 15 and 75 mmHg (2 and 10 kPa). The reason that all patients do not respond is probably due to differences in permeability of the membranes and myometrial sensitivity.

There is no significant transfer of prostaglandin $F_{2\alpha}$ from the uterus to the blood stream for at least 6 hours and the increase in plasma $F_{2\alpha}$ found after that time (Anderson *et al.*, 1972a) may well be due to endogenous production in the uterus. Such production is stimulated by both spontaneous contractions (Vane and Williams, 1973) and those induced by oxytocin or angiotensin (Baudouin-Legros *et al.*, 1974).

Brenner *et al.* (1972a) reported a successful abortion rate of 70% with a single injection of 15 mg of prostaglandin $F_{2\alpha}$, but Mackenzie *et al.* (1974) had little success with this dose. There are conflicting views about the use of 25 mg of $F_{2\alpha}$: some authors (Brenner *et al.*, 1972a) find that it produces a 90% abortion rate within 48 hours, while others think it is an inadequate dose (Roberts *et al.*, 1972). The proportion of successful abortions using a single injection of 40 mg of $F_{2\alpha}$ is in the range of 76% (Wiqvist *et al.*, 1973) to 89% (Elder, 1974), while with a single injection of 50 mg an abortion rate as high as 96% has been reported (Brenner *et al.*, 1973). Using 100 mg the abortion rate in one small series was 100% (Craft, 1973).

The injection-abortion interval varies from patient to patient. For those aborting, either completely or incompletely, with doses up to 25 mg the mean time is 20 hours with a range of 7–56 hours (Toppozada *et al.*, 1971). Similar mean injection-abortion times have been recorded using 40 mg and 50 mg doses (Anderson *et al.*, 1972a; Fraser and Brash, 1974). Our experience has been that the mean time using 40 mg of $F_{2\alpha}$ is 15.2 ± 8.6 hours in those having a successful abortion. The delay interval is shorter in multiparous patients than in primiparous patients. The mean injection-abortion interval for all patients receiving 100 mg prostaglandin $F_{2\alpha}$ was 17.3 hours (Craft, 1973).

A relation between the time of day at which the injection of intra-amniotic prostaglandin $F_{2\alpha}$ is given and the injection-abortion interval has been reported from Australia (Smith and Shearman, 1974). We have confirmed that there is a significant reduction in the injection-abortion interval when the initial injection is given at a specific time (Elder *et al.*, 1976). The optimum time in our experience is different, 12.00 to 14.00 hours compared to the 18.00 hours found by Smith and Shearman (1974), and the timing is not quite so specific. The reasons for these findings are as yet obscure, but may be related to a diurnal variation in endogenous prostaglandin $F_{2\alpha}$ levels (Jubiz *et al.*, 1972) or to oestrogen and progesterone levels affecting the myometrial response. If these results are confirmed it is desirable that intra-amniotic injections of prostaglandin $F_{2\alpha}$ should be given at the optimum time.

The proportion of complete to incomplete abortions varies from one study to another, but it is our experience that a complete abortion occurs in only about one-sixth of patients. Consequently routine surgical evacuation of the uterus under anaesthetic is desirable. If it is thought that abortion is complete, ultrasound B-scanning of the the uterus, as described by Stone and Elder (1974), can be carried out to verify that this is the case.

An alternative method of administering prostaglandin $F_{2\alpha}$ into the amniotic cavity is the repetition of smaller doses using an indwelling catheter. Brenner *et al.* (1972a, 1973) reported favourably on the use of 25 mg prostaglandin $F_{2\alpha}$ given up to 4 times within 30 hours if necessary. This resulted in a higher incidence of complete abortion, a lower incidence of incomplete abortion, and a shorter injection-abortion interval. A disadvantage of the method is the need for a larger bore needle with which to perform amniocentesis, so that a catheter can be threaded down its lumen, and the increased risk of intra-uterine infection from the presence of such a catheter.

Unwanted Effects of Intra-amniotic Prostaglandin $F_{2\alpha}$

The incidence of side-effects, of which vomiting is the commonest, is generally considered acceptable with respect to mid trimester abortion. Vomiting occurs in one-third to one-half of the patients and diarrhoea in only a few (Craft, 1973; Mackenzie *et al.*, 1974; Elder, 1974). A systemic reaction can occur if the prostaglandin solution is inadvertently injected into a uterine venous sinus. This takes the form of severe diarrhoea, vomiting, bradycardia, hypotension and bronchospasm. If the placental site is localised by sonar, and a small test dose is given initially, inadvertent intravenous injection should be a rare occurrence. The reaction passes off within 15—20 minutes. A pyrexial reaction is not uncommon and may not always be due to infection.

There is doubt about the effects of intra-amniotic prostaglandin $F_{2\alpha}$ on blood coagulation parameters. Anderson *et al.* (1972a) found no effect on platelets, prothrombin time, fibrinogen or fibrin and fibrinogen degradation products. Dillon *et al.* (1974) found a small increase in platelet count, fibrinogen and factors V and VIII, reaching a maximum 6 hours after the injection. Electroencephalographic changes are common but convulsions are rare. They have been reported after a dose of 30 mg (Lyneham *et al.*, 1973). Mackenzie *et al.* (1974) found that major convulsions occurred in 5 out of 320 cases. Two patients of

Lyneham *et al.* (1973) had histories of epilepsy but the use of prostaglandins does not seem to be contra-indicated in well-controlled epileptics.

The incidence and full extent of cervical damage during mid trimester abortions induced with prostaglandin is probably under-reported, though rupture of the cervix has been described (Bradley-Watson *et al.*, 1973; Wentz *et al.*, 1973; Mackenzie *et al.*, 1974). The injudicious use of too much oxytocin to expedite prostaglandin abortions may be contributory. Similarly, the proportion of patients with an incomplete abortion who eventually develop pelvic inflammatory disease is unrecorded. The lack of documentation on long-term sequelae must be regarded as a significant failure on the part of those performing the abortions.

Methyl Analogues of Prostaglandin $F_{2\alpha}$

Methyl analogues of prostaglandin $F_{2\alpha}$ are effective in doses 10 times less than the parent compound, 2.5–5.0 mg as a single intra-amniotic injection. These doses give an abortion rate of 95–98% (Wiqvist *et al.*, 1973). The injection-abortion interval is not significantly shorter, but the incidence of vomiting, which seems to be dose dependent, is probably reduced (Bygdeman, Béguin *et al.*, 1972; Wiqvist *et al.*, 1973). The more gradual build up of uterine action following a latent period of several hours suggests that the 15-methyl prostaglandin $F_{2\alpha}$ derivative permeates the membranes more slowly when given by the intra-amniotic route and has a less sudden ischaemic effect on the myometrium, but a more prolonged effect. The slower rate of action may be the reason why abortion with the methyl derivative is less painful than with a equiactive dose of the parent compound (Wiqvist *et al.*, 1973). There is still a troublesome incidence of vomiting and diarrhoea associated with the use of 15-methyl-prostaglandin $F_{2\alpha}$ methyl ester to induce mid trimester abortion.

Ancillary Manoeuvres

Two measures have been suggested which may expedite the effects of intra-amniotic prostaglandins in inducing abortion. The introduction of a laminaria tent into the cervix 14–18 hours before the prostaglandin is injected (Eaton *et al.*, 1972) results in cervical dilation to 10–12 mm in most patients and reduces the average time to abortion to about 14 hours (Stubblefield *et al.*, 1976). This procedure did not appear to cause infection on a short-term basis, but must surely increase the potential for infection if used on a large scale. The other measure which may shorten the duration of the abortion is to inject urea (80 g) intra-amniotically in combination with the prostaglandin E_2 (2.5 mg). Craft (1975) obtained a mean abortion time of 11 hours in this way. Clements and Khunda (1976) had similar results but recorded a number of complications, including a ruptured uterus in a grande multipara and a patient who developed haemoglobinuria, probably after an accidental intravesical infusion of hypertonic urea.

EXTRA-AMNIOTIC PROSTAGLANDINS

First Trimester

Prostaglandin E_2 was tested by the extra-amniotic route by Embrey and Hillier (1971). They obtained complete abortions in 4 first trimester patients with instillations of 50–200 μg at one or two hourly intervals, up to total doses of 600–1675 μg. Roberts *et al.* (1971) had no complete success in 20 cases, using injections of 20–60 μg every 2 hours up to a maximum dose of 2900 μg. Using prostaglandin $F_{2\alpha}$ by the extra-amniotic route in the first trimester a certain degree of success has been reported. Csapo *et al.* (1972a) reported 7 abortions from 12 cases, using an infusion of 2–4 mg/hour up to a maximum total dose of 58 mg.

Middle Trimester

Prostaglandin E_2 has been used by continuous infusion into the extra-amniotic space to procure abortion. This involves the insertion of a Foley gauge 12 (o.d. 4 mm) catheter through the cervix using an aseptic technique, though of course some organisms from the cervix are bound to be carried into the uterine cavity. The balloon of the catheter is distended with 15–20 ml of sterile water to retain it in position. The suggestion that the presence of the balloon of the Foley catheter in the cervical canal may be at least partly responsible for inducing myometrial activity has been refuted (Embrey and Hillier, 1972). Prostaglandin E_2, diluted with normal saline to concentrations varying between 25 and 100 μg/ml is instilled, using a constant rate infusion pump, or intermittent administration from a manually operated syringe. Using the latter method Miller *et al.* (1972) found that 90% of patients aborted after receiving a total dose of 2.5 mg prostaglandin E_2 during a mean infusion period of 16 hours. Fraser and Brash (1974) reported very similar results, 89% of patients having aborted within 36 hours. The mean dose of prostaglandin E_2 used was 2.69 mg and the mean infusion time 16.2 hours. Midwinter *et al.* (1973) found that the optimum rate of infusion of prostaglandin E_2 was 66.5 μg/hour and that at this rate the mean infusion time was similar − 16.7 hours − and the total dose of prostaglandin E_2 was halved to 1.15 mg.

The incidence of side-effects such as nausea and vomiting is dose-dependent. Most authors find that about one-third of patients are affected by these gastro-intestinal side-effects, and this was the experience of Midwinter *et al.* (1973) using a dose of 66.5 μg/hour.

In the series of Miller *et al.* (1972), 9 out of 60 patients lost more than 200 ml of blood, and 5 of these needed blood transfusions. All these cases had retained products removed under general anaesthesia.

The majority of abortions that occur are incomplete. Should abortion not have occurred within 24 hours or should the membranes rupture then intravenous oxytocin should be administered in doses of the order of 80 mu/min, if necessary to secure continuing uterine contractions.

The method requires supervision of the constant infusion pump or repeated instillations of prostaglandin E_2, 200 μg, 2-hourly or, $F_{2\alpha}$, 750 μg, 2-hourly. The catheter may fall out, requiring re-insertion if the cervix is not dilated adequately for abortion to occur. Mackenzie *et al.* (1974) found that 31 out of 101 patients given extra-amniotic E_2 needed evacuation of the uterus for incomplete expulsion of the products of conception compared with only 7 out of 42 who had intra-amniotic E_2. The presence of a foreign body in the cervical canal and uterus for many hours is a potential source of infection but the long-term incidence of subsequent pelvic inflammatory disease is unknown.

Prostaglandin $F_{2\alpha}$, in contrast to prostaglandin E_2, gives rise to a high incidence of nausea, vomiting and diarrhoea when instilled extra-amniotically and seems to be less effective as an ecbolic (Mackenzie *et al.*, 1974). For this reason the extra-amniotic use of $F_{2\alpha}$ for the induction of abortions after 12 weeks' gestation (Miller *et al.*, 1972; Fraser and Brash, 1974) has been limited. In patients 13 to 15 weeks' pregnant Shapiro (1975) used $F_{2\alpha}$, 3 mg every 1 to 3 hours. Nineteen out of 20 patients aborted with an average induction-abortion interval of 18 hours, but half of them had nausea and vomiting and 6 had retained products of conception.

The 15-methyl analogue of prostaglandin $F_{2\alpha}$ acts more rapidly initially (Laumas *et al.*, 1974) but has a more prolonged effect. Preliminary studies indicate that most patients abort after one extra-amniotic injection of 200–400 μg but some patients may need up to 5 such injections. In a small study of 17 patients Bygdeman, Béguin *et al.* (1972) found that all patients aborted, with a mean injection-abortion interval of 14.5 hours (range 6.3 to 27.7 hours), but Mackenzie *et al.* (1974) reported a mean interval of 25.1 hours (range 4 to 68 hours).

INTRA-VAGINAL PROSTAGLANDINS

First Trimester

The number of cases reported using intra-vaginal prostaglandin pessaries or tablets to induce abortion early in pregnancy is relatively small. Prostaglandins E_2 (0.5–40 mg) or $F_{2\alpha}$ (2.5–200 mg) have been used intra-vaginally for 'menstrual regulation', with varying degrees of success (Csapo, 1974; Shalita, 1975). Using vaginal doses of 20 mg of E_2 or 50 mg of $F_{2\alpha}$ every 2½ hours, Karim and Sharma (1971b) recorded a complete abortion rate of 90% in first and second trimester abortions, with only 7 out of 45 patients experiencing untoward gastro-intestinal side-effects but Brenner *et al.* (1972b) were less successful. The vaginal route has no advantage over those already described except that administration is easy and the procedure might be useful for large-scale use with minimal medical supervision.

Bygdeman, Borell *et al.* (1976) have reported on the use of triglyceride vaginal pessaries containing 15(S)15-methyl-prostaglandin $F_{2\alpha}$ methyl ester to induce abortion. Vaginal doses of 1–2 mg every 3 hours resulted in plasma concentrations of 400–500 pg/ml of the methyl derivative. After a latent period of 30 minutes there was a gradual increase in uterine tone and then coordinated uterine contractions developed over the next hour or two. The procedure has been used for 'menstrual regulation' within 14 days of when the missed menstrual period was expected. Thirty-five pregnant patients started bleeding within a few hours and aborted; the loss continued for an average of 9 days, and curettage was only performed in 2 patients because it continued for more than 14 days.

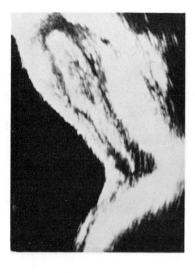
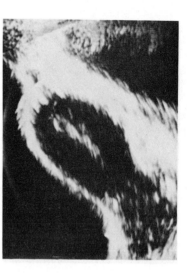
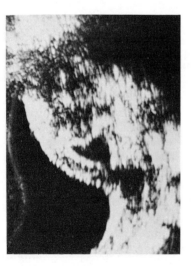
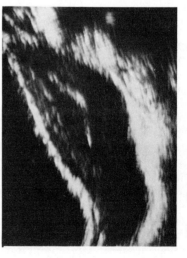

Figure 13.1 (a) Ultrasonic picture of distorted gestation sac with blood clot behind it during the early stages of expulsion. (b) Uterus after expulsion of the sac; a large amount of placental tissue and blood clot is retained 3 days later. (c) and (d) Empty uterus; the uterine cavity shows as a white shadow 9 days after the abortion, the retained products having been expelled piecemeal.

One of these patients had retained products of conception. Fifty per cent of the patients experienced vomiting or diarrhoea. Most required analgesics; five needed intramuscular pethidine (meperidine). Of 40 patients between 4 and 8 weeks' pregnant given vaginal 15(S)15-methyl prostaglandin $F_{2\alpha}$ methyl ester by Zoremthangi *et al.* (1976), only 27 aborted.

Our experience of the use of single pessary of 3 mg 15-methyl-prostaglandin $F_{2\alpha}$ methyl ester in 18 patients has been that 17 of them aborted completely. The 18th patient did not react at all and required vacuum termination. The mean gestation was less than 7 weeks. Pain and bleeding started within 6 hours and at this time the gestation sac is being dislodged and expelled (*Figure 13.1a*). Bleeding, usually no heavier than a period, continued for between 6 and 13 days. *Figures 13.1b, c* and *d* illustrate emptying of the uterus during that time. Gastrointestinal side-effects occurred in more than half the patients. In some cases these were severe, but they usually lasted only 6 hours, and all but 2 of the patients were able to go home the same evening (Dutt, T.P. *et al.*, 1979).

Between 9 and 13 weeks' maturity, Bygdeman, Borell *et al.* (1976) found that vaginal 15-methyl-prostaglandin $F_{2\alpha}$ methyl ester caused abortion within 18 hours in 57 out of 58 patients, but the abortion was complete in only half this number. One patient required blood transfusion. Vomiting was not a problem but oral diphenoxylate chloride (Retardin, Lomotil), 5 mg, and atropine, $50\,\mu g$ was needed to prevent diarrhoea and 6 patients needed intramuscular analgesics. Half the patients develop low-grade pyrexia without evidence of infection (Bygdeman, Martin *et al.*, 1974).

This approach to therapeutic abortion is of interest but until analogues are developed with a better therapeutic ratio − a more potent ecbolic action and proportionately less gastro-intestinal side-effects − the method will not be suitable for general use. There may then be a prospect of a simple self administered medical method of inducing early abortion. At present it seems that the earlier the method is used the more likely is it to be successful. The success rate at 6 weeks is about 95% (Bygdeman and Bergström, 1976).

Middle Trimester

Béguin *et al.* (1972) used 20 mg of prostaglandin E_2 intravaginally in 10 patients, of whom 7 aborted completely. Repeated doses of E_2, 20 mg every 2½ hours (*Figure 13.2*), gave an increased success rate (Karim and Sharma, 1971b).

Single or repeated doses of 50 mg of prostaglandin $F_{2\alpha}$ vaginally were relatively unsuccessful (Béguin *et al.*, 1972; Brenner *et al.*, 1972b). Only a few patients aborted but there was a high incidence of gastro-intestinal side-effects. Wentz *et al.* (1973) obtained better results using lactose tablets of prostaglandin $F_{2\alpha}$ inserted intravaginally at hourly intervals. The abortion time was less than 29 hours in 19 out of 20 patients, the average time being 16 hours. There were many untoward side-effects such as vomiting, diarrhoea and fever.

If prostaglandin used by the vaginal route must be absorbed into the bloodstream before being effective there is no chance that this method will reduce the incidence of gastro-intestinal side-effects compared with other methods of administration. It appears that the composition of the pessaries used and their rate of disintegration is important. There is a difference of opinion regarding the relative merits of E_2 and $F_{2\alpha}$. The introduction of more potent methyl analogues, impregnated in a Silastic or wax base to produce a slow release

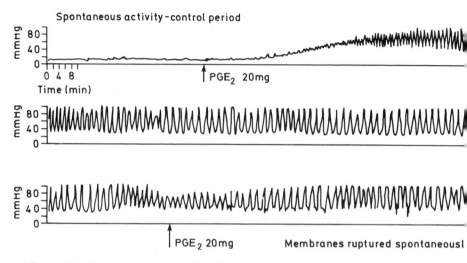

Figure 13.2 Continuous record of the effect of vaginal administration of prostaglandin E₂ on the pregnant human uterus in a nulliparous patient, aged 18, 14 weeks pregnant, induction—abortion interval 7 hours. (Karim and Sharma, 1971b).

provides the best hope for the future use of this method of prostaglandin administration to induce mid trimester abortions. The release of tritiated $F_{2\alpha}$ from a polyvinyl insertion tube has been studied by Lau *et al.* (1974) using rabbits. It was found that of 3 mg of $F_{2\alpha}$ in the Silastic-polyvinyl tube only 50% remained 3 hours after insertion into the vagina of a pregnant rabbit. All animals studied aborted within 48 hours.

Vaginal pessaries containing 15(S)15-methyl-prostaglandin $F_{2\alpha}$ methyl ester, 1–2 mg every 3 hours (Borell *et al.*, 1976) or 16,16-dimethyl-prostaglandin E_2, 1 mg every 3 hours (Martin *et al.*, 1976) have been used to procure mid trimester abortions. The latter compound caused fewer unwanted gastro-intestinal effects but 5 out of 30 patients developed temporary pyrexia. Half the patients retained the placenta for at least 2 hours, when it was removed surgically; doubtless many of the others had some retained products of conception.

INTRA-AMNIOTIC HYPERTONIC SALINE

The injection of hypertonic saline into the amniotic cavity has been the commonest method of inducing mid trimester abortions and is still widely used in the United States of America. The risks of severe illness or death due to hypernatraemia, haemolysis and sepsis, however rare these may be, and the belief that prostaglandins are safer, has caused most gynaecologists in Great Britain to cease to use the procedure over the last few years.

In a direct comparative study, Lauersen *et al.* (1974) found no difference between the success rate of intra-amniotic saline or prostaglandin $F_{2\alpha}$. The endocrine changes were similar, suggesting that both procedures cause damage to the feto-placental site, but with late abortions induced with prostaglandins the fetus is sometimes born alive. In a large-scale controlled trial conducted by the Joint Program of the Study of Abortion (Center for Disease Control, 1977), the comparative risks of mid trimester abortion (13 to 20 weeks' maturity) were studied. It was found that fever, endometritis, retained products of conception and convulsions were all less frequent in association with intra-amniotic saline than with prostaglandin $F_{2\alpha}$. Lengths of hospital stay were similar for the two groups (mean 2.1 days) although intra-amniotic saline produced longer mean induction to abortion intervals; 29 hours against 25 hours. On the other hand, the saline treated patients were less likely to need re-admission to hospital. It is not possible to make valid comparisons of mortality at given durations of gestation from the data so far presented.

Mortality seems to us to be the overriding consideration. Most of the deaths reported in Japan during the late 1940's and early 1950's were probably due to abortions being performed by relatively unskilled personnel (Wagatsuma, 1965). Berger *et al.* (1974) reported that widespread use of hypertonic saline for therapeutic abortion in New York State has resulted in 11 deaths in 56 274 cases (19.5 per 100 000), some 8 times the mortality associated with suction or sharp curettage. It is of the same order as the overall mortality for abortions performed at 13 weeks' maturity (21.1 per 100 000; Schiffer *et al.*, 1973) and that for all intra-uterine instillations in the United States of America (17.7 per 100 000; Center for Disease Control, 1977). It must be accepted that both these last figures are biased upwards by the inclusion of high proportions of saline abortions and the former by the inclusion of terminations of pregnancy by hysterotomy or hysterectomy which carry a much higher mortality due to associated risks. The data presented by Cates *et al.* (1977), suggest that intra-uterine instillations of prostaglandins or hypertonic saline are more dangerous in the middle trimester than surgical evacuation of the uterus *per vaginam*.

Until the position with respect to mortality is clarified we shall continue to use prostaglandins in preference to hypertonic saline. We do feel that much of the risk associated with the latter procedure can be obviated by the use of the vaginal technique described on p. 289, with replacement of amniotic fluid by saline, free vaginal drainage to avoid increases in basal intra-uterine pressure, and abandoning the procedure if any difficulty is encountered in penetrating the amniotic cavity without bleeding.

Mode of Action

Weiss, R.R. *et al.* (1972) found it desirable to achieve a sodium concentration of 2200 mEq/litre in the amniotic fluid to ensure abortion within 48 hours. In Kerenyi and Muzsnai's (1975) study the initial concentration of sodium achieved after intra-amniotic injection of hypertonic saline was between 1200 and 3300 mEq/litre in cases where abortion eventually resulted. The wide variation reflected differences in the amount of amniotic fluid originally present and the amount drained. The infusion itself adds to the amount of fluid present increasing uterine volume. Over the next one to three hours there is an increase in amniotic fluid volume of the order of 25% (Gochberg and Reid, 1966; Wagner, 1971; Kerenyi and Muzsnai, 1975). This is an osmotic effect (Goodlin and Kresch, 1968) and the amniotic fluid sodium concentration falls. After 8 to 10 hours the sodium level has fallen to 25% of its peak value because of escape into the bloodstream and renal excretion. Half the salt injected has been excreted in the urine within 36 hours (Wong *et al.*, 1972). Changes in amniotic fluid chloride are parallel to those of sodium.

Both overall increases in uterine volume and sodium concentration are directly related to the production of abortion (Bengtsson and Csapo, 1962; Kerenyi and Muzsnai, 1975). The two factors are complementary but the volume increase is more important in earlier pregnancies. Presumably distension of the uterus, consequent stimulation of the myometrium and impairment of the utero-placental circulation, impairment of placental function and infarction of the placenta all play a part in the induction of abortion.

The normal uterus in mid pregnancy is relatively inactive, the intra-amniotic pressure being about 4 mmHg (0.5 kPa), and even doses of oxytocin as large as 100 mu/min, whilst increasing the intra-amniotic pressure, do not induce contractions as strong as those of abortion caused by intra-amniotic saline or those of normal labour (Bengtsson and Csapo, 1962). This inactivity and insensitivity to stimuli is thought to be at least in part due to high myometrial progesterone levels. Within one or two hours of the intra-amniotic injection there is a spontaneous increase in uterine activity, but much of the early activity is inefficient and characterised by high frequency, low amplitude contractions. This is probably the myometrial response to the osmotic increase in uterine volume. These contractions do not significantly increase the intra-amniotic pressure. The myometrium is now much more sensitive to oxytocin and if this drug is infused intravenously a transition to a pattern of more efficient, low frequency, high amplitude contractions results. The addition of intravenous oxytocin thus results in a shorter interval between the injection of hypertonic saline and abortion.

Amniotic pressure between contractions increases so that after 16 to 22 hours, when the amniotic fluid is no longer hypertonic, it rises to 30 mmHg (4 kPa). With contractions, this pressure then rapidly increases to 70–120 mmHg (9–16 kPa), higher than that experienced during the contractions of normal labour. With contractions like this the cervix takes up and dilates and abortion rapidly ensues.

The hypertonic saline causes the placenta to become oedematous and widespread congestion and thrombosis occur in its vessels; there is necrosis of chorionic villi and decidua. The fetal heart usually disappears at this stage. The increase in uterine activity has been said to be due to reduction in the amounts of progesterone produced by the damaged placenta (Csapo, 1966; Wiest *et al.*, 1966; Csapo *et al.*, 1969). The induction-abortion interval can be prolonged by administration of the synthetic progestagen dydrogesterone (Gennser *et al.*, 1968). This theory has been criticised because Fuchs *et al.* (1965) found that uterine activity began before the progesterone levels of uterine venous blood had begun to fall and Osborn *et al.* (1968) found that the onset of uterine activity was not coincidental with a significant change in placental output of progesterone. Also the most significant drop in plasma progesterone may not occur until the placenta separates in the course of the actual abortion (Lurie *et al.*, 1966; Laumas *et al.*, 1974). It seems probable that although a fall in myometrial progesterone levels as a result of death of the feto-placental unit may not initiate uterine action, it may be a factor in permitting the increase and maintenance of such activity. Other hormones produced by the placenta such as oestradiol, oestrone, oestriol, chorionic gonadotrophin and placental lactogen have been shown to drop by 50 to 70%, 45%, 65%, 27% and by up to 50%

respectively, during the injection-abortion interval (Gennser *et al.*, 1968; Laumas *et al.*, 1974; Jayaraman *et al.*, 1975). Laumas *et al.* (1974) found the drop in plasma oestradiol to be associated with the initiation of abortion. In addition, it is known that the injection-abortion interval is shorter in cases of intra-uterine fetal death (Csapo *et al.*, 1963). This is consistent with the view that reduction in hormone output facilitates the process of abortion but it also suggests that hypertonic saline can stimulate uterine contractions after the placental influence has been withdrawn.

It has been suggested that there is a coincident release of oxytocin from the posterior pituitary gland and this may play a role (Gaitonde *et al.*, 1974).

Another hypothesis on the mode of action of hypertonic saline instilled intra- or extra-amniotically suggests that the salt tends to localise in the decidual cells, allowing leakage of lysosomal enzymes which damage further cells (Gustavii, 1974, 1975). The onset of uterine contractions, by causing hypoxia and ischaemia of the lysosomal membrane, can also contribute to this process. Lysosomes contain phospholipase A_2 (Franson *et al.*, 1971) which acts as a trigger for prostaglandin synthesis by releasing prostaglandin precursors from the membrane phospholipids. It may be that the increased synthesis of prostaglandins stimulates the uterus to contract. The fact that plasma oestradiol falls promptly (Laumas *et al.*, 1974) but plasma progesterone, placental lactogen and cystine aminopeptidase levels take longer to fall after hypertonic saline than after injections of prostaglandin $F_{2\alpha}$ are consistent with the view that the former procedure acts indirectly on the placenta with some delay.

Systemic Effects of Intra-amniotic Hypertonic Saline

It would be surprising if the injection of such a large amount as 200 ml of hypertonic saline containing 684 mmol (40 g) of sodium chloride into a body compartment did not have widespread effects. It has been shown that there is an antidiuretic response after the intra-amniotic injection, comparable to that caused by intravenous hypertonic saline (Anderson and Turnbull, 1968). The water retention results in a slight increase in blood volume with a fall of 3–4% in haematocrit. With normal renal function it takes about 12 hours for half of the injected sodium to be accounted for by urinary excretion (American College of Obstetricians and Gynecologists, 1976).

To reduce the transfer of sodium from the amniotic cavity, which might be harmful to high risk patients such as those with heart disease, it has been suggested that all the amniotic fluid be aspirated 45 minutes after completing the injection of hypertonic saline. This reduces the salt load to 18% of that induced by the standard procedure, without altering the abortifacient efficacy (Perry *et al.*, 1974).

Plasma sodium is increased slightly, this rise commencing soon after the injection, and reaching a peak after 2 to 4 hours. The mean increase was 4.4 mEq/l (Easterling *et al.*, 1972). Plasma chloride and potassium levels are not significantly altered. The haematocrit has been found to be decreased but never by more than 10% (Anderson and Turnbull, 1968).

There is some evidence that intra-amniotic hypertonic saline causes intravascular coagulation as there is a reduced level of fibrinogen, a reduced platelet count, and an increase in fibrin and fibrinogen degradation products (Brown *et al.*, 1972; Beller *et al.*, 1972; Weiss, A.E. *et al.*, 1972).

Contra-indications

This method of inducing abortion is contra-indicated in patients who are likely to be intolerant of an abortion procedure which lasts many hours, may be painful and results in visible expulsion of the products of conception, and also in patients where difficulty in abdominal amniocentesis or complications therefrom are predictable.

High risk patients include women with sickle-cell disease, moderate to severe anaemia and cardiac or cardiovascular disorders including hypertension and renal disease.

Procedures

Before 13 weeks' maturity the amniotic fluid volume is less than 100 ml and it is difficult to penetrate the amniotic sac with a needle. Sixteen weeks is the optimum time for transabdominal amniocentesis − by then the volume is 150−250 ml (Reiss, 1969).

General anaesthesia is contra-indicated because of the risk of undetected intravenous infusion of hypertonic saline. It is also unreasonable to take the risks of anaesthesia for the injection and then let the patient wake up to undergo having an abortion during the next day or two, perhaps followed by another general anaesthetic to evacuate retained products of conception. Some workers premedicate the patient with diazepam or chlorpromazine, but in general premedication is best avoided so that the patient can report any symptoms accurately. Transabdominal amniocentesis is then performed under local anaesthesia and at least 100 ml of amniotic fluid drained. Aspiration is best avoided as it may collapse the amniotic cavity before it has been fully drained. Between 100 and 300 ml of 20% saline is then injected. A detailed account of the technique is given by Menzies and Hawkins (1968). Blood-stained taps suggest that the needle has entered a blood vessel, a placental sinus or the uterine wall, and contra-indicate injection. They do not bar a further attempt a week later. Whilst the saline is being injected, the occurrence of severe pain suggests accidental injection into tissue or peritoneum; sudden onset of loin pain, headache, flushing, thirst or numbness of the fingers suggest intravascular absorption of saline. In either event, the procedure is at once abandoned, and an intravenous infusion of 5% dextrose in water given.

The average injection-abortion interval derived from many studies using up to 200 ml of hypertonic saline is about 35 hours, but if the volume is increased to 300 ml the injection-abortion interval is shortened to an average of 23 hours. It has been suggested by Weiss, R.R. *et al.* (1972) that a more rapid abortion rate is associated with a higher sodium concentration in the amniotic fluid. Sixty-eight of their 80 patients aborted within 48 hours. The mean amniotic fluid sodium concentration was 3049 mEq/l, that for 12 patients whose abortions lasted for more than 48 hours being 1613 mEq/l. Other authors have been unable to demonstrate any relationship between the quantity of amniotic fluid removed, or the amount of hypertonic saline injected, and the injection-abortion interval. Menzies and Hawkins (1968) found that the more mature the pregnancy, the less likely was failure, and it has since been found that as gestation advances, the same concentration of sodium will produce larger increases in uterine volume osmotically and the induction-abortion interval depends on this (Kerenyi and Muzsnai, 1975). This is an important finding since it means it is not usually necessary to increase the quantity of hypertonic saline injected if the uterus is larger. The injection-abortion interval is apparently un- related to the age of the patient (Bracken *et al.*, 1972). Some authors have found that the injection-abortion interval was longer in primigravid patients when compared with multiparous patients (Berk *et al.*, 1971) while others could show no effect of parity (Menzies and Hawkins, 1968; Bracken *et al.*, 1972; Stim, 1972).

The Vaginal Approach

The use of this route for intra-amniotic injection has been reported, employing a needle inserted through the cervical canal (Menzies and Hawkins, 1968) or through the anterior fornix, passing below the bladder into the uterus to pene- trate the amniotic sac (Wagner *et al.*, 1962; Ruttner, 1966).

The vaginal route is advantageous in pregnancies of less than 16 weeks' maturity, if difficulty is encountered with transabdominal injection, in the obese patient or if uterine fibromyomata are present. We have been more con- cerned with reducing the risk of the relatively rare but potentially fatal compli- cations of intravenous hypertonic infusion. In the two fatal cases from Great Britain reported in detail by Cameron and Dayan (1966), the abdominal route was employed. One patient had the injection performed under general anaes- thesia and was therefore unable to report the early symptoms of intravenous leakage; in the other 200 ml of amniotic fluid was removed and 400 ml of hypertonic saline replaced.

If a pregnancy of between 14 and 18 weeks' maturity is to be terminated by the intra-amniotic injection of hypertonic saline, the following procedure is therefore recommended. Having emptied the bladder the patient is lightly sedated with diazepam and put in the lithotomy position. With aseptic and antiseptic precautions, the cervix is grasped with a tenaculum and the ball-ended guide of a paracervical block needle or an Iowa trumpet inserted through the cervix and used to penetrate the amniotic sac. The needle itself is only inserted if the sac cannot be penetrated with the guide alone, the position of the uterus being verified bimanually first. When amniotic fluid drains, its volume is measured, and an equivalent volume of 20% saline run in from a drip bottle. The procedure of drainage and replacement is repeated twice more. If uterine con- tractions are not initiated within 12 hours, an oxytocin drip is set up, starting with 10 u/l at 20–40 drops/min (10–25 mu/min), and increasing the dose hourly, up to 100 u/l (100–250 mu/min) if necessary, until effective uterine contractions start. If frank bleeding is encountered during the operative pro- cedure the method is abandoned. The pregnancy may then be terminated by inducing general anaesthesia and performing vaginal or abdominal hysterotomy. Alternatively, the following day hypertonic urea, mannitol or a prostaglandin may be introduced into the amniotic cavity *per abdomen*.

With pregnancies between 14 and 18 weeks' maturity we have found replacement of the amniotic fluid with hypertonic saline and an intravenous oxytocin drip as effective as using the abdominal approach. With avoidance of over-distension of the uterus and free drainage from below the risk of hypertonic infusion is clearly diminished.

In pregnancies of over 16 weeks' maturity, if termination with a hypertonic solution is elected, we prefer to use urea or mannitol by the abdominal route and an oxytocin drip, rather than inject hypertonic saline into a closed uterine cavity.

Immediate onset of effective uterine contraction occurs in a few women. If this happens, placental abruption should be suspected, oxytocin avoided and close observation of the patient, and of her urinary output, instituted.

The membranes occasionally rupture during the injection, sometimes later. No special measures are needed but vaginal interference should be avoided to reduce the risk of infection.

Management

Uterine contractions usually start within one or two hours but effective uterine action is often only appreciated after 24 hours, when analgesia with pethidine (meperidine) or morphine may be needed. If there are no significant contractions after 24 hours, an intravenous oxytocin infusion may be used, starting with a small dose (5 mu/min) and increasing the concentration hourly until effective contractions begin, though there is little evidence that it really speeds the process. Care is taken to adjust concentrations so that fluid intake is limited.

The abortion is usually spontaneous; the cervix should be inspected for lacerations and ergometrine (ergonovine) given intramuscularly. Anti-D immuno-globulin is given to rhesus negative women. The placenta is sometimes retained, requiring removal under general anaesthesia.

If the patient fails to abort within 48 hours of the saline injection and the fetal heart is present, multiple gestation may be suspected.

In the event of failure of the abortion, the simplest procedure is the intra-amniotic injection of a prostaglandin, which is nearly always successful, or to repeat the saline injection a week later. Alternatively, and particularly if the patient is distressed, she may be taken to the operating theatre and the uterus evacuated vaginally under general anaesthesia, dilating the cervix and removing the products with ovum forceps and a blunt spoon curette or by suction curet-tage. If this is done it will be found that blood loss is usually small, much less than would be expected from a comparable gestation without a previous saline injection.

Complications of Intra-amniotic Hypertonic Saline

Injection Difficulties

In general, when real difficulties are encountered with the amniocentesis it is best to consider an alternative method of terminating the pregnancy. When the abdominal route is employed, it is possible unwittingly to inject hypertonic saline into the bladder. This can result in haematuria or more serious bladder damage and infection requiring continuous drainage and antibiotics (Menzies and Hawkins, 1968). It is possible to damage intestine or the uterus itself with the needle, but these complications are rare.

Hypernatraemia

This can arise from (a) an injection of hypertonic saline directly into a blood vessel, (b) leakage through the uterus into the peritoneal cavity and subsequent rapid absorption of sodium, (c) leakage from the amniotic cavity into the maternal circulation through a tear in the membranes, (d) rapid absorption through the fetal membranes or (e) an impairment of renal excretion of sodium. The incidence of hypernatraemia is unknown but it is probable that mild asymptomatic episodes are common. Plasma sodium levels of 160 mEq/l have been reported in a symptomless patient (Anderson and Turnbull, 1968).

It is essential that the patient receiving an intra-amniotic hypertonic saline injection should not be heavily sedated or under general anaesthesia if the early symptoms of an intravenous leak are to be recognised. These are agitation, headache, discomfort or pain in the abdomen or pelvis, tingling and warmth in the fingers or lips, and a diffuse sense of warmth together with peripheral flushing. Thirst is a very common symptom but the early appearance of severe thirst is a sign that serious hypernatraemia is present or imminent. These symptoms may appear during the injection in which case it should be stopped at once; they may appear subsequently. The patient should be given a rapid intravenous infusion of 1 litre of 5% dextrose in water.

Sudden severe hypernatraemia produced by the entry of a bolus of hypertonic saline into the circulation can lead to hypotension, bradycardia, apnoea, cardiac arrest and unconsciousness. These symptoms are thought to be due initially to the effect of the hypertonic saline on the reflex system of the pulmonary vasculature (Johnson *et al.,* 1966). A more gradual severe hypernatraemia leads to thirst, headache, hypertension, intravascular haemolysis and central nervous system abnormalities. Severe hypernatraemia will lead to death in more than 50% of cases, usually in those with central nervous system signs. The pathology in these cases has been suggested as initially brain shrinkage and negative cerebrospinal fluid pressure due to hypernatraemia (Luttrell *et al.,* 1959) followed by cerebral oedema during the treatment phase. These changes may lead to intracranial haemorrhage and thrombosis. Cameron and Dayan (1966) found acute haemorrhagic infarction of the amygdaloid nuclei and adjacent structures and Y-shaped infarcts in the pons in their two fatal cases, together with diffuse cortical damage. They considered this was likely to be due to dehydration of the brain by the hypertonic infusion.

Water Intoxication and Electrolyte Disturbance

Excessive intake of intravenous fluid following the use of intra-amniotic hypertonic saline can lead to hypernatraemia and *grand mal* seizures. An accessory factor is the concurrent use of large doses of oxytocin, which have an anti-diuretic effect (Theobald, 1934). Water intoxication has occurred after only 3000 ml of intravenous fluid containing 60 u of oxytocin over 23 hours (Lilien, 1968). Fluid intake should be restricted when infusion rates of oxytocin exceed 20 mu/min. Maintenance of intake-output records and appropriate control of fluid balance should prevent the problem. If fluid overload occurs, then the situation will resolve if the intravenous oxytocin infusion is stopped, provided renal function is normal.

It has been suggested that intravenous oxytocin can be given safely in a balanced electrolyte (Ringer-lactate) solution at rates up to 167 mu/min solution. The duration of the administration should not exceed 36 hours and plasma electrolytes should be checked if urinary output decreases during the infusion (Lauersen and Birnbaum, 1975).

Haemorrhage

Serious haemorrhage is not a common complication of this technique of inter-rupting pregnancy. Only 1–4% of patients require a blood transfusion, but a few more need evacuation of retained products of conception if bleeding continues.

Minor changes in coagulation factors are common with a fall in plasma fibrinogen and platelets, and the appearance of fibrin deposition in the damaged placenta. Cohen and Ballard (1974) found 10 cases of serious coagulopathy in 5000 saline abortions. The risk is increased by early oxytocin infusion. If severe disseminated intravascular coagulation leading to haemorrhage occurs, replace-ment of blood and fluids, observation, prompt operative evacuation of the uterus and exhibition of oxytocin, ergometrine or both and observation and maintenance of urinary output are required. If a haemorrhagic state persists, treatment with intravenous heparin, and either fresh blood or blood supple-mented with platelet-rich plasma and fibrinogen may be needed. The precise aetiology of disseminated intravascular coagulation in these patients is not clear, but it may follow amniotic fluid infusion with the introduction of tissue thrombo-plastin into the maternal circulation from the placenta or amniotic fluid.

Infection

This is the commonest cause of death after therapeutic abortion with hypertonic saline (Schiffer *et al.*, 1973). The febrile morbidity recorded from many studies is 5–10%, as with most other methods of terminating pregnancy. It is uncertain if these are always due to bacterial infections, as organisms are not often cultured from the blood. Fever may be caused by tissue necrosis in the uterus, and is sometimes due to pyrogens in the saline. A potential source of infection is an ascending infection from the vagina during a protracted abortion. It is safest to presume that the cause is infective and to institute an intramuscular or intravenous antibiotic regimen, providing for Gram-positive, Gram-negative and anaerobic pathogens. Any retained products of conception should be evacuated from the uterus.

Damage to the Cervix

Laceration of the cervix can occur during the abortion. The cervix can be torn posteriorly in the region of the isthmus, the fetus delivering through the posterior fornix. The cervix should always be inspected and repaired under general anaesthesia if necessary.

OTHER INTRA-AMNIOTIC SOLUTIONS

The history of the use of intra-amniotic injections to procure abortion was fully reviewed by Kerr *et al.* (1966). Some substances for this purpose have been studied since that time.

Alcohol

Gomel and Carpenter (1973) reported on intra-amniotic injection of 100–170 ml of 47.5% ethyl alcohol after removal of the same amount of amniotic fluid. Complete abortion resulted in 12 out of 12 patients but the injection-abortion interval was longer than would have been expected with the use of hypertonic saline.

Urea

To avoid the complications of hypertonic saline, hypertonic urea has been injected into the amniotic cavity to induce abortion. The amniotic fluid may be drained and replaced with urea, 80 g in 150 or 200 ml of 5% dextrose. The injection-abortion intervals are longer than those with hypertonic saline, ranging from 30 to 100 hours (Greenhalf and Diggory, 1971). Intravenous oxytocin (140–330 mu/min) has been used to shorten the mean interval (Pugh *et al.*, 1971), but it is desirable to restrict the fluid intake or use frusemide 40 mg i.m. after 24 hours to avoid water intoxication (Craft and Musa, 1971; Burnett *et al.*, 1975). The effectiveness of hypertonic urea is less than that of saline, but when combined with intravenous oxytocin it is relatively effective and safe. With pregnancies of greater than 16 weeks' maturity the fetus may show the signs of life after the abortion. Despite the absence of clinical problems there is some laboratory evidence of intravascular coagulation with a fall in platelet count and plasma fibrinogen in most of the patients, and the appearance of fibrin and fibrinogen degradation products in the plasma in about one-third (Burnett *et al.*, 1975). Plasma urea increases and in patients with renal conditions the use of intra-amniotic prostaglandins or mannitol is to be preferred to that of urea, to avoid confusion of interpretation of renal function tests.

Glucose

Wood *et al.* (1962) described the use of intra-amniotic 50% dextrose to induce labour in cases of intra-uterine death of the fetus, but this was followed by reports of maternal deaths due to infection. The combination of necrotic tissue and dextrose provided a culture medium for organisms such as *Clostridium welchii* (Peel, 1962). Brosset (1958) used replacement of as much amniotic fluid as possible with 50% dextrose containing oxytetracycline to induce mid trimester abortion in 54 patients; 51 aborted with an average induction-abortion interval of 38 hours. The other 3 cases developed a missed abortion and the uterus had to be emptied surgically. Comparative studies between the use of hypertonic dextrose and saline indicate that saline is better because of a shorter injection-abortion interval, and a lower incidence of subsequent need for curettage (Menzies and Hawkins, 1968; Droegmueller and Greer, 1970). Despite the use of prophylactic antibiotics to reduce the risks of infection the method is not recommended.

Fructose

Intra-amniotic 40 or 50% dextrose can be painful. This problem does not arise with 40% fructose but any simple sugar makes a good bacteriological culture medium. For this reason, fructose is no longer used.

Mannitol

Craft and Musa (1971) drained the amniotic fluid from 15 to 20 weeks' pregnancies and replaced it with 200 ml of 25% mannitol. Abortion occurred in 6 out of 12 cases. This method is not recommended with a live fetus past 16 weeks as the fetus is commonly aborted alive.

EXTRA-AMNIOTIC INJECTIONS

We have already referred to the use of prostaglandins introduced into the extra-amniotic space. Other substances are sometimes employed by this route to procure abortion. With late mid trimester abortions induced by this procedure the fetus may show the signs of life for a short while.

Ethacridine Lactate

This, (6,9-diamino-2-ethoxy-acridine lactate, Acrinal, Rivanol), is a derivative of acridine, a yellow dye with an antiseptic action. A soft catheter (gauge 8–12, o.d. 3–4 mm) is inserted through the cervical canal and then between the uterus and the membranes until it reaches the uterine fundus. Thirty to 50 ml of a 0.1% solution of ethacridine is introduced and the end of the catheter clamped to prevent reflux. Manabe (1969) recommended a repeat injection after 24 hours, and the use of intravenous oxytocin to encourage uterine action. Because of the antiseptic action of ethacridine the risk of infection was said to be negligible. Manabe (1969) reported on the successful induction of abortion with ethacridine in 39 out of 40 patients. The induction-abortion time varied from 8 to 58 hours. Despite its widespread use in Japan, it is not clear if the procedure is effective merely by stripping membranes or by virtue of an irritant action of absorbed ethacridine on the myometrium. In Manabe's (1969) patients most fetuses were aborted alive, suggesting that placental destruction is not involved.

Soft Soaps

There are various formulae for soft soap pastes, which were widely used to induce mid trimester abortions between 1930 and 1950. The essentials of the recipe are an oil and water suspension which is highly alkaline, due to the presence of sodium hydroxide, and which contains various chemicals such as chlorocresol (0.05%), benzoic acid (1.33%) or potassium iodide (2.0%).

These pastes were instilled very slowly and gently through a narrow tube inserted through the internal cervical os. The volume used was recommended as 5 ml plus 1 ml for each week of pregnancy, making a total of up to 20 ml (Barns, 1947).

The method is potentially dangerous because of the risk of fat emboli which can be fatal. Effectiveness is greatest between 13 and 16 weeks' maturity when in Barns' (1947) study all patients aborted, completely or incompletely, with a mean injection-abortion interval of 43.5 hours (range 13 to 375 hours). In a more recent report Lachelin and Burgess (1968) found that 44% of patients aborted within 24 hours and that 75% aborted within 48 hours. They did not find that the parity or the maturity of the pregnancy, between 9 and 20 weeks, had any significant effect on the injection-abortion interval. Before 13 weeks' maturity Barns (1947) found that while the method was successful in 92% of cases, the average time to abortion was shorter, being 27.7 hours. After 17 weeks the method was very ineffective (Barns, 1947). Although soap pastes are relatively effective for the induction of early mid trimester abortions a long time may be needed to effect expulsion of the products of conception. The total stay in hospital required was found to be between 3 and 16 days (Lachelin and Burgess, 1968). The risks of such toxic substances entering the blood stream causing haemolysis or embolism, or of infection, or chemical damage to the fallopian tube make the method unsuitable for present day practice. This experience is borne out in a study by Sood (1971) who recorded pyrexia lasting for more than 3 days in 12 out of 83 women. Three of these developed septicaemia, and there was one death due to uterine rupture.

Extra-amniotic Hypertonic Saline

Several investigators have used the extra-ovular injection of hypertonic saline to induce abortion, with slow infusion through a Foley catheter. The method is not so effective as intra-amniotic saline (Chaudry *et al.*, 1976) and is predictably more dangerous from the point of view of intravascular infusion of hypertonic saline. The incidence of intravascular leakage is 3% (Llewellyn-Jones *et al.*, 1975) compared with 0.5% for intra-amniotic saline injection (Brenner, 1975).

Gustavii and Green (1972) have shown that amniotic fluid prostaglandin $F_{2\alpha}$ levels rise after the extra-ovular instillation of hypertonic saline, suggesting that prostaglandin release is involved in the mechanism of action.

Oxytocin

Oxytocin instilled by the extra-amniotic route was not found to be effective in causing abortion by Seppala and Vara (1972), but Halbrecht and Blum (1974) used an extra-amniotic instillation of isotonic saline supplemented by the intravenous infusion of oxytocin 20 u/l in 5% dextrose, with success in abortions at 16 to 23 weeks' maturity.

ABORTION INDUCED BY THE BOUGIE OR METREURYNTER

After the second World War Japan experienced a population explosion which was kept in check by the use of therapeutic abortions — many of which were performed in the middle trimester. Intra-amniotic hypertonic saline was widely used but because the method was employed by unskilled personnel there were a number of deaths (Wagatsuma, 1965). This resulted in a reversion to the use of the traditional German method of inducing labour, which involved the insertion of a rubber catheter between the uterus and membranes.

The bougie is made of gum elastic with a diameter of 0.5—1.0 cm and a length of 30—45 cm. Two catheters are inserted between the decidua and the membranes so that their tips are at the uterine fundus. The cervical dilatation required is only to Hegar 8 (8 mm), and the technique is simple. Excess bougie is cut off at the cervix and intravenous oxytocin is usually administered.

The abortifacient effect may be due to trauma of decidual cells releasing lysosomal enzymes which cause the synthesis and liberation of prostaglandins and hence uterine contractions (Gustavii, 1974). Uterine action starts after some time — occasionally as long as 33 hours — but thereafter abortion usually follows within 12 hours. There is no change in the urinary excretion of oestriol or pregnanediol during the procedure, and the fetuses are born alive (Manabe, 1968). Ninety per cent of patients abort, but many have a pyrexia.

Induction of abortion using the metreurynter method involves dilating the cervix to Hegar 12—16 (12—16 mm). The metreurynter is a rubber balloon ended tube, like a Foley catheter. It is inserted through the cervical canal, and filled with 100—300 ml of normal saline. Weights of 300—800 g are attached to the end of the tube and hung over the bed, so that a steady traction is exerted by the balloon on the already partially dilated cervix. Intravenous oxytocin is usually administered as well, at least until regular uterine contractions are established. Once the cervix is sufficiently dilated to expel the balloon, abortion of the fetus occurs within 1 to 2 hours. In some cases there is a gradual increase in uterine activity, while in others the activity of the uterus remains low initially, increasing after 10 hours (Manabe, 1967). Once established, uterine action increases progressively throughout the abortion process. The abortion time can be as long as 4 to 5 days, but 80% of patients will abort (Manabe, 1969). There is no alteration in the urinary excretion of oestrogen and pregnanediol throughout abortion procured with a metreurynter (Manabe, 1967). No signs of acute infection of the placenta are found histologically, although infection has been noted if the abortion period is prolonged.

Both bougie and metreurynter methods are simple to perform and require little equipment. They are still effective once the membranes have ruptured. Because of the presence of an indwelling foreign body, often for periods of time of up to 4 days, there is a risk of infection and so prophylactic antibiotics are advisable. Intravenous oxytocin may also help by reducing the induction-abortion interval.

A combination of dilatation of the cervix with laminaria tents and the insertion of a metreurynter has been described as a better method than direct evacuation of uterine contents, after 15 weeks' maturity (Manabe and Nakajima, 1972). Abortion occurs within 5 to 24 hours, with concomitant therapy including quinine, papaverine and antibiotics.

There is no doubt that by present-day standards bougie and metreurynter methods are inadequate, for they require cervical dilatation, they are slow to induce abortion, they probably lead to a higher incidence of infection, and the fetus is sometimes delivered alive. They have no real advantages in present-day practice, although at the time during which they were introduced in Japan, their associated morbidity was preferable to the mortality associated with other methods.

CYTOTOXIC AGENTS

The range of nucleotoxic and cytotoxic drugs is large. It includes (a) anti-metabolites such as aminopterin, mercaptopurine (Puri-nethol) and methotrexate, (b) alkylating agents such as nitrogen mustard, chlorambucil (Leukeran), and cyclophosphamide (Endoxana, Cytoxan), (c) antimitotic agents such as colchicine and actinomycin D (Cosmegen) and (d) alkaloids such as vinblastine (Velbe, Velban).

In 1952, Thiersch studied the effect of 6–12 mg of oral aminopterin as an abortifacient in women with cancer or other serious illnesses. Fetal death and spontaneous abortion occurred in some patients, but in others the fetus survived and was found to be malformed when evacuated surgically. Nucleotoxic compounds such as podophylline and colchicine derivatives are consistently capable of causing abortion without being toxic to the mother (Didcock *et al.*, 1956). Antimetabolites such as mercaptopurine are almost inactive in causing abortion in mice and monkeys once pregnancy is well established, but are more active during the earlier stages of pregnancy.

An orally active synthetic uridine derivative, triacetyl-6-azauridine, has been tried in monkeys (Van Wagenen *et al.*, 1970) and was effective as an abortifacient, without any evidence of maternal toxicity.

The observed toxicity, the potential teratogenic effect on surviving fetuses, and the unknown effects on future pregnancies limit the clinical use of the large number of cytotoxic agents that are available.

ABORTIFACIENT DRUGS

Many drugs of vegetable origin have been claimed to cause abortion and various preparations have been sold to the public with the implication that they will have this effect. Hawkins (1965) reviewed these products and concluded that although none of them contained ingredients which, in the recommended doses, are known specifically to cause abortion, on the other hand, something between 1 in 20 and 1 in 3 women taking them will subsequently miscarry.

Most of these abortions would have occurred spontaneously but perhaps a few were due to the moderate or severe systemic effect of the ingredients ingested in large doses by some women. Sometimes there may be reflex stimulation of uterine contractions, secondary to violent intestinal activity. In cases where abortion occurs in consequence of severe systemic illness, the mechanism may be one of temporary interference with the utero-placental circulation from direct or neurogenic vascular spasm and congestion. In a few cases where massive doses of a substance like quinine are ingested, the drug may actually pass the placenta and cause direct damage to the fetus. In either event, if the pregnancy continues there is a chance of an abnormal baby resulting.

It is possible that some agents have an emmenogogue action in some women, that is they can cause uterine bleeding without necessarily inducing abortion, though the evidence is largely anecdotal. Examples are oil of juniper (present in gin) and some preparations of aloes.

Most 'female pills' contain mild laxatives; some contain enough iron to cause gastro-intestinal effects; some have enough pulegium oil to cause vascular congestion in the pelvis; a few contain powerful purgatives such as aloes, apiol, colocynth or dihydroxyanthraquinone in amounts which could cause serious illness if an overdose such as the whole box were taken. Some contain agents such as cajuput or ergot, an overdose of which might have cardiovascular effects; others have cimicifuge or quinine which in large amounts might affect the patient's nervous system.

We were unable to induce therapeutic abortion in patients scheduled for surgical termination of pregnancy by giving them increasing doses of norethynodrel with mestranol and then withdrawing the hormones at the time a menstrual period would have been due (Hawkins *et al.*, 1974). Now that there is a suspicion that a continuing pregnancy after such treatment might lead to an abnormal fetus, the 'hormone withdrawal' approach would seem to be undesirable; even if termination by another method was planned in the event of failure there is always a chance that the patient might equivocate after the medical approach had failed.

Potts (1970) has reviewed some of the other agents which have been used in the attempt to find a medical abortifacient.

OPERATIVE TERMINATION OF THE MID TRIMESTER PREGNANCY

There are occasions when an operative approach is indicated for the termination of a mid trimester pregnancy. An example is the management of a patient whose medical or psychiatric status is such that operative abortion under general anaesthesia is preferable to the prolonged stress of an abortion induced with prostaglandins or hypertonic saline. Other situations where operation may be preferred are when difficulty has been encountered with an injection procedure. Blood draining through the needle inserted into the uterus *via* the abdomen or the vagina, and difficulty in entering the gestation sac are examples. If abortion fails to follow administration of prostaglandins or hypertonic saline operation may be preferred to repeated attempts.

The need for tubal sterilisation is no longer universally regarded as an indication for the use of abdominal hysterotomy to terminate a mid trimester pregnancy. The report of the Committee on the Working of the Abortion Act

(1974) cited a mortality of 27.8 per 100 000 for hysterotomy and sterilisation, compared with 3.0 per 100 000 for termination of pregnancy alone by vacuum curettage with a pregnancy of less than 13 weeks' maturity. In fact, comparison of these figures is meaningless, as they are based on 2 deaths in 7204 cases and 2 deaths in 131 279 cases, respectively, bearing in mind that sterilisation is more likely to be performed on patients who have medical indications for avoiding pregnancy. Nonetheless, it seems reasonable to avoid hysterotomy in the first trimester when the pregnancy can be terminated vaginally. Some gynaecologists consider the right approach is to terminate the pregnancy vaginally with an injection procedure, by vacuum evacuation or by curettage. They check that the abortion is complete by exploration of the uterus under general anaesthesia and perform sterilisation laparoscopically or by open abdominal operation. Any increase in mortality associated with the combination of procedures is probably attributable to associated medical conditions in some patients being sterilised (Committee on the Working of the Abortion Act, 1974). The alternative is to bring the patient back six weeks later for an 'interval' sterilisation. This can be inconvenient for the patient and some may not return until they have another unwanted pregnancy.

Dilatation and Curettage, Vacuum Aspiration

A few gynaecologists feel competent to terminate a pregnancy at 14 to 18 weeks' maturity by dilatation of the cervix and evacuation of the products of conception with the aid of ovum forceps and a blunt spoon curette used alternatively until the uterus is empty. Ergometrine (ergonovine), one or two doses of 0.5 mg intravenously, perhaps supplemented with oxytocin, 5 u intravenously, may be given to assist expulsion of the products, and control haemorrhage by stimulating contraction and retraction of the uterus. Some use an intravenous ergometrine infusion, 2 mg in 500 ml of saline, or an oxytocin infusion containing 20 u/l, throughout the procedure. Hegar dilators up to No. 20 (diameter 2 cm) should be available in case digital exploration is necessary to control haemorrhage. We disapprove of the use of hot (40 °C) intra-uterine 0.9% saline douches to arrest haemorrhage: they can wash debris up into the fallopian tubes and peritoneal cavity, their effect may be only temporary and they may conceal the occurrence of uterine rupture.

Termination of the 14 to 18 week pregnancy should not be attempted by dilatation and curettage without general or epidural anaesthesia, supplies of cross-matched blood on the spot and the facilities of adequate staff and a fully equipped operating theatre. Occasionally the uterus may be ruptured, or haemorrhage so severe as to require emergency hysterectomy may occur.

Most gynaecologists feel that the hazards of causing an incompetent cervix, of haemorrhage, of uterine rupture and of incomplete evacuation with subsequent infection are such that dilatation and curettage is not a reasonable procedure for terminating the mid trimester pregnancy. On the other hand, the study made by the Joint Program for the Study of Abortion (Center for Disease Control, 1977) concluded that cervical dilatation and suction together with the use of crushing forceps or sharp curettage, in mid trimester abortions, carried a major complication rate of only 0.69 per 100 cases, compared with 1.81 and 2.90 for hypertonic saline and prostaglandin $F_{2\alpha}$ abortions respectively. Surgical evacuation of the uterus by the vaginal route also had the lowest mortality (Cates *et al.*, 1977).

Hysterotomy

The removal of fetus and placenta from the uterus by hysterotomy was, until a few years ago, the standard method of terminating a mid trimester pregnancy. The operation can be performed by the abdominal or vaginal approach.

Abdominal Hysterotomy – Operative Technique

The commonest incision in the uterus is vertical, in the body of the uterus, resembling the incision for classical Caesarean section. In this situation the myometrium is thick, and there is maximum mobility of the sutured edges as well as maximum involution. The result of this is to loosen the sutures and lead to a weak wound united by fibrous tissue. This is made worse by the presence of any infection. Such a hysterotomy scar can rupture during a subsequent pregnancy or confinement.

The other problem with the vertical fundal incision is the potential for the formation of omental, intestinal and abdominal scar adhesions to the uterine scar. The peritoneum is intimately adherent to the myometrium of the fundus which precludes its use to bury the suture line. It is difficult to secure haemostasis with completely buried interrupted catgut sutures. The superficial layer may be repaired with a buried continuous suture but even this leaves the line of junction in proximity with loops of intestine.

These risks may be much reduced by employing a low transverse approach. The body of the uterus is retracted upwards with one hand to expose the uterovesical pouch. It is then possible to incise the loosely adherent peritoneum and make a transverse incision in the lower part of the uterus, 2–3 cm above the level of the internal os, holding the knife as nearly horizontal as the symphysis pubis will permit, in order to enter the cavity of the uterus. It is debatable whether or not this cut is in the anatomical lower segment. The myometrium in this situation is thinner, and uterine motility during the process of involution will be reduced and the scar should be less fibrotic and stronger. Provided care is taken to avoid the uterine vessels at the lateral ends of the incision, this approach is recommended. The suture line is buried in peritoneum at the bottom of the utero-vesical fold. The transverse incision is much better than a vertical incision in the lower segment of the uterus, as the latter may involve the internal cervical os, and it is difficult to re-cover the uterine wound with peritoneum without pulling the bladder upwards.

The injection of 5 u of oxytocin directly into the myometrium at the site of the proposed incision is recommended. After two or three minutes there will be local blanching and the blood loss will be markedly diminished. The transverse incision also tends to reduce haemorrhage at operation because it is in the same anatomical plane as the course of the branches of the uterine vessels.

The wound should be sutured with interrupted chromic catgut sutures, in two layers, and then re-peritonised. It is preferable to exclude the decidua from the inner layer of sutures, as its inclusion may weaken the scar.

The death rate in Great Britain from abdominal hysterotomy performed during the second trimester of pregnancy is between 48 and 70 deaths per 100 000 abortions, for women aged 10 to 29 and 30 to 49, respectively. This makes it many times more dangerous than vacuum aspiration, the figures for which range between 3 and 9 deaths per 100 000 abortions, for ages 10 to 29 and 30 to 49 respectively (Committee on the Working of the Abortion Act, 1974). The principal causes of death after hysterotomy are haemorrhage and infection.

Complications

Haemorrhage This is defined as a blood loss of more than 500 ml and is a relatively common complication of hysterotomy, occurring in about 15% of patients (Stallworthy *et al.*, 1971). Stewart and Goldstein (1972) noted that significant haemorrhage occurred in as many as 30% of patients. Blood transfusions may be required in between 10% and 20% of patients having abdominal hysterotomy. Haemorrhage is primarily due to bleeding at operation but may also be secondary to retained products, which can require re-evacuation of the uterus after as many as 11% of hysterotomies (Sood, 1971).

Infection Pyrexia after operation, defined as a temperature of 38°C for at least 12 hours, can occur in as many as 40% of patients (Stallworthy *et al.*, 1971; Stewart and Goldstein, 1972). In these studies it was mainly due to genital tract infections, which were introduced at the time of operation or were secondary ascending infections of the uterus and tubes. Occasionally infection may become severe, leading to peritonitis or septicaemia, but usually the more obvious clinical signs disappear with antibiotic treatment. The long-term problems of chronic pelvic infection and infertility are less well documented, and their incidence may be very much higher than is currently appreciated. All gynaecologists are aware of the wife allegedly complaining of primary infertility who turns out to have had an abortion in the past which was apparently uneventful post-operatively. Only the silently damaged tubes bear testimony to the potential risks of the procedure.

Implantation Endometriosis This can occur in the uterine scar, the peritoneal cavity or the abdominal wound following abdominal hysterectomy. Some gynaecologists consider it can be avoided by surrounding the uterus with packs before opening the cavity and taking scrupulous care to avoid inclusion of decidua in uterine and abdominal wounds. Higgenbotham (1973) found endometriotic nodules in the abdominal scar of 4 out of 242 patients who had had an abdominal hysterotomy. It may be a rare complication but it can lead to considerable trouble with monthly pain. Local excision, electrocautery or cryosurgery of the implanted nodules is the recommended treatment.

Uterine Rupture in a Subsequent Pregnancy Russel and Hewlett (1969) found at hysterography that in approximately half of the patients who had had a hysterotomy the uterine scar was deformed. These authors recommended that the midline corpus incision be used if sterilisation is also to be carried out, but that in other patients a low transverse scar is better. Better wound healing probably ensues if the decidua are excluded from the sutures used to repair the uterine incision, but the evidence for this is not conclusive.

In a study of the clinical outcome after hysterotomy Clow and Crompton (1973) found that the outcome of labour and mode of delivery was the same as that found in a comparative series of patients who were pregnant after a caesarean section. These authors examined the scar by inspection or palpation in 31 cases and found it to be thin in 14 cases, with rupture or impending rupture in 3 cases. The remaining 17 scars were intact. From this series the risk of uterine rupture in a subsequent pregnancy due to a hysterotomy scar is 8%. This risk is increased if there has been a post-operative wound infection.

Vlies and Dewhurst (1975) recommend great caution in the use of oxytocic drugs in labour in patients with a hysterotomy scar. They consider that the use of epidural anaesthesia may mask rupture of the scar and it should be avoided. They also advocate routine palpation of the hysterotomy scar after a vaginal delivery.

The immediate post-operative morbidity, chiefly due to haemorrhage and infection, and the long-term morbidity of infertility and the risks of uterine rupture in a subsequent pregnancy make abdominal hysterotomy an operation to be avoided where possible. The advent of relatively safer methods of inducing mid trimester abortions has made it uncommon.

Vaginal Hysterotomy Sometimes it is desired to perform hysterotomy to terminate a pregnancy of between 14 and 20 weeks' maturity surgically without resort to laparotomy. Particular indications are the presence of extensive pelvic inflammatory disease or adhesions from multiple previous laparotomies, and intestinal disorders such as Crohn's disease, ulcerative colitis or diverticulitis where laparotomy conveys some hazard. Few gynaecologists would now resort to the classical vaginal hysterotomy, incising the whole length of the cervix up to and including the internal os, and then attempting a repair which does not heal well. The procedure described below is one which was employed successfully for many years by the late Professor W.C.W. Nixon and his assistants. It is singularly free from complications and leaves the uterus competent to carry a pregnancy and effect normal vaginal delivery. With a little experience of the procedure, the gynaecologist may find that it is an acceptable alternative to abdominal hysterotomy, with reduced morbidity, reduced hospital stay, and cosmetic superiority.

Under general anaesthesia with the patient in the lithotomy position, the cervix is drawn down with vulsella and a horizontal incision made in the skin of the anterior fornix below the bladder reflection. The fascia is incised down to the cervix, and the bladder displaced upwards. A retractor is inserted to maintain the bladder up and away from the cervix and the lower part of the body of the uterus. The lower part of the *corpus* is incised vertically in the midline, just above the level of the internal os, cutting down on a No. 7 Hegar dilator lying in the cervical canal. With a 14 week pregnancy the incision need only be 2–3 cm long; with more mature pregnancies a slightly longer incision may be necessary to permit evacuation of the fetus. Products of conception are then evacuated with ovum forceps and a blunt spoon curette alternately until the cavity is empty, using ergometrine to assist uterine contraction. The completeness of the abortion is readily confirmed by digital exploration. Tissue forceps are placed on both sides at the upper extremity of the incision in the uterus to cause eversion and facilitate repair with one or two layers of interrupted chromic catgut sutures. The skin incision is repaired using interrupted catgut; if the sutures incorporate the fascia below the skin incision haemostasis is usually good. The patency of the cervical canal is confirmed by passing a No. 7 dilator.

Using this procedure very few complications have been seen. On one occasion failure to retract the bladder adequately and to secure direct vision of the uterine incision with tissue forceps led to a suture penetrating the bladder, and eventually a small vesico-vaginal fistula. No cases of endometriosis in the uterine incision such as those reported in Sweden (Lindahl, 1959) were encountered.

REFERENCES

AMERICAN COLLEGE OF OBSTETRICIANS AND GYNAECOLOGISTS (1976). Hypertonic saline amnio-infusion for termination of second trimester pregnancy. *ACOG Technical Bulletin,* number 37

AMY, J.J., KARIM, S.M.M. and SIVASAMBOO, R. (1973). Intra-amniotic administration of prostaglandin 15(S)15 methyl-E_2 methyl ester for termination of pregnancy. *J. Obstet. Gynaec. Br. Commonw.,* **80**, 1017–1020

ANDERSON, G.G., HOBBINS, J.C., RAJKOVIC, V., SPEROFF, L. and CALDWELL, B.V. (1972a). Midtrimester abortion using intra amniotic prostaglandin $F_{2\alpha}$. *Prostaglandins,* **1**, 147–155

ANDERSON, G.G., HOBBINS, J.C., SPEROFF, L. and CALDWELL, B.V. (1972b). The induction of therapeutic abortion using intravenous prostaglandin $F_{2\alpha}$. *Contraception,* **5**, 303–311

ANDERSON, A.B.M. and TURNBULL, A.C. (1968). Changes in amniotic fluid, serum and urine following the intra-amniotic injection of hypertonic saline. *Acta obstet. gynec. scand.,* **47**, 1–21

ANDOLŠEK, L. (1974). Operative events. In *The Ljubljana Abortion Study, 1971–1973,* pp. 15–16. Ed. Andolšek, L. National Institutes of Health Center for Population Research, Bethesda, Maryland

ANDOLŠEK, L., CHENG, M., HREN, M., OGRINC-OVEN, M., NG, A., RATNAM, S., BELSEY, M., EDSTRÖM, K., HEINER, P., KINNEAR, K. and TIETZE, C. (1977). The safety of local anaesthesia and outpatient treatment: a controlled study of induced abortion by vacuum aspiration. *Stud. fam. Plann.,* **8**, 118–124

ATIENZA, M.F., BURKMAN, R.T., KING, T.M., BURNETT, L.S., LAU, H.L., PARMLEY, T.H. and WOODRUFF, J.D. (1975). Menstrual extraction. *Am. J. Obstet. Gynec.,* **121**, 490–495

BALLARD, C.A. and SLAUGHTER, L. (1976). Second trimester abortion with intramuscular injections of 15-methyl prostaglandin $F_{2\alpha}$. *Contraception,* **14**, 541–549

BARNS, H.H.F. (1947). Therapeutic abortion by means of soft-soap pastes. *Lancet,* **ii**, 825–827

BAUDOUIN-LEGROS, M., MEYER, P. and WORCEL, M. (1974). Effects of prostaglandin inhibitors on angiotensin oxytocin and prostaglandin $F_{2\alpha}$ contractile effects on the rat uterus during the oestrous cycle. *Br. J. Pharmac.,* **52**, 393–399

BÉGUIN, F., BYGDEMAN, M., TOPPOZADA, M. and WIQVIST, N. (1972). The response of the midpregnant human uterus to vaginal administration of prostaglandin suppositories. *Prostaglandins,* **1**, 397–405

BELLER, F.K., ROSENBERG, M., KOLKER, M. and DOUGLAS, G.W. (1972). Consumptive coagulopathy associated with intra-amniotic infusion of hypertonic salt. *Am. J. Obstet. Gynec.*, **112**, 534–543

BENGTSSON, L.P. and CSAPO, A.I. (1962). Oxytocin response; withdrawal, and reinforcement of defense mechanism of the human uterus at midpregnancy. *Am. J. Obstet. Gynec.*, **83**, 1083–1093

BERGER, G.S., TIETZE, C., PAKTER, J. and KATZ, S.H. (1974). Maternal mortality associated with legal abortion in New York State: July 1, 1970 – June 30, 1972. *Obstet. Gynec., N.Y.*, **43**, 315–326

BERIĆ, B. and KUPRESANIN, M. (1971). Vacuum aspiration, using paracervical block, for legal abortion as an outpatient procedure up to the 12th week of pregnancy. *Lancet*, **ii**, 619–621

BERIĆ, B., KUPRESANIN, M. and HULKA, J.F. (1972). The Karman catheter: a preliminary evaluation as an instrument for termination of pregnancies up to 12 weeks of gestation. *Am. J. Obstet. Gynec.*, **114**, 273–275

BERK, H., ULLMAN, J. and BERGER, J. (1971). Experience and complications with the use of hypertonic intra-amniotic saline solution. *Surgery Gynec. Obstet.*, **133**, 955–958

BIENARZ, J., HUNTER, G. and SCOMMEGNA, A. (1974). Efficacy and acceptability of 15(S)-15-methyl-prostaglandin E_2-methyl ester for midtrimester pregnancy termination. *Am. J. Obstet. Gynec.*, **120**, 840–843

BORELL, U., BYGDEMAN, M., LEADER, A., LUNDSTRÖM, V. and MARTIN, J.N. Jr. (1976). Successful first trimester abortion with 15(S)15-methyl-prostaglandin $F_{2\alpha}$-methyl ester vaginal suppositories. *Contraception*, **13**, 87–94

BRACKEN, M.B., HACHAMOVITCH, M. and GROSSMAN, G. (1972). Factors associated with instillation-abortion time during saline-instillation abortion. *Am. J. Obstet. Gynec.*, **114**, 10–12

BRADLEY-WATSON, P.J., BEARD, R.J. and CRAFT, I. (1973). Injuries of the cervix after induced midtrimester abortion. *J. Obstet. Gynaec. Br. Commonw.*, **80**, 284–285

BRENNER, W.E. (1972). Intravenous prostaglandin $F_{2\alpha}$ for therapeutic abortion: the efficacy and tolerance of three dosage schedules. *Am. J. Obstet. Gynec.*, **113**, 1037–1045

BRENNER, W.E. (1975). Second trimester interruption of pregnancy. In *Progress in Gynecology, Volume 6*, pp. 421–444. Ed. Taymor, M.L. and Green, T.H. Grune and Stratton, New York

BRENNER, W.E., DINGFELDER, J.R., STAUROVSKY, L.G., KUMARASMY, T. and GRIMES, D.A. (1974). Intramuscular administration of 15(S)-15 methyl prostaglandin E_2-methyl ester for induction of abortion. *Am. J. Obstet. Gynec.*, **120**, 833–836

BRENNER, W.E., HENDRICKS, C.H., BRAAKSMA, J.T., FISHBURNE, J.I., KRONCKE, F.G. and STAUROVSKY, L. (1972a). Intra-amniotic administration of prostaglandin $F_{2\alpha}$ to induce therapeutic abortion. Efficacy and tolerance of two dosage schedules. *Am. J. Obstet. Gynec.*, **114**, 781–787

BRENNER, W.E., HENDRICKS, C.H., BRAAKSMA, J.T., FISHBURNE, J.I. Jr. and STAUROVSKY, L.G. (1972b). Vaginal administration of prostaglandin $F_{2\alpha}$ for inducing therapeutic abortion. *Prostaglandins*, **1**, 455–467

BRENNER, W.E., HENDRICKS, C.H., FISHBURNE, J.I., BRAAKSMA, J.T., STAUROVSKY, L.G. and HARRELL, L.C. (1973). Induction of therapeutic abortion with intra-amniotically administered prostaglandin $F_{2\alpha}$. *Am. J. Obstet. Gynec.*, **116**, 923–930

BROSSET, A. (1958). The induction of therapeutic abortion by means of a hypertonic glucose solution injected into the amniotic sac. *Acta obstet. gynec. scand.*, **37**, 519–525

BROWN, F.D., DAVIDSON, E.C. and PHILLIPS, L.L. (1972). Coagulation changes after hypertonic saline infusion for late abortions. *Obstet. Gynec., N.Y.*, **39**, 538–543

BURNETT, L.S., KING, T.M., ATIENZA, M.F. and BELL, W.R. (1975). Intra-amniotic urea is a mid-trimester abortifacient: clinical results and serum and urinary changes. *Am. J. Obstet. Gynec.*, **121**, 7–16

BURNHILL, M.S., GAINES, J.A. and GUTTMACHER, A.F. (1962). Concentrated oxytocin solution for therapeutic interruption of mid trimester pregnancy. A preliminary report. *Obstet. Gynec., N.Y.*, **20**, 94–100

BYGDEMAN, M., BÉGUIN, F., TOPPOZADA, M., WIQVIST, N. and BERGSTRÖM, S. (1972). Intrauterine administration of 15(S)-15-methyl prostaglandin $F_{2\alpha}$ for induction of abortion. *Lancet*, **i**, 1336–1337

BYGDEMAN, M. and BERGSTRÖM, S. (1976). Clinical use of prostaglandins for pregnancy termination. *Population Reports*, series G, number 7, 65–75

BYGDEMAN, M., BORELL, U., LEADER, A., LUNDSTRÖM, V., MARTIN, J.N., Jr., ENEROTH, P. and GREEN, K. (1976). Induction of first and second trimester abortion by the vaginal administration of 15-methyl-$PGF_{2\alpha}$ methyl ester. *Advances in Prostaglandin and Thromboxane Research*, **2**, 693–704

BYGDEMAN, M., MARTIN, J.N., WIQVIST, N., GRÉEN, K. and BERGSTRÖM, S. (1974). Reassessment of systemic administration of prostaglandins for induction of midtrimester abortion. *Prostaglandins*, **8**, 157–169

CALDEYRO-BARCIA, R. and SERENO, J.A. (1961). The response of the human uterus to oxytocin throughout pregnancy. *Oxytocin. Proceedings of an International Symposium held in Montevideo, 1959*, pp. 177–200. Ed. Caldeyro-Barcia, R. and Heller, H. Pergamon, Oxford

CAMERON, J.M. and DAYAN, A.D. (1966). Association of brain damage with therapeutic abortion induced by amniotic fluid-replacement: report of two cases. *Br. med. J.*, **i**, 1010–1013

CATES, W. Jr., GRIMES, D.A., SMITH, J.C. and TYLER, C.W. Jr. (1977). The risk of dying from legal abortion in the United States, 1972–1975. *Int. J. Gynaecol. Obstet.*, **15**, 172–176

CENTER FOR DISEASE CONTROL (1977). *Abortion Surveillance, 1975.* p. 49. U.S. Department of Health, Education and Welfare, Public Health Service, Center for Disease Control, Atlanta, Georgia

CHAUDRY, S.L., HUNT, W.B. II and WORTHMAN, J. (1976). Pregnancy termination in mid trimester — review of major methods, *Population Reports*, series F, number 5, 65–83

CHENG, M., ANDOLŠEK, L., NG, A., RATNAM, S., HREN, M., OGRINC-OVEN, M., BELSEY, M., EDSTRÖM, K., HEINER, P., KINNEAR, K. and TIETZE, C. (1977). Complications following induced abortion by vacuum aspiration: patient characteristics and procedures. *Stud. fam. Plann.*, **8**, 125–129

CLEMENTS, R.V. and KHUNDA, S. (1976). Mid-trimester termination. *Br. med. J.*, **ii**, 587

CLOW, W.M. and CROMPTON, A.C. (1973). The wounded uterus: pregnancy after hysterotomy. *Br. med. J.*, **i**, 321–323

COHEN, E. and BALLARD, C.A. (1974). Consumptive coagulopathy associated with intraamniotic saline instillation and the effect of intravenous oxytocin. *Obstet. Gynec., N.Y.*, **43**, 300–303

COLTART, T.M. and COE, M.J. (1975). Intravenous prostaglandins and oxytocin for mid-trimester abortion. *Lancet*, **i**, 173–174

COMMITTEE ON THE WORKING OF THE ABORTION ACT (1974). *Report*, volume I, p. 45. Her Majesty's Stationery Office, London

CRAFT, I. (1973). Intra amniotic prostaglandin E_2 and $F_{2\alpha}$ for induction of abortion: a dose response study. *J. Obstet. Gynaec. Br. Commonw.*, **80**, 46–47

CRAFT, I. (1975). Intra-amniotic urea and low-dose prostaglandin E_2 for mid trimester termination. *Lancet*, **i**, 1115–1116

CRAFT, I.L. and MUSA, B.D. (1971). Induction of mid-trimester therapeutic abortion by intra-amniotic urea and intravenous oxytocin. *Lancet*, **ii**, 1058–1060

CSAPO, A.I. (1974). 'Prostaglandin impact' for menstrual induction. *Population Reports*, series G, number 4, 33–40

CSAPO, A.I. (1966). The termination of pregnancy by the intra-amniotic injection of hypertonic saline. *Year Book of Obstetrics and Gynecology, 1966–1967 Series*, pp. 126–163. Ed. Greenhill, J.P. Year Book Medical Publishers, Chicago

CSAPO, A.I., JAFFIN, H., KERENYI, T., MATTOS, C.E.R. and SOUSA-FILHO, M.B. (1963). Fetal death *in utero*. *Am. J. Obstet. Gynec.*, **87**, 892–905

CSAPO, A.I., KIVIKOSKI, A., PULKKINEN, M.O. and WIEST, W.G. (1972a). First trimester abortions induced by the extraovular infusion of prostaglandin $F_{2\alpha}$. *Prostaglandins*, **1**, 295–303

CSAPO, A.I., KIVIKOSKI, A. and WIEST, W.G. (1972b). Mid trimester abortions induced by intraamniotic prostaglandin $F_{2\alpha}$ treatment. *Prostaglandins*, **1**, 305–319

CSAPO, A.I., KNOBIL., E., PULKKINEN, M., VAN DER MOLEN, H.J., SOMMERVILLE, I.F. and WIEST, W.G. (1969). Progesterone withdrawal during hypertonic saline-induced abortions. *Am. J. Obstet. Gynec.*, **105**, 1132–1134

DIDCOCK, K., JACKSON, D. and ROBSON, J.M. (1956). The action of some nucleotoxic substances on pregnancy. *Br. J. Pharmac. Chemother.*, **11**, 437–441

DILLON, T.F., PHILLIPS, L.L., RISK, A., HORIGUCHI, T., MOHAJER-SHOJAI, E. and MOOTABAR, H. (1974). The efficacy of prostaglandin $F_{2\alpha}$ in second-trimester abortion. *Am. J. Obstet. Gynec.*, **118**, 688–699

DROEGEMUELLER, W. and GREER, B.E. (1970). Saline versus glucose as a hypertonic solution for abortion. *Am. J. Obstet. Gynec.*, **108**, 606–609

DUTT, T.P., BLAIR, M. and ELDER, M.G. (1979). Ultrasound assessment of uterine emptying in first trimester abortions induced by intravaginal 15-methyl $PG5_{2\alpha}$ methyl ester. *Am. J. Obstet. Gynec.*, in press

EASTERLING, W.E. Jr., WEISS, A.E., ODOM, M.H. and TALBERT, L.M. (1972). Plasma volume, electrolyte and coagulation factor changes following intra-amniotic hypertonic saline infusion. *Am. J. Obstet. Gynec.*, **113**, 1065–1071

EATON, C.J., COHN, F. and BOLLINGER, C.C. (1972). Laminaria tent as a cervical dilator prior to aspiration-type therapeutic abortion. *Obstet. Gynec., N.Y.*, **39**, 533–537

ELDER, M.G. (1974). Induction of abortion by a single intra-amniotic injection of 40 mg prostaglandin $F_{2\alpha}$. *Contraception*, **10**, 6, 607–616

ELDER, M.G., STONE, M. and DUTT, T.P. (1976). Chronoperiodicity in response to the intra-amniotic injection of PGF$_{2\alpha}$. *Contraception*, **13**, 95–100

EMBREY, M.P. (1970). Induction of abortion by prostaglandins E$_1$ and E$_2$. *Br. med. J.*, **ii**, 258–260

EMBREY, M.P. (1971a). PGE compounds for induction of labour and abortion. *Ann. N.Y. Acad. Sci.*, **180**, 518–523

EMBREY, M.P. (1971b). Induction of abortion by prostaglandins E (PGE$_1$ and PGE$_2$). *J. reprod. Med.*, **6**, 15–18

EMBREY, M.P. and HILLIER, K. (1971). Therapeutic abortion by intrauterine instillation of prostaglandins. *Br. med. J.*, **i**, 588–590

EMBREY, M.P. and HILLIER, K. (1972). Abortion with extra-amniotic prostaglandins. *Lancet*, **ii**, 654–655

FRANSON, R., WAITE, M. and LA VIA, M. (1971). Identification of phospholipase A$_1$ and A$_2$ in the soluble fraction of rat liver lysosomes. *Biochemistry, N.Y.*, **10**, 1942–1946

FRASER, I.H. and BRASH, J.H. (1974). Comparison of extra- and intra-amniotic prostaglandins for therapeutic abortion. *Obstet. Gynec., N.Y.*, **43**, 97–103

FUCHS, F., FUCHS, A.R., SHORT, R.V. and WAGNER, G. (1965). Uterine motility and concentrations of progesterone in uterine venous blood after intra-amniotic injection of hypertonic saline. *Acta obstet. gynec. scand.*, **44**, 63–70

GAITONDE, A., MEHTA, A.C. and PURANDARE, B.N. (1974). Hypertonic saline for termination of pregnancy in the second trimester. In *Medical Termination of Pregnancy and Sterilization*, pp. 26–29. Ed. Talwalker, C.V. C.V. Talwalker, Bombay

GENNSER, G., KULLANDER, S. and LUNDGREN, N. (1968). Studies of therapeutic abortions induced by injection of hypertonic saline. *J. Obstet. Gynaec. Br. Commonw.*, **75**, 1058–1062

GOCHBERG, S.H. and REID, D.E. (1966). Intra-amniotic injection of hypertonic saline for termination of pregnancy. *Obstet. Gynec., N.Y.*, **27**, 648–654

GOLDTHORP, W.O. (1977). Ten-minute abortions. *Br. med. J.*, **ii**, 562–564

GOLDSMITH, S. and MARGOLIS, A.J. (1971). Aspiration abortion without cervical dilation. *Am. J. Obstet. Gynec.*, **110**, 580–582

GOMEL, V. and CARPENTER, C.W. (1973). Induction of mid-trimester abortion with intrauterine alcohol. *Obstet. Gynec., N.Y.*, **41**, 455–458

GOODLIN, R.C. and KRESCH, A.J. (1968). Amniotic fluid osmolality following intra-amniotic injection of saline. *Am. J. Obstet. Gynec.*, **100**, 839–842

GREENHALF, J.O. and DIGGORY, P.L.C. (1971). Induction of therapeutic abortion by intra-amniotic injection of urea. *Br. med. J.*, **i**, 28–29

GREER, B.E., DROEGEMUELLER, W. and ENGEL, T. (1975). Preliminary experience with 15(S)15-methyl prostaglandin F$_{2\alpha}$ for midtrimester abortion. *Am. J. Obstet. Gynec.*, **121**, 524–527

GUSTAVII, B. (1974). Sweeping of the fetal membranes by a physiologic saline solution: effect on decidual cells. *Am. J. Obstet. Gynec.*, **120**, 531–536

GUSTAVII, B. (1975). The distribution within the placenta, myometrium and decidua of ^{24}Na-labelled hypertonic saline solution following intra-amniotic or extra-amniotic injection. *Br. J. Obstet. Gynaec.*, **82**, 734–739

GUSTAVII, B. and GREEN, K. (1972). Release of prostaglandin F$_{2\alpha}$ following injection of hypertonic saline for therapeutic abortion: a preliminary study. *Am. J. Obstet. Gynec.*, **114**, 1099–1100

HALBRECHT, I. and BLUM, M. (1974). Induction of mid-trimester abortion by means of extra-amniotic infusion of an isotonic saline solution combined with intravenous oxytocin drip infusion. *Contraception*, **10**, 637–643

HALL, W.J. and PICKLES, V.R. (1963). The dual action of menstrual stimulant A2 (prostaglandin E_2). *J. Physiol., Lond.*, **169**, 90–91

HAWKINS, D.F. (1965). Reports on some preparations for female ills. In *Survey of Abortifacient Drugs*, appendix 2, pp. 8–12. Abortion Law Reform Association, Birmingham

HAWKINS, D.F., MENZIES, D.N. and HERHEIMER, A. (1974). Cited in *Obstetric Therapeutics*, pp. 49–50. Ed. Hawkins, D.F. Baillière Tindall, London

HIGGENBOTHAM, J. (1973). Termination of pregnancy by abdominal hysterotomy. *Lancet*, **i**, 937–938

HILLIER, K. and EMBREY, M.P. (1972). High dose intravenous administration of prostaglandin E_2 and $F_{2\alpha}$ for the termination of mid-trimester pregnancies. *J. Obstet. Gynaec. Br. Commonw.*, **79**, 14–22

HODGSON, J.E. and PORTMAN, K.C. (1974). Complications of 10,453 consecutive first-trimester abortions: a prospective study. *Am. J. Obstet. Gynec.*, **120**, 802–807

HORSKÝ, J. (1971). Induced abortions: their relation to demographical indexes and health. *VII World Congress on Fertility and Sterility, Tokyo/Kyoto 17–25 October 1971. Excerpta Medica International Congress Series No. 234*, pp. 146–147. Excerpta Medica, Amsterdam

HOWIE, P.W., CALDER, A.A., FORBES, C.D. and PRENTICE, C.R.M. (1973). Effect of intravenous prostaglandin E_2 on platelet function, coagulation, and fibrinolysis. *J. clin. Path.*, **26**, 354–358

JAYARAMAN, S., SINHA, M.K., RAGHAVEN, K.S., MATHUR, V.S., RASTOGI, G.K. and DEVI, P.K. (1975). Effect of prostaglandin $F_{2\alpha}$ and hypertonic saline on the placental function during midtrimester abortion. *Am. J. Obstet. Gynec.*, **121**, 528–530

JOHNSON, J.W.C., CUSHNER, I.M. and STEPHENS, N.L. (1966). Hazards of using hypertonic saline for therapeutic abortion. *Am. J. Obstet. Gynec.*, **94**, 225–229

JUBIZ, W., FRAILEY, J. and BARTHOLOMEW, K. (1972). Prostaglandins of the F group (PGF): assessment by radioimmunoassay of their role in human physiology. *Clin. Res.*, **20**, 178

KARIM, S.M.M. and FILSHIE, G.M. (1970). Use of prostaglandin E_2 for therapeutic abortion. *Br. med. J.*, **iii**, 198–200

KARIM, S.M.M. and FILSHIE, G.M. (1972). The use of prostaglandin E_2 for therapeutic abortion. *J. Obstet. Gynaec. Br. Commonw.*, **79**, 1–13

KARIM, S.M.M. and SHARMA, S.D. (1971a). Second trimester abortion with single intra amniotic injection of prostaglandins E_2 or $F_{2\alpha}$. *Lancet*, **ii**, 47–48

KARIM, S.M.M. and SHARMA, S.D. (1971b). Therapeutic abortion and induction of labour by the intravaginal administration of prostaglandins E_2 and $F_{2\alpha}$. *J. Obstet. Gynaec. Br. Commonw.*, **78**, 294–300

KARIM, S.M.M., SHARMA, S.D. and FILSHIE, G.M. (1972). Termination of pregnancy with 15-methyl analogues of prostaglandins E_2 and $F_{2\alpha}$. *J. reprod. Med.*, **9**, 383–391

KARMAN, H. and POTTS, M. (1972). Very early abortion using syringe as a vacuum source. *Lancet*, **i**, 1051–1052

KERENYI, T.D. and MUZSNAI, D. (1975). Volume and sodium concentration studies in 300 saline-induced abortions. *Am. J. Obstet. Gynec.*, **121**, 590–595

KERR, M.G., ROY, E.J., HARKNESS, R.A., SHORT, R.V. and BAIRD, D.T. (1966). Studies of the mode of action of intra-amniotic injection of hypertonic solutions in the induction of labour. *Am. J. Obstet. Gynec.*, **94**, 214–224

KERSLAKE, D. and CASEY, D. (1967). Abortion induced by means of the uterine aspirator. *Obstet. Gynec., N.Y.*, **30**, 35–45

KOLSTAD, P. (1957). Therapeutic abortion. A clinical study based on 968 cases from a Norwegian Hospital, 1940–53. *Acta obstet. gynec. scand.*, **36**, supplement 6, p. 57

KOTASEK, A. (1971). Artificial termination of pregnancy in Czechoslovakia. *Int. J. Gynaecol. Obstet.*, **9**, 118–119

LACHELIN, G.C.L. and BURGESS, D.E. (1968). Therapeutic abortion using utus paste. *J. Obstet. Gynaec. Br. Commonw.*, **75**, 1173–1175

LAU, I.F., SAKSENA, S.K. and CHANG, M.C. (1974). Intravaginal insertion of a dimethylpolysiloxane-polyvinyl-pyrrolidone-prostaglandin $F_{2\alpha}$ tube for midterm abortion in rabbits. *Am. J. Obstet. Gynec.*, **120**, 837–839

LAUERSEN, N.H. and BIRNBAUM, S.J. (1975). Water intoxication associated with oxytocin administration during saline-induced abortion. *Am. J. Obstet. Gynec.*, **121**, 2–6

LAUERSEN, N.H. and WILSON, K.H. (1975). Midtrimester abortion induced by serial intramuscular injections of 15(S)-15-methyl-prostaglandin $F_{2\alpha}$. *Am. J. Obstet. Gynec.*, **121**, 273–276

LAUERSEN, N.H., WILSON, K.H., BELING, C.G. and FUCHS, F. (1974). Comparison of prostaglandin $F_{2\alpha}$ and hypertonic saline for induction of midtrimester abortion. *Am. J. Obstet. Gynec.*, **120**, 875–889

LAUMAS, K.R., RAHMAN, S.A., HINGORANI, V., PURI, C.P., BALIGA, N. and LAUMAS, V. (1974). Hormonal changes in patients undergoing therapeutic abortion with prostaglandin $F_{2\alpha}$, 15(S)15-methyl prostaglandin $F_{2\alpha}$ and hypertonic saline. *Contraception*, **10**, 617–636

LEE, L.T. and PAXMAN, J.M. (1975). Legal aspects of menstrual regulation: some preliminary observations. *J. Family Law*, **14**, 181–221

LEWIS, S.C., LAL, S., BRANCH, B. and BEARD, R.W. (1971). Outpatient termination of pregnancy. *Br. med. J.*, **iv**, 606–610

LILIEN, A.A. (1968). Oxytocin-induced water intoxication. A report of a maternal death. *Obstet. Gynec., N.Y.*, **32**, 171–173

LINDAHL, J. (1959). In *Somatic Complications Following Legal Abortion*. Heinemann, London

LIU, D.T.Y. and HUDSON, I. (1974). Karman cannula and first-trimester termination of pregnancy. *Am. J. Obstet. Gynec.*, **118**, 906–909

LLEWELLYN-JONES, D., O'TOOLE, V., REYNOLDS, J. and SALEH, Y. (1975). Extraovular hypertonic saline for the induction of abortion in the second quarter of pregnancy. *Aust. & N.Z. J. Obstet. Gynaecol.*, **15**, 31–35

LOUNG, K.C., BUCKLE, A.E.R. and ANDERSON, M.M. (1971). Results in 1000 cases of therapeutic abortion managed by vacuum aspiration. *Br. med. J.*, **iv**, 477–479

LURIE, A.O., REID, D.E. and VILLEE, C.A. (1966). The role of the fetus and placenta in maintenance of plasma progesterone. *Am. J. Obstet. Gynec.*, **96**, 670–675

LUTTRELL, N., FINBERG, L. and DRAWDY, L.P. (1959). Haemorrhagic encephalo-
pathy induced by hypernatraemia. II. Experimental observations on hyper-
osmolarity in cats. *Archs Neurol.*, **1**, 153—160

LYNEHAM, R.C., LOW, P.A., McLEOD, J.G., SHEARMAN, R.P., SMITH, I.D. and
KORDA, A.R. (1973). Convulsions and electroencephalogram abnormalities
after intra-amniotic prostaglandin $F_{2\alpha}$. *Lancet*, **ii**, 1003—1005

MACKENZIE, I.Z., EMBREY, M.P. and HILLIER, K. (1974). Intra-amniotic prostaglandin for induction of abortion: an improved regime using prostaglandin
E_2. *J. Obstet. Gynaec. Br. Commonw.*, **81**, 554—557

MANABE, Y. (1967). Metreurynter-induced abortions at midpregnancy. The
changes in uterine contractility and in urinary output of pregnanediol and
estrogen. *Am. J. Obstet. Gynec.*, **99**, 557—561

MANABE, Y. (1968). Urinary excretion of oestriol and pregnanediol during
bougie-induced abortion in mid-pregnancy. *J. Endocr.*, **42**, 331—335

MANABE, Y. (1969). Artificial abortion at midpregnancy by mechanical stimulation of the uterus. A review of 20 years' experience with current methods
in Japan. *Am. J. Obstet. Gynec.*, **105**, 132—146

MANABE, Y. and NAKAJIMA, A. (1972). Laminaria-metreurynter method of
midterm abortion in Japan. *Obstet. Gynec., N.Y.*, **40**, 612—615

MARTIN, J.N., BYGDEMAN, M., RAMADAN, M., GRÉEN, K., LEADER, A.,
LUNDSTRÖM, V. and WIQVIST, N. (1976). Vaginally administered 16,16-
dimethyl-PGE_2 for the induction of midtrimester abortion. *Prostaglandins*,
11, 123—132

MATTHEWS, C.D. and MATTHEWS, A.E.B. (1969). Transplacental haemorrhage in
spontaneous and induced abortion. *Lancet*, **i**, 694—695

MENZIES, D.N. and HAWKINS, D.F. (1968). Therapeutic abortion using intra-
amniotic hypertonic solutions. *J. Obstet. Gynaec. Br. Commonw.*, **75**,
215—218

MIDWINTER, A., SHEPHARD, A. and BOWEN, M. (1973). Continuous extra-amniotic
prostaglandin E_2 for therapeutic termination and the effectiveness of various
infusion rates and dosages. *J. Obstet. Gynaec. Br. Commonw.*, **80**, 371—373

MILLER, A.W.F., CALDER, A.A. and MacNAUGHTON, M.C. (1972). Termination of
pregnancy by continuous intra-uterine infusion of prostaglandins. *Lancet*, **ii**,
5—7

OSBORN, R.H., GOPLERUD, C.P. and YANNONE, M.E. (1968). Response of peripheral plasma progesterone concentration to intra-amniotic hypertonic
saline. *Am. J. Obstet. Gynec.*, **101**, 1073—1077

PAKTER, J., HARRIS, D. and NELSON, F. (1971). Surveillance of abortion program
in New York City. *Bull. N.Y. Acad. Med.*, **47**, 8, 853—874

PEEL, J. (1962). Inducing labour by intra-amniotic injection. *Br. med. J.*, **ii**,
1397—1398

PERRY, G., SCHULMAN, H. and WONG, T.-C. (1974). Modified saline abortion for
medically high-risk patients. *Obstet. Gynec., N.Y.*, **44**, 571—578

POTTS, D.M. (1970). Termination of pregnancy. *Br. med. Bull.*, **26**, 65—71

PUGH, M., KHUNDA, S. and BALDWIN, R. (1971). Induction of therapeutic abortion
with urea. *Br. med. J.*, **i**, 345

REGISTRAR GENERAL (1969—1972). *Statistical Review of England and Wales.
Supplements on Abortion.* Her Majesty's Stationery Office, London

REISS, H.E. (1969). Methods and dangers of termination of pregnancy. *Proc. R.
Soc. Med.*, **62**, 832—833

ROBERTS, G., CASSIE, R. and TURNBULL, A.C. (1971). Therapeutic abortion by intrauterine instillation of prostaglandin E_2. *J. Obstet. Gynaec. Br. Commonw.*, **78**, 834–837

ROBERTS, G., GOMERSALL, R., ADAMS, M. and TURNBULL, A.C. (1972). Therapeutic abortion by intra-amniotic injection of prostaglandins. *Br. med. J.*, **iv**, 12–14

RUSSELL, A.J. and HEWLETT, P.M. (1969). A hysterographic study of the abdominal hysterotomy scar. *J. Obstet. Gynaec. Br. Commonw.*, **76**, 721–723

RUTTNER, B.T. (1966). Termination of mid-trimester pregnancy by transvaginal intra-amniotic injection of hypertonic solution. *Obstet. Gynec., N.Y.*, **28**, 601–605

SCHIFFER, M.A., PAKTER, J. and CLAHR, J. (1973). Mortality associated with hypertonic saline abortion. *Obstet. Gynec., N.Y.*, **42**, 759–764

SCHULMAN, H., KAISER, I.H. and RANDOLPH, G. (1971). Out-patient saline abortion. *Obstet. Gynec., N.Y.*, **37**, 521–526

SEPPALA, M. and VARA, P. (1972). Prostaglandin-oxytocin enhancement. *Br. med. J.*, **i**, 747

SHALITA, R. (1975). Prostaglandins promise more effective fertility control. *Population Reports*, series G, number 6, 57–62

SHAPIRO, A.G. (1975). Extraovular prostaglandin $F_{2\alpha}$ for early midtrimester abortion. *Am. J. Obstet. Gynec.*, **121**, 333–336

SMITH, I.D. and SHEARMAN, R.P. (1974). Circadian aspects of prostaglandin $F_{2\alpha}$-induced termination of pregnancy. *J. Obstet. Gynaec. Br. Commonw.*, **81**, 841–848

SOOD, S.V. (1971). Some operative and postoperative hazards of legal termination of pregnancy. *Br. med. J.*, **iv**, 270–273

SPARKS, R.M. and LEE, C.M. (1973). Clinical use of PGs in fertility control. *Population Reports*, series G, number 1, 1–15

STALLWORTHY, J.A., MOOLGAOKER, A.S. and WALSH, J.J. (1971). Legal abortion: a critical assessment of its risks. *Lancet*, **ii**, 1245–1249

STEWART, G.K. and GOLDSTEIN, P. (1972). Medical and surgical complications of therapeutic abortions. *Obstet. Gynec., N.Y.*, **40**, 539–550

STIM, E.M. (1972). Saline abortion. *Obstet. Gynec., N.Y.*, **40**, 247–251

STONE, M. and ELDER, M.G. (1974). An evaluation of sonar in the prediction of complications after vaginal termination of pregnancy. *Am. J. Obstet. Gynec.*, **120**, 890–894

STONE, M., MORRIS, N. and BLAIR, M. (1977). Factors influencing morbidity following termination of pregnancy. *Eur. J. Obstet. Gynaec. reprod. Biol.*, **7**, 69–72

STRAUSZ, I.K. and SCHULMAN, H. (1971). 500 outpatient abortions performed under local anaesthesia. *Obstet. Gynec., N.Y.*, **38**, 199–205

STRINGER, J., ANDERSON, M., BEARD, R.W., FAIRWEATHER, D.V.I. and STEELE, S.J. (1975). Very early termination of pregnancy (menstrual extraction). *Br. med. J.*, **iii**, 7–9

STUBBLEFIELD, P., NAFTOLIN, F., FRIGOLETTO, F.D. and RYAN, K.J. (1976). Laminaria augmentation of intra-amniotic prostaglandin $F_{2\alpha}$ for midtrimester pregnancy termination. *Advances in Prostaglandin and Thromboxane Research*, **2**, 977

THEOBALD, G.W. (1934). The repetition of certain experiments on which Molitor and Pick base their water-centre hypothesis, and the effect of afferent nerve stimuli on water diuresis. *J. Physiol., Lond.*, **81**, 243–254

THIERSCH, J.B. (1952). Therapeutic abortions with folic acid antagonist, 4-aminopteroylglutamic acid (4-amino P.G.A.) administered by oral route. *Am. J. Obstet. Gynec.*, **63**, 1298–1304

TOPPOZADA, M., BYGDEMAN, M. and WIQVIST, N. (1971). Induction of abortion by intra amniotic administration of prostaglandin $F_{2\alpha}$. *Contraception*, **4**, 293–303

TOPPOZADA, M., BYGDEMAN, M., PAPAGEORGIOU, C. and WIQVIST, N. (1973). Administration of 15-methyl-prostaglandin $F_{2\alpha}$ as a pre-operative means of cervical dilatation. *Prostaglandins*, **4**, 371–379

VAN DER VLUGT, T. and PIOTROW, P.T. (1973a). Menstrual regulation – what is it? *Population Reports,* series F, number 2, 9–23

VAN DER VLUGT, T. and PIOTROW, P.T. (1973b). Uterine aspiration techniques. *Population Reports,* series F, number 3, 25–48

VAN DER VLUGT, T. and PIOTROW, P.T. (1974). Menstrual regulation update. *Population Reports,* series F, number 4, 49–64

VAN WAGENEN, G., DECONTI, R.C., HANDSCHUMACHER, R.E. and WADE, M.E. (1970). Abortifacient and teratogenic effects of triacetyl-6-azauridine in the monkey. *Am. J. Obstet. Gynec.*, **108**, 272–281

VANE, J.R. and WILLIAMS, K.I. (1973). The contribution of prostaglandin production to contractions of the isolated uterus of the rat. *Br. J. Pharmac.*, **48**, 629–639

VLIES, P.R. and DEWHURST, C.J. (1975). Pregnancy and labour following hysterotomy. *Int. J. Gynaecol. Obstet.*, **13**, 162–164

WAGATSUMA, T. (1965). Intra-amniotic injection of saline for therapeutic abortion. *Am. J. Obstet. Gynec.*, **93**, 743–745

WAGNER, G. (1971). Intrauterine volume after intraovular instillation of hypertonic saline. *Acta obstet. gynec. scand.*, **50**, supplement 9, 44

WAGNER, G., KARKER, H., FUCHS, F. and BENGTSSON, L.P. (1962). Induction of abortion by intraovular instillation of hypertonic saline. *Dan. med. Bull.*, **9**, 137–142

WEISS, A.E., EASTERLING, W.E., Jr., ODOM, M.H., McMILLAN, C.W., JOHNSON, A.M. and TALBERT, L.M. (1972). Defibrination syndrome after intra-amniotic infusion of hypertonic saline. *Am. J. Obstet. Gynec.*, **113**, 868–874

WEISS, R.R., NEUWIRTH, R.S. and FRIEDMAN, M.M. (1972). Effect of intra-amniotic sodium concentration on saline induced abortion. *Obstet. Gynec., N.Y.*, **40**, 243–246

WENTZ, A.C., AUSTIN, K. and KING, T.M. (1973). Abortifacient efficacy of intra-vaginal prostaglandin $F_{2\alpha}$. *Am. J. Obstet. Gynec.*, **115**, 27–32

WIEST, W.G., KERENYI, T. and CSAPO, A.I. (1966). Progesterone and the induction of labor with hypertonic solutions. *Obstet. Gynec., N.Y.*, **27**, 589

WIQVIST, N., BYGDEMAN, M. and TOPPOZADA, M. (1971). Induction of abortion by the intravenous administration of prostaglandin $F_{2\alpha}$. *Acta obstet. gynec. scand.*, **50**, 381–389

WIQVIST, N., BYGDEMAN, M. and TOPPOZADA, M. (1973). Intra-amniotic prostaglandin administration – a challenge to the currently used methods for induction of mid trimester abortion. *Contraception*, **8**, 113–131

WONG, TING-CHAO, PALAV, A.B., BUM JOO KIM and TRICOMNI, V. (1972). Changes in serum and urinary electrolytes. *N.Y. St. J. Med.*, **72**, 564–577

WOOD, C., BOOTH, R.T. and PINKERTON, J.H.M. (1962). Induction of labour by intra-amniotic injection of hypertonic glucose solution. *Br. med. J.*, **ii**, 706–709

WRIGHT, C.S.W., CAMPBELL, S. and BEAZLEY, J. (1972). Second-trimester abortion after vaginal termination of pregnancy. *Lancet*, **ii**, 1278–1279

ZOREMTHANGI, B., AGARWAL, N., PURI, C.P., LAUMAS, K.R. and HINGORANI, V. (1976). Evaluation of 15(S)15-methyl-PGF$_{2\alpha}$ methyl ester suppositories with a two dose schedule for termination of early pregnancy. *Contraception*, **14**, 519–527

Part V
Sterilisation

14 Sterilisation Counselling

Perspective on the indications for operative sterilisation of the female has changed considerably during the last two decades. The definitive medical indications – conditions in which it is possible to advise a patient that if she becomes pregnant again her life is at serious risk – have become very few in number. Standards of medical care have improved to such an extent that the severity of medical complications in women of reproductive age is rarely such as to support firm advice that a pregnancy will cause permanent damage to health. Obstetric knowledge and care have also improved so that the obstetrician now confidently approaches patients with conditions that formerly caused trepidation.

In contrast, there has been a very great increase in the number of patients requesting sterilisation as a means of family limitation. The reasons for this may be primarily economic. In developed countries the strain of raising a large family is increasing, and women are demanding greater social freedom and a sexual life free from the chance of pregnancy. The pressure of world population problems, relaxation of legal restrictions and reduced risk of anaesthetic and operative complications have combined to encourage physicians to comply with this demand. In many countries there is now little objection to sterilisation on request provided the patient has a full understanding of the implications, and equivocation or potential for psychiatric complications can be excluded. Although physician and patient must accept the irreversibility of the procedure it would be purblind to deny that both may have some knowledge of recent developments in procedures for reanastomosis of the fallopian tubes.

As a result the incidence of operative sterilisation has risen considerably in Great Britain, the United States of America and many other countries. Sampling 12 areas in Great Britain, Cartwright showed that the sterilisation rate has increased from 2% to 5% of recently delivered mothers between the years 1967 and 1970 (Diggory, 1971), and there is little doubt that the rate has continued to approximate to the higher of these two figures. In the United States of America, Nichols (1969) estimated that 180 000 female sterilisations were carried out in 1968, and the Association for Voluntary Sterilisation suggested that 265 000 were performed in 1971 (Schwyhart and Kutner, 1973). Shepard (1974) has reviewed the literature on these trends. The rate seems to have continued at about the higher level during succeeding years.

The majority of sterilisations carried out today in Great Britain are for social reasons and fall into the category of 'on request'. Many couples in their late 20s or 30s who have completed their families do not wish to continue using contraceptive methods for the next 20 years, or find that current contraceptive

317

techniques are unsatisfactory and so request sterilisation. In 1967 the American College of Obstetricians and Gynecologists abandoned recommendations relating approval of elective sterilisation to the patient's age and to the number of her existing children and also suggested dissolution of hospital committees for appraising patients requesting sterilisation. It is now a widely held view that age and parity are immaterial, provided the couple fully understand the nature of the operation and its implications. It is desirable that both partners are interviewed, either together or individually and there must be no doubt of the irreversibility of the procedure. Good counselling ensures that few patients subsequently regret the operation and obviates the need for a patient to fulfil arbitrary criteria relating to her age and parity before being considered for sterilisation.

LEGAL ASPECTS

Very few countries have specific legislation allowing voluntary sterilisation, which defines the precise conditions under which the operation may be carried out. Under the code of civil law sterilisation is allowed, with varying restrictions, in the following countries: Czechoslovakia, Denmark, Finland, East and West Germany, Honduras, Iceland, Iran, Japan, Norway, Panama, Puerto Rico, Saudi Arabia, Singapore, Sweden, Thailand, the United Kingdom and some of the United States of America. These restrictions may preclude the operation being carried out for eugenic reasons, or allow it only after a specified number of pregnancies.

Criminal prosecution is applicable to voluntary contraceptive sterilisation in many countries in Europe and Latin America, particularly those in which Roman Catholicism is the predominant religion. These include: Argentine, Austria, Bulgaria, Bolivia, Brazil, Chile, Columbia, Costa Rica, Ecuador, Eire, France, Guatemala, Hungary, Italy, Malta, Poland, Portugal, Spain, Switzerland, South Vietnam, Uruguay and Venezuela.

Many other countries in Africa and Asia have a criminal law applicable but there are clauses stating that the operation is permissible if it is carried out in good faith for the benefit of the patient. These countries include: Burma, Ethiopia, Ghana, India, Malawi, Malaysia, Nepal, Nigeria, Pakistan, Sri Lanka, Tanzania, the Union of Soviet Socialist Republics and Zambia.

Despite the great variation in laws and the confusion surrounding their interpretation there have been very few prosecutions. In Jamaica the law implies that performing sterilisation is causing grievous bodily harm. Despite this, thousands of sterilisations are performed annually in Government hospitals, free of charge. The laws of most countries do not differentiate between male and female sterilisation.

In the United Kingdom, the situation at present is that sterilisation, for whatever reason, social, medical or eugenic, is lawful, provided that the patient has given full and valid consent, knowing the implications of the operation (British Medical Journal, 1960; Medical Defence Union, 1974). This means that sterilisation of a mentally defective individual (Addison, 1967) or a minor (British Medical Journal, 1975) is unlawful. These comments are applicable equally to males and females. It is advisable that when sterilisation is performed solely as a convenient method of birth control, the written consent of the patient and his or her spouse, if they are living together, should be obtained. Legal opinion is that a man may have a legal right to the opportunity of having children by his wife and that if his wife has undergone an operation with the primary purpose of sterilisation without his consent, then he might successfully claim damages against the surgeon. Should sterilisation be desirable on medical grounds, then the spouse's permission is not essential. There is, however, a body of legal opinion which states that both wives and husbands can undergo sterilisation without the consent of their spouses. To date, there has not been a case in the United Kingdom in which a husband has instituted a claim for damages against a surgeon for having sterilised his wife against his wishes, and so the difference of opinion is academic at the moment. In 1972 in the United Kingdom the National Health Service (Family Planning) Amendment Act mentioned a voluntary vasectomy service. The word 'voluntary' presumably confirms the legal view that sterilisation can be authorised by either spouse against the other's wishes. By virtue of this Act, the British Parliament has given approval to the principle at least, of voluntary human sterilisation.

In Scandinavia, laws allow for voluntary sterilisation and Sweden has a National Board of Health and Welfare which will authorise sterilisation with written consent, on medical, eugenic or social grounds. In June 1973 Denmark passed a new law which allows anyone over the age of 25 years to be sterilised, with special precautions for the mentally ill. Sterilisation procedures must be carried out in public hospitals, and the patients must be fully informed of the attendant risks.

The motion adopted by Le Conseil National in France in 1955 forbade the use of sterilisation as a purely contraceptive measure. It is permissible in exceptional circumstances provided the doctor notifies his reasons to the Conseil Départemental de l'Ordre, without mentioning the patient by name. In 1964, the rules were amended so that a sterilisation can be performed if the patient has given written consent, provided that 3 medical practitioners agree and the Conseil Départemental de l'Ordre is notified (unless the case is of especial urgency).

In Germany the legal position is not so clear. The State Court of Justice in judgement on 27th October, 1964, decided that sterilisation carried out by a doctor when the patient has consented, after adequate explanation, is not punishable and that carrying out a sterilisation procedure is not a criminal act. The necessity of having a medical indication for operation is abolished and even the consent of an expert Committee is not necessary. However, it is legally still possible for the State Prosecutor to initiate proceedings on the grounds that the decision of the Court of Justice is incorrect. Such proceedings have not occurred so far, but perhaps because of fear of such legal action, doctors have a certain reluctance to perform sterilisation operations. The position regarding voluntary consent is also uncertain. On several occasions, a medical expert committee has decided that voluntary consent is an added requisite for the carrying out of sterilisation, but a standard procedure has not been developed.

A similar situation exists in Czechoslovakia where a written application is submitted to a Board on which sit the doctor in charge of the District Institute of Public Health, a senior gynaecologist and a senior physician. However, sterilisation in Czechoslovakia is only available on medical and eugenic grounds and it differs from some other Eastern European countries in not allowing sterilisation for multiparity and for social reasons.

In the United States of America the laws vary from state to state. Twenty-eight states have laws on sterilisation and of these 26 permit compulsory sterilisation to be performed on mentally ill patients maintained in mental hospitals. This is in direct contrast to the situation in the United Kingdom. Until 1971 it was illegal in Connecticut to sterilise anyone unless for eugenic or medical reasons but now all restrictions on voluntary sterilisation have been lifted. In Utah, the Supreme Court ruled in May 1974 that voluntary sterilisation was permissible for social reasons and that the law on eugenic sterilisation in no way overlapped. In this State, doctors were afraid to sterilise women on social grounds until the Supreme Court's ruling had been given. Virginia is another State in which the law has recently been changed. Any person over 21 years of age can be sterilised if that person makes a request in writing and has the written consent of a spouse, if there is one. There is a 30 day waiting period for both men and women before sterilisation may be carried out, but it does not apply in the puerperium. Statutes in Georgia, North Carolina and Oregon authorise voluntary sterilisation for non-medical reasons.

There are no Federal laws in the United States of America on sterilisation and the absence of laws in many States allows the physician a good deal of discretion, but also causes a lot of uncertainty. Full voluntary consent from the patient is necessary and the consent of the spouse is desirable, but not essential. As in the United Kingom, the question as to whether an individual has some protected interest in the procreative abilities of his or her spouse has not been tested in the courts.

Hong Kong has no specific legislation of its own and they follow the practice of the United Kingdom in that, where possible, the husband's consent should be obtained.

The situation in India and Sri Lanka is basically similar. There is no law on the statute book regarding sterilisation but it has been the practice since early 1972 for the person offering himself or herself for sterilisation to give written consent and to produce a signed statement from his or her spouse consenting to the operation.

Singapore has a complex procedure. Boards are set up consisting of a District Judge, two doctors, one of whom is in the public service, and two members appointed by the Minister of Health, one of whom is a professionally qualified Social Worker. The person wishing sterilisation must be over 21 years of age and must apply in writing on a prescribed form to the Board giving consent to such treatment. The spouse's consent is also necessary. Sterilisation is available on medical, eugenic or social grounds. Thirty days must elapse between applying for sterilisation and consideration of the application by the Board, during which time the applicant may withdraw. The Board may examine the applicant medically. If the application is approved, sterilisation may be carried out by any medical practitioner. The operating doctor and the Board are immune from legal action. This is an unusual and rather bureaucratic approach to the problem, but nevertheless, it is hard to see many loopholes in such a system.

STERILISATION COUNSELLING IN PRACTICE

Opinions differ as to who is the best person to discuss the possibility of a sterilisation operation with the patient and her husband. It is best if they have the opportunity to consult both an individual who knows their circumstances well, such as their family practitioner, and also to have the benefit of a more objective discussion with a specialist gynaecologist who is not so closely involved with their environment and their problems. For patients who have a known psychiatric history or are suspected to be psychologically unstable it is desirable also to seek the advice of a psychiatrist at the hospital at which the operation is to be performed. If there is any acute psychiatric reaction after the operation, he is then already acquainted with the patient and in the best position to treat it.

Discussion of proposed sterilisation will of course vary according both to the needs and circumstances of the patients and their medical and psychological status and also to the attitudes and experience of the physician. Nonetheless there are certain topics which we feel should always be considered.

Reason for Request

Full discussion of this not only leads to fuller understanding of the circumstances but also brings out misconceptions that the patient may have about her obstetric and medical status, about the functions of sterilisation and about possible alternative contraceptive procedures.

Nature of Operation

Even if they work in hospitals, patients often have the strangest ideas about the nature of sterilising procedures! It is essential to convey a rough idea of the pelvic anatomy and of the nature of the possible operative procedures and their effects. The probable length of hospital stay and eventual cosmetic results should be included in the discussion. If it is the custom of the surgeon to perform curettage in association with interval sterilisation to exclude the presence of an undiagnosed early pregnancy, this should be explained, or the patient may be upset when she is presented with a consent form which includes curettage.

Preservation of Menstrual and Sexual Function

Many patients do not appreciate that tubal sterilisation preserves menstrual function. This can be a source of grave concern to patients for whom menstruation is of cultural importance. Only a few patients may be under the impression that libido is suppressed by sterilisation but many have some idea that it may be affected adversely. It is helpful to refer to the many women whose sex lives are greatly improved after the operation has relieved fears of pregnancy and the inconvenience of contraception.

Relative Irreversibility

Some patients who have hitherto appeared to understand completely the nature of sterilisation will still be found to be nursing the belief that it can be readily reversed if their circumstances change. Equivocation may well be demonstrated when it is made clear that reversal is not a very successful procedure and is in general only undertaken when the circumstances are exceptional.

Consequences of Marital Breakdown

It is necessary to be quite blunt about this even to the extent of quoting current divorce figures. When discussing an operation which will prejudice 10–15 years of a woman's reproductive life, she should be prepared to express an opinion as to what her feelings would be about future fertility if her marriage did break up and she remarried.

Consequences of Loss of Children

Similarly, she should face up to how she would feel if anything happened to her existing children.

Psychological Sequelae

The occasional occurrence of loss of libido and even amenorrhoea after tubal sterilisation is distressing. Most patients can understand that defeminisation reactions sometimes occur after the operation and that from the nature of the operation the reactions cannot be of physical origin. They also readily appreciate the psychological mechanisms involved. Discussion of this potential problem usually prevents its occurrence.

Physical Sequelae

Whether or not these should be discussed is a moot point. It is our opinion that the incidence of disturbances of menstruation during the years after tubal sterilisation is now known to be sufficiently great that the possibility should be mentioned to patients. We feel that if there is a psychological component to the phenomenon, and there is a little evidence that this is so, then frank mention of the problem before the operation should tend to put it in perspective and perhaps prevent its occurrence. Others may feel that inappropriate mention of the matter might predispose to its occurrence. With patients who are already subject to irregular and heavy menstruation and who are absolutely convinced of the need for a completely irreversible procedure, the possibility of sterilisation by hysterectomy should be discussed.

Failure Rate

Medicolegal proceedings in the United Kingdom have made it fairly clear that a surgeon who did not inform the patient of the failure rate before or shortly after the operative procedure could be held liable should the patient subsequently become pregnant. There ought to be no difficulty in conveying the failure rate to the patient if the matter is put in perspective. Most patients appreciate that no surgical procedure is always perfect and that they have to be told for medico-legal reasons although the real chance of failure is remote. They may even be flattered by the thought that occasionally a woman is so fertile that she can overcome the barrier created! If they are told that the odds against ever conceiving again are 100 or 200 to 1, that this is very much safer than any known contraceptive procedure, and that no one would suggest there is any need for additional precautions, they seldom have any further queries. The fact that the patient has been informed of the failure rate should be recorded in the case notes as an *aide-mémoire* in case the point is ever raised.

Detection of Equivocation

Not infrequently during the interview the physician will suspect equivocation. This must always be explored. Frank discussion of the problem involved, even if it leads to postponement or cancellation of the proposed operation, is the key to avoidance of untoward psychiatric sequelae.

Vasectomy as an Alternative

It is not our custom to raise this topic when a request for female sterilisation has been made, unless the couple are totally unaware of the possibility of male sterilisation, or there is a medical hazard associated with operative procedures on the wife or a genetic factor on the husband's side which is contributing to the request for sterilisation. Cultural influences are such in Great Britain that if vasectomy is acceptable to the couple, it will usually be mentioned by them. Vasectomy may be a more minor surgical procedure than female sterilisation, but the former operation is in general concerned with a considerably longer period of reproductive ability than is tubal ligation. We have seen domestic conflict ensue from raising these issues and from intrusion into a marital decision which has already been made. In many of the cases where we have volunteered the possibility of vasectomy it has been disclosed that the decision for female sterilisation was the wife's. Exploration has revealed that she has a basic fear of her husband's infidelity and is worried about the future of her marriage if he were to have a vasectomy.

Special Cases

The Young Woman

In general the younger the individual the more likely she is to change her mind, and the less sure she will be of her marriage and her existing children. No arbitrary age limit should be set for sterilisation, but most gynaecologists would agree that patients below the age of 25 require very careful consideration. This means careful counselling of both partners to ensure that they have a full understanding of the implications of their actions. Young patients have a higher risk of upsetting their libido, and of developing other psychosomatic problems as a result of being sterilised. These potential problems should be fully discussed before operation. Any suggestions of equivocation, or that the patient is trying to defeminise herself, should be an indication for not proceeding.

There is some evidence that women sterilised under the age of 30 are particularly susceptible to subsequent gynaecological problems (Adams, 1964; Whitehouse, 1971; Donaldson *et al.*, 1975). With this in mind, one of us (Hawkins, unpublished observations) has studied a series of patients under 30 years of age who were requesting sterilisation. Twenty-three of the patients were sent for a psychiatric evaluation before the operation, with a request that particular attention be paid to the possibility of equivocation and the risk of subsequent defeminisation. There was no benefit in terms of gynaecological sequelae — eight of the patients have since returned with gynaecological problems, whilst in a control series not seen by the psychiatrist only 6 out of 30 have been back with such difficulties. What was of interest was that 5 of the 23 patients interviewed did not come in for the sterilisation operation and that 2 of the 30 who did not have a psychiatric interview have since returned requesting reversal of the sterilisation.

The Single Woman

Many gynaecologists balk at the idea of sterilisation of an unmarried female, but it must be accepted that a woman's body is her own property, and that the principle of voluntary sterilisation is acceptable in the United Kingdom and some other countries. In the rare event of the nulliparous patient's making such a request there is nearly always a psychiatric component to the situation. The advice of a psychiatrist should be sought. Should he find the patient mentally stable, to have full understanding of the situation, to have sound reasons for the request, to have no fear of equivocation and predict no ill-consequences then it may be reasonable to proceed with the operation. More common is the presentation of the single parent under the age of 30 with one or two children, often living in relatively poor circumstances. If the physician is confident of the patient's full understanding of the irreversibility of the procedure and that she will not regret her decision should her circumstances change, he may proceed to operate. There is a distinct risk that this type of patient will present with a request for reversal some time in the future. With a woman of 35 or over who is certain that she will remain single but continues to run the risk of pregnancy, or a single woman with several children and a stable relationship request sterilisation, this request may be acceded to with more confidence.

Minors

In our opinion sterilisation of a child under the age of sixteen is unethical. The fact that in 1973 and 1974, 13 boys and 38 girls under the age of 18 were sterilised in Great Britain (British Medical Journal, 1975) is a matter of grave concern. It is widely accepted that a child under the age of 16 is incapable of giving 'informed consent' to an irreversible surgical procedure not of a therapeutic nature, and to conduct such an operation without such consent is unequivocally unethical and, in most countries, illegal. In general, such procedures as have been performed have been instigated for eugenic indications by well-meaning, though often emotionally charged, individuals. In civilised communities it should always be possible to wait until a child has reached an age when it fully appreciates not only the implications of sterilisation, but also the potential fallibility of the best current medical opinion on the transmission of genetically-determined disorders. The use of long-acting contraceptive steroids administered by injection or intra-uterine devices until the age of consent is reached has been suggested (Royal College of Obstetricians and Gynaecologists, 1975). This pronouncement still implies the imposition of contraceptive manoeuvres. Ordinary contraceptive counselling and procedures are adequate for the needs of most teenagers with or without a genetically transmitted disorder, until the 'age of understanding', rather than just the 'age of consent' is reached. As with any other teenager who appreciates the need for prevention of pregnancy but is incapable of employing other contraceptives for medical, psychiatric or social reasons, use of an injectable contraceptive or an intra-uterine device is reasonable.

The Mentally Incompetent

However desirable on medical and social grounds it might appear to be to sterilise a severely mentally deficient or disturbed individual we are in no doubt that it is unethical if that individual is incapable of understanding the meaning and full implications of the operation. Pressures applied by the patient's family or the psychiatric and social services suggesting that sterilisation would be for the patient's own protection must be resisted if she cannot give full 'informed consent'. If the situation is that of a serious risk of an unwanted pregnancy then the answer is to improve the patient's environment, not to perform involuntary sterilisation.

MEDICAL INDICATIONS

Definitive Medical Indications for Sterilisation

There are still a few heart and kidney conditions in which the patient can be advised unequivocally that pregnancy and confinement convey a serious risk of maternal death.

Cyanotic Congenital Heart Disease

Severe congenital malformations with major septal defects which are unlikely to be operable in the foreseeable future provide a firm indication for sterilisation. Operative sterilisation itself carries some risk to the life of such patients, and the best advice may be vasectomy for the husband. On the other hand a realistic appraisal of the prognosis for the wife may decide the couple to elect female sterilisation, to preserve the husband's fertility should the wife die.

An example of this situation is a fully developed Eisenmenger's syndrome, with an atrial or ventricular septal defect, a patent ductus arteriosus and pulmonary hypertension. Once the last component is established nothing short of a heart and lung transplant could correct the situation. The circulatory adjustments of pregnancy cause progressively increasing cyanosis. If the patient survives to the confinement, the rapid shifts of blood volume occurring after either normal delivery or caesarean section cause a fatal degree of reversal of the shunt. Similar considerations can apply to severe cases of Fallot's tetralogy, the Ebstein malformation and severe coarctation of the aorta. In all these three conditions very careful appraisal must be made, firstly of the severity of the condition and secondly of the potential for operative repair. We have seen patients with Fallot's or Ebstein's complex and a number of cases of coarctation of the aorta survive pregnancy and the confinement without deterioration, as well as two women whose severe Fallot's tetralogy has been dealt with surgically and who went through entirely uncomplicated pregnancies and normal deliveries.

Severe Rheumatic Valvular Heart Disease

Patients with a degree of heart failure due to severe valvular disease which has failed to respond to cardiac surgery and medical treatment are best advised to be sterilised. These women often have a double valvular lesion and atrial fibrillation. Even if techniques for surgical management of these conditions are developed in the future, there is little doubt that the rheumatic process will have caused further deterioration in the meantime. These patients must be carefully distinguished from those in whom valvotomy or open heart surgery has not been attempted. In this group the prognosis for a successful pregnancy is quite good after cardiac surgery.

Systemic Lupus Erythematosus with Severe Renal Damage

The chances for a successful pregnancy are small if kidney function is severely affected, in spite of adequate steroid therapy. Even so, renal damage alone is not always an insoluble problem. There is a chance that a patient with this condition can be maintained by dialysis and eventually proceed to transplant and carry a pregnancy. If, on the other hand, systemic lupus erythematosus is progressing in spite of adequate steroid therapy, it is unlikely that the patient will ever be fit enough to survive a pregnancy and confinement.

Conclusion

Clearly there are other medical conditions of such severity that sterilisation can be confidently advised on the grounds that pregnancy is likely to lead to maternal death, but in developed countries such patients with such conditions are few and far between. The great majority of women for whom sterilisation is considered on medical grounds are those for whom pregnancy would be associated with a small, statistically definable, risk to life or health. At the one extreme is the situation where the physician would suggest sterilisation unless it is quite clear that the patient is prepared to accept a real risk to her life in order to have the chance of producing a baby. At the other is the asymptomatic cardiac patient, the latent diabetic, or the woman with recurrent low grade hyptertension during her pregnancies. In this group it is reasonable to suggest sterilisation when the family is complete, on the grounds that further pregnancies, in association with increasing age, might possibly play an adverse role in the course of this disease.

Relative Indications for Sterilisation

Counselling in these cases involves two processes. One is the presentation to the patient of a realistic prognosis for the medical condition, which must take into account possible developments during the patient's potential reproductive life. The other is a careful appraisal of the patient's own values. Only when these assessments have been fully accomplished is the physician in a position to advise. These attitudes represent a major change in his role. Two or three decades ago he was expected to deliver an impartial judgement on a medical indication for sterilisation. Today's patient is far more knowledgeable about her medical problems, far more competent to come to terms with an accurate prognosis and far more desirous of making her own decisions as to what are the most important factors in her life. This reduces the function of the physician to those of providing technical information and of advising on the best means of fulfilling the patient's wishes. This advice may be presented as a formal medical opinion or merely as apparent compliance with the patient's wishes, according to her degree of understanding of the situation.

These general considerations are capable of application to nearly all the medical conditions, except certain psychiatric disorders in which the patient's judgement and ability to appraise her own values may be impaired. In these cases, much great responsibility for giving firm advice lies with the physician. For this reason, if no other, he should take the greatest pains to assess the potential for possible future improvement in the patient's psychiatric status and circumstances. Even though there are firm opinions that the psychiatric problem will not deteriorate or that it may improve as an immediate consequence of a sterilising operation, consideration should be given to the possibility that the procedure may lay the foundations for further psychiatric problems in the future. A patient may have been sterilised years before as a result of a valid judgement and have subsequently, or perhaps consequently, improved, often in association with changes in her domestic situation. She may then present a request for a reversal against a background of acute emotional stress arising from her inability to bear children.

A history of a psychiatric disorder apparently provoked by pregnancy or of puerperal psychosis may be considered a relative indication for sterilisation, but it is by no means absolute. With good psychiatric support the condition may not recur in relation to a subsequent pregnancy. If complete resolution occurred after one confinement, the same result may be anticipated after another, should the condition recur.

Severe chronic psychiatric illness presents the greater ethical problem of ensuring that the patient completely comprehends the nature of the operation and its consequences. Should this be the case, then the physician may feel justified in recommending sterilisation in a wide range of chronic psychiatric illness, ranging from chronic schizophrenia or chronic depression to milder situations such as intermittent depression, inadequate personality and general 'inability to cope'.

Apart from heart disease, there are a number of medical conditions where the possible deleterious effects of pregnancy have been misunderstood and the prognosis made unduly pessimistic. In other conditions improvements in management have led to an improved prognosis for pregnancy. The risks are usually such that the patient may or may not find them acceptable.

Haematological Disorders

The mere fact that a patient has a major haemoglobinopathy such as sickle-cell disease (haemoglobin S/S) or haemoglobin S/C disease does not mean that fatal crises will occur if she becomes pregnant. If the patient has a history of a number of major crises, it is possible that these may recur in pregnancy; if she has never had crises, it is possible she might get one in pregnancy. If she has been through a previous pregnancy without crises, it is likely she will repeat the performance. The hazards can be reduced by good medical care. The risk to the fetus can be much reduced by monitoring for placental insufficiency and by delivery before term. The risk of a sickling crisis in relation to the confinement can be minimised by elective caesarean section in crisis-prone patients who have not proved their ability to deliver vaginally, as well as by good anaesthesia and postoperative care.

It may be thought that in considering the haemoglobinopathies genetic considerations should predominate. In practice, even patients with haemoglobin S/S are often resistant to the thought that sterilisation may be justified on the grounds that their child will, at the least, inherit the trait. The alternative of antenatal blood sampling from the fetus at 16 weeks, with a view to therapeutic abortion if the fetus is homozygous, may be discussed. Even this is often rejected if it is explained that currently available procedures may be associated with a risk of abortion as high as 20%. Nevertheless, every effort must be made to secure knowledge of the nature of the husband's haemoglobin and the family history and to provide the patient with an accurate genetic prognosis. Very few patients with sickle cell trait (haemoglobin A/S) will accept the idea of sterilisation on the basis that their child might carry the trait.

Coagulopathies convey some hazard if haemorrhage occurs, but they do not mean that the patient will inevitably have a postpartum haemorrhage. In fact, provided the third stage is well managed, and retained products of conception or an atonic uterus avoided, haemorrhage is unusual.

Thromboembolic disorders such as a history of pulmonary embolism in relation to a pregnancy or to oral contraception do not necessarily contra-indicate a further pregnancy, though the patient may require anticoagulant therapy. Well managed anticoagulants, given for this or other reasons, can be used throughout a pregnancy and confinement successfully, employing low-dose subcutaneous heparin during the first trimester, warfarin during the middle trimester and intravenous heparin for a week or two before the confinement. The level of anticoagulation can then be much reduced during labour; the third stage can be closely supervised, and full anticoagulation instituted in the puerperium. In practice it is rare that such a full regimen is needed.

Patients have gone through pregnancy successfully with leukaemia and similar conditions, under treatment with mercaptopurine or Busulphan and steroids, provided methotrexate and some of the alkylating agents can be avoided. The main risk is of a virus infection such as cytomegalovirus affecting the fetus.

Cardiovascular Disorders

Some authorities still consider that pregnancy has a harmful effect on the long-term prognosis of patients with severe essential hypertension, and that the fetal prognosis is so bad as to justify termination of a pregnancy and sterilisation. In fact, with modern management using well chosen and well controlled hypotensive therapy and good obstetric care, it should be possible to avoid harm to the mother and the outlook for a successful pregnancy is quite encouraging. Of course the risks are greater if there is renal damage leading to albuminuria and nitrogen retention, but deterioration in renal function can occur in such women whether or not they are pregnant and the remedy for renal failure is the same — haemodialysis.

Systemic lupus erythematosus undoubtedly gives rise to some risk to the mother, an increased abortion rate and an increased perinatal mortality (Grigor *et al.*, 1977). On the other hand, provided there is no serious renal involvement, many such patients have had a successful pregnancy with the aid of adequate steroid therapy.

Congenital cerebral vascular abnormalities such as berry aneurysms, cerebral haemangiomas or a history of subarachnoid haemorrhage are potentially dangerous in pregnancy. On the other hand they might be amenable to surgery, and their risks can be reduced by treatment of elevated blood pressure and avoidance of any stress during the confinement.

Pulmonary Disease

Chronic chest conditions such as asthma, bronchiectasis, chronic bronchitis or tuberculosis are by no means a bar to pregnancy. Asthma and basal bronchiectasis are sometimes improved during pregnancy and the drugs employed in managing all these conditions have not been clearly shown to have any deleterious effect on the fetus. What must be assessed by the parous patient is her ability to cope with any hospitalisation that might be necessary during the pregnancy and the care of additional children. It should be possible to manage the medical situation with reasonable safety.

Renal Conditions

Severe renal disease conveys an increased hazard of abortion and placental insufficiency and an increased perinatal mortality. The condition of some patients with severe renal disease may deteriorate during pregnancy and renal failure develops. This is no longer necessarily a lethal situation and patients have been carried through pregnancy with the aid of peritoneal dialysis until the fetus is mature. Pregnancy is rare in patients who are maintained on haemodialysis, and if it does occur it is usually followed by spontaneous abortion. On the other hand many women with renal transplants have completed successful pregnancies without significant deterioration. The patient with chronic renal disease who desires sterilisation should obviously be accommodated, but there is little case for telling the woman who is aware of the 'high risk' category of future pregnancies that she 'must be sterilised'.

Gastro-intestinal Disorders

Malabsorption syndromes may require special management and hospitalisation during pregnancy. Coeliac disease, Crohn's disease and ulcerative colitis are all associated with increased spontaneous abortion and perinatal mortality rates and may undergo exacerbations requiring hospital management. On the other hand they all present situations which require carefully informed appraisal by the patient, rather than medical advise that sterilisation is indicated.

Having once undergone cholestatic jaundice of pregnancy, a woman may well come to the conclusion that she is unwilling to tolerate it again, although the risk of complete hepatic failure is small. Hiatus hernia and peptic ulceration may give rise to much discomfort and need careful symptomatic management but actual perforation of a peptic ulcer is extremely rare during pregnancy.

Neurological Disease

Epilepsy managed on anticonvulsants may carry a calculated risk of fetal abnormality of up to 6% (Smithells, 1976) but it is probable that this can be much reduced by folic acid supplements started before conception, use of barbiturates alone where possible and careful regulation of the anti-convulsant dose. From the point of view of the woman who wants another baby, the chance of a successful pregnancy is at least 17 to 1.

Multiple sclerosis was believed to be subject to exacerbations in pregnancy, but it is now realised that they are no more likely than in the non-pregnant woman. Otosclerosis was thought sometimes to progress rapidly during pregnancy. It is a condition which sometimes progresses rapidly in any woman in the reproductive age group, pregnant or not.

The overriding considerations with respect to sterilisation in these conditions are adequate counselling of the patient with respect to her medical condition, the extent of her desire for another pregnancy, and her assessment of her ability to cope with another child.

Endocrine Disorders

It is widely accepted that women with established diabetes mellitus should be carefully counselled as to the complications and management of their diabetes during pregnancy, but it is seldom suggested that they be sterilised until they decide they have completed their family. Adequately treated thyroid disorders, particularly thyrotoxicosis which has been treated by partial thyroidectomy, require only careful management to enable the patient to have the family she wishes. Many obstetricians and physicians now have sufficient experience of the management of patients on steroid therapy to ensure a good prognosis if pregnancy is desired. Successful pregnancy is possible in well managed diabetes insipidus.

Skeletal Disorders

Any medical advice which may be needed with respect to sterilisation in such conditions as rheumatoid or osteo-arthritis, congenital bone disease, ankylosing spondylitis or congenital and skeletal acquired deformities should be based on the patient's projected mobility and ability to cope with her future family.

Malignant Disease

Many patients who have been treated with extensive radiotherapy, and some who have had extensive chemotherapy, may find themselves infertile. If this is not the case, then there is no clear evidence that any apparently successfully treated malignant condition is ever reactivated as a direct consequence of pregnancy. This should be made clear if such patients request sterilisation, though of course their wishes will be given appropriate consideration.

Obstetric Considerations

Though repeated caesarean section may be technically more difficult after about the third, this should not be the primary consideration in the decision for or against sterilisation. It is really a matter of whether or not the patient's desire for another baby enables her to tolerate another operative delivery, and to accept the slightly increased operative risks involved.

Recurrent severe pre-eclampsia is sometimes cited as an indication for sterilisation. In fact pre-eclampsia tends to recur with decreasing severity and improving obstetric prognosis, provided pregnancies are not distributed over so many years that the increasing age of the patient predisposes her to hypertension. If a woman suffers from hypertension of earlier onset or greater severity in a subsequent pregnancy, it is likely that the underlying condition is essential hypertension.

Recurrence of eclampsia in another pregnancy is extremely rare. It is not clear if this is a primary phenomenon or a consequence of intensified antenatal care. Again, there is no categorical obstetric indication for sterilisation unless this is what the patient wants.

Genetic Problems

Severe rhesus isoimmunisation is much rarer since the prophylactic use of anti-D immunoglobulin was introduced, but such patients are still encountered. The fetal prognosis is still poor, even if intra-uterine transfusion of the fetus or plasmapheresis are employed. Patients whose husbands are homozygous rhesus positive, and who are immunised sufficiently for their babies to need intra-uterine transfusions or several exchange transfusions should be offered sterilisation as the prognosis can only worsen. It may be that vasectomy is thought appropriate by some couples who wish to consider artificial insemination from a rhesus-negative donor in due course.

A woman who has had a congenitally abnormal child or who has a family history of congenital abnormality may well request sterilisation and in such a case it is essential that genetic counselling on the chance of a recurrence be provided. In the great majority of such cases, the chance of recurrence is small, and it is necessary to emphasise that from the point of view of the patient a 5%

recurrence rate means 20 to 1 odds that her next baby will be normal. In a few situations such as neural tube defects, sex-linked congenital disorders and some congenital metabolic diseases the possibility of amniocentesis early in pregnancy and therapeutic abortion if the baby is affected, can now be offered as an alternative to sterilisation.

Bobrow (1976) gives a summary of the techniques of genetic counselling, with the emphasis on conveying information, not on dictating a course of action. It must be realised that a request for sterilisation on the basis of a risk of having a congenitally abnormal baby is compounded of many factors, of which the actual magnitude of the risk may be the least important. We have seen a number of patients in whom there is no increased risk of an abnormal baby who have preferred to link their request for sterilisation to the overall 2% chance of having a grossly abnormal baby, rather than admit to the emotional, marital or social difficulties which are the real basis for the request. On the other hand we have seen women who have had more than one grossly abnormal baby which has died, in whom the chance of a normal baby is only 1 in 4, but who are determined to proceed with their childbearing career until they achieve a normal child.

The extent of this problem is illustrated by Bobrow's (1976) data on patients with a genetic risk of greater than 1 in 10; only 68% decided after genetic counselling to have no further babies. In fact a proportion of this group did not implement their decision, the subsequent mean pregnancy rate for these couples being 0.49.

In practice, patients requesting sterilisation on genetic grounds should be managed with considerable care, however clear these grounds may seem at first sight. The essence of the matter is time — opportunity for the patients to consider their motives and their values after they have been presented with the facts. This often requires lengthy discussions with both partners, while several other individuals — family practitioner, gynaecologist, paediatrician, genetic counsellor, psychiatrist and clergyman — may all be involved. Often, procrastination for several months, with the provision of adequate contraception, is needed to achieve a valid decision. A ten-minute interview in a postnatal ward or a busy gynaecological clinic is the worst basis for arriving at an effective conclusion.

Relative Indications — Conclusion

With all the above medical conditions, it should be clear that any decision about sterilisation should be a value judgement made by the patient after she has been well counselled with respect to the nature, implications and prognosis of her medical condition.

We have noted two new features in the attitudes of some patients in recent years. The first is that many women with major medical disorders are extremely well informed about their condition, its management, its complications and its prognosis, including that with respect to pregnancy. It is advisable to *listen* to these patients with great care. They have often arrived at soundly reasoned judgements and merely require comments on any minor misapprehensions and agreement with their decisions. The second situation that must be recognised is that of the patient who is well aware that she may have a limited life-expectancy, even though she rightly lives in the hope that this may be improved. Years ago these patients would usually favour sterilisation on the basis that they might not live to bring up a child. It is not uncommon now to meet such women with the view that their role is to produce a healthy child, and to care for it as long as they are able; having had a good start in life they feel that the child will then do well and proceed to justify its own existence. Again, the physician's function may be merely to listen to the patient's value judgements with respect to sterilisation, rather than to provide formal advice.

THE SEQUELAE OF STERILISATION

Psychological Problems

The great majority of patients who are sterilised are well satisfied with the consequences, even though a proportion attribute some physical consequences to the operation. Whitehouse (1969) found that whilst about 25% reported deterioration in their sex lives an equal number reported improvement. Few expressed dissatisfaction with the operation on this account, accepting it as a price for security from pregnancy. In most series something under 18% of patients regret having had the operation (Whitehouse, 1969; Schwyhart and Kutner, 1973; Winston, 1977), but only a proportion of these actually request reversal.

The degree to which patients are satisfied with the results of a sterilisation procedure varies with their environment and culture (Presser, 1970). The pressure of government sponsored population control programmes may have an adverse effect on outcome by encouraging sterilisation of individuals who have not been fully counselled and for whom the operation may not be the best solution to problems (Nakra and Gaind, 1973). In the North of England, Donaldson *et al.* (1975) found that the incidence of regret after the operation fell from 38% in women sterilised under the age of 25 to nil in those aged 30 to 40 when they had the operation. They also found that regret was subsequently expressed by 31% of Roman Catholics, compared with 14% of patients belonging to the Church of England and 7% to other Protestant denominations. Schwyhart and Kutner (1973) found that women whose parity was less than 4 were more likely to regret the operation.

Gynaecological Problems

A significant proportion of women having tubal sterilisation subsequently develop abnormalities of the menstrual cycle or other gynaecological troubles. The commonest problem is menorrhagia, the onset usually being at least a year after the operation (Wheeless, 1975). Estimates of the incidence of physical sequelae of sterilisation vary widely (*Table 14.1*). Between 38% and 50% of the patients who return with complaints require further gynaecological treatment and between 18% and 43% of those who return come to hysterectomy (Haynes and Wolfe, 1970; Muldoon, 1972; Roe *et al.*, 1972).

Kasonde and Bonnar (1976) were unable to demonstrate increased menstrual flow after tubal sterilisation by measuring the loss, but they only followed the patients for one year after the operation. Neil *et al.* (1975) confirmed the reality

Table 14.1 LATE SEQUELAE OF TUBAL STERILISATION

Source	Cases followed up	Subsequent gynaecological complaints		Subsequent menstrual disturbances		Eventually needed hysterectomy
		Total	Needing treatment	Total	Needing treatment	
Williams *et al.*, 1951	200	–	24%	–	15%	2%
Prystowsky and Eastman, 1955	1022	–	9%	5%	–	–
Jensen and Lester, 1957	{406	43%	–	24%	–	–
	{472	–	8%	–	–	1%
Powell, 1962	112	–	12%	35%	–	4%
Lu and Chun, 1967	1055	–	–	–	–	1%
Black and Sclare, 1968	168	–	17%	–	4%	–
Lang and Richardson, 1968	198	–	–	–	3%	1%
Kroener, 1969	143	–	13%	–	–	5%
Neill, 1969	100	–	–	30%	–	–
Whitehouse, 1969	95	–	–	47%	–	6%
Haynes and Wolfe, 1970	489	72%	36%	10%	–	13%
Houseman, 1971	302	27%	–	14%	–	3%
Smith and Symmonds, 1971	161	–	–	–	4%	2%
Muldoon, 1972	374	–	43%	–	20%	19%
Roe *et al.*, 1972	235	23%	8%	12%	–	3%
Akhter, 1973	200	16%	–	7%	–	–
Tappan, 1973	221	–	–	41%	3%	–
Wilson, 1973	60	–	–	–	–	2%
Little, 1975	3306	–	3%	–	–	–
Average		36%	17%	22%	8%	5%

of the problem by comparing the incidence of reported increased menstrual loss in patients after laparoscopic sterilisation (39%), after interval sterilisation by laparotomy (22%) and after the husband had a vasectomy (13%). They also confirmed an increased incidence of dysmenorrhoea in women who had been sterilised, though the group with increased menstrual pain were not the same group as those who complained of increased menstrual loss. Donaldson *et al.* (1975) obtained similar results with respect to menstrual abnormality in another controlled study.

Physical sequelae seem to occur after both interval and postpartum sterilisation and after tubal ligation and resection, after laparoscopic fulguration and after clip sterilisation (Wilson, 1973; Neil *et al.*, 1975; Hulka, 1975). According to Williams *et al.* (1951), Lu and Chun (1967) and Muldoon (1972) definitive uterine pathology is subsequently found only in between 2 and 13% of patients who have been sterilised. The overall incidence of untoward sequelae is thought to be higher in younger women of low parity (Adams, 1964; Whitehouse, 1971; Donaldson *et al.*, 1975) and in grande multiparae and women with a scarred uterus (Muldoon, 1972).

The main difficulty in the assessment of the incidence and aetiology of gynaecological sequelae of sterilisation lies in the nature of the data in the literature (*see* Schwyhart and Kutner, 1973). Most series reported include patients who have had previous gynaecological or psychiatric sequelae; many are based only on those who return with complaints to the gynaecologist who performed the operation. Follow-up rates are low, and duration of follow-up restricted. We therefore undertook a study of 285 women sterilised at Hammersmith Hospital between 7 and 10 years previously, excluding patients who had any history of gynaecological or psychiatric problems before the operation (Houseman and Hawkins, unpublished observations). We adopted a stratified sampling approach (Sims, 1973). The first sample consisted of patients who had returned to the hospital with complaints. The second group replied to a letter and the third group, who did not reply, were reached by a home visit. We were thus able to estimate the incidence of complaints in patients who did not return to us and compute estimates of the overall incidence of sequelae.

Table 14.2 SEQUELAE OF TUBAL STERILISATION IN 285 WOMEN (HOUSEMAN AND HAWKINS, UNPUBLISHED DATA)

	Returned with complaints (Number of patients)	*Complaints in patients who did not return*	*Estimated total complaints*
Menorrhagia	19	42%	41%
Irregular periods	13	16%	18%
Dysmenorrhoea	8	23%	21%
Premenstrual pain	10	17%	17%
Other*	19	2%	9%
Any complaint	54	48%	59%

*Pseudocyesis, dyspareunia, vaginal discharge, prolapse, depression, pregnancy, request for reversal

It will be seen from *Table 14.2*, that although only 19 patients who had developed menorrhagia and 8 who had developed dysmenorrhoea returned to the gynaecological clinic, the overall incidences of these complaints, developing *de novo* after tubal sterilisation, were 41% and 21% respectively. In all, no fewer than 59% of women had developed gynaecological complaints within 7 to 10 years after the operation. This result may be compared with that of Haynes and Wolfe (1970); they found that 72% of patients they followed up for 3½ years had returned with gynaecological complaints.

Analysis of the data from patients who actually returned proved unprofitable, but when the total incidence was examined a number of facts emerged. Although there were very few women under 30, the average age at the time of operation in those who developed complaints (33 years) was less than that for patients with no complaints (36 years). This was not due to the intervention of the menopause as only 5 women out of the 285 had reached the age of 45 by the time the follow-up period was completed. No relationship to parity could be detected but there were few patients of low parity. Complaints were commonest (69%) among those who had been sterilised at the time of caesarean section, less common (46%) with interval sterilisation and least common (34%) with puerperal sterilisation. The Madlener operation seemed to give rise to more complaints (69%) than Pomeroy or other procedures (50%). The religion of the patients was of considerable interest (*Table 14.3*). There was no difference between the proportions of adherents to the different religions amongst those who returned with complaints, but when the total incidence was examined, post-sterilisation sequelae were considerably more common amongst the Roman Catholics. It seems that these women tend to accept the subsequent gynaecological problems after sterilisation, rather than return to the gynaecologist to complain about them.

It therefore seems that gynaecological complaints, occurring during the years after tubal sterilisation, are much commoner than has been appreciated. Particular care should be taken to counsel young women whose religion conflicts with their wishes, in this respect. The cause of the sequelae, which are nearly all functional in nature, is unknown. It is likely that there is a psychological contribution. The fact that complaints are commoner in young women who have abandoned their reproductive function and in those whose religion conflicts

Table 14.3 RELIGION AND SEQUELAE OF TUBAL STERILISATION (HOUSEMAN AND HAWKINS, UNPUBLISHED DATA)

	Cases	Returned with complaints	Total with complaints
Church of England	122	10%	54%
Roman Catholic	96	12%	71%*
Other	67	15%	53%

*Differs significantly (P<0.01)

with the operation suggests this; the finding parallels that of Donaldson *et al.* (1975) on the incidence of regret after having the operation. Interference with the blood supply to the ovary may be involved, particularly in women whose ovaries obtain much of their supply through the broad ligament anastomosis with the uterine artery. It may be that the Madlener operation as it used to be performed or laparoscopic fulguration are more likely to interfere with the vascular arcade. There is no evidence of interference with ovarian hormone production, but it is conceivable that there is interruption of some local endocrine effect, such as a prostaglandin action on luteolysis. Silent postoperative pelvic inflammatory disease might play a part, but in Great Britain there is seldom evidence of pelvic inflammation in patients whose symptoms are so severe as to justify hysterectomy.

Pelvic inflammatory disease in the tubal remnants is certainly a problem in some parts of the world where the disease is rife. A much rarer late complication is a tubal ectopic pregnancy (Thelin and van Nagell, 1972).

REQUESTS FOR REVERSAL OF TUBAL STERILISATION

The request for reversal of a sterilisation procedure implies a failure of sterilisation counselling. It is therefore instructive to consider the characteristics of a series of patients requesting reversal. Of a series of 29 such women, 5 were aged 20–24, 19 were aged between 25 and 29 and 5 between 30 and 34 when they were sterilised. Eight of the women had fewer than three children when they were sterilised. Three-quarters of them were still under 35 years of age by the time they requested reversal. The primary reasons for which they were sterilised seem unremarkable (*Table 14.4*); the secondary reasons are of interest — 5 patients had psychiatric disorders and in 6 more there was known to be marital disharmony. A clear majority of the patients requested reversal because their marriage had broken down and they wished for a child with a new partner. With two of the cases there was some suspicion that the sterilisation had actually contributed to the breakdown of the marriage, by means of regrets, recriminations and effects on libido. Two other patients attributed subsequent

Table 14.4 REQUESTS FOR REVERSAL OF TUBAL STERILISATION IN 29 CASES
(HAWKINS, UNPUBLISHED)

Reasons for sterilisation	Cases
Primary indications:	
Parity alone	10
Parity plus husband's wishes	3
Parity plus obstetric problems	7
Parity plus contraceptive problems	7
Parity plus medical problems	2
Secondary indications:	
Psychiatric disorder	5
Marital disharmony	6
Reasons for requesting reversal	
Marital breakdown; remarriage	24
Depression attributed to sterilisation	2
Gynaecological problems attributed to sterilisation	1
Loss of child	1
Regrets decision	1

depression to the operation. The lesson is clear; the mistakes are made with younger women with emotional disorders or with an unstable marital situation. The compliance of a psychiatrist seems to convey no protection, and sterilisation never repaired an unstable marriage.

Winston (1977) has studied a larger series of requests for reversal. He makes the point that many of the women had never received adequate contraceptive advice before sterilisation was decided on. Thirty-three per cent of the patients had been on anti-depressant drugs before they were sterilised and no fewer than 76% emphasised that their marriage had been so unhappy that they decided to cease childbearing. Nine patients said that their husband threatened to leave them unless they were sterilised, but in each of these cases the marriage broke up after the operation. Six other patients blamed the breakdown of their marriage to sexual and other difficulties following the sterilisation. Most patients claimed they had had inadequate counselling — the subsequent course of events can only be taken as validating this claim. Many had been sterilised by methods which precluded any attempt at reversal.

MORTALITY OF TUBAL STERILISATION

Reports of large-scale studies were accumulated by Presser (1970). There were 5 deaths in 20 058 sterilisations, a rate of 25 per 100 000. As this figure is based on publications in the literature and not statutory registrations, it must be regarded as an under-estimate.

VASECTOMY

The indication for vasectomy is essentially the same as that for female sterilisation, completion of the family, with or without associated medical or social reasons. In addition, some couples who do not fall into any of these categories will ask for vasectomy simply as a substitute for contraception. In the current climate of opinion and with the world's present overpopulation, there seems to be no reason why vasectomy should not be added to the armamentarium of population control. It should be stressed that proper counselling is necessary to reduce to a minimum the psychological side-effects, which form the major complications of the operation.

Type of Patient

Any man may be considered for vasectomy, but from published studies it seems that most men having this operation are aged between 25 and 40 (Tauber, 1973), approximately 20% being over 40 years of age.

The incidence of vasectomy may be related to social class and financial and educational status, but the association varies according to the population studied. In most developed countries the availability of vasectomy as a routine service is extremely variable and data on this point may be misleading.

It has been suggested that vasectomy tends to be chosen by couples who had previously used sheaths as their contraceptive of choice, in other words male contraceptive users (Howard, G., personal communication, 1973). On the other hand Lear (1972) and Kohli (1973) found that only 14% of patients requesting vasectomy were previous condom users. The incidence of condom usage in the various populations must be considered. Howard is quoting from Great Britain where the use of the condom is proportionately twice as high as the United States of America where Kohli's survey was based.

Psychological problems following vasectomy have been extensively studied. In general, retrospective studies indicate that vasectomy does not lead to much trouble, but Wolfers (1970), in her series, found some psychological problem arising in 12% of patients. Vasectomy can cause some psychological disturbance because of its confusion with castration and subsequent loss of potency. Ziegler, Rodgers and Kriegsman (1966) and Ziegler, Rodgers and Prentiss (1969) concluded that vasectomy had an underlying demasculinising effect. This was subconsciously compensated for by an increased frequency of sexual intercourse after the operation, as a result of which sexual performance was reduced to the extent of temporary impotence in some cases (Ziegler, Rodgers and Prentiss, 1969). There seems to be no doubt that the chances of emotional sequelae are low provided that the simplicity and minor nature of the operation are explained to the patient, and that emphasis is laid on the exact physiological effect. This is that the operation does not alter androgen production, scarcely affects the ejaculate volume, and in no way physically alters potency or coital sensation.

The operation should be performed only when the man is involved in a long-standing stable relationship and on no account should it be performed on a man with hypochondriacal tendencies or doubts about his masculinity. Careful counselling is necessary to establish this point, to ensure that the man is not being coerced into the operation and to ascertain that there are no background sexual problems.

With careful selection and explanation vasectomy is a minor surgical procedure and its main hazards are psychological. There is no compelling evidence to indicate widespread or severe emotional sequelae.

Severe sequelae can occur in vasectomised subjects who already had pre-existing difficulties of personalities or relations with the opposite sex, either within or without marriage. The proportion of men unsuited to vasectomy for psychological reasons is small, probably about 3% (Lear, 1972).

Legal Aspects

It is desirable to obtain informed consent from both husband and wife before carrying out vasectomy. Informed consent entails a personal interview with both parties involving a full explanation of the nature, effects and complications of the operation. It is vital that both husband and wife realise that sterility is not immediate and that two negative seminal analyses are necessary before this assumption can reasonably be made. It is also essential for both parties to realise that the operation is not 100% effective and also that in most cases it is irreversible. Having fulfilled these conditions the signatures of both parties agreeing to the operation should be obtained. There has so far been no test case in Great Britain to settle the question of the legality or otherwise of the operation of vasectomy, but if the conditions outlined above are complied with, and the operation carried out in good faith, in an accepted manner, it is unlikely that a successful litigation could be brought.

In the event of a single man wishing vasectomy, there would seem to be no legal barrier to performing the operation, provided the conditions described were adhered to. This request is unlikely, and most surgeons would be reluctant to comply.

REFERENCES

ADAMS, T.W. (1964). Female sterilization. *Am. J. Obstet. Gynec.*, **89**, 395–401
ADDISON, P.H. (1967). Legal aspects of sterilization and contraception. *Med.-leg. J. Lond.*, **35**, 164–167
AKHTER, M.S. (1973). Vaginal versus abdominal tubal ligation. Study at Victoria General Hospital. *Am. J. Obstet. Gynec.*, **115**, 491–496
BLACK, W.P. and SCLARE, A.B. (1968). Sterilization by tubal ligation – a follow-up study. *J. Obstet. Gynaec. Br. Commonw.*, **75**, 219–224
BOBROW, M. (1976). Genetic counselling: a tool for the prevention of some abnormal pregnancies. *J. clin. Path.*, **29**, supplement 10, 145–149
BRITISH MEDICAL JOURNAL (1960). Legality of sterilisation: a new outlook. *Br. med. J.*, **ii**, 1516–1518
BRITISH MEDICAL JOURNAL (1975). Sterilization of minors. *Br. med. J.*, **iii**, 775–777
DIGGORY, P. (1971). Place and timing of contraception and sterilization. *Proc. R. Soc. Med.*, **64**, 955–958
DONALDSON, R.J., MATHIE, I.K., BROWN, S. and BYRNE, M.R. (1975). *Aspects of Female Sterilisation – a Teeside Survey*, p. 86. Teeside Health Department Research Unit
GRIGOR, R.R., SHERVINGTON, P.C., HUGHES, G.R.V. and HAWKINS, D.F. (1977). Outcome of pregnancy in systemic lupus erythematosus. *Proc. R. Soc. Med.*, **70**, 99–100

HAYNES, D.M. and WOLFE, W.M. (1970). Tubal sterilization in an indigent population. Report of fourteen years' experience. *Am. J. Obstet. Gynec.,* **106**, 1044–1053

HOUSEMAN, R.J. (1971). Sterilization of young wives. *Br. med. J.,* **iii**, 184

HULKA, J.F. (1975). Irregular bleeding following laparoscopy. *Ob-Gyn Collected Letters,* **16**, 182–183

JENSEN, F. and LESTER, J. (1957). Ten years of tubal sterilization by the Madlener method. *Acta obstet. gynec. scand.,* **36**, 324–339

KASONDE, J.M. and BONNAR, J. (1976). Effect of sterilization on menstrual blood loss. *Br. J. Obstet. Gynaec.,* **83**, 572–575

KOHLI, K.L. (1973). Motivational factors and socio-economic characteristics of vasectomised males. *J. biosoc. Sci.,* **5**, 169–177

KROENER, W.F. (1969). Surgical sterilization by fimbriectomy. *Am. J. Obstet. Gynec.,* **104**, 247–254

LANG, L.P. and RICHARDSON, K.D. (1968). The implications of a rising female sterilization rate. *J. Obstet. Gynaec. Br. Commonw.,* **75**, 972–975

LEAR, H. (1972). Psychological characteristics of patients requesting vasectomy. *J. Urol.,* **108**, 767–769

LITTLE, W.A. (1975). Current aspects of sterilization. The selection and application of various surgical methods of sterilization. *Am. J. Obstet. Gynec.,* **123**, 12–18

LU, T. and CHUN, D. (1967). A long term follow-up study of 1055 cases of postpartum tubal ligation. *J. Obstet. Gynaec. Br. Commonw.,* **74**, 875–880

MEDICAL DEFENCE UNION (1974). *Consent to Treatment,* pp. 9–10. Medical Defence Union, London

MULDOON, M.J. (1972). Gynaecological illness after sterilization. *Br. med. J.,* **i**, 84–85

NAKRA, B.R.S. and GAIND, R. (1973). Psychiatric aspects of sterilization. *Br. med. J.,* **iii**, 168–169

NEIL, J.R., HAMMOND, G.T., NOBLE, A.D., RUSHTON, L. and LETCHWORTH, A.T. (1975). Late complications of sterilization by laparoscopy and tubal ligation. *Lancet,* **ii**, 699–700

NEILL, J.G. (1969). A follow-up study of one hundred cases of sterilization by tubal ligation. *Ulster med. J.,* **38**, 119–122

NICHOLS, D.H. (1969). Vaginal hysterectomy versus tubal ligation: considerations pertaining to the sterilization of multiparous patients with pelvic relaxation. *Obstet. Gynec., N.Y.,* **34**, 881–882

POWELL, L.C. (1962). Cesarean section sterilization — hysterectomy or tubal ligation? *Obstet. Gynec., N.Y.,* **19**, 387–396

PRESSER, H.B. (1970). Voluntary sterilization: a world view. *Reports on Population/Family Planning,* number 5, 1–36

PRYSTOWSKY, H. and EASTMAN, N.J. (1955). Puerperal tubal sterilization. Report of 1830 cases. *J. Am. med. Ass.,* **158**, 463–467

ROE, R.E., LAROS, R.K. Jr. and WORK, B.A. Jr. (1972). Female sterilization. I. The vaginal approach. *Am. J. Obstet. Gynec.,* **112**, 1031–1036

ROYAL COLLEGE OF OBSTETRICIANS AND GYNAECOLOGISTS (1975). Sterilization of children under 16 years of age. *President's Newsletter,* October, pp. 2–3

SCHWYHART, W.R. and KUTNER, S.J. (1973). A reanalysis of female reactions to contraceptive sterilization. *J. nerv. ment. Dis.,* **156**, 354–370

SHEPARD, M.K. (1974). Female contraceptive sterilization. *Obstetl gynec. Surv.,* **29**, 739–787

SIMS, A.C.P. (1973). Importance of a high tracing-rate in long-term medical follow-up studies. *Lancet,* **ii**, 433–435

SMITH, R.A. and SYMMONDS, R.E. (1971). Vaginal salpingectomy (fimbriectomy) for sterilization. *Obstet. Gynec., N.Y.,* **38**, 400–402

SMITHELLS, R.W. (1976). Environmental teratogens of man. *Br. med. Bull.,* **32**, 27–33

TAPPAN, J.G. (1973). Kroener tubal ligation in perspective. *Am. J. Obstet. Gynec.,* **115**, 1053–1057

TAUBER, A.S. (1973). A long term experience with vasectomy. *J. reprod. Med.,* **10**, 147–149

THELIN, T.J. and VAN NAGELL, J.R. Jr. (1972). Ruptured ectopic pregnancy after bilateral tubal ligation. *Obstet. Gynec., N.Y.,* **39**, 589–590

WHEELESS, C.R. (1975). Irregular bleeding following laparoscopy. *Ob-Gyn Collected Letters,* **16**, 181–182

WHITEHOUSE, D.B. (1969). Tubal ligation. A follow-up study. *Adv. Fert. Contr.,* **4**, 22–26

WHITEHOUSE, D.B. (1971). Sterilization of young wives. *Br. med. J.,* **ii**, 707

WILLIAMS, E.L., JONES, H.E. and MERRILL, R.E. (1951). The subsequent course of patients sterilized by tubal ligation. A consideration of hysterectomy for sterilisation. *Am. J. Obstet. Gynec.,* **61**, 423–426

WILSON, P.C.M. (1973). Female sterilization by the laparoscope in small suburban hospitals in Sydney. *Med. J. Aust.,* **i**, 893–894

WINSTON, R.M.L. (1977). Why 103 women asked for reversal of sterilisation. *Br. med. J.,* **ii**, 305–307

WOLFERS, H. (1970). Psychological aspects of vasectomy. *Br. med. J.,* **iv**, 297–300

ZIEGLER, F.J., RODGERS, D.A. and KRIEGSMAN, S.A. (1966). Effect of vasectomy on psychological functioning. *Psychosom. Med.,* **28**, 50–63

ZIEGLER, F.J., RODGERS, D.A. and PRENTISS, R.J. (1969). Psychosocial response to vasectomy. *Archs gen. Psychiat.,* **21**, 46–54

15 Methods of Operative Sterilisation

ELECTIVE TUBAL STERILISATION

Tubal Ligation With or Without Partial Salpingectomy

If sterilisation is to be conducted as an interim procedure, other than immediately following a confinement, curettage of the uterus should be performed initially to exclude an early intra-uterine pregnancy, however reliable the patient's history may seem. Although mistakes may be uncommon, there are few patients more distressed than those who find themselves pregnant shortly after a sterilisation procedure.

Most surgeons prefer a small suprapubic Pfannenstiel incision for an interim sterilisation or a small midline subumbilical incision for a puerperal sterilisation. Subcuticular polyglycolic or catgut sutures can be used to close the skin; if sutures or clips are employed the patient can usually be discharged from hospital on the third postoperative day. She may then return in a week for removal of sutures or have her family practitioner remove them. Uchida (1975) describes a 1 cm midline incision which is retracted with hooks, drawing up the loop of the tube into the incision with another hook. A semicircular incision around the lower margin of the umbilicus, dissecting down the midline without extending the skin incision, can also be made for puerperal sterilisation.

Whilst cosmetic results with 'keyhole' incisions may be excellent, this must be weighed against the very small risk of failure to identify structures correctly and the risk of failing to observe pelvic pathology. Provided the fimbrial end of the tube is visualised there should be no mistakes regarding the structure ligated. Acute anteversion of the uterus with an intra-uterine sound and the insertion of a proctoscope or a Cusco speculum facilitates visualisation and access to the fallopian tube through a small transverse suprapubic incision. Even without the proctoscope excellent results have been obtained using small incisions with only local anaesthesia (Chowdhury and Chowdhury, 1975).

The classical sterilisation operation involving ligation of a loop of the fallopian tube was described by Madlener (1919). He picked up the fallopian tube in its mid portion, crushed the lower parts of both limbs of the loop, and ligated them with non-absorbable suture material, either silk or thread. The method was criticised by Bishop and Nelms (1930) on the grounds that recanalisation can occur because the non-absorbable suture can cut through the crushed tissue. They describe the method probably used first by Pomeroy. A loop of

343

tube in the loose mid portion is grasped, ligated with absorbable suture material and resected. The base of the loop is not crushed before ligation. The method is simple, rarely leads to infection or haemorrhage and is claimed to have a higher success rate than the Madlener procedure. The absence of crushing and the use of absorbable suture material reduces the chance of a fistula forming between the two limbs of the loop. Once the suture material is absorbed, the two cut ends of the tube tend to splay apart, joined by a fibrous cord, and the peritoneum grows over them, preventing recanalisation. Some gynaecologists believe that catgut encourages eventual fibrosis, and use several turns of this material for ligation.

The Pomeroy procedure is probably the commonest method of female sterilisation in use at the present time. It is unpopular in some areas in the United States of America where pelvic inflammatory disease is common and patients tend to return with peritoneal cysts or acute and chronic inflammation in the tubal remnants. Hysterectomy is sometimes preferred as a sterilising procedure in these areas and it is often accompanied by bilateral salpingo-oophorectomy and oestrogen replacement therapy.

In recent years we have had to consider both the high incidence of post-sterilisation menstrual problems among young women, and the increasing minority of patients whose marriages break up and who are aware of the potential that microsurgical techniques offer for reanastomosis of the tubes (Winston, 1977). In sterilising women under the age of 30 we are therefore inclined to resect a relatively small loop of tube and take some pains to avoid damaging the vascular arcade of the mesosalpinx.

Variations in Technique

Köhler (1927) described looping the tube in its mid portion, ligating the base of the loop with silk sutures and excising the loop. He used non-absorbable suture material and did not crush the tube, but cut off the loop as in the Pomeroy procedure. Peitman (1926) carried out a sub-serous partial tubal excision. In this operation the tube is ligated with silk in two places about 2 cm apart, the peritoneum is split, exposing the tube, and a section is excised between the ligatures before recovering with peritoneum. The technique is similar to that described by Uchida (1961; *see also* Overstreet, 1964) except that in the Uchida operation the distal end is ligated with the open fringe or serosa and left unburied. Rabinowitsch (1927) carried out the same operation as Peitman except that he ligated the ends of the tube with silk and buried the proximal end of the tube into the myometrium. Irving (1924) described a method for sterilisation after caesarean section, involving double ligation of the tube with chromic catgut and its division about 4 cm from the uterine cornu. The proximal portion is dissected free from its mesosalpinx and buried in the myometrium. The distal portion of the tube is buried within the leaves of the broad ligament. The operation is completed by the approximation of all the peritoneal surfaces. Planner (1927) doubly ligated the tube with silk, cut between the ligatures, sewed the ends with silk and buried the proximal stump in the broad ligament. Hofbauer (1927) cut the tube, ligated the proximal end with silk and joined the round and ovarian ligaments over the stump. Williams, E.A. (1971) secures the proximal tubal stump behind the round ligament and the distal stump in front of it.

Failure Rates of Orthodox Tubal Sterilisation Procedures

Most failure rates reported for sterilisation procedures are under-estimates. Should the operation fail the pregnant patient will often go to another hospital because of a lack of confidence in the surgeon. She may also wish to conceal the pregnancy, or go elsewhere to have an abortion. Few studies have planned follow-up programmes, and even these are of little value unless a very high rate of tracing is maintained for many years. Discrepancies in the follow-up procedure from one centre to another often render direct comparison of different methods impossible. These difficulties are in part responsible for the differences between clinical experience on the one hand and the results of many published series on the other.

The chief advantage of the Madlener procedure is its simplicity, but the tubal crushing involved can cause a haematoma, and ligation of the tube using a non-absorbable suture can cause recanalisation. It is therefore less effective than the Pomeroy or other more complicated techniques. Dees (1961) reported a failure rate of 3.7% among 566 patients having Madlener operations. On the other hand Knight (1946) in a collected series of nearly 5000 patients, reported a pregnancy rate of only 0.6%. Haynes and Wolfe (1970) found that in a mixed series of cases of sterilisation the Madlener technique produced the worst results. There would seem to be little reason for using this technique as the Pomeroy method is nearly as simple and has a lower failure rate.

Low failure rates have been recorded in large series using the Pomeroy procedure. Lull and Mitchell (1950) reported a failure rate of 0.25% from 1550 cases. White (1966) recorded a failure rate of 0.17% from 1146 cases, and Knight (1946) a rate of 0.3% in a series of 1262 cases. However, in a small series of 100 patients Fort and Alexander (1966) found a failure rate of 2%. It is the experience of most gynaecologists that about 0.6% of patients report failures with the Pomeroy technique. It must be accepted that a proportion of patients who have failures will go elsewhere when pregnant, and so a small series of well followed up patients may give a more accurate result than a large series with poor follow-up. The morbidity rate for the Pomeroy procedure is low.

Irving and Uchida Procedures

Large studies using tubal ligation, excision and burying the ends of the tubes have been reported. Garb (1957) recorded 1056 cases of Irving's sterilisation with no failures. Uchida himself claimed 20 000 operations without a failure (Uchida, 1975). These reports seem to be a good advertisement but it must be accepted that the figures tend to be unrepresentative since the series are not comparative and there is no evidence of a thorough follow-up of patients. Procedures involving tubal ligation with excision seem to be safer than those involving merely ligation; burying the cut ends of the tube may further reduce the failure rate of the procedure, but the evidence for this is not clear. Burying the tubes beneath the peritoneum or in the myometrium as described in the Irving technique inevitably adds to the operative time and to the risks of complications such as haemorrhage. It is the feeling in Great Britain that the unproven possibilities of a small additional reduction in failure rate is not justified by the additional operative time and risk of complications, and so the Pomeroy technique is the method of choice of most gynaecologists.

STERILISATION BY THE VAGINAL ROUTE

Most of these forms of tubal surgery can be carried out vaginally as well as transabdominally. The vaginal procedures have not achieved much popularity, partly because access is sometimes difficult and partly because of the higher chance of introducing infection into the peritoneal cavity. In Great Britain there have been few enthusiasts for vaginal tubal ligation and excision, but in the United States of America a number of publications have described these techniques (*see* Wortman and Piotrow, 1973). The approach is usually through a small transverse incision in the posterior vaginal fornix (Morris, 1969). A finger is inserted, the pelvis explored and the tubes located. Tissue forceps are used to grasp and deliver them through the incision one at a time. Some surgeons find it easier, if the uterus is anteverted, to work through the anterior fornix, displacing the bladder upwards and opening the utero-vesical pouch. If there is difficulty delivering the tubes into the colpotomy incision, a round ligament may be grasped with sponge-holding forceps; traction then makes it easy to reach the tube on the same side. This technique can be useful if the uterus is somewhat bulky. Any of the standard techniques such as Pomeroy, Madlener or fimbriectomy can then be performed easily. The failure rates for these operations were found to be somewhat higher than for the abdominal approach by Cheng *et al.* (1977), mistaken identification of the tube being more common, but Tatum and Schmidt (1977) reported lower failure rates with the vaginal operations, and very few of the failures resulted in ectopic gestations. The morbidity rate associated with the vaginal approach seems to be higher. Lee *et al.* (1951) reported 1169 cases of vaginal Madlener type interval sterilisation with a morbidity rate of 11.5%, while Soglow (1971) recorded a morbidity rate of 10% and Tappan (1973) a rate as high as 20%. It is claimed that if the culdoscope is employed by well-trained surgeons to visualise the tubes, under local anaesthesia, the complication rate can be much reduced (*see* Wortman, 1976).

Should hysterectomy be the method of choice for sterilisation then if there is utero-vaginal prolapse and the uterus is not excessively large the vaginal route is preferable. Vaginal hysterectomy in capable hands, with good patient selection, can result in a low post-operative morbidity rate with little discomfort, early mobility, and little trouble with intestinal atony.

In the absence of utero-vaginal prolapse there are no strong grounds for preferring the vaginal to the abdominal route, and so in most cases the decision will be one for the surgeon's particular skills and preference.

Chemicals

Richart *et al.* (1971) have described sterilisation by the vaginal route using retrograde injection of silver nitrate through the fimbrial ends of the tubes at culdoscopy to cause tubal occlusion. It is difficult to see the benefits of this technique. The silver nitrate tends to spill out of the tubes into the peritoneal cavity and the patients subsequently suffer abdominal discomfort (Richart, 1976). Other methods of sterilisation by the vaginal route involve the injection of sclerosing chemicals into the upper part of the uterus through an intra-uterine catheter. Quinacrine has been used in this way to occlude the uterotubal junctions. The failure rate is extremely high with up to 55% of cases with subsequent tubal patency (Zipper *et al.*, 1975; Israngkun *et al.*, 1976). Infusion of the chemical under direct vision using a hysteroscope does not reduce the failure rate (Alvarado *et al.*, 1974).

Conclusion

It would appear that the vaginal approach has few advantages over the trans-abdominal approach except those of reduction of post-operative discomfort, shortening of hospital stay, and the operator's preference. The risks of failure and of post-operative complications would seem, at least in relatively inexperienced hands, to be significantly higher.

LAPAROSCOPIC STERILISATION

Method for Laparoscopy

Laparoscopic sterilisation, though it shortens the patient's stay in hospital, is not particularly economical of operating theatre time. It usually involves a general anaesthetic, a basic technique for which has been described by Alexander *et al.* (1969). The procedure can also be performed under local anaesthesia using an operating laparoscope which requires only a single incision, there being separate channels for the fibreoptic system and the instruments. Local anaesthesia is obtained by a paracervical block performed vaginally with 1% lignocaine, local infiltration of the periumbilical tissues down to the peritoneum and instillation of 20 ml of 1% lignocaine to bathe the uterus and tubes under direct vision (Penfield, 1974).

A guarded Verres needle is inserted sub-umbilically into the peritoneal cavity and 3–4 litres of carbon dioxide instilled, to distend the anterior abdominal wall. With the patient in a steep Trendelenburg position, a small sub-umbilical incision is made down to and including the rectus sheath. The trochar and cannula of the laparoscope is pushed gently through the rectus sheath and peritoneum, the trochar removed, and the fibreoptic laparoscope introduced through the cannula.

The commonest method of laparoscopic sterilisation involves the insertion of a Palmer's coagulation biopsy forceps through a separate incision either in the midline or in one iliac fossa. The tubes are then coagulated in two places with or without division. Though the operating laparoscope allows the procedure to be carried out with only one incision (Wheeless and Thompson, 1973; Penfield, 1974) complication rates are higher with this instrument (Confidential Enquiry into Gynaecological Laparoscopy, 1978e).

Transvaginal insertion of the laparoscope has been described after the production of a pneumo-peritoneum by the abdominal route. The introduction of infection is more likely than with the abdominal route; the field of vision is not so good and access to the tubes is more difficult. This approach is not used widely in Great Britain.

Tubal Coagulation and Division

Using the abdominal route laparoscopic sterilisation is usually effected by tubal coagulation with or without division of the tube. The proximal site of coagulation and division should be 1—2 cm from the uterotubal junction, with a distal site of coagulation 1 cm beyond this. The reason that these points are chosen is that the fallopian tube is narrowest in this area. Coagulation should be carried out for about 30 seconds at each site, irrespective of how soon the outside of the tube blanches. This is because a high temperature applied for a short time will not always penetrate and cause full-thickness tissue destruction. It has been found that avulsion of part of the tube followed by recauterisation of the stumps reduces the pregnancy rate (Wheeless and Thompson, 1973) and reduces the proportion of ectopic gestations in the failures that do occur (Tatum and Schmidt, 1977).

Division of the tube may be undertaken either by electrocoagulation with the biopsy forceps or with scissors. It is possible to tear the mesosalpinx with biopsy forceps and so cause post-operative haemorrhage (Peterson and Behrman, 1971).

It is the view of most authors that division of the tubes after coagulation leads to fewer failures. The process of division can cause bleeding but this is not a major problem. Steptoe (1972) found that laparotomy was necessary to ligate a blood vessel in 1.75% of cases. Wheeless and Thompson (1973), noted bleeding in 58 from a total of 3600 cases (1.6%). The bleeding was usually recoagulated through the laparoscope. Liston *et al.* (1970) felt that coagulation alone was safer because of the risks of haemorrhage and subsequent haematoma formation.

Application of Clips

As an alternative to electrocautery and division of the tubes several workers in recent years have applied occlusive clips made of various substances to the tubes. Tantalum clips have been used but unless the tube is completely blocked, which is not always the case, then failures will occur (Davidson and Donald, 1972). The method has been said to be reversible, as removal of these clips several months after their application in animals resulted in restoration of fertility (Neumann and Frick, 1961).

Spring-loaded (Hulka-Clemens) clips made of plastic, with a steel spring to keep the jaws closed, have been developed (Wortman, 1976). These are applied to the tube, approximately 2 cm from the uterus, through a specially adapted operating laparoscope. The spring maintains adequate pressure on the clip and its teeth prevent slipping. The clips cause atrophy of about 4 mm of the tube, which is adequate to prevent recanalisation. This occludes the lumen of the tube completely. Thirty-six weeks after sterilisation histological examination of the tubes reveals complete occlusion under the clip but normal epithelium on either side. It seems that reversal of this operation by excising the atrophic area and reanastomosing the ends is feasible.

Application of Silicone Rubber Bands

Recently Yoon, Wheeless and King (1974) have described a technique for placing a silicone rubber band around a loop of fallopian tube by means of a laparoscope. The band is loaded into a special applicator which incorporates a forceps attachment for grasping the tube. The laparoscope is inserted in the usual way, the loop of tube grasped about 2 cm from the uterotubal junction, and is drawn up into the inner sleeve of the applicator. The band is then pushed down into place around the base of the loop.

The complication rate with the use of the bands is higher than those with laparoscopic sterilisation using either electrocoagulation or application of clips (Confidential Enquiry into Gynaecological Laparoscopy, 1978d).

Failure Rates

With routine use laparoscopic tubal coagulation and division failure rates are probably rather higher than those for the Pomeroy method (Hughes and Liston, 1975; Hutchins and Curpen, 1975; Cheng *et al.*, 1977). With experienced laparoscopists, results are often better. Liston *et al.* (1970) reported only 9 pregnancies among 760 patients (1.2%) of which 4 were due to operative failure, whilst 5 women may have been pregnant at the time of sterilisation. Steptoe (1976), reporting information from the Association of American Laparoscopists based on 146 976 sterilisations, gave a pregnancy rate of 0.46% if the surgeon had done less than 100 such operations, but only 0.16% thereafter. In another study a failure rate in the region of 0.3% was found (Black, 1971). The duration of follow-up in this study was up to 4 years. These results are supported by a large series of 3600 cases in which one to three coagulations were performed on each tube. The total subsequent pregnancy rate was 0.7% (Wheeless and Thompson, 1973). It was felt that only half of these failures were due to surgical errors, the other half of the patients being already pregnant at the time of sterilisation. Amongst 1600 cases in whom a segment of tube was removed and the stumps recoagulated there were no failures. Recent studies comparing coagulation alone with coagulation and division of the tube suggest that the latter is more effective in preventing pregnancy. A pregnancy rate of 1.1% due to failure to occlude the tube by simple coagulation has been compared with a series in which the tube was clearly divided as well as coagulated and the only failure due to recanalisation gave a rate of 0.15% (Wheeless, 1976).

Failure rates with tantalum clips vary from 1% to 27% (Wortman, 1976; Tatum and Schmidt, 1977). The rate following the application of Hulka spring clips has been recorded as 24 out of 907 patients (2.6%). Eleven of these failures were because of application of the clips to the wider ampulla rather than the narrower isthmus of the tube or to application to the round ligament and three to defective clips (Hulka *et al.*, 1975). The use of silicone rubber bands in 100 patients studied for periods of up to 12 months was initially said not to have led to any pregnancies (Yoon *et al.*, 1974), but a few failures (0.3–4%) have since been reported (Wortman, 1976; Phillips *et al.*, 1977). Of 15 failures reported with this procedure by Phillips *et al.* (1977) 9 were ectopic pregnancies, and on this basis we are at present reluctant to recommend the use of the silicone bands. The limited duration of follow up in these studies is inadequate for definite conclusions to be formed.

There are two common reasons for failure or laparoscopic sterilisation. One is the electrocoagulation of some structure other than the fallopian tube, usually the round ligament. The other is residual patency of the tubes after coagulation or coagulation and division. Jordan *et al.* (1971) carried out 443 hysterosalpingograms 6 weeks post-operatively, one-third of which showed spill of the dye indicating incomplete tubal occlusion. Two-thirds of these patent tubes were unilateral and one-third bilateral. Fibrosis and tubal occlusion is not complete at six weeks and injection of dye at that time under pressure will cause patency. There was a higher incidence of patency among those who had had the tubes divided (19 out of 42) than in those who had not had tubal division (3 out of 18). If an x-ray is carried out to confirm tubal obliteration it should not be performed until at least three months post-operatively. It is not recommended as a routine procedure.

Advantages

With laparoscopic sterilisation the patient need be in hospital for only 24–48 hours. Provided the tubes are divided as well as coagulated it is as safe as any other standard sterilisation procedure. Other methods such as the application of clips or rubber bands to the tubes do not significantly reduce the failure rate but may reduce the incidence of operative complication rate as there is no risk of intestinal burns.

If only a single coagulation division is performed or clips are used the potential for reversing the operation is probably slightly better than with the Pomeroy method and is much better than with the more destructive methods of sterilisation. Extensive coagulation of the tube produces irreparable damage.

Finally, laparoscopy has the advantage that it can be performed under local anaesthesia as an outpatient procedure (Alexander *et al.*, 1973; Wheeless and Thompson, 1973). If local anaesthesia is being used it should be remembered that the P_{CO_2} in the blood rises because of absorbed carbon dioxide from the pneumoperitoneum and because of mild respiratory depression due to narcotic sedation. In these cases it is advisable to encourage the patient to hyperventilate (Alexander *et al.*, 1973).

Disadvantages

Steptoe (1976) cites the death rate as 8 per 100 000. Other estimates include one of 2.5 per 100 000 in the United States of America and one of 10.4 per 100 000 from Great Britain (Confidential Enquiry into Gynaecological Laparoscopy, 1978f).

The creation of a pneumoperitoneum and the Trendelenburg position of the patient renders the diaphragm partially or completely immobile. This, together with the absorption of carbon dioxide from the peritoneum, can lead to acidosis and cardiac arrhythmia (Peterson and Behrman, 1971). The progressive increase in intra-abdominal pressure is accompanied by increased intra-thoracic pressure and central venous pressure and by mild tachycardia and hypertension (Smith *et al.*, 1971). It has been suggested that increased intra-abdominal pressure might lead to a reduction in cardiac output, by reducing the venous return. Smith *et al.* (1971) found no evidence for this with intra-abdominal pressures of less than 30 cm of water, but the most efficacious treatment of either bradycardia or hypotension is rapid deflation of the abdomen (Confidential Enquiry into

Gynaecological Laparoscopy, 1978b). On the whole, the procedure is best avoided in patients with cardiac or respiratory insufficiency.

Laparoscopy can be difficult in obese patients and is contra-indicated in patients with diaphragmatic, abdominal, umbilical, inguinal or femoral hernias, in case the abdominal organs are forced through the hernial orifice in the first mentioned, or in case there are troublesome adhesions associated with the other types of hernia. Patients with a history of previous laparotomy or peritonitis should be laparoscoped with great care, if at all, because of adhesions and the increased risk of perforating the bowel with either the Verres needle or the laparoscope.

Problems associated with the passage of the laparoscope include bleeding from the abdominal wall or the perforation of a major intra-abdominal vessel. A trochar inserted into the iliac fossa for insertion of the biopsy forceps may rupture the inferior epigastric vessels but incision with a small knife with trans-illumination from the laparoscope should preclude this. Cases of perforation of the abdominal aorta or iliac vessels have been recorded with fatal results. Fortunately this extremely uncommon complication can be avoided by rendering the abdomen tense by an adequate pneumoperitoneum before the insertion of the trochar. Perforation of the bowel is a more common hazard and occurs for the same reason or because the bowel is adherent to the anterior abdominal wall. Jordan *et al.* (1971) recorded bowel damage in 0.3% of cases. Other complications that may arise include gas embolism, parietal and mediastinal emphysema and the injection of gas into the intra-abdominal viscera, particularly the omentum.

Complications of the sterilisation procedure itself include burns and local haemorrhage. Skin or viscera can be burnt by an inadequately insulated and earthed endoscope. Burns to the viscera can occur when an endoscope, earthed by the metal-sheath of its fibre-optic light source, is positioned near the active diathermy electrode; the possibility that there is an electrical connection between the diathermy apparatus and the plate electrode; or the fact that the diathermy was on when the operator did not realise it. These risks can be eliminated by using an insulated sheath or bush for the light guide and by ensuring that metal parts of the sheath do not touch other metal objects. The incorporation of an audible signal to indicate that the diathermy output is being energised will prevent it being on without the knowledge of the operator. A comprehensive account of safety procedures is given by Corson *et al.* (1973).

Finally, the placing of the two electrodes within the prongs of the instrument which grasps the tube is a further safety feature. This means that the current passed is local and if the instrument is made of nylon, with only the insulated electrodes made from steel, there is no chance of sparking (Rioux and Cloutier, 1974). Burns to the gastro-intestinal tract were recorded in 0.3% of cases, and burns to the skin and abdominal wall in 0.2% of cases (Wheeless and Thompson, 1973) but somewhat higher rates have been found in other surveys (Confidential Enquiry into Gynaecological Laparoscopy, 1978c and f).

Local haemorrhage, associated with division of the tubes, is also a significant complication (Liston *et al.*, 1970), occurring in about 1.6% of cases (Wheeless and Thompson, 1973). Most of these can be managed adequately by further coagulation through the laparoscope.

The incidence of anaesthetic complications and sepsis are not significant provided routine precautions are taken. Subsequent menstrual problems seem to be more common in patients having laparoscopic sterilisation than after Pomeroy sterilisation (Neil *et al.*, 1975), but the reason for this is obscure.

HYSTEROSCOPY

Hysteroscopy as described by Semm and Rimkus (1974) allows for the coagulation of the uterotubal junction. The advantages of this method over laparoscopy are the elimination of intra-peritoneal dangers such as haemorrhage, intestinal damage, or infection, together with a reduction in anaesthetic and other problems caused by the pneumoperitoneum. It is necessary to visualise the tubal orifices, to introduce an electrode into the tube and to coagulate up to 4 cm of its interstitial portion and isthmus under direct vision (Quinonas *et al.*, 1973; Richart *et al.*, 1973).

Dilatation of the cervix is carried out under intracervical or paracervical block and the uterus is distended with 30% dextran (average mol. wt. 40 000, 10% solution; Dextran 40, Gentran 40, Rheomacrodex) under a pressure of 70–150 mmHg or with carbon dioxide (100 ml/min). A Teflon mesh plug can be inserted into the tubal ostia in addition to coagulation. Hysterosalpingograms performed after 3 months showed that 7 patients from 44 still had tubal patency (Richart *et al.*, 1973).

The potential advantages of the procedure warrant further exploration, but so far results have not been encouraging. In the collaborative study reported by Darabi and Richart (1977) tubal patency was tested after hysteroscopic cautery. Of 524 cases so tested 175 had patent tubes and 11 others had become pregnant. Even after a repeat hysteroscopic cauterisation, there was failure of the tubes to close in 18% of cases. Complications in a series of 773 cases included 7 perforations of the uterus, 7 cases of bowel or peritoneal damage, 8 subsequent ectopic gestations and 2 episodes of pelvic infection. Bleeding (28 cases) and pelvic pain (5 cases) also occurred.

OTHER OPERATIONS FOR STERILISATION

Cornual Resection

Williams, J.W. (1928) described cornual resection. He excised the proximal end of the tube from the uterine cornu by a wedge-shaped incision, oversewed the uterine defect, and ligated the distal stump of tube. Garb (1957) recorded a failure rate of 2.9% in a series of 311 such cases. Post-operative complications, particularly haemorrhage, are much commoner than with simple tubal surgery. It is for these reasons that the operation is now seldom performed.

Salpingectomy

This operation has also been used as a method of sterilisation, by ligation of the proximal tubal stump with absorbable suture material, and excision of the tube. There is a risk of impairment of blood flow to the ovary in some women who derive much of their ovarian supply from the uterine artery *via* the broad ligament anastomosis. It has been suggested that the method leads to a 5% incidence of ovarian cysts, but this is not very different from the incidence of symptomless ovarian cysts found incidentally at laparotomy.

Salpingectomy is not widely performed for sterilisation and there is not a large body of literature from which to derive failure rates. On anatomical principles salpingectomy should have the disadvantages of increased haemorrhage and haematoma formation. When compared with the Pomeroy method, it should be a more effective method of sterilisation.

Fimbriectomy

The distal part of the tube is doubly tied with silk and the fimbrial end excised. Kroener (1969) reported a 100% success rate in over 1000 bilateral fimbriectomies performed by his associates, while Tappan (1973) recorded a failure rate of 0.5% in 256 patients. We have seen several failures, working in a general hospital where the procedure was employed by some of the gynaecologists for a few years. We have also seen some distressed patients, requesting reanastomosis of their tubes, for whom nothing could be done.

Hysterectomy

Abdominal and vaginal hysterectomy provide the most certain methods of sterilising women. They have the advantage that the risk of subsequent uterine pathology is eliminated though the chance of this is small, between 2.5% (Williams, E.L. *et al.*, 1951) and 5.5% (Muldoon, 1972). There are no late sequelae such as menorrhagia. The incidence of gynaecological symptoms after tubal ligation may be high, but only in a proportion of patients is the symptomatology severe enough or prolonged enough to justify hysterectomy. Smith and Symmonds (1972) found four patients in 161 who subsequently needed hysterectomy after fimbriectomy, and Houseman (1971) and Muldoon (1972) reported that 3% and 19%, respectively, needed hysterectomy after tubal ligation.

The arguments against hysterectomy as a primary sterilisation procedure are that it substitutes a major operation for a relatively minor one with a corresponding increase in morbidity and mortality (Hibbard, 1972). The failure rates of standard methods of sterilisation are so low that the advantage of eliminating sterilisation failures becomes theoretical, whilst the elimination of a chance of subsequent uterine or ovarian pathology does not in general justify the routine use of major surgery. It is in the younger age group that tubal ligation is most likely to produce sequelae. These are the very patients from whom gynaecologists are reluctant to remove the uterus, because of the chance of subsequent physical and psychological problems; the possibility of a request for reversal of the sterilisation cannot be ignored. Again, the group of patients in which one can be most confident of the need for permanence, namely those with major medical indications for the procedure, is the very group in which the chance of the increased morbidity of a hysterectomy is best avoided.

The psychological consequences of hysterectomy must not be underestimated. It is not infrequent for women to regret having been sterilised and these patients have a chance of subsequently developing psychosomatic gynae-cological symptoms. Post-sterilisation problems may well be in part a reflection of poor patient selection. In such cases substituting a hysterectomy for tubal ligation will merely shift the site of such psychosomatic symptoms, and in some cases might lead to an even greater difficulty in adjusting to the sterile state. On the other hand, apparent menorrhagia following tubal ligation may be due to increased awareness of blood loss occurring as a result of the sterile state and in these occasional patients hysterectomy removes the nagging monthly reminder of this. In a comparison of the psychological aftermath of hysterectomy and tubal ligation Hampton and Tarnasky (1974) were unable to detect any signifi-cant difference between the operations.

In conclusion, hysterectomy as a primary sterilising procedure is reasonable in patients with uterine pathology such as fibromyomata, and in patients who suffer from menorrhagia or other menstrual abnormalities and who fully appreciate that the operation is quite irrevocable. It may also be appropriate in communities where pelvic inflammatory complications are common after tubal sterilisation. The use of hysterectomy on relatively trivial gynaecological grounds is sometimes considered for sterilisation in environments where primary sterilising procedures have a religious or cultural stigma.

STERILISATION IN RELATION TO PREGNANCY

Puerperal sterilisation can be performed either a few days after vaginal delivery or abortion or at the time of caesarean section or hysterotomy.

The methods commonly used are conventional tubal ligation and division, particularly the Pomeroy method, laparoscopic sterilisation, or hysterectomy.

Advantages

The advantages of sterilisation at the time of operation are that it saves a second operation, with its slight but inevitable risk, and that it is convenient for the patient. A mother with a new baby and other small children will often find it difficult to return to hospital several weeks later for interval sterilisation. In some cases pregnancy may occur again before sterilisation can be carried out. Additional advantages of hysterectomy for sterilisation are that the failure rate is eliminated and an actual or potential site of pathology is removed.

Disadvantages

The disadvantages of sterilisation immediately after a pregnancy are medical and psychological.

The main medical disadvantages are higher failure and morbidity rates. The higher morbidity rate is partly due to an increased risk of thrombo-embolism. During later pregnancy and the puerperium there is an increase in the numbers of platelets and in their adhesiveness and aggregation properties, together with a rise in plasma coagulation factors and fibrinogen. Prystowsky and Eastman (1955) in their series of 1022 puerperal Pomeroy sterilisations reported three deaths (0.3%), two due to pulmonary embolism and one due to a subsequent ruptured ectopic pregnancy.

The main psychological problem of sterilisation in the puerperium or after abortion is regret at having the operation done. Pregnancy is a bad time to make a decision regarding further pregnancies because of the profound effect it can have on the mood of the patient. Additionally the baby may die or be discovered to have a previously unsuspected congenital abnormality during the neonatal period. Mowat (1974) reported that 11 of the 75 patients who had requested sterilisation during pregnancy had changed their minds within three months of the confinement.

In the majority of patients who request therapeutic abortion and sterilisation, a separate approach to the two problems seems more sensible. The combination of tubal sterilisation with therapeutic abortion may convey an increased risk of operative complications (Shepard, 1974) though this is not the case with laparoscopic sterilisation (Confidential Enquiry into Gynaecological Laparoscopy, 1978a). Where social and medical circumstances permit, consideration should be given to terminating the pregnancy and performing the tubal ligation three months later. In a few patients, termination hysterectomy may be the operation of choice. If hysterectomy is employed, the chance of creating emotional trauma by performing the operation either at caesarean section or in association with therapeutic abortion is high unless patient selection is excellent. This means that there is a good medical reason for removing the uterus, or that the patient is certain that she wishes hysterectomy.

Pomeroy Method

This method is commonly used during the puerperium or at the time of caesarean section or hysterotomy, because it is quick and simple. In a series of 400 cases studied by Prystowsky and Eastman (1955) the failure rate of Pomeroy sterilisation performed at caesarean section or hysterotomy was 1.8%, which is six times higher than when the operation was performed electively in the puerperium. This may be because the increased vascularity of the tissues makes recanalisation more likely. On the other hand, Shepard's (1974) review did not confirm the magnitude of the difference. The average failure rates were 0.3% with sterilisation at caesarean section and 0.2% in the puerperium. All these figures may be misleading as follow-up was defective in most of the series. The complication and morbidity rates for the combination of caesarean section and tubal ligation are of course higher than those for tubal ligation alone, but there is no evidence that simple tubal ligation adds to the complications of caesarean section.

The failure rate of the Pomeroy procedure in the puerperium may be higher than in the non-pregnant patient (Prystowsky and Eastman, 1955) though in Shepard's (1974) accumulation from the literature, the reverse appeared to be the case. Uchida (1975) recommended that tubal section should be supplemented by fimbriectomy, performed by excising the whole distal ends of the tubes. This seems reasonable with sterilisation at caesarean section, if the surgeon is absolutely confident there will be no request for reversal of the operation.

The morbidity rate of puerperal tubal ligation is probably higher than that of interval sterilisation. The performance of more complex sterilisation procedures such as Irving's method reduces the failure rate but because of the vascularity of the uterus and broad ligament it significantly increases the morbidity due to haemorrhage and haematoma formation.

Laparoscopic Sterilisation in the Puerperium

This can be carried out during the puerperium, or at the time of a therapeutic abortion. There is no difference from the standard technique for the passage of the laparoscope, nor from the techniques of sterilisation already described. There is an increased risk of haemorrhage from the mesosalpinx on division of the tube. The site of tubal division should be carefully observed for continuing haemorrhage, but this should be controllable by further coagulation. If not then laparotomy will be necessary.

Hysterectomy

Sterilisation by hysterectomy has been advocated either at the time of caesarean section or during the puerperium by many authors (Hallat and Hirsch, 1958; Brenner *et al.,* 1970; Bazley and Crisp, 1974). Wilson *et al.* (1973) found that the morbidity of postpartum hysterectomy is three times that of postpartum tubal ligation.

Caesarean hysterectomy has been advocated as a means of sterilisation and it has been suggested that the post-operative complications are no greater than those following caesarean section alone (Barclay, 1969). The main problem was blood loss due to the increased vascularity of the tissues. Sterilisation was the indication for hysterectomy at the time of caesarean section in 269 patients; there was one maternal death — due to a transfusion reaction. Wilson *et al.* (1973) confirmed that the average blood loss at caesarean hysterectomy was nearly double that with caesarean section and tubal ligation, and 33% of patients needed transfusion during the former procedure, compared with 4% during the latter. In experienced hands caesarean hysterectomy may have an acceptably low rate of complications. Nonetheless, the inevitable mortality and serious complications which must occur, particularly with less experienced surgeons, seems too high a price to pay for the elimination of the small failure rate of tubal ligation.

Termination Hysterectomy has also been advocated as a method of sterilisation at the time of therapeutic abortion (Lewis and Williams, 1970). Vaginal termination hysterectomy has been used successfully by Laufe and Kreutner (1971).

Reaction to the concept of hysterectomy for termination of pregnancy and sterilisation is often emotionally charged. Schulman (1972) lays much emphasis on the mortality of hysterectomy, which he cites as 164 per 100 000 patients. Tubal ligation alone carries a mortality of 17 to 25 per 100 000 patients (Lu and Chun, 1967; Presser, 1970) and this can be increased if the operation is combined with termination of pregnancy (Ottosson, 1971; Registrar General, 1969–1972). In England and Wales in 1969 to 1972 the overall mortality from all methods of therapeutic abortion combined with tubal sterilisation was 56 per 100 000; that of termination hysterectomy was 134 per 100 000 (Registrar General, 1969–1972).

Termination hysterectomy has been recommended either by the abdominal route (Lewis and Williams, 1970) or vaginally (Laufe and Kreutner, 1971; Ballard, 1974). The latter authors preferred the vaginal route because the overall morbidity rate was less than 20%, and the absence of a scar prevented the patient from being reminded of an event which she probably wished to forget.

It is easy to under-estimate the psychological effects of termination hysterectomy. The inevitable emotional state of mind associated with termination of pregnancy makes this a bad time to take a decision as irrevocable as sterilisation, especially if it entails losing the uterus as well. On the other hand, in Peck's (1973) follow-up of 29 patients who had termination hysterectomy, 3 had regrets about the termination, but none regretted the hysterectomy.

The disadvantages of termination hysterectomy and caesarean hysterectomy are obvious. Apart from the possibility of psychological trauma, there is the increased morbidity of a major operation compared with two simpler ones. The increase in morbidity has not been considered a major problem by some authors (Hallatt and Hirsch, 1958) but others have found that the morbidity at caesarean hysterectomy was such as to make it an unjustifiable procedure unless in exceptional circumstances (Brenner *et al.*, 1970). These authors found that there was an overall complication rate of 28.7%. Bazley and Crisp (1974) found a major complication rate of less than 3% for puerperal sterilisation and 4–6% for hysterectomies done at caesarean section. The need for blood transfusion at and after caesarean hysterectomy is greater than with hysterectomy performed for a gynaecological reason. On the other hand hysterectomy for procuring therapeutic abortion does not seem to lead to an excessively high morbidity, though it is doubtful whether vaginal hysterectomy for therapeutic abortion in a nation-wide series would give such good results as those obtained by Laufe and Kreutner (1971). The combination of two simple procedures would probably carry a lower morbidity rate.

Conclusion

It is our view that if sterilisation is to be performed in association with delivery then it should be either by the Pomeroy or laparoscopic method, carried out about the third day. Laparoscopic sterilisation at the time of vaginal termination of pregnancy is a safe procedure in experienced hands. Should the patient be having a caesarean section then the advantages of a Pomeroy tubal ligation and division outweigh the disadvantage of any increase in failure rate when the procedure is conducted at this time, but the failure rate must be borne in mind when assessing the situation. Except in the occasional case where there is obvious uterine pathology, and where hysterectomy would have had to be carried out in the near future, there are major medical and psychological disadvantages to removing the uterus at the time of abortion or caesarean section or during the puerperium.

REVERSIBLE FEMALE STERILISATION: OPERATIVE CONTRACEPTIVE PROCEDURES

Should sterilisation be truly reversible then it could be considered as an operative contraceptive procedure. In general it is essential that a woman who wishes to be sterilised has a clear idea of what the operation entails, and its effect on her reproductive and endocrine state. If she requests reversible sterilisation it may be that her mind is not completely made up, and she should be given the opportunity to review other contraceptive procedures in depth before she is committed to an operative procedure with its possible risks and inadequately defined potential for reversal.

Sometimes a woman who has tried conventional contraceptive techniques and found them either to fail or to be totally unsatisfactory requests reversible sterilisation. On questioning she expresses the fear that permanent sterilisation would diminish her libido. The primary approach to tnis problem should be to secure psychiatric support for her, but this is sometimes unavailable or unacceptable. If she is made irreversibly sterile she is likely to develop not only loss of libido but also other psychosomatic symptoms. It may be that a potentially reversible sterilising procedure is then indicated. The woman who wishes that her sterilisation operation might be reversed only in unpredictable circumstances, such as the death of her children or re-marriage, is usually more resigned to her state and less likely to have psychosomatic symptoms specifically related to her consequent infertility.

One approach to reversible sterilisation involves prevention of the release of ova. This can be done by burying the ovary within the leaves of the broad ligament. Patients who have had this operation often develop pelvic pain and dysmenorrhoea. Reversal of the operation can be difficult because of adhesions (Morris, N.F., personal communication, 1972). There were no pregnancies in a small series of 6 such operations or in 6 patients who had their ovaries encased in a Silastic bag (Wood and Leeton, 1969). A similar operation, burying the ovary in the broad ligament, has been carried out by Lindemann (1970) in a larger series of 54 patients. He followed up these patients, whose average age was 34 years, for a total of 813 cycles during which time there were no pregnancies. Five patients developed small transient ovarian cysts, and 8 complained of pain at the time of ovulation. This is the most successful series to date, but it would seem that the side-effects of this type of reversible sterilisation make it inappropriate for routine use. It is possible that thickening of the ovarian capsule may make subsequent ovulation difficult.

Reversal of Tubal Sterilisation

This depends very much on the way in which the sterilisation procedure was carried out. To make subsequent anastomosis easier Williams (1971) recommended excising only 5 mm of tube at a point close to the uterus, securing the medial cut end behind the round ligament and the lateral end in front of it. If there is an adequate length of tube proximal and distal to the excised portion and if the fimbriae are healthy, then tubal anastomosis may be a simple procedure. Should the proximal portion of the tube be very short then tubal implantation into the uterus must be carried out if microsurgical procedures are not available. Should the sterilisation procedure have been a fimbriectomy then salpingostomy with or without the use of a Silastic prosthesis (Mulligan, 1966) is the operation of choice but success is unlikely.

Of the laparoscopic methods of sterilisation, electrocoagulation and division of the tubes in two places does not lend itself to reanastomosis. The recent use of Hulka clips (Hulka *et al.*, 1975), which necrose only 4 mm of tube, makes the chance of successful reanastomosis quite good.

The use of plastic rods inserted into the tube and held in place by tantalum clips applied to the outside of the tube (Steptoe, 1974) may provide a good and easily reversed method of sterilisation, but neither its efficacy nor its reversibility has yet been assessed adequately.

Tubal reanastomosis is carried out using fine polythene rod splints to support the ends of the tubes. The rods are usually left *in situ* and removed per abdomen or through the cervix six weeks later. Fine needles and 4/0 catgut or 4/0 silk are used to suture the tubes. Siegler and Perez (1975) have reported 46 cases of tubal reanastomosis, some their own, others from the literature. Seventeen women (39%) became pregnant; one of these had a tubal pregnancy.

A newer approach which has been developed in experimental work on rabbits and applied to humans is the use of microsurgical techniques for the reanastomosis (Winston, 1975, 1977). Adhesions are divided using a very fine electrocautery probe, to reduce bleeding to an absolute minimum. The tubal remnant is identified in the uterine cornu and reanastomosis performed with 8/0 nylon sutures under an operating microscope. This technique, which is highly specialised, resulted in extremely good results in experimental animals, and 11 of the 16 women in whom it has been used have had normal intra-uterine pregnancies (Winston, 1977). With this technique fibrosis at the operation site is minimal.

Uterotubal implantation (Green-Armytage, 1952) is in general a fairly successful operation for restoring tubal patency when the tubes have been blocked at the cornual end. Some gynaecologists use a reamer to make tunnels in the uterine cornua (Green-Armytage, 1957; Johnstone, 1959; Williams, G.F.J., 1973); others prefer to cut the tunnels with a small scalpel; Stallworthy (1963) used an open transverse fundal incision in the uterus. Some use polythene splints, withdrawing them six weeks later; others who do not use splints at all obtain much the same results. Green-Armytage (1957) reported 14 term pregnancies (36%) in a series of 38 patients having implantations for cornual obstruction. Palmer (1960) reported a 75% patency rate after tubal implantation; Peel (1964) found a 55% patency rate.

When the operation is employed to reverse tubal sterilisation, the results are probably not so good as this. Often, only the ampullary end of the tube is available to implant and this may leave only 2 or 3 cm of extra-uterine tube. Siegler and Perez (1975) collected 124 cases, of whom 24 (19%) became pregnant; these included 17 normal pregnancies, 4 abortions, and 2 ectopic gestations.

VASECTOMY

Operative Procedure

Usually the operation can be carried out under a local anaesthetic. The patient should bath and shave the scrotal skin before presenting himself for operation. Preoperative sedation with oral diazepam, 10 mg, is desirable. The skin should be cleaned with any suitable surgical skin preparation. Approximately 5 ml of 0.5% lignocaine is injected intradermally at the antero-lateral part of the scrotum over the vas deferens and then into the tissues surrounding the vas itself. Too much local anaesthetic can make localisation of the vas difficult. A small incision is made in the skin and subcutaneous tissues over the vas which is held between finger and thumb. It is then picked up in tissue forceps, the surrounding layers of the spermatic cord dissected off gently, and two catgut ligatures placed on the vas 3—4 cm apart. The intervening segment is removed. The remaining ends should be ligated again and then folded back on themselves and sutured into position so that the cut ends face away from each other. This reduces the risk of recanalisation as it is extremely difficult, if not impossible, to occlude the lumen of the vas totally by simple ligation. The dartos muscle in the cord can tend to approximate the cut ends and recanalisation may occur unless the ends are folded back or unless a very long segment is removed. The latter course precludes reanastomosis at a future date. The skin and subcutaneous layers are sutured in one layer, care being taken to secure haemostasis lest a haematoma form. Catgut is used by most surgeons to ligate the vas, but in attempts to reduce the inflammatory response and risk of recanalisation, silk (Freund and Davis, 1969), thread (Vyas and Trivedi, 1967) and tantalum clips (Moss, 1972) have been employed.

A simpler method has been described by Tauber (1973) involving coagulation of the cut ends after a 1 cm segment has been excised. Tantalum clips are applied and the ends allowed to retract. The skin is not sutured. The results are apparently good, but this method seems more liable to recanalisation of the vas (Schmidt, 1972).

Schmidt (1966) described an alternative method involving high interruption of the vas without resection of a segment. To prevent the recanalisation he destroys the lumen of the vas for 1—2 mm from the incision by electrocautery, and then interposes a layer of fascia between the two ends. This was found to be a safe method with the possibility of an easy reanastomosis should this be necessary.

A scrotal support reduces postoperative discomfort, and this should be worn for about one week. Intercourse, with contraceptive precautions, can take place as soon as desired after vasectomy, although it has been suggested that ejaculation too soon may cause excessive pressure on the newly ligated vas. This seems to be a theoretical problem.

Advantages and Disadvantages

The advantages of vasectomy over female sterilisation are its simplicity and the fact that it can be carried out as an out-patient procedure using local anaesthesia. It has therefore been suggested that vasectomy is a suitable operation in general practice in this country (Hobbs, 1972) and as an office procedure in the United States of America (Tauber, 1973). The operation has been performed many times, safely and well, by general practitioners, but even the simplest of operations can give rise to problems. There can be difficulty in finding the vas, hypotension may be caused by traction on the vas, difficulty may be found in tracing a retracted cut end, and a haematoma may form postoperatively. Extensive dissection may be required to find the vas in men with a short spermatic cord and thick scrotal skin and in those who have had previous surgery in that area such as inguinal herniorrhaphy. Some men have a double vas, both parts of which are small, and this makes location difficult. Vasectomy in predictably difficult cases should only be attempted under a general anaesthetic.

One disadvantage of vasectomy is that sterility is not immediate and so other adequate contraceptive methods are necessary until at least two negative seminal analyses are obtained. The time taken for the seminal vesicles to empty varies with the number of ejaculations and the patient is encouraged to have intercourse as often as possible and, if necessary, to masturbate. After 30 ejaculations it will be found that the seminal analysis is nearly always negative. Hanley (1971) found that the lowest and highest number of ejaculations to attain azoospermia after vasectomy were 6 and 32 respectively. Rees (1973) states that only 8 ejaculations are required to empty the seminal vesicles. This figure seems low and it is our practice to advise 30 ejaculations before carrying out seminal analyses to ensure azoospermia. The use of the number of ejaculations rather than an arbitrary time interval after operation is more reliable and should make it clear to the patient that it is the seminal vesicles and ampullae that need to be emptied before vasectomy can be pronounced successful. Some surgeons advise that sterility is attained once no further motile spermatozoa are seen in a fresh specimen of semen. The possibility of error in such a situation is great, as motility is dependent on many factors. It is desirable to wait until there are no spermatozoa, motile or non-motile, in three centrifuged specimens.

Irrigation of the seminal vesicles at operation should be helpful in washing out the spermatozoa, but Blandy (1973) found difficulty in dislodging water soluble contrast media from the seminal vesicles and many spermatozoa may remain despite the irrigation procedure. There is also the added risk of introducing chronic infection in the seminal vesicles and epididymis, which is difficult to eradicate.

Vasectomy is often irreversible. In carrying out the procedure many surgeons compromise between making the operation successful and leaving the vas in such a situation that reanastomosis could be carried out. Excision of a long length of vas, say more than 5 cm, makes reunion without severe tension impossible and conveys irreversibility. Excision of only a small segment predisposes to recanalisation. For this reason, the excision of 2–3 cm, together with looping back of the ends, is advocated. The problem of reanastomosis is finding the cut ends, mobilising them, and their subsequent reanastomosis without excessive tension. Given a favourable situation, reanastomosis may be possible in as many as 70% of patients (Hanley, 1971). Phadke and Phadke (1967) found that only 55% of men whose vasa had been rejoined produced children. The incidence of successful reanastomosis is greater than the incidence of subsequent pregnancies. This may be due to the production of sperm-immobilising and sperm-agglutinating antibodies after vasectomy.

Although it is inevitable that some men will change their mind about sterility, probably because of re-marriage, it must be stressed that vasectomy should not be performed if there is any doubt in the patient's mind and the patient should be clear that essentially the operation must be regarded as irreversible.

Failures and their Reasons

Spontaneous recanalisation is more likely in the presence of excessive granulation tissue (Pugh and Hanley, 1969). This is produced after haematoma formation, infection or foreign body reaction. Excision of an inadequate segment of vas deferens, and failure to turn back the cut ends or to insert fascial tissue between them, will increase the chance of spontaneous recanalisation. Other reasons for failures include ligation of a blood vessel instead of the vas, or the presence of an undiagnosed double vas. The excised segments should be examined microscopically by a histopathologist to confirm their identity.

Complications

A detailed review of complications has been presented by Wortman (1975). Operative complications include scrotal haematoma and bruising. A small amount of bruising is relatively common after vasectomy; haematoma formation is not, though Rees (1973) found haematoma in 10.5% of patients. In the Margaret Pyke series of 1000 vasectomies (Barnes *et al.,* 1973) the incidence of minor haematoma was 3.5% of which 0.7% required further treatment. To discourage haematoma formation and to reduce postoperative discomfort, a tight scrotal support is useful. Haematoma may become infected. In the scrotum the consequences can be severe and dangerous leading to severe tissue necrosis, and so strict asepsis at operation is essential. Rees (1973) found an overall infection rate of 2.6% but epididymitis occurred in only 0.8% of patients. A painful foreign body granuloma may form at the cut end of the vas due to a foreign body reaction induced by spermatozoa. These granulomata may form discrete tender nodules.

Leakage of spermatozoa can be due to absorption of ligatures before the cut ends of the vas are fibrosed, to inadequate occlusion at operation, to tight ligatures which necrose the vas or to an excessive build-up of pressure behind the ligature caused by ejaculatory peristalsis.

Vasectomy is said to cause an autoimmune response to spermatozoa trapped in the seminiferous tubules. Blocking the vas deferens causes the reabsorption of spermatozoa, and subsequently sperm-immobilising and sperm-agglutinating antibodies develop in a proportion of men. Two per cent of normally fertile men have circulating antibodies against their own spermatozoa (Rumke, 1967); in men who have had vasectomies this figure can rise to as high as 54% for sperm-agglutinating antibodies, and 31% for sperm-immobilising antibodies (Ansbacher, 1971). It is probable that absorption of nucleoproteins from spermatozoa with the initiation of an autoimmune response may account for the formation of these antibodies. This theory is substantiated by the fact that intraluminal phagocytosis is involved in the disposal of dead spermatozoa (Phadke, 1964) and that other generalised autoimmune conditions, such as arthritis, may develop as remote sequelae of a vasectomy (Roberts, 1970). It is likely that these circulating antibodies can cause a reduction in subsequent fertility, despite successful reanastomosis of the vas deferens.

Reversal of Vasectomy

The technique of reanastomosis of the vas deferens or vaso-vasotomy involves identifying and dissecting free the fibrosed ends of the vas. Minimal mobilisation of about 3 mm of vas from the underlying fascia (Schmidt, 1975) is employed to reduce the chances of vascular injury and of subsequent avascular necrosis at the anastomosis site. The ends of the vas are cut to expose healthy lumen and after ensuring patency an end-to-end anastomosis is usually performed. Sutures of 5/0 or 6/0 monofilament nylon are used to join the adventitial and muscular layers only but recently sutures through the mucosa have been advocated to diminish the risk of leakage of spermatozoa (Schmidt, 1975). The use of an operating microscope will aid the correct positioning of sutures. Closed splints of nylon or fine polythene and open splints of polythene tubing have been used. Solid splints are removed between 4 and 14 days after operation; tubular splints remain *in situ* permanently (Bradshaw, 1976).

The success rate of these procedures, as defined by the reappearance of sperm in the ejaculate, can be as high as 92% (Bradshaw, 1976) but pregnancy only occurs in 50% or less of these cases. Reasons for anatomical failure include the formation of a spermatic granuloma at the anastomosis site due to leakage of spermatozoa (Johnson, 1972), excessive fibrosis or difficulty in reanastomosis because of the previous excision of a long segment of vas.

Functional failure after reanastomosis may be due to damage to the sympathetic nerves, inhibiting transport of spermatozoa (Hulka and Davis, 1972), to problems antedating the operation such as a relatively low sperm count or subfertility in the wife, or to the production of sperm agglutinating or immobilising antibodies which seem to be more prevalent in patients who have redeveloped a spermatic granuloma (Schmidt, 1975).

Vasectomy in dogs leads to progressive arrest of spermatogenesis and degenerative changes in the epithelium of the seminiferous tubules (Joshi *et al.*, 1972). In the dogs with complete arrest of spermatogenesis there is hypertrophy of the Leydig cells. In bilaterally vasectomised men spermatogenesis is normal on testicular biopsy. It is not known whether these apparently normal spermatozoa are always capable of fertilisation.

If an autoimmune response impairing fertility is a significant problem after vasectomy, then the concept of temporary vasectomy is a false hope. Although spermatogenesis may continue, fertility could be diminished. In addition Bunge (1972) has shown that there is no increase of plasma testosterone levels after vasectomy, which suggests that functional hypertrophy of the Leydig cells does not occur in humans. The fact that there is no significant alteration in plasma testosterone has been confirmed by Purvis *et al.* (1976). These authors found that vasectomy was associated with significant decreases in plasma pregnenolone, dehydroepiandrosterone and androstenedione, and significant increases in dihydrotestosterone, oestrone and probably oestradiol (Purvis *et al.*, 1976). The long-term significance of these hormonal changes is obscure and needs to be evaluated in a large study. There is no evidence that levels of follicle stimulating hormone or luteinising hormone are increased.

REFERENCES

ALVARADO, A., QUINONES, R. and AZNAR, B. (1974). Tubal instillation under hysteroscopic control. *Hysteroscopic Sterilisation. Proceedings of a Workshop on Hysteroscopic Sterilisation, Minneapolis. June 22–24, 1973.* Stratton Intercontinental, New York

ALEXANDER, G.D., NOE, F.E. and BROWN, E.M. (1969). Anaesthesia for pelvic laparoscopy. *Anesth. Analg.*, **48**, 14–18

ALEXANDER, G.D., GOLDRATH, M., BROWN, E.M. and SMILER, B.G. (1973). Outpatient laparoscopic sterilization under local anaesthesia. *Am. J. Obstet. Gynec.*, **116**, 1065–1068

ANSBACHER, R. (1971). Sperm-agglutinating and sperm immobilizing antibodies in vasectomized men. *Fert. Steril.*, **22**, 629–632

BALLARD, C.A. (1974). Therapeutic abortion and sterilization by vaginal hysterectomy. *Am. J. Obstet. Gynec.*, **118**, 891–896

BARCLAY, D.L. (1969). Cesarean hysterectomy at the Charity Hospital in New Orleans – 1000 consecutive operations. *Clin. Obstet. Gynec.*, **12**, 635–651

BARNES, M.N., BLANDY, J.P., ENGLAND, H.R., GUNN, Sir GEORGE, HOWARD, G., LAW, B., MASON, B., MEDAWAR, J., REYNOLDS, C., SHEARER, R.J., SINGH, M. and STANLEY-ROOSE, D.G. (1973). One thousand vasectomies. *Br. med. J.*, **iv**, 216–221

BAZLEY, W.S. and CRISP, W.E. (1974). Postpartum hysterectomy for sterilization. *Am. J. Obstet. Gynec.*, **119**, 139–145

BISHOP, E. and NELMS, W.F. (1930). A simple method of tubal sterilization. *N.Y. St. J. Med.*, **30**, 214–216

BLACK, W.P. (1971). Sterilization by laparoscopic tubal electrocoagulation: an assessment. *Am. J. Obstet. Gynec.*, **111**, 979–983

BLANDY, J. (1973). Vasectomy. *Br. J. hosp. Med.*, **9**, 319–324

BRADSHAW, L.E. (1976). Vasectomy reversibility – a status report. *Population Reports*, series D, number 3, 41–60

BRENNER, P., SALL, S. and SONNENBLICK, B. (1970). Evaluation of cesarean section hysterectomy as a sterilization procedure. *Am. J. Obstet. Gynec.*, **108**, 335–339

BUNGE, R.G. (1972). Plasma testosterone levels in man before and after vasectomy. *Invest. Urol.*, **10**, 9

CHENG, M.C.E., WONG, Y.M., ROCHAT, R.W. and RATNAM, S.S. (1977). Sterilization failures in Singapore: an examination of ligation techniques and failure rates. *Stud. fam. Plann.*, **8**, 109–114

CHOWDHURY, S. and CHOWDHURY, Z. (1975). Tubectomy by paraprofessional surgeons in rural Bangladesh. *Lancet*, **ii**, 567–569

CONFIDENTIAL ENQUIRY INTO GYNAECOLOGICAL LAPAROSCOPY (1978, a, b, c, d, e and f). *Gynaecological Laparoscopy*, pp. 30, 102, 114, 122, 131 and 152 respectively. Ed. Chamberlain, G. and Brown, J.C. Royal College of Obstetricians and Gynaecologists, London

CORSON, S.L., PATRICK, H., HAMILTON, T. and BOLOGNESE, R.J. (1973). Electrical considerations of laparoscopic sterilization. *J. reprod. Med.*, **11**, 159–164

DARABI, K.F. and RICHART, R.M. (1977). Collaborative study on hysteroscopic sterilization procedures. Preliminary report. *Obstet. Gynec., N.Y.*, **49**, 48–54

DAVIDSON, A.C. and DONALD, I. (1972). Female sterilisation. *Scott. med. J.*, **17**, 210–213

DEES, D.B. (1961). Should hysterectomy replace routine tubal sterilization? *Am. J. Obstet. Gynec.*, **82**, 572–577

FORT, A.T. and ALEXANDER, A.M. (1966). Vaginal Pomeroy sterilisation. A description of technic and a review of 100 cases. *Obstet. Gynec., N.Y.*, **28**, 421–424

FREUND, M. and DAVIS, J.E. (1969). Disappearance rate of spermatozoa from the ejaculate following vasectomy. *Fert. Steril.*, **20**, 163–170

GARB, A.E. (1957). A review of tubal sterilization failures. *Obstetl. gynec. Surv.*, **12**, 291–305

GREEN-ARMYTAGE, V.B. (1952). Tubo-uterine implantation. *Br. med. J.*, **i**, 1222–1224

GREEN-ARMYTAGE, V.B. (1957). Tubo-uterine implantation. *J. Obstet. Gynaec. Br. Emp.*, **64**, 47–49

HALLATT, J.G. and HIRSCH, H. (1958). Total hysterectomy for sterilization following caesarean section. *Am. J. Obstet. Gynec.*, **75**, 396–400

HAMPTON, P.T. and TARNASKY, W.G. (1974). Hysterectomy and tubal ligation: a comparison of the psychological aftermath. *Am. J. Obstet. Gynec.*, **119**, 949–952

HANLEY, H.G. (1971). Male sterilization. *Br. J. hosp. Med.*, **6**, 156–158

HAYNES, D.M. and WOLFE, W.M. (1970). Tubal sterilization in an indigent population. Report of fourteen years' experience. *Am. J. Obstet. Gynec.*, **106**, 1044–1053

HIBBARD, L.T. (1972). Sexual sterilization by elective hysterectomy. *Am. J. Obstet. Gynec.*, **112**, 1076–1083

HOBBS, J.J. (1972). Vasectomy in general practice. *Jl R. Coll. gen. Pract.*, **22**, 583–589

HOFBAUER, J. (1927). The utilization of the round ligaments in tubal sterilization. *Surgery Gynec. Obstet.*, **44**, 829–831

HOUSEMAN, R.J. (1971). Sterilization of young wives. *Br. med. J.*, **iii**, 184

HUGHES, G. and LISTON, W.A. (1975). Comparison between laparoscopic sterilization and tubal ligation. *Br. med. J.*, **iii**, 637–639

HULKA, J.F. and DAVIS, J.E. (1972). Vasectomy and reversible vas occlusion. *Fert. Steril.*, **23**, 683–696

HULKA, J.F., OMRAN, K.F., PHILLIPS, J.M., Jr., LEFLER, H.T., Jr., LIEBERMAN, B., LEAN, H.T., PAI, D.A., KOETSAWANG, S. and CASTRO, V.M. (1975). Sterilization by spring clip: a report of 1000 cases with a 6-month follow-up. *Fert. Steril.*, **26**, 1122–1131

HUTCHINS, C.J. and CURPEN, N.C. (1975). Comparison between laparoscopic sterilization and tubal ligation. *Br. med. J.*, **iii**, 764

IRVING, F.C. (1924). A new method of ensuring sterility following cesarean section. *Am. J. Obstet. Gynec.*, **8**, 335–337

ISRANGKUN, C., PHAOSAVADI, S., NEUWIRTH, R.S. and RICHART, R.M. (1976). Clinical evaluation of quinacrine hydrochloride for sterilization of the human female. *Contraception*, **14**, 75–80

JOHNSON, D.S. (1972). Reversible male sterilisation: current status and future directions. *Contraception*, **5**, 327–338

JOHNSTONE, J.W. (1959). Implantation of the fallopian tubes for sterility. *J. Obstet. Gynaec. Br. Commonw.*, **62**, 410–416

JORDAN, J.A., EDWARDS, R.L., PEARSON, J. and MASKERY, P.J.K. (1971). Laparoscopic sterilisation and follow-up hysterosalpingogram. *J. Obstet. Gynaec. Br. Commonw.*, **78**, 460–466

JOSHI, K.R., RAMDEO, I.N., SACHDEV, K.N. and BHARADWAJ, T.P. (1972). Effects of vasectomy on testes. *Int. Surg.*, **57**, 711–713

KNIGHT, R.V.D. (1946). Tubal sterilization. *Am. J. Obstet. Gynec.*, **51**, 201–209

KÖHLER, M. (1927). Zur vereinfachung der technik der tubaren sterilisation. *Zentbl. Gynäk.*, **51**, 1589–1590

KROENER, W.F. (1969). Surgical sterilization by fimbriectomy. *Am. J. Obstet. Gynec.*, **104**, 247–254

LAUFE, L.E. and KREUTNER, A.K. (1971). Vaginal hysterectomy: a modality for therapeutic abortion and sterilization. *Am. J. Obstet. Gynec.*, **110**, 1096–1099

LEE, J.G., Jr., RANDALL, J.H. and KEETTEL, W.C. (1951). Tubal sterilization: a review of 1169 cases. *Am. J. Obstet. Gynec.*, **62**, 569–575

LEWIS, A.C.W. and WILLIAMS, E.A. (1970). Termination hysterectomy. *J. Obstet. Gynaec. Br. Commonw.*, **77**, 743–744

LINDEMANN, H.J. (1970). Transpositio ovarii extraperitonealis. *Geburtsh. Frauenheilk.*, **30**, 845–847

LISTON, W.A., DOWNIE, J., BRADFORD, W. and KERR, M.G. (1970). Female sterilisation by tubal electrocoagulation under laparoscopic control. *Lancet*, **i**, 382–383

LU, T. and CHUN, D. (1967). A long-term follow-up study of 1055 cases of post-partum tubal ligation. *J. Obstet. Gynaec. Br. Commonw.*, **74**, 875–880

LULL, C.B. and MITCHELL, R.M. (1950). The Pomeroy method of sterilization. *Am. J. Obstet. Gynec.*, **59**, 1118–1123

MADLENER, M. (1919). Über sterilisierenden operationen an den tuben. *Zentbl. Gynäk.*, **43**, 380–384

MORRIS, J.A. (1969). *Posterior colpotomy.* Thomas, Springfield, Illinois

MOSS, W.M. (1972). A sutureless technic for bilateral partial vasectomy. *Fert. Steril.*, **23**, 33–37

MOWAT, J. (1974). Delayed postpartum sterilization. *Br. med. J.*, **ii**, 306–308

MULDOON, M.J. (1972). Gynaecological illness after sterilization. *Br. med. J.*, **i**, 84–85

MULLIGAN, W.J. (1966). Results of salpingostomy. *Int. J. Fert.*, **11**, 424–430

NEIL, J.R., HAMMOND, G.T., NOBLE, A.D., RUSHTON, L. and LETCHWORTH, A.T. (1975). Late complications of sterilisation by laparoscopy and tubal ligation. *Lancet*, **ii**, 699–700

NEUMANN, H.H. and FRICK, H.C., II (1961). Occlusion of the fallopian tubes with tantalum clips. *Am. J. Obstet. Gynec.*, **81**, 803–806

OTTOSSON, J-O. (1971). Legal abortion in Sweden: thirty years' experience. *J. biosoc. Sci.*, **3**, 173–192

OVERSTREET, E.W. (1964). Techniques of sterilization. *Clin. Obstet. Gynec.*, **7**, 109–125

PALMER, R. (1960). Salpingostomy – a critical study of 396 personal cases operated upon without polythene tubing. *Proc. R. Soc. Med.*, **53**, 357–359

PECK, J.E. (1973). Reaction to termination hysterectomy. *Contraception*, **9**, 33–38

PEEL, Sir JOHN (1964). Utero-tubal implantation. *Proc. R. Soc. Med.*, **57**, 710–714

PEITMAN, H. (1926). Zur technik der tubaren sterilisation. *Zentbl. Gynäk.*, **50**, 1720–1721

PENFIELD, A.J. (1974). Laparoscopic sterilization under local anesthesia. *Am. J. Obstet. Gynec.*, **119**, 733–736

PETERSON, E.P. and BEHRMAN, S.J. (1971). Laparoscopic tubal sterilization. *Am. J. Obstet. Gynec.*, **110**, 24–29

PHADKE, A.M. (1964). Fate of spermatozoa in cases of obstructive azoospermia and after ligation of vas deferens in man. *J. Reprod. Fert.*, **7**, 1–12

PHADKE, G.M. and PHADKE, A.G. (1967). Experiences in the reanastomosis of the vas deferens. *J. Urol.*, **97**, 888–890

PHILLIPS, J., HULKA, B., HULKA, J., KEITH, D. and KEITH, L. (1977). Laparoscopic procedures: the American Association of Gynecologic Laparoscopists, membership survey for 1975. *J. reprod. Med.*, **18**, 227–232

PLANNER, O. (1927). Beitrag zur tubaren sterilisation. *Zentbl. Gynäk.*, **51**, 1829–1830

PRESSER, H.B. (1970). Voluntary sterilisation: a world view. *Reports on Population/Family Planning*, number 5, 1–36

PRYSTOWSKY, H. and EASTMAN, N.J. (1955). Puerperal tubal sterilisation. Report of 1830 cases. *J. Am. med. Ass.*, **158**, 463–467

PUGH, R.C.B. and HANLEY, H.G. (1969). Spontaneous recanalisation of the divided vas deferens. *Br. J. Urol.*, **41**, 340–347

PURVIS, K., SAKSENA, S.K., CEKAN, Z., DICZFALUSY, E. and GINER, J. (1976). Endocrine effects of vasectomy. *Clin. Endocrinol.*, **5**, 263–272

QUINONAS, G.R., ALVARADO, D.A. and AZNAR, R.R. (1973). Tubal occlusion by electrocoagulation under hysteroscopy. *Int. J. Fert.*, **18**, 167–173

RABINOWITSCH, K.N. (1927). Zur technik der tubaren sterilisation. *Zentbl. Gynäk.*, **51**, 634–635

REES, R.W.M. (1973). Vasectomy: problems of follow up. *Proc. R. Soc. Med.*, **66**, 52–54

REGISTRAR GENERAL, THE. *Statistical Review of England and Wales for the Years 1969, 1970, 1971 and 1972, respectively. Supplements on Abortion.* Her Majesty's Stationery Office, London

RICHART, R. (1976). Cited by Wortman, J. (1976), *Population Reports*, series C, number 7, 88

RICHART, R.M., GUTIERREZ-NAJAR, A.J. and NEUWIRTH, R.S. (1971). Transvaginal human sterilization: a preliminary report. *Am. J. Obstet. Gynec.*, **111**, 108–110

RICHART, R.M., NEUWIRTH, R.S., ISRANGKUN, C. and PHAOSAVASDI, S. (1973). Female sterilization by electrocoagulation of tubal ostia using hysteroscopy. *Am. J. Obstet. Gynec.*, **117**, 801–804

RIOUX, J.E. and CLOUTIER, D. (1974). A new bipolar instrument for laparoscopic tubal ligation. *Am. J. Obstet. Gynec.*, **119**, 737–739

ROBERTS, H.J. (1970). Letter to the Editor. *Perspect. Biol. Med.*, **14**, 176–178

RÜMKE, P. (1967). Sperm-agglutinating autoantibodies in relation to male infertility. *Proc. R. Soc. Med.*, **61**, 275–278

SCHMIDT, S.S. (1966). Technics and complications of elective vasectomy. *Fert. Steril.*, **17**, 467–482

SCHMIDT, S.S. (1972). Vas reanastomosis procedures. *Human Sterilisation. Proceedings of the Conference, Cherry Hill, New Jersey, October 28–31, 1969*, pp. 76–85. Ed. Richart, R.M. and Prager, D.J. Thomas, Springfield, Illinois

SCHMIDT, S.S. (1975). Vas anastomosis: a return to simplicity. *Br. J. Urol.*, **110**, 309–314

SCHULMAN, H. (1972). Editorial. Major surgery for abortion and sterilization. *Obstet. Gynec., N.Y.*, **40**, 738–739

SEMM, K. and RIMKUS, V. (1974). Technische bemerkungen zur CO_2–hysteroskopie. *Geburtsh. Frauenheilk.*, **34**, 451–460

SHEPARD, M.K. (1974). Female contraceptive sterilization. *Obstetl. gynec. Surv.*, **29**, 739–787

SIEGLER, A.M. and PEREZ, R.J. (1975). Reconstruction of fallopian tubes in previously sterilized patients. *Fert. Steril.*, **26**, 383–392

SMITH, R.A. and SYMMONDS, R.E. (1971). Vaginal salpingectomy (fimbriectomy) for sterilization. *Obstet. Gynec., N.Y.*, **38**, 400–402

SMITH, I., BENZIE, R.J., GORDON, N.L.M., KELMAN, G.R. and SWAPP, G.H. (1971). Cardiovascular effects of peritoneal insufflation of carbon dioxide for laparoscopy. *Br. med. J.*, **iii**, 410–411

SOGLOW, S.R. (1971). Vaginal tubal ligation at time of vacuum curettage for abortion. *Obstet. Gynec., N.Y.*, **38**, 888–892

STALLWORTHY, J.A. (1963). In *British Obstetric and Gynaecological Practice*, 3rd edn, p. 756. Ed. Bourne, A. and Claye, Sir Andrew. Heinemann, London

STEPTOE, P.C. (1972). Problems of laparoscopic sterilisation. *Lancet*, **i**, 1115

STEPTOE, P.C. (1974). Intratubal devices for reversible sterilization. In *Gynaecological Laparoscopy. Principles and Techniques*, pp. 304–314. Ed. Phillips, J.M. and Keith, L. Stratton Intercontinental, New York

STEPTOE, P.C. (1976). Further experience in gynaecological endoscopy. *Proc. R. Soc. Med.*, **69**, 143

TAPPAN, J.G. (1973). Kroener tubal ligation in perspective. *Am. J. Obstet. Gynec.*, **115**, 1053–1057

TATUM, H.J. and SCHMIDT, F.H. (1977). Contraceptive and sterilization practices and extrauterine pregnancy: a realistic perspective. *Fert. Steril.*, **28**, 407–421

TAUBER, A.S. (1973). A long term experience with vasectomy. *J. reprod. Med.*, **10**, 147–149

UCHIDA, H. (1961). Uchida's abdominal sterilization technique. *Proceedings of the 3rd World Congress on Obstetrics and Gynecology, Vienna*, I. item 26

UCHIDA, H. (1975). Uchida tubal sterilisation. *Am. J. Obstet. Gynec.*, **121**, 153–158

VYAS, B.K. and TRIVEDI, D.R. (1967). A single handed method of vasectomy. *J. Indian med. Ass.*, **49**, 28–29

WHEELESS, C.R. (1976). The past, present and future use of the laparoscope in female sterilisation. In *Advances in Female Sterilization Technology*, pp. 30–36. Ed. Sciarra, J.J., Droegemueller, W. and Spiedel, J.J. Harper and Row, Hagerstown, Maryland

WHEELESS, C.R., Jr. and THOMPSON, B.H. (1973). Laparoscopic sterilization. Review of 3600 cases. *Obstet. Gynec., N.Y.*, **42**, 751–758

WHITE, C.A. (1966). Tubal sterilization: a 15 year survey. *Am. J. Obstet. Gynec.*, **95**, 31–39

WILLIAMS, E.A. (1971). Reversible sterilization in the female. *Br. med. J.*, **iv**, 297

WILLIAMS, E.L., JONES, H.E. and MERRILL, R.E. (1951). The subsequent course of patients sterilized by tubal ligation. *Am. J. Obstet. Gynec.*, **61**, 423–426

WILLIAMS, G.F.J. (1973). Fallopian tube surgery for reversal of sterilisation. *Br. med. J.*, **i**, 599–601

WILLIAMS, J.W. (1928). Indications for therapeutic sterilization in obstetrics. When is advice concerning prevention of conception justifiable? *J. Am. med. Ass.*, **91**, 1237–1242

WILSON, E.A., DILTS, P.V., Jr. and SIMPSON, T.J. (1973). Comparative morbidity of postpartum sterilization procedures. *Am. J. Obstet. Gynec.*, **115**, 884–889

WINSTON, R.M.L. (1975). Microsurgical reanastomosis of the rabbit oviduct and its functional and pathological sequelae. *Br. J. Obstet. Gynaec.*, **82**, 513–522

WINSTON, R.M.L. (1977). Microsurgical tubocornual anastomosis for reversal of sterilisation. *Lancet*, **i**, 284–285

WOOD, C. and LEETON, J. (1969). Sterilisation by ovariotexy. A reversible technique. *Lancet,* **ii**, 1213–1215

WORTMAN, J. (1976). Vasectomy. What are the problems? *Population Reports,* series D, number 2, 25–39

WORTMAN, J. (1976). Tubal sterilization. Review of methods. *Population Reports,* series C, number 7, 73–95

WORTMAN, J. and PIOTROW, P.T. (1973). Colpotomy. The vaginal approach. *Population Reports,* series C, number 3, 29–44

YOON, I.B., WHEELESS, C.R. and KING, T.M. (1974). A preliminary report on a new laparoscopic sterilization approach. The silicone rubber band technique. *Am. J. Obstet. Gynec.,* **120**, 132–136

ZIPPER, J., STACCHETTI, E. and MEDEL, M. (1975). Transvaginal chemical sterilization: clinical use of quinacrine plus potentiating adjuvants. *Contraception,* **12**, 11–21

Part VI
Family Planning
Counselling, Clinical Trials

16 Motivation and Contraception

Many factors may influence individual behaviour in connection with the use of methods of fertility regulation. Whether the reader's main interest is in the improvement of the quality of life for specific families or persons, or in the problem of world over-population, he must appreciate that the behaviour of the individual is fundamental to the success of birth control. No amount of family planning services or reliable methods of contraception are of value unless they are used effectively by individuals.

When the means are available for individuals to regulate their fertility but are not used effectively, this is often referred to as a problem of motivation. To consider women who fail to prevent pregnancies as lacking in motivation is a great over-simplification. It is not possible to attribute a specific human act to one motive alone, any behaviour may be the result of several interacting motives. Successful fertility regulation involves many different acts and many different kinds of behaviour, and the motives for these vary in strength and from time to time. The desire to prevent a pregnancy may be uppermost when contraceptive supplies are procured but other factors may override this in the context of the sexual relationship. Much motivation is unconscious and may be in conflict with expressed wishes. Motives can be personal and unique to an individual or common to an entire population. All one can assume is that there is a complexity of motivation involved in all aspects of individual fertility regulation.

Bogue (1967) applied a general theory of motivation to the specific problem of family planning by developing a classification of motives operating towards high fertility on the one hand, and low fertility on the other hand. These ranged from personality needs to individual concern for community and national needs. The important point that Bogue makes is that both sets of motives, those favouring high fertility and those favouring low fertility, are operating at the same time. When people have large families it does not mean that they lack desires that would be satisfied by prevention of pregnancy but that other different needs are being satisfied by large families. In the same way, when women state that they wish to prevent a pregnancy and then fail to utilise the services and methods available there may be one or a number of factors involved in their lives that give meaning to their behaviour.

The Occurrence of Unwanted Pregnancies

In the present context the term 'unwanted' refers to a conception that was consciously unwanted before and at the time that it occurred. The complexity and variation in meaning of the word 'unwanted' when applied to birth control is fully discussed by Pohlman (1969).

A great number of unwanted conceptions occur when methods of fertility regulation are used inconsistently or incorrectly. This phenomenon has been referred to as 'WEUP' — wilful exposure to unwanted pregnancy. The term was originated by Lehfeldt (1959) after his study of 24 patients who, often repeatedly, exposed themselves to unwanted pregnancy when they had an adequate contraceptive method available. The exposure was usually related to conflicting motives. The WEUP studies were later extended to include newer methods of contraception such as oral contraceptives (Lehfeldt, 1965; Lehfeldt and Guze, 1966). Despite adequate instruction of patients, pills are often taken erratically and irregularly. Many of the women in the WEUP studies were prone to repeated 'accidents' in the use of contraception despite being fully aware of how the methods worked and the risks they were taking.

Ineffective use of methods of fertility regulation can be seen as a conflict of emotions or ambivalence towards pregnancy. Although a woman on one level knows that another child would create all sorts of problems for her, on another level she desires a pregnancy and will expose herself to the possibility of conceiving for one or a number of motives. The ambivalence may be unconscious and the woman herself unaware of it. Her behaviour may be affected by aspects of her own individual nature or perhaps more commonly by influences from her relationships with other people and by cultural attitudes.

Proof of Fertility

One motive suggested for exposure to unwanted pregnancy is the need to prove fertility. For females, pregnancy is proof of womanhood. Even if a woman does not want to have a child she may like to feel that she could have one if she so desired. Ability to conceive can be a matter of social status where women take a pride in their ability to conceive. Rainwater (1966) describes the 'Caribbean marriage' in which women go through several common-law unions and have a number of children before marrying. Legal marriage occurs later in their sexual and procreative lives when their fertility has been well established.

On the man's part fertility may be confused with virility. When a man is the proud father of several children this is often regarded as overt proof of his sexual prowess and the possibility that he has been irresponsible in regard to the use of contraception is of secondary importance. The desire of men for large families to prove their masculinity is part of a complex of male sex role expectations called machismo which includes dominance in relationships with women. Attempts have been made to examine machismo as one of the factors influencing the failure of contraception in certain cultures (Hill *et al.,* 1959). These studies carried out in the Caribbean found little evidence for any association with fertility but, as Back and Hass (1973) suggest, what may be important is that the women believe that their husbands want a lot of children even if the men do not.

Rewards for Childbearing Versus Contraception

The instinctive nature of motherhood or fatherhood may make a birth rewarding in itself, but there are many other personal and social rewards for procreation.

Many women are already tied to the home with children or may never have had the chance to develop alternatives to a full-time mothering role. If they go out to work the job is likely to be something convenient for shopping or collecting the children from school and not of a particularly interesting or skilled nature. For them, having another baby is the most obvious means of achieving self-esteem or expressing creativity. In some marriage relationships pregnancy is the time when the woman receives the most care, attention and tenderness from her husband. Rainwater (1960) observes '. . . . many women indicated that the only time they really felt their husbands close to them and deeply interested in them was when they were pregnant. When this is the case, it is easy to see that motivation to limit pregnancies is reduced'. In a social sense, having a baby is more often than not highly celebrated, parents are much congratulated and the event is generally approved of and given much attention. Regular visits to the family planning clinic do not have such social rewards and may be embarrassing to talk about, as the visits are an overt admission of plans for sexual intercourse.

The mass media may also exert an influence on the success of fertility regulation. Pregnancies, births and attempts to conceive are much more interesting news and of greater dramatic and romantic content than the use of birth control. A brief viewing of a 'life situation' television series will prove the point. When birth control does receive publicity this often emphasises the dangers of various methods. In addition television commercials are apt to over-glamourise babies and children, showing large families, all very happy, well housed, well fed and nicely dressed. The reality of too many children is often vastly different.

Contraception still does not have the respectability of motherhood, and the rewards for its use are less obvious. When a woman chooses to limit her births it is often for economic reasons, to improve or maintain the quality of life for the family, to enable her to go out to work or to be involved in more activities out of the home. There is thus some reward for continued attention to contraception, but it is indirect and negative — take a pill and nine months later there is no new baby to look after.

There may be social attitudes towards not having enough children. Rainwater (1965) in an analysis of rationales for family size, found it possible to extract one central norm: 'one shouldn't have more children than one can support, but one should have as many children as one can afford'. He found that to have fewer children than one had the means to keep was regarded as an expression of selfishness. We have frequently encountered the attitude that it is one's duty to have children if one can find the money.

The Decision to Practise Contraception

Decision-making is relevant: successful birth control starts off with a disadvantage because it implies that a conscious decision must be made and deliberate action taken. Pregnancy, on the other hand, often results from an avoidance of making a firm decision or postponement of the necessary behaviour. In other words, it is easier to do nothing. Some methods of contraception require that the decision be made for each sexual act, which sets stringent requirements for consistency of habit in a matter as impulsive and intimate as sex. Also, for some couples who do little planning for the future in a general sense, living from one pay packet to another or from one social security cheque to the next, planning for children or planning to go to the family planning clinic may be alien to their way of life.

Attributes of Fertility Regulating Methods

Other factors operating against the effective use of contraception are concerned with the attributes of the method itself. Side-effects such as changes in menstrual patterns may be frightening or disconcerting to women who do not fully understand the functioning of their bodies. Side-effects may also have social implications. For example, the lack of success of intra-uterine devices and low-dose progestagen oral contraceptives in India is partly due to the fact that they can cause prolonged and irregular bleeding and religious strictures forbid a menstruating woman to prepare food and engage in sexual activity. For some women who are inhibited about touching their own bodies, the use of certain methods may create guilt feelings and conflict if they have been brought up to consider such behaviour as bad. There is no doubt that feeling for threads of an intra-uterine device or inserting a cap is a distasteful experience for many women who attend family planning clinics seeking assistance in pregnancy prevention. Crowded living accommodation with lack of privacy or bathroom facilities may make it awkward for more modest women to use barrier methods of contraception. Such attributes of methods may produce feelings that counteract a strong desire to facilitate fertility regulation.

The use of many methods including oral contraception involve clinical procedures that can be a source of anxiety and embarrassment, such as pelvic examinations and answering questions about bleeding and sexual intercourse. The logistics of provision of a method, such as transport to the clinic, what to do with the children on clinic visits and having to take time off work to get there, are all relevant to the use of contraception.

What is important to a woman who wishes to prevent conception is how a method is used; who provides it, where and when it is provided and what is involved in its continued use? — all these factors may be more important than the theoretical effectiveness of the method in preventing a pregnancy or the side-effects and safety factors. It is not the objective properties of the contraceptive method but the individual's perception of the method that is likely to determine birth control behaviour.

Communication and Birth Control

An important factor considered in many studies investigating the determinants of fertility regulating behaviour is the matter of communication between sexual partners (Stycos *et al.*, 1956; Hill *et al.*, 1959; Rainwater, 1965; Cartwright, 1970). It may seem strange but there is much evidence to suggest that many couples, although they engage in sexual intercourse, cannot or do not talk to each other about anything to do with it. Embarrassment or distance between sexual partners make communication about birth control difficult.

When a girl exposes herself to the risk of pregnancy with a casual acquaintance it is often because she does not know how to approach such a practical subject as contraception in an impulsive or emotional situation. In a study of the sexual behaviour of American negro adolescents it was found that many of the girls had a fairly sophisticated knowledge of methods of birth control, but that one of the factors operating against effective use was their embarrassment over discussing sexual matters with their boyfriends (Hammond and Ladner, 1969).

Even in the marriage relationship the co-operation necessary for the effective use of contraception may be lacking. Many husbands and wives find it difficult to talk to each other about the number of children they would like, methods of birth control and general sexual matters. This often means that the weight of responsibility for decision and action falls on only one partner.

Social and Psychological Influences and the Intra-uterine Device

Many of the psychological factors that can interfere with successful prevention of pregnancy are of more obvious relevance to barrier methods of contraception which are closely associated with the sexual act. More modern methods such as the intra-uterine device are not immune.

When the intra-uterine device was reintroduced on a large scale as a result of an international conference in 1962 (Tietze, 1962) it seemed to be a highly suitable method, its theoretical effectiveness and effectiveness in practice being the same. The method is independent of the sexual act; the device is fitted and removed by a third party; and no repetitive action is required by the user. Nearly all other methods of birth control allow for more influence from social and psychological factors as far as continued motivation is concerned. However, the intra-uterine device may be removed for a variety of reasons other than desired pregnancy and this occurs at rates which vary widely between different clinics. Spontaneous expulsions also occur with different frequencies and may apparently be unnoticed by the user. Side-effects acceptable to one user may justify its removal to another. Wide variations have been found in the use-effectiveness of the intra-uterine device related to attributes both of the clinic or personnel who provide the device and of the users themselves (Tietze and Lewit, 1970; Bernard, 1970). Even pregnancy rates show mysterious inconsistencies. In a British study of intra-uterine device use it was found that clinics in different towns with patients of similar age and parity using the same intra-uterine device and served by the same doctor showed very different pregnancy rates (Snowden, 1972). The more research carried out to evaluate intra-uterine devices the more the interrelationships between 'provider related', 'culture related' and 'user related' variables are seen to be complex.

In any evaluation study, events that may occur after the fitting of a device, such as pregnancy, expulsion and removal, are known to the provider, but a number of patients will be classified as lost to follow-up and for this group such event rates will be unknown. This means that recorded event rates are minimum estimates, and the actual event rates may be higher (Hawkins, 1969). Vaginal discharge, menstrual disturbance and pelvic pain may be associated with the use of an intra-uterine device. There is always the possibility that these are symptoms of medical complications such as cervical erosion, vaginal infection, menstrual disorder, pelvic inflammatory disease, perforation of the uterus or cervical cancer. If not dealt with at clinic check-ups the patient may require admission to the acute gynaecological unit of a hospital and the provider of the contraceptive service will remain in ignorance. The relevance of not knowing what has happened to some women is pointed out by Hawkins (1970) who stresses the necessity for tracing and visiting defaulters from clinics for their own safety as well as for accurate statistical evaluation of devices. When a patient fails to return to the clinic it may be that nothing is wrong but is is easy for an expulsion to remain unnoticed by the user with resulting pregnancy. Adherence to follow-up procedures is of importance for the effective use of an intra-uterine device.

Factors Relating to Clinic Attendance for the Intra-uterine Device

We have been examining attributes of the marital relationship of family planning patients that might affect successful fertility regulating behaviour (Whitlock, Z. and Hawkins, D.F., unpublished observations). All the women in the study had expressed a desire to prevent conception and had elected to use the intra-uterine device. Many did not keep their follow-up appointments and failed to return even when a reminder letter was sent. This variation in attendance behaviour made it possible to select groups of good and poor attenders for comparison.

The emphasis in our study was on the extent of emotional support and solidarity in patients' relationships with their husbands. Emotional support was assessed in terms of the amount of perceived 'togetherness' or 'jointness' as opposed to perceived isolation or segregatedness in the way that the couples carried out their marital roles. Domestic activities can be shared, interchangeable or carried out by one partner. Decisions can be made jointly or separately with or without discussion. The amount of perceived understanding can vary, as can ease of communication between partners. An extensive home interview and questionnaire was completed for each of the 188 women in the study, in order to assess their conjugal relationships.

It was found that good attendance at the clinic was associated with emotional support in various different areas of marital activity. Distributions of good and poor attender responses for a few selected questionnaire items are shown in *Tables 16.1–5*. In the area of domestic decision making (*Table 16.1*) it can be seen that among good attenders there was a greater proportion of 'both equally' responses indicating joint decision making. In the poor attender group, there was a greater proportion of 'husband always' and 'wife always' responses indicating more segregation of roles. *Table 16.2* shows an example of one domestic task, washing-up. As one would expect it was rare for the husband to always do the washing-up. The difference between groups is shown by a greater proportion of 'both equally' responses in the good attender group, indicating more sharing on the part of the husband in the wife's work. *Table 16.3* shows one aspect of the sexual relationship where good attendance is associated with more mutuality of pleasure. The item shown in *Table 16.4* assesses the extent of intimate communication between conjugal partners. Discussion about menstruation is of particular relevance to the intra-uterine device method of contraception as typical side-effects are increased pain and bleeding. A response of 'Yes, I can talk to my husband about period pain and bleeding' was much more common among good attenders. *Table 16.5* shows a direct measure of emotional support for attending the family planning clinic. A greater proportion of the husbands

Table 16.1 DOMESTIC DECISIONS AND FAMILY PLANNING CLINIC ATTENDANCE
Who usually decides what you will do on holiday?

	Husband always	Husband more	Both equally	Wife more	Wife always	Number of respondents
Good attenders	11%	3%	77%	3%	6%	95
Poor attenders	31%	5%	50%	1%	13%	92

Table 16.2 DOMESTIC TASKS AND FAMILY PLANNING CLINIC ATTENDANCE
Who usually does the washing-up?

	Husband always	Husband more	Both equally	Wife more	Wife always	Number of respondents
Good attenders	1%	0%	25%	10%	64%	95
Poor attenders	1%	0%	11%	9%	79%	92

Table 16.3 THE SEXUAL RELATIONSHIP AND FAMILY PLANNING CLINIC ATTENDANCE
Who do you think gets the most pleasure out of sex?

	Husband always	Husband more	Both equally	Wife more	Wife always	Number of respondents
Good attenders	11%	14%	75%	0%	0%	95
Poor attenders	56%	10%	34%	0%	0%	92

Table 16.4 THE SEXUAL RELATIONSHIP AND FAMILY PLANNING CLINIC ATTENDANCE
Can you talk to your husband about period pain and bleeding?

	Yes	No	Number of respondents
Good attenders	88%	12%	95
Poor attenders	48%	52%	92

Table 16.5 HUSBAND SUPPORT FOR FAMILY PLANNING CLINIC ATTENDANCE
Does your husband ask how you got on at the clinic?

	Always	Sometimes	Never	Number of respondents
Good attenders	64%	17%	19%	95
Poor attenders	38%	32%	30%	92

of good attenders appear always to enquire about clinic visits whereas the husbands of poor attenders are more likely never to ask.

The tables show only a few examples of the different facets of marital interaction and the theme demonstrated in these results was typical throughout the study.

In the present study the conjugal relationship was assessed purely from interviews with wives. Thus responses are the wife's report of her perception of the actual behaviour that takes place with the domestic situation. This does not affect the conclusions drawn from results as what is important for assessment of emotional support is the way that the woman perceives her relationship.

Conclusion

There are many social and personal factors that may influence the success of attempts to regulate fertility other than a desire to prevent conception. Some of those mentioned still lack validation and are in the form of hypotheses. It can be assumed however that for every aspect of birth control behaviour there is a complex structure of psychological influences dependent on the individual user and his or her social environment.

Particular attention has been paid to emotional support factors in the marital relationship of women who want to prevent conception. Studies previous to our own have found similar associations between joint organisation of marital roles and behaviour to affect fertility regulation (for example: Hill *et al.*, 1959; Blood and Wolfe, 1960; Rainwater, 1960 and 1965; Chilmar, 1968; Mitchell, 1972). Some of these studies were carried out before the widespread use of intra-uterine contraception and it is interesting that marital interaction appears to play such an important part in the use of methods that superficially appear to have little need for male cooperation. One reason for this may be concerned with the attributes of family planning clinics. To many women visiting a clinic is a frightening and anxiety-provoking experience or at least an unpleasant duty. In this context it is not surprising that emotional support from the husband may be a crucial factor in determining whether a woman will return at regular intervals for her necessary examinations and supplies.

REFERENCES

BACK, K.W. and HASS, P.H. (1973). Family structure and fertility control. In *Psychological Perspectives on Population*, pp. 75–105. Ed. Fawcett, J.T. Basic Books, New York

BERNARD, R.P. (1970). IUD performance patterns – a 1970 world view. *J. Int. Fed. Gynecol. Obstet.,* 8, 926–940

BLOOD, R.O. and WOLFE, D.M. (1960). *Husbands and Wives: the Dynamics of Married Living.* Free Press of Glencoe, New York

BOGUE, D. (1967). What are the motives for and against birth control in various cultures? *Mass Communication and Motivation for Birth Control. Proceedings of Summer Workshop at the University of Chicago,* pp. 21–25. Ed. Bogue, D.J. Community and Family Study Centre, University of Chicago

CARTWRIGHT, A. (1970). *Parents and Family Planning Services*, pp. 140–157. Routledge and Kegan Paul, London

CHILMAN, C. (1968). Fertility and Poverty in the United States: Some implications for family planning programs, evaluation, and research. *J. Marriage Fam.,* 30, 207–227

HAMMOND, B.E. and LADNER, J.A. (1969). Socialization into sexual behaviour in negro slum ghetto. In *The Individual, Sex and Society*, pp. 41–51. Ed. Broderick, C.B. and Bernard, J. Johns Hopkins Press, Baltimore

HAWKINS, D.F. (1969). Complications with IUDs. *Br. med. J.,* ii, 381

HAWKINS, D.F. (1970). Intra-uterine contraception. *Practitioner,* 205, 20–29

HILL, R., STYCOS, J.M. and BACK, K. (1959). *The Family and Population Control.* University of North Carolina Press, Chapel Hill

LEHFELDT, H. (1959). Willful exposure to unwanted pregnancy (WEUP).

Psychological explanation for patient failures in contraception. *Am. J. Obstet. Gynec.*, **78**, 661–665

LEHFELDT, H. (1965). Psychological aspects of planned parenthood. *J. Sex Research*, **1**, 97–103

LEHFELDT, H. and GUZE, H. (1966). Psychological factors in contraceptive failure. *Fert. Steril.*, **17**, 110–116

MITCHELL, R.E. (1972). Husband-wife relations and family-planning practices in urban Hong Kong. *J. Marriage Fam.*, **34**, 139–146

POHLMAN, E.H. (1969). *Psychology of Birth Planning*, pp. 177–197. Schenkman, Cambridge, Massachusetts

RAINWATER, L. (1960). *And the Poor Get Children: Sex, Contraception and Family Planning in the Working Class*, p. 84. Quadrangle Books, Chicago

RAINWATER, L. (1965). *Family Design: Marital Sexuality, Family Size and Contraception*. Aldine, Chicago

RAINWATER, L. (1966). Crucible of Identity: the negro lower class family. *J. Am. Acad. Arts Sci.*, **95**, 172–216

SNOWDEN, R. (1972). Social and personal factors involved in the use-effectiveness of the I.U.D. *Proceedings of the Family Planning Research Conference, a Multidisciplinary Approach. Exeter, England, September 27–28, 1971. International Congress Series No. 260*, pp. 74–81. Ed. Goldsmith, A. and Snowden, R. Excerpta Medica, Amsterdam

STYCOS, J.M., BACK, K. and HILL, R. (1956). Problems of communication between husband and wife on matters relating to family limitation. *Human Relations*, **9**, 207–215

TIETZE, C. (1962). Intrauterine contraceptive rings: history and statistical appraisal. *Intrauterine Contraceptive Devices. Proceedings of the Conference, April 30–May 1, 1962, New York City. Excerpta Medica, International Congress Series No. 54*, pp. 9–20. Ed. Tietze, C. and Lewit, S. Excerpta Medica, Amsterdam

TIETZE, C. and LEWIT, S. (1970). Evaluation of intrauterine devices: ninth progress report of the Co-operative Statistical Program. *Stud. Fam. Plann.*, **55**, 1–40

17 Special Groups of Patients

TEENAGERS

With physical and psychological maturity occurring progressively earlier and the age of marriage getting later it is inevitable that more and more adolescents experiment with sex or have regular sexual experiences outside marriage. In countries in Asia, South America and Africa pregnancy among adolescent girls is quite common, with 10–20% of total births being to women under 20 years of age. There has not been a notable increase in these figures during the last decade. In contrast there has been a marked increase in the United States of America and in Europe. For example, between 1963 and 1972 the percentage of total births to women under the age of 20 in the United States of America rose from 14.5 to 19.3%, in the German Democratic Republic from 13.6 to 23% and in Yugoslavia from 8.3 to 14.4% (Hunt, 1976). It is interesting to note that in Denmark and Sweden, where sexual freedom occurred much earlier, the figures have dropped from 11.8% and 11.7% respectively in 1963 to 6.8% and 7.5% respectively in 1972.

Among girls who are under 16 years of age, pregnancy has always been relatively common in cultures such as those found in Asia where early marriage is prevalent. In Europe and North America the incidence of pregnancy in this group, although low, is rising. In England and Wales in 1976 there were 1428 births and 3412 legal abortions performed on girls under 16 years of age.

The reasons for increasing sexual activity among the young are the pressures of urbanised society in which sexual prowess or more subtle sexuality is stressed as being important, and earlier physical maturation and onset of puberty. The social consequences of pregnancy among teenagers are many, and include interrupted education of the mother and reduced job opportunities with consequent financial problems. Unplanned teenage pregnancies make a notable contribution to the numbers of single parent families, either directly or by causing stress leading to a broken marriage. Consequently the children are also at risk of psychological and social maladjustment. The obstetric risks of pregnancy in young teenagers include a higher incidence of maternal death (Efiong and Banjoko, 1975), pre-eclamptic toxaemia (Russell, 1968), complications of labour, prematurity and low birth weight infants (Roopnarinesingh, 1970). Medical complications may include an increased risk of developing squamous cell carcinoma of the cervix in later life.

For these many reasons it is desirable to prevent unwanted pregnancy among sexually active teenagers. The delivery of family planning services to this group is difficult. They are considered to be minors in many countries and the provision of contraception may therefore be illegal or allowed only to married patients with their husbands' consent. For example, in Hungary intra-uterine devices may not be fitted in girls under the age of 18 years. In Great Britain it is illegal for a male to have sexual intercourse with a female who is under 16 years of age, although the police do not usually prosecute unless the girl is under 14. A doctor prescribing contraceptives for such a girl might conceivably be accused of 'aiding and abetting' in this crime. It is advisable that a doctor seeks the permission of the girl's parents, provided that she is willing for this to be done. Should this consent not be given, then it is up to the individual medical practitioner to decide whether to prescribe contraception or not. It is unlikely that a doctor is at legal risk if he provides contraceptive advice for a girl under 16 years of age if he acts in good faith to protect the girl against the potentially harmful effects of sexual intercourse (Medical Defence Union, 1974).

In the United States of America the exact legal position varies from State to State. The Committee on Education in Family Life, set up by the American College of Obstetricians and Gynecologists, recommended that when necessary, the physician should provide contraceptive advice without the parents' knowledge. The physician should seek consultation with a colleague when he has doubts about a minor's responsibility and maturity, but the minor involved in sexual activity should have the right to contraceptive services, with or without parental consent. In California, there is the concept of 'emancipated minors', aged 15 or over, living away from home and managing their own affairs. Minors who are emancipated, married, divorced or serving in the armed services may consent to all types of medical care, and those in receipt of Welfare payments are cited by the law as able to give their own consent to family planning services.

Knowledge of contraceptive methods is poor among the young despite an increase in sex education in schools. Teenagers are also often unaware of the availability of services and they can easily be put off by patronising or moralising attitudes among clinic staff. Even though psychological maturity lags behind physical maturity, the teenager seeking contraceptive advice feels mature and emancipated and needs to be treated as such. When information about contraception or the provision of a method is sought, the sexual partner ought also to be involved where possible and other conditions such as venereal disease discussed at the same time as contraceptive advice is given. With teenagers coitus is often unplanned and may be infrequent. Motivation to prevent pregnancy may be less in teenage males than in females and in some situations, with a socially irresponsible male or a girl who wants to get married, such motivation may be entirely absent. Deliberate 'risk-taking' is a well-known phenomenon. Whilst the mortality associated with the use of any form of contraception by teenagers is very low, much lower than that from the consequences of unprotected intercourse (Tietze, 1977), some problems arise with the use of each form of contraception by teenagers. With these considerations in mind what contraceptive methods are most suitable for teenagers?

Oral Contraception

Though extremely effective this relies on regular pill-taking, which requires motivation and a planned sex life. To use oral contraceptives implies a premeditated intention to indulge in sexual intercourse which many young girls do not have, as well as the ability and motivation to take the pills regularly. Another problem is the development of the 'whore syndrome'. When boy-friends discover that a girl is taking the pill, they tend to take acquiescence to a request for intercourse for granted — a situation which is unacceptable to many teenage girls. Some teenagers react adversely to the minor side-effects which often occur in the first one or two cycles. Such factors can combine to give a patient failure rate of as high as 15% (Tietze and Lewit, 1971). Another dis-advantage for the adolescent is that suppression of ovulation with oral contra-ceptive steroids before the menstrual cycle has become regularly established may increase the chance of eventually developing post-pill amenorrhoea (*see* Hunt, 1976, for references). Finally, there is a small chance that the administra-tion of contraceptive pills containing oestrogen to girls who have not completed growth might accelerate epiphyseal closure. This risk should be given particular consideration with growth-retarded girls.

Intra-uterine Devices

The insertion of an intra-uterine device reduces the problem of poor motivation, but complication rates are in general increased in young nulliparous patients, making follow-up visits important for safety. It is possible to insert the smaller copper devices in such patients without too much difficulty, but expulsion rates are relatively high (Snowden *et al.*, 1977a and b; Weiner *et al.*, 1978). Pregnancy rates for intra-uterine devices in these patients are increased but they may well be lower than with a combined oral contraceptive taken irregularly. Recent suggestions that the intra-uterine device may predispose to pelvic inflammatory disease provide a cause for concern in nulliparous girls, particularly among those who may already be at increased risk for pelvic infection because of sexual promiscuity. Again, the fitting of an intra-uterine device and regular follow-up implies a premeditated and regular sex life which is contrary to the usual sexual pattern of teenagers.

Barrier Methods

Diaphragms

This method of contraception is effective (Vessey and Wiggins, 1974) provided it is used carefully. One problem is that nulliparous teenage girls often find the gynaecological procedures of fitting a diaphragm daunting. Use of a diaphragm requires preparation for each act of intercourse, practice at insertion, privacy for this to be carried out, and facilities for washing and storing the diaphragm. Despite these potential disadvantages a recent study from the United States among young girls of low social class reported a high rate of contraceptive effectiveness and continuation (Lane *et al.*, 1976).

Condoms

These should be especially suitable for unmarried teenagers because their use does not require any preparation or long term planning and they are available from many retail outlets. Provided they are always used correctly they probably provide the safest contraceptive measure, with a significant degree of protection from venereal disease, which may be common among sexually active teenagers (Barlow, 1977). Evidence that the development of atypical squamous metaplasia with its neoplastic potential is more prevalent among sexually promiscuous adolescents (Singer, 1975) suggests that the use of a condom might protect the cervix from the aetiological factor associated with intercourse, whether it be seminal fluid or a virus which is introduced at that time.

It would appear that condoms might be the best protection for teenagers who may become involved in occasional, irregular and unpremeditated intercourse. Unfortunately, these are the very circumstances in which they are most likely to fail. Unfamiliarity with the sexual partner, embarrassment, haste and inhospitable physical surroundings all predispose to inadequate application, detumescence, displacement or abandoning of the condom, and failure to retain it in place until withdrawal is completed. It is in the stable liaison, or with the experienced woman who is always prepared to provide a condom and insist on its application and correct use, that these devices are most successful. Although it may be good advice to teenagers always to carry condoms, in practice this is only feasible for those who are sexually emancipated and can accept the possibility of adverse comment from peer groups or parents.

Postcoital Contraception

This is only of use when a single episode of unprotected intercourse has taken place at a time of the menstrual cycle when conception is possible. The use of high doses of oestrogen or progestagens (Chapter 4, pp. 114–118) or the insertion of a copper intra-uterine device (Gravigard or Gynae-T) have both been shown to be effective. The disadvantages of nausea and vomiting with oestrogens, and the risks of infection and perforation associated with the insertion of an intra-uterine device, make these methods suitable only on an occasional basis.

Contraceptive Counselling for Teenagers

Teenagers who have a relatively stable sexual relationship or a regular and premeditated sex life either come for contraceptive counselling or can be reached by the social agencies and counselling made available. The form of contraception best suited to their needs — oral contraceptives, intra-uterine devices, diaphragms or condoms — can then be provided.

Young people who are irregularly promiscuous often either realise the risk they are taking and present for advice, or come to a physician for related or unrelated reasons. In our opinion the opportunity should not be lost to enquire tactfully, in the absence of the parents and the presence of a chaperone, as to the teenager's sexual activities and possible need for advice. From time to time this may incur parental wrath. The competent physician should readily develop manoeuvres to deal with this situation. If he finds himself in difficulty he can always cite the various governmental health agencies and professional oragnisations which advocate education of teenagers in these matters.

The most difficult group of all are those most likely to acquire an unwanted pregnancy — the 'good' boys and girls. In developed countries the scene is seldom set by ignorance. The usual background is either thoughtlessness, with failure to face up to the fact that intercourse may take place, or the misplaced confidence that it will not occur. In practice, it does occur, conditioned by powerful emotional involvement, an unrecognised sexual drive, a persuasive partner or over-indulgence in alcohol. Moral precepts are best taught by example — didactic instruction on the virtues of celibacy does not help the boys and girls presented with these situations. Basic sex education in schools and education on the risks of unwanted pregnancy are essential. Sex education of the young requires very considerable ability to strike the balance between science, emotion and practicality appropriate to the group under instruction, without encouraging salaciousness, experimentation or reduction of sex to a simple physiological function. The example of those they respect and the fear of unwanted pregnancy may be the only supportive factors to protect the boy or girl placed in an adverse situation. Only realisation of the personal risk of conception may stimulate the teenager to seek contraceptive advice. It is therefore necessary to adopt a forthright and realistic attitude to this risk, although for some this involves the difficulty of accepting that their moral precepts are going to be broken. It must be conceded that the morality of this situation is decided by the individual, even if that individual is a teenager, if progress is to be made in preventing unwanted pregnancies. Formation of teenage morality is a matter for years of subtle influence and example, not formal instruction in moral codes of conduct.

THE OLDER WOMAN

It is not widely realised that the sexual potential of the human female is at its greatest between the ages of 35 and 45 (Kinsey *et al.*, 1953). The practical expression of this sexuality is limited by convention, social and economic pressures and the demands of motherhood and marriage. The consequent conflict can sometimes result in unanticipated bouts of considerable sexual activity by women in this age group.

Until recently contraception for women over 35 years of age was considered by most doctors in the same light as for younger women. The risks of long term use of combined oral contraceptives and the significantly increased risks of cardiovascular disease among women over 40 are now documented, and the particular risk to smokers in this group has been recognised. This has led to a general reappraisal of methods of fertility control for the older woman. In 1977 Tietze published estimates of mortality associated with fertility control methods which showed that for women under 30 years of age the risk of death associated with use of combined oral contraceptives, the intra-uterine device, barrier methods or first trimester abortion was very similar. The calculated annual risk of 1—2 fatalities per 100 000 women under 30 years of age was lower than the maternal mortality rate in women where no contraception was used. After the age of 40 women who smoked and who were on combined oral contraceptives had 2½ times the mortality risk associated with unprotected intercourse, the figures being 58 and 23 deaths per 100 000 women per year respectively. Women over 40 who used other methods of contraception and pill users who were non-smokers, had a mortality rate which was lower than the maternity mortality rate. Other studies have demonstrated an increase in death rates from cardiovascular disease among women on the pill when compared with other contraceptive methods, and particularly among those women who are over 35 years of age and who smoke (Mann *et al.*, 1976; Vessey *et al.*, 1977). For all ages the lowest mortality rate associated with contraception was found among users of barrier methods who resorted to early abortion in the event of failure, but it should be remembered that sterilisation is safer still.

Oral Contraceptives

As cardiovascular changes take place gradually and the actual magnitude of the risk is small there is time for adequate discussion about alternative methods of contraception. In general it is unwise for women over the age of 35 who smoke to continue on the combined oral contraceptive pill and certainly after the age of 40 there is an appreciable risk to smokers. If the patient is a non-smoker and not obese or hypertensive the risks are lower and should the patient so wish it is reasonable to continue with oral contraception if there are good reasons for preferring the pill to medically safer alternatives.

Should an older woman prefer oral contraception to other methods there is a good case for changing to the progestagen-only pills, which do not have the metabolic side-effects of oestrogen-containing preparations. The overall method failure rate for older women is 3—4 pregnancies per 100 woman-years, which is similar to that of the intra-uterine device or barrier methods. In older women the failure rates are relatively less because of declining fertility due partly to a higher proportion of naturally occurring anovulatory cycles and partly to less frequent opportunities for intercourse. An additional advantage of progestagen may be a reduction in premenstrual tension. A disadvantage is the difficulty in differentiating between the irregular bleeding which may occur with continuous progestagen therapy and that possibly due to gynaecological pathology. The daily ingestion of a steroid to prevent pregnancy when intercourse is becoming less frequent may not be an acceptable idea to many women.

Barrier Methods

These methods, which are related specifically to each act of intercourse, are particularly suitable for the older couple, whose coital frequency may be declining. Provided the methods are acceptable, the motivation among older women to use the diaphragm and among men to use the condom regularly and properly is high. The failure rate in this group for the diaphragm is 2—3 per 100 woman-years (Vessey and Wiggins, 1974) and less than 1 per 100 woman-years for condoms lubricated with a spermicide (Potts and McDevitt, 1975). These methods are at least as effective as the intra-uterine device or the progestagen-only pill and cause no side-effects. Lubricated condoms can be helpful if the vagina is dry. Barrier methods may cause problems with the application of the condom or insertion of the diaphragm if sexual problems are becoming manifest but skilful sexual counselling can lead to their incorporation in a successful ritual. Significant utero-vaginal prolapse in older women can make use of a diaphragm difficult or ineffective.

Abortion

Although the use of barrier methods, with early abortion in cases of failure, has been found to be medically the safest in terms of mortality, many older women find the thought of abortion particularly repugnant. Should this not be a problem a combination of barrier methods with abortion if needed should be considered as a method for the older woman. Whilst we would not wish to see any patient influenced to have an operation she does not want, in terms of objective logic where there is a case for abortion in these women there is nearly always an equally good case for sterilisation, possibly at the same time.

If menstrual irregularities occur in the older woman pregnancy may not be diagnosed until week 10 or 12 by which time the risks of termination of pregnancy have increased.

Intra-uterine Devices

This method, requiring no day-to-day motivation, gives an overall failure rate of 3—5 pregnancies per 100 woman-years. Among older women this figure is lower (Snowden *et al.*, 1977c). Many women who are changing from the pill seek a female orientated method of contraception and request insertion of a device. This procedure should be conducted with particular care — perforation rates are higher in older women. Menstrual flow may have been artificially reduced by the use of combined oral contraceptives, and if these are discontinued and an intra-uterine device inserted, unacceptable menorrhagia may ensue. This is more likely among women in the peri-menopausal years who are prone to suffer from heavy periods due to hormone dysfunction. The incidence of uterine fibromyomata is higher among older women and if large, fibroids may cause difficulty in insertion and limit the efficiency of an intra-uterine device. Fibroids may also exacerbate menorrhagia caused by an intra-uterine device.

Sterilisation

Many older women who have completed their families and wish to stop taking the pill seek sterilisation as the best method of fertility control. Since the reports about the risks of combined oral contraceptives, requests for sterilisation have increased markedly in Great Britain. This is a logical sequence of events and if the couple have relied on female contraception it is usually the woman who requests tubal ligation. Nevertheless it is important during counselling to mention vasectomy and in addition to emphasise that either procedure is in effect irreversible. Should the woman have menorrhagia with an intra-uterine device *in situ*, her cycle may need to be assessed after removal of the device. Should she continue to have heavy periods it should be emphasised that tubal sterilisation, however it is performed, may even exacerbate this symptom. If there is severe menorrhagia, particularly in association with any uterine abnormality such as fibroids, a hysterectomy is the appropriate operation for sterilisation.

Summary

The older woman should be encouraged to consider alternative methods to the combined oral contraceptives, though there is usually no need for an abrupt change. Sterilisation or the barrier methods probably offer the medically safest and most reliable alternatives, but full consideration must be given to the individual's requirements, sex life and life-style.

POSTPARTUM ORAL CONTRACEPTION

Combined Oral Contraceptives

Use of the combined pill during the immediate puerperium has led to anxiety that it may interfere with lactation, that it may increase the risks of thrombo-embolic episodes, and that it may mask causes of amenorrhoea such as posterior pituitary necrosis or the Chiari-Frommel syndrome.

Shulman (1972) did not find any cases of thrombosis or pulmonary embolism in 495 patients who started taking the combined pill during the immediate puerperium. The effect of combined pills on blood clotting during the early puerperium warrants further study before definite conclusions on safety can be drawn but the increased risk is probably very small. The incidence of postpartum pituitary damage is so very small as to constitute a theoretical rather than a practical consideration.

The combined pill can bring about diminution or cessation of lactation in some women (Bhiralens *et al.,* 1970; Miller and Hughes, 1970; Borglin and Sandholm, 1971). It has been suggested that the 19-nortestosterone compounds can be absorbed by the baby from the breast milk and this might lead to increased skeletal age in the infant (Breibart *et al.,* 1963) but Kates *et al.* (1969) found no such alteration among women taking sequential pills. Laumas *et al.* (1967), administering tritiated norethynodrel and mestranol to women having stillbirths, found only 1.1% of the isotope in the breast milk. Nilsson *et al.* (1977) found a plasma-milk ratio of about 7 with *d*-norgestrel and calculated that only 0.1% of the dose reached the baby and that this did not accumulate. Saxena *et al.* (1977) found a plasma-milk ratio of 10 for norethis-terone, again corresponding to about 0.1% of the dose reaching the baby. It seems unlikely that the amount of steroid the baby receives is of significance.

There are several advantages to starting combined oral contraception in the immediate puerperium. The risk of a pregnancy within the first two months of delivery is eliminated. This risk has been estimated as 5.6% by Sever (1971) and as 10.3% by Batts (1971). There is a more rapid return to cyclical bleeding than would be expected in the normal course of events (Wentz *et al.,* 1966). There is also some reduction in the lochia and the first postpartum menstrual loss tends to be reduced (Sands, 1966; Rech and Schwarz, 1966). Uterine involution, as assessed clinically, is in general unaltered, but Frank *et al.* (1969) did note that there was some histological evidence of delayed involution as shown by persistence of haemosiderin and inflammatory cell infiltrates in the myometrium. Four weeks postpartum, the effect of the oral contraceptive on the endometrium is to reduce the number and size of the glands and to render it atrophic, with minimal secretory activity.

The incidence of the usual side-effects of the combined pill, such as nausea and breakthrough bleeding, is low in the puerperium, nausea being recorded in only 17 out of 706 cycles by Rech and Schwarz (1966) and in 4 out of 106 patients by Kates *et al.* (1969). On the other hand breakthrough bleeding occurred in 47 out of 706 cycles and 5 out of 106 patients. Unwanted effects tend to occur more commonly during the first cycle of oral contraceptive use and their incidence in fact may be less than in the non-parturient oral contraceptive user.

A woman who starts oral contraceptives immediately after delivery does not seem to increase her chance of ovulatory failure when the pill is stopped.

Conclusion

The immediate postpartum use of combined oral contraceptives is a safe and effective means of contraception at an otherwise unpredictable time in the woman's reproductive life, when contraceptive methods such as diaphragms or intra-uterine devices may not be particularly applicable.

Low-dose Progestagen Preparations

An advantage of starting to take a low-dose progestagen preparation daily during the puerperium is that lactation is unaffected (Guiloff *et al.*, 1974). The amounts of progestagen reaching a breast fed baby are very small indeed, ranging from about $0.03\,\mu g$/day with *d*-norgestrel to about $0.3\,\mu g$/day with norethisterone (from data of Nilsson *et al.*, 1977 and Saxena *et al.*, 1977). The progestagens are suitable for patients in whom combined oral contraceptives are contraindicated. They do not usually inhibit ovulation. Their disadvantages are that they do not control the onset of menstruation in the same way as the combined preparations, and that episodes of irregular bleeding are likely to occur in the early puerperium. In one of our controlled studies using norethisterone, $0.35\,\mu g$ daily, discontinuations for bleeding problems were 14.7 per 100 woman-years when this progestagen was started one week postpartum, compared with 7.5 per 100 woman-years when it was started 6 or more weeks after the confinement (Hawkins, D.F. and Tothill, A.U., unpublished observations). In general the higher pregnancy rate renders continued use of progestagen-only preparations undesirable unless the woman is merely anxious to postpone the next pregnancy for a few months.

There have been relatively few studies of the use of low-dose progestagen preparations in the postpartum patient. Moggia *et al.* (1972) used $300\,\mu g$ of quingestanol acetate. This study involved 652 patients, 80% of whom were postpartum, and they were followed up for a total of 6201 cycles. Sixteen pregnancies resulted, of which seven appeared to be due to method failure – a rate of 1.2 per 100 woman-years. However, 80% of patients were on the progestagen preparation during the relatively infertile period of postpartum amenorrhoea, which lasted on average for 2.5 months.

Quingestanol acetate tends to increase menstrual flow and also to increase the mean length of the menstrual cycle during the first few months of treatment. These rapidly return to normal. The average cycle length is close to the pre-treatment value, but there are approximately 20% of short cycles ($\leqslant$24 days) and 20% of long cycles ($\geqslant$34 days). Breakthrough bleeding is a problem in that 35% of patients have some intermenstrual bleeding during 7% of all the cycles. These figures are comparable to those found with the use of quingestanol in the non-puerperal woman. Some patients consider that there is a slight reduction in lactation. No other significant side-effects were recorded.

In our own studies (Hawkins and Benster, 1977) we were concerned with a rather unreliable suburban London population, the majority of the patients being a few weeks postpartum. The overall pregnancy rates with low-dose progestagens were 5–6 per 100 woman-years, of which about half were method failures, the remainder being clearly attributable to omitting to take the pills. The progestagens were most successful when they were used on a short-term basis by women who merely intended to postpone the next pregnancy for a few months; considerably higher pregnancy rates resulted when the analysis was confined to women who intended to take the progestagen pill for a year or more. The ectopic gestation rates with these three compounds were 0.8–0.9 per 100 woman-years, which suggests that although the progestagens do not cause ectopic gestation, they do not prevent it. Most discontinuations for bleeding problems occurred in the first three months; the incidence of abnormal bleeding was least with norethisterone, 0.35 mg daily, and somewhat greater with chlormadinone acetate, 0.5 mg or megestrol acetate, 0.5 mg in oil. There were very few other side-effects, and patients with varicose veins or a history of thrombophlebitis or liver disease took the progestagens without ensuing complications. In another study (Hawkins, D.F. and Tothill, A.U., unpublished observations) norethisterone, 0.35 mg, used as a postpartum oral contraceptive did not interfere with lactation.

A new chloro-substituted derivative of chlormadinone, started one week postpartum, was tested by McEwan *et al.* (1977). The effectiveness of the progestagen did not differ significantly from that of norethisterone, but the incidence of bleeding problems was higher with the new compound than with norethisterone. There was no interference with lactation.

Conclusion

Low-dose progestagen oral contraceptives are particularly useful postpartum on a temporary basis for lactating women, for the relatively infertile and for women in whom combined oral contraception is contra-indicated. With long-term use there is a greater risk of pregnancy and of menstrual abnormality than with combined oral contraceptives.

Barrier Methods

Condoms

These are a particularly suitable method for the puerperium. They have no side-effects, lactation is unaffected and as fertility is low they provide very adequate protection against another pregnancy. The protection of cervical cells undergoing metaplasia from spermatozoa and seminal plasma during and immediately after the first pregnancy may be a factor in preventing carcinoma of the cervix (Coppleson and Reid, 1967). Condoms provide this protection.

Diaphragms

The progressive involution of the vagina makes fitting unsatisfactory during the immediate puerperium and this method should only be considered about two months after delivery.

Intra-uterine Devices

In general, the expulsion rate of routine devices inserted either at delivery or in the early puerperium is sufficiently high as to be discouraging (Phatak and Vishwaneth, 1966; Swartz *et al.*, 1967; see Zatuchni, 1970; Banharnsupawat and Rosenfield, 1971; Diamond and Freeman, 1973; Shervington, 1974). On the other hand, some enthusiasts working with specialised devices such as the Birnberg bow (Burnhill and Birnberg, 1966) and the Dalkon shield (Emens, 1973) have obtained better results. The Petal (Lem) device (Rashbaum and Wallach, 1971) which contains copper and has legs that should fold up during the involution process was designed for postpartum patients but it is not widely used as there are fairly high rates of expulsions and removals for pain or bleeding. The Combined Multiload CU-250 is currently being tested for postpartum use (Emens, J.M., personal communication).

The rates of uterine perforation are bound to be increased in relation to postpartum insertion. Disappearance of the threads is also a problem (Phatak and Chandorkar, 1970). It is difficult to know if irregular bleeding is due to retained products of conception or to the device.

Injectables

The use of a single injection of medroxyprogesterone acetate (150 mg) or norethisterone oenanthate (200 mg) is particularly useful in the puerperium. It does not affect involution of the genital tract and gives good protection against pregnancy for about 8 weeks until a decision as to future use of contraception can be taken.

It has been found that medroxyprogesterone acetate passes freely into breast milk, with a 1:1 concentration gradient from maternal plasma (Saxena *et al.*, 1977). In these circumstances, depot injections for contraceptive purposes are best avoided in lactating women.

CONTRACEPTION AFTER LEGAL ABORTION

It is important that arrangements for effective contraception should be instituted at the time of the abortion, before the patient leaves hospital, if repetition of the problem is to be avoided. Many patients do not keep follow-up appointments, and to refer them elsewhere for contraceptive advice invites default. Barrier methods are not in general suitable as the patient has already demonstrated her lack of the sort of motivation which is necessary to use condoms or diaphragms reliably. In practice the choice of method usually lies between an intra-uterine device inserted at the time of the operation, a combined oestrogen—progestagen oral contraceptive started a day or two after the abortion, a progestagen injection and sterilisation. It is necessary to discuss the choice with the patient before the abortion.

Intra-uterine devices inserted directly the uterus has been evacuated are quite successful (*see* Chapter 10, p. 202). The devices are not so commonly expelled as after a confinement, but devices such as a Lippes loop D or an Antigon, which are less liable to expulsion, should be used. Infection is not a common problem but it is desirable to see the patient after one or two weeks to check that infection has not occurred and after one month to verify that the device is still in place. Combined oral contraceptives may be started the day after the abortion, or five days later, without interfering with the redevelopment of a regular menstrual cycle. A long acting progestagen injection may be given immediately after the abortion and arrangements made for a nurse to visit the patient at home and repeat the injection or make arrangements for alternative contraception eight weeks later. If the patient considers that sterilisation is the best solution to her problems, then either a device may be inserted or a progestagen injection given, and a date fixed for readmission for sterilisation. In certain cases it may be concluded that the only realistic solution is sterilisation in conjunction with the abortion, but sometimes this approach is best avoided (*see* Chapter 15, pp. 354—357).

For the young nullipara the choice will usually lie between oral contraception and an intra-uterine device. If it is felt that the pills will be taken reliably, or under reliable supervision, then the eventual risk of post-pill amenorrhoea and its consequences is relatively small in a girl who has already shown her ability to conceive. An intra-uterine device requires less patient motivation but conveys a small risk of infection and interference with fertility at some later date.

Conclusion

The parous woman is well served by an intra-uterine device inserted at the time of the abortion, oral contraception being a reasonable alternative. Long-acting progestagen injections are desirable for those with poor memories for pills or follow-up appointments, if home visits can be arranged.

For the older woman, sterilisation is the most appropriate manoeuvre; an intra-uterine device may suffice if sterilisation is not acceptable.

REFERENCES

BANHARNSUPAWAT, L. and ROSENFIELD, A.G. (1971). Immediate postpartum IUD insertion. *Obstet. Gynec., N.Y.,* **38**, 276—285
BARLOW, D. (1977). The condom and gonorrhoea. *Lancet,* **ii**, 811—813
BATTS, J.A. (1971). Hospital-based family planning program. *Am. J. Obstet. Gynec.,* **110**, 49—53
BHIRALENS, P., CHIEMPRASERT, T. and KOETSAWANG, S. (1970). Effects of oral gestagens upon lactation. In *Post-partum Family Planning. A Report on the International Program,* pp. 345—356. Ed. Zatuchni, G.A. McGraw-Hill, New York

BORGLIN, N.E. and SANDHOLM, L.E. (1971). Effect of oral contraceptives on lactation. *Fert. Steril.*, **22**, 39–41

BREIBART, S., BONGIOVANNI, A.M. and EBERLEIN, W.R. (1963). Progestins and skeletal maturation. *New Engl. J. Med.*, **268**, 255

BURNHILL, M.S. and BIRNBERG, C.H. (1966). Contraception with an intrauterine bow inserted immediately post partum. An interim report. *Obstet. Gynec., N.Y.*, **28**, 329–331

COMMITTEE ON EDUCATION IN FAMILY LIFE (1976). *The Management of Sexual Crises in the Minor Female.* American College of Obstetricians and Gynecologists

COPPLESON, M. and REID, B.L. (1967). *Preclinical Carcinoma of the Cervix Uteri*, p. 93. Pergamon Press, Oxford

DIAMOND, R.A. and FREEMAN, D.W. (1973). Insertion of intrauterine devices in the early postpartum period. *Minn. Med.*, **56**, 49–50

EFIONG, E.I. and BANJOKO, M.O. (1975). Obstetric performance of Nigerian primigravidae aged 16 and under. *Br. J. Obstet. Gynaec.*, **82**, 228–233

EMENS, J.M. (1973). Insertion of the Dalkon shield post-partum. *Dalkon Shield Symposium, London, October 11th, 1972*, pp. 18–21. Ed. Templeton, J.S. A.H. Robins, Horsham, Sussex

FRANK, R., ALPERN, W.M. and ESHBAUGH, D.E. (1969). Oral contraception started early in the puerperium. *Am. J. Obstet. Gynec.*, **103**, 112–118

GUILOFF, E., IBARRA-POLO, A., ZANARTU, J., TOSCANINI, C., MISCHLER, T.W. and GOMEZ-ROGERS, C. (1974). Effect of contraception on lactation. *Am. J. Obstet. Gynec.*, **118**, 42–45

HAWKINS, D.F. and BENSTER, B. (1977). A comparative study of three low-dose progestogens, chlormadinone acetate, megestrol acetate and norethisterone, as oral contraceptives. *Br. J. Obstet. Gynaec.*, **84**, 708–713

HUNT, W.B. II (1976). Adolescent fertility – risks and consequences. *Population Reports*, series J, number 10, 157–175

KATES, R.B., GOSS, D.A. and TOWNES, P.J. (1969). Immediate postpartum use of sequential oral contraceptive therapy. *Sth. med. J.*, **62**, 694–696

KINSEY, A.C., POMEROY, W.B., MARTIN, C.E. and GEBHARD, P.H. (1953). *Sexual Behaviour in the Human Female*, p. 519. Saunders, Philadelphia and London

LANE, M.E., ARCEO, R. and SOBRERO, A.J. (1976). Successful use of the diaphragm and jelly by a young population: report of a clinical study. *Fam. Plann. Perspect.*, **8**, 81–86

LAUMAS, K.R., MALKANI, P.K., BHATNAGAR, S. and LAUMAS, V. (1967). Radioactivity in breast milk of lactating women after oral administration of ^{3}H-norethynodrel. *Am. J. Obstet. Gynec.*, **98**, 411–413

MANN, J.I., INMAN, W.H.W. and THOROGOOD, M. (1976). Oral contraceptive use in older women and fatal myocardial infarction. *Br. med. J.*, **ii**, 445–447

McEWAN, J.A., JOYCE, D.N., TOTHILL, A.U. and HAWKINS, D.F. (1977). Early experience in contraception with a new progestogen. *Contraception*, **16**, 339–350

MEDICAL DEFENCE UNION (1974). *Consent to Treatment.* London

MILLER, G.H. and HUGHES, L.R. (1970). Lactation and genital involution effects of a new low-dose oral contraceptive on breast feeding mothers and their infants. *Obstet. Gynec., N.Y.*, **35**, 44–50

MOGGIA, A.V., MISCHLER, T., BERMAN, E., BEAUQUIS, A., TORRADO, M. and KOREMBLITT, E. (1972). Evaluation of the contraceptive efficacy of quingestinol acetate (W 4540) when administered as an oral low-dose contraceptive in the puerperium. *J. reprod. Med.*, **8**, 169–173

NILSSON, S., NYGREN, K.-G. and JOHANSSON, E.D.B. (1977). *d*-Norgestrel concentrations in maternal plasma, milk, and child plasma during administration of oral contraceptives to nursing women. *Am. J. Obstet. Gynec.*, **129**, 178–184

PHATAK, L. and CHANDORKAR, K. (1970). A. Experience with immediate postpartum and post-abortal IUD insertions. B. Disappearance of IUD threads. In *Post-partum Family Planning. A Report on the International Program*, pp. 229–306. Ed. Zatuchni, G.A. McGraw-Hill, New York

PHATAK, L.V. and VISHWANETH, S. (1966). The use of intrauterine contraceptive devices during the immediate postpartum period (preliminary report). *Am. J. Obstet. Gynec.*, **96**, 587

POTTS, M. and McDEVITT, J. (1975). A use effectiveness trial of spermicidally lubricated condoms. *Contraception*, **11**, 701–710

RASHBAUM, W.K. and WALLACH, R.C. (1971). Immediate post-partum insertion of a new intrauterine contraceptive device. *Am. J. Obstet. Gynec.*, **109**, 1003–1004

RECH, F.M. and SCHWARZ, R.H. (1966). Post-partum oral contraception. A clinical evaluation. *Fert. Steril.*, **17**, 556–558

ROOPNARINESINGH, S.S. (1970). Young negro primigravida in Jamaica. *J. Obstet. Gynaec. Br. Commonw.*, **77**, 424–426

RUSSELL, J.K. (1968). Advances in obstetrics and gynaecology. *Practitioner*, **201**, 568–574

SANDS, R.X. (1966). Induction of the first menstruation after childbirth. *Obstet. Gynec., N.Y.*, **28**, 32–36

SAXENA, B.N., SHRIMANKER, K. and GRUDZINSKAS, J.G. (1977). Levels of contraceptive steroids in breast milk and plasma of lactating women. *Contraception*, **16**, 605–613

SEVER, J.L. (1971). Rubella immunization risk postpartum. *J. Am. med. Ass.*, **217**, 697

SHERVINGTON, P.Y. (1974). Cited by Elder, M.G. and Hakim, C.A. (1974). The puerperium. In *Obstetric Therapeutics*, p. 548. Ed. Hawkins, D.F. Baillière Tindall, London

SHULMAN, J.J. (1972). Contraception provision in the immediate post-partum period. *Obstet. Gynec., N.Y.*, **40**, 403–408

SINGER, A. (1975). The uterine cervix from adolescence to the menopause. *Br. J. Obstet. Gynaec.*, **82**, 81–99

SNOWDEN, R., WILLIAMS, M. and HAWKINS, D. (1977a, b and c). *The IUD. A Practical Guide*, pp. 53, 67 and 70–73 respectively. Croom Helm, London

SWARTZ, D.P., BULLARD, T.H., BOONE, P.A. and HOELSCHER, E.W. (1967). Early postpartum intra-uterine device insertion. A preliminary report. *Advances in Planned Parenthood, Excerpta Medica International Congress Series No. 138*, pp. 164–167. Ed. Sobrero, A.L. and Lewit, S. Excerpta Medica, Amsterdam

TIETZE, C. (1977). Induced abortion: 1977 supplement. *Report on Population/ Family Planning, number 14*, second edition, supplement, pp. 1–19

TIETZE, C. and LEWIT, S. (1971). Use-effectiveness of oral and intrauterine contraception. *Fert. Steril.*, **22**, 508–513

VESSEY, M. and WIGGINS, P. (1974). Use-effectiveness of the diaphragm in a selected family planning clinic population in the United Kingdom. *Contraception*, **9**, 15–21

VESSEY, M.P., McPHERSON, K. and JOHNSON, B. (1977). Mortality among women participating in the Oxford Family Planning Association/contraceptive study. *Lancet,* **ii**, 731–733

WEINER, E., BERG, A.A. and JOHANSSON, I. (1978). Copper intrauterine contraceptive devices in adolescent nulliparae. *Br. J. Obstet. Gynaec.,* **85**, 204–206

WENTZ, W.B., JAFFE, R.M. and FOXX, R.M. (1966). Marginal-dose contraception in the puerperium. *Obstet. Gynec., N.Y.,* **28**, 369–372

ZATUCHNI, G.I. (1970). Editor, *Post-partum Family Planning. A Report on the International Program.* See Chapters 18, 19 and 24. McGraw-Hill, New York

18 Contraception in Patients with Medical Disorders

Contraception in patients with medical disorders is an area in which the roles of the internal medicine specialist and the gynaecologist or family planning doctor overlap. Consequently it is a no man's land. Medical specialists in general know little about contraception, except perhaps from their own personal experiences, whilst the average gynaecologist or family planning doctor has a fairly sketchy knowledge of the more serious medical conditions. Because of the rarity of many of the more debilitating diseases, no one individual is likely to have wide experience of the effects of various contraceptive methods in that particular disease state.

Contraception for someone who is already ill and who may well have a reduced life expectancy can be a difficult problem. The risks of pregnancy if contraception is not used, the risks inherent in the contraceptive method itself, and the risks of pregnancy as a result of failure of the method must all be considered within the context of the patient's social and medical state. Every action in life has a finite risk, be it crossing the road, driving a car, gardening, having sexual intercourse, using contraception or having a baby. When the relative risks of contraception and pregnancy resulting from its failure are assessed together the most effective contraceptive, the combined pill, is not necessarily the safest from the medical point of view.

It has been suggested that distribution of the combined pill might become the responsibility of family planning clinic nurses, and even that there should be free access or sale of the pill to the general public. This idea has been strongly advocated and practised in the underdeveloped countries, but up to now it has been resisted in Great Britain and the United States of America where prescription of oral contraceptives is still under the control of a doctor. In a country where the life expectancy of the population is low, due to starvation and disease, the additional hazards of a contraceptive method such as the combined pill are small compared with the benefits to be gained. In the developed countries it is acceptable to prescribe potent drugs that carry a small inherent risk, provided that they are necessary to cure disease. Oral contraceptives are potent drugs affecting many body functions, and they are *not* necessary for the maintenance of life, to cure disease, or even to prevent pregnancy. It is therefore imperative that all precautions are taken lest a healthy woman be converted into a sick one, when other methods of contraception are available. In a group already at risk from a medical disorder, the additional risks may become less important, relative to the need for preventing pregnancy.

Consideration of the appropriate contraceptive involves deciding whether it is merely desirable to postpone pregnancy or whether it would be disastrous should the patient become pregnant again. If the problem is the postponement of pregnancy for a year or two, then the full range of contraceptive methods can be available, within the limitations of the disease itself. If it is extremely undesirable for the woman to have another pregnancy, then the methods available are limited, and it is in these cases that the possibility of sterilisation becomes important.

Sterilisation carried out for purely medical reasons, when the patient would have a high chance of dying were she to have a pregnancy, is rare. The conditions concerned include severe congenital cardiac abnormalities such as Eisenmenger's syndrome, which is pulmonary hypertension together with an atrial or ventricular septal defect and a patent ductus arteriosus or an aortic pulmonary septal defect, and severe disseminated lupus erythematosis with renal involvement. Sterilisation has its own operative hazards, but there are no medical disorders where sterilisation is more dangerous than pregnancy.

In most of the severe medical disorders pregnancy can be negotiated with a mortality rate of less than 5%, and so there is no absolute indication for sterilisation. Assessment of the patient's own values is necessary in order to decide if these risks of death due to pregnancy or the risks of a contraceptive method, or its failure, are such as to warrant sterilisation. Sterilisation is always justified as an alternative to available contraceptive methods provided the couple involved fully understand and accept the implications of the operation.

There are a very few disease states where it is better to postpone a first pregnancy for a few years than to proceed with having a baby as soon as possible. These are situations where treatment such as renal dialysis or the surgical relief of conditions such as hydronephrosis or valvular heart disease can significantly improve the patient's general health. Most patients with moderately severe medical disorders should have their families as soon as possible. If they are then sterilised in perhaps their mid or late 20s psychiatric symptoms related to their loss of fertility may ensue. To avoid this, these patients should be counselled beforehand and the sterilisation procedure should be clearly related to the welfare of the existing family as well as to the individual's own health. In the uncommon situation where pregnancy must be avoided at all costs and sterilisation is not acceptable, then the combined pill is the next most efficient method of preventing pregnancy. In some of these women the pill is contra-indicated, including those with latent diabetes, previous thrombo-embolism, hypertension or liver damage. Despite the contra-indications, there is a small group of women who will accept the small risk of sudden death rather than curtail their sex life or use another method of contraception.

The medically safest methods of contraception, the barrier methods, are those which require the greatest motivation on the part of the patient. It might be considered unreasonable to expect that this degree of motivation will be maintained in all patients from the mid twenties to the menopause, but it is our experience in recent years that women with major medical disorders who are fully acquainted with their situation often demonstrate great reliability. Given sufficient motivation, barrier methods provide very much safer contraception than is generally appreciated. Recent large studies in patients with a real desire to plan their families have found failure rates of 1.9–2.4 per 100 woman-years for diaphragm (Vessey and Wiggins, 1974; Lane *et al.*, 1976) and 0.9–4.0 per 100 woman-years for condoms (John, 1973; Glass *et al.*, 1974).

A compromise is a combination of the medically safe low-dose progestagen pills, which have a failure rate of 6 per 100 woman-years, and a barrier contraceptive – 'a belt and braces' effect. This approach has been used with good results with a number of women who were most anxious to avoid pregnancy and who were unable to take the combined pill. Again, a considerable degree of motivation is required, and although most of these patients have this many may prefer sterilisation. The use of intramuscular progestagens, such as medroxyprogesterone or norethisterone oenanthate, given every 8–12 weeks, may provide effective contraception, without many of the metabolic side effects of the combined pill.

An intra-uterine device is not adequate protection for someone who must avoid pregnancy at all costs. There is evidence that, despite the usually quoted failure rates of between 1 and 3%, a 98–100% follow-up rate rather than the usual 90% will demonstrate a considerably higher failure rate (*see Figure 9.2*, p. 174). The additional use of a barrier method of contraception or spermicide at mid cycle may reduce the failure rate.

Cardio-vascular Disorders

In Great Britain the incidence of rheumatic heart disease has declined six-fold during a period of 20 years, so that the incidence among pregnant women between 1968 and 1971 was as low as 0.3% (Barnes, 1974). The natural history of rheumatic heart disease is such that a patient should ideally have her family as early as is reasonable. Limited spacing of pregnancies should pose few problems because barrier methods or low-dose progestagen pills can be used. Congenital heart disease still has an incidence of about 0.1% of all pregnant patients.

The combined pill and the intra-uterine device both convey significant risks to patients with heart disease. Oestrogen-containing oral contraceptives increase the risks of thrombosis, salt and fluid retention and hypertension. Thrombosis, either intracardiac or peripheral, is the least predictable of these complications and presents the greatest risk to the patient. Salt and water retention or hypertension will be noticed before they can do any harm, provided the patient is followed up weekly, at least initially. The effect of the low-dose 30 μg oestrogen pills on these parameters is as yet unknown, but it is unlikely that complications will be much reduced.

An intra-uterine device is potentially dangerous for patients with either right-sided heart lesions or a septal defect, because of the risk of pelvic sepsis and subsequent septic emboli from the pelvis lodging in the heart and causing bacterial endocarditis. For these reasons someone with heart disease and a past history of pelvic inflammatory disease should not use an intra-uterine device.

For patients with heart disease who are on anticoagulants the combined pill should be safer, as the chance of thrombosis is much reduced, but the risks of hypertension and fluid retention are still present. The combined pill should not be prescribed for patients with a history of myocardial infarction, as there is now evidence that, even in healthy women over 35, there is an increased incidence of infarction in pill users. Menorrhagia can be a problem for a few patients on anticoagulants if they have an intra-uterine device.

Hypertension

Well-controlled severe essential hypertension or hypertension due to renal disease has a less harmful effect on pregnancy, and *vice versa*, than was thought some years ago. Nonetheless, if the diastolic blood pressure is greater than 110 mmHg and there are cardiac and retinal changes present, pregnancy is best avoided. Combined oral contraceptives are undesirable in these patients because of their potentiating effects on the production of plasma renin substrate and hence on the blood pressure. The 'belt and braces' technique of a barrier method with a low-dose progestagen pill, or an intra-uterine device, or barrier methods alone, should be used by these patients. The prognosis for patients with renal complications is improving, and so sterilisation should not be advised unless this is what the patient really wants.

Haematological Disorders

It is sometimes advised that patients with a bleeding diathesis such as thrombo-cytopenic purpura should have ovulation and menstruation suppressed by regular injections of a progestagen, which also provides effective contraception. Over a period of years this can be a recipe for major problems, as sooner or later heavy breakthrough bleeding can occur. Similar considerations occur in patients being treated with cytotoxic drugs for leukaemia and other blood dyscrasias. Continuous daily administration of a combined oral contraceptive containing $50-100 \mu g$ of oestrogen and 2–4 mg of norethisterone or norethynodrel is one way of suppressing menstruation, but even then there is a risk of breakthrough bleeding. The primary approach to this problem should be to use a combined oral contraceptive cyclically, increasing the progestagen content in stages until the menstrual loss is much attenuated, but with some withdrawal bleeding still occurring.

Respiratory Disorders

Diseases of the respiratory system do not pose contraceptive problems, except for the recently reported increased failure of the combined pill when used in patients with tuberculosis who are being treated with rifampicin (Mumford, 1974). This antibiotic increases the rate of enzyme activity responsible for the metabolism of the oral contraceptive steroids, thereby reducing their efficacy.

Alimentary Disorders

Patients with malabsorption syndromes have a reduced absorption of the oral contraceptive steroids with consequent reduction in their effectiveness. These conditions include steatorrhoea, coeliac disease, ulcerative colitis, Crohn's disease and intestinal hurry following partial or total gastrectomy. The patients should be advised that the pill may be ineffective, especially during an exacerbation of their disease. An acute attack of gastro-enteritis lasting two or three days may have the same effect as forgetting the pills, and so other precautions should be taken during and immediately after such an attack.

Liver Disorders

During active liver disease the combined pill is contra-indicated because of the cholestatic effect of oestrogens. Patients who have had liver disease such as infective hepatitis should have liver function tests carried out before commencing oral contraception, then after two months, and thereafter at longer intervals. If these tests are abnormal then barrier methods, a low-dose progestagen or a combination of the two can be used. Otherwise, an intra-uterine device may be fitted. Low-dose progestagen pills have been used in many women with abnormal liver function tests without harmful effects. Oestrogen-containing pills should not be used except under strict supervision. Should the liver function tests remain normal, then any method may be used.

Patients with known or suspected gall-bladder disease are well advised to avoid oral contraceptives containing oestrogen, because of the increased risk of cholesterol gall stones.

Diabetes Mellitus

Potential or latent diabetics should not take oestrogen-containing oral contraceptives. For the well-controlled overt diabetic, reliable avoidance of pregnancy may be more important than a minor change in carbohydrate tolerance, and the combined pill is probably a reasonable contraceptive provided diabetic control is reviewed. Although diabetes is traditionally an infertility factor, many diabetic patients seem to fall pregnant with remarkable facility, and the increased risk of contraceptive failure with barrier methods or intra-uterine devices may not be acceptable. The increased risk of pelvic sepsis with the devices may also make their use in diabetics undesirable.

Chronic Renal Failure

When haemodialysis coincides with ovulation, bleeding may occur from a ruptured follicle because of the effect of heparin. The suppressant action of the combined pill on ovulation can make it a useful method of treatment for these patients. Women who have had renal transplants can go through pregnancy without major problems, and in these patients there is no particular contra-indication to any contraceptive method.

Central Nervous System

Patients with a history of cerebral thrombosis or symptoms suggestive of cerebral arterial spasm during pregnancy should not take the combined pill because of the risks of precipitating a severe or fatal stroke.

Patients who suffer from migraine, especially if it is related to the menstrual cycle, should probably not take the combined pill. Pill-induced migraine may be due to cerebral arteriolar hypertrophy (Grant, 1968) and this may in turn increase the risk of the rare complication of cerebral arterial thrombosis. In practice, migraine sufferers often find that their headaches are more frequent and severe while on the combined oral contraceptive, and do not wish to continue. We have recently encountered patients with menstrual migraine who have been advised to take a $50\,\mu g$ oestrogen pill continuously for eight weeks at a time, reducing the incidence of withdrawal bleeding and migraine to every second month. There is no clear understanding of the mechanism of menstrual migraine; should Grant's (1968) views be correct then the advice is dangerous.

Epileptics should avoid oestrogen-containing pills because their salt and water retaining properties may make the epilepsy more difficult to control. Some anti-convulsants such as phenytoin potentiate enzyme activity and increase the rate of breakdown of contraceptive steroids, making the pill unreliable. Epileptics are sometimes unreliable and forgetful people, who may increase the risk of contraceptive failure by not taking the pill regularly. An intra-uterine device may be the contraceptive method of choice, but regular verification of its presence is required. Alternatively, the well-motivated use of condoms by the husband may be the best answer.

Otosclerosis is sometimes cited as a condition which may be exacerbated by oral contraceptives but there seems to be little evidence on this point.

The use of combined oral contraception has been said to be contra-indicated in patients with depression (British Medical Journal, 1969). This is not un-reasonable, but there is a great individual variation in the aetiology and degree of depression. The oestrogen component of a combined pill reduces the bio-logical availability of pyridoxine, which acts as a co-enzyme in tryptophan metabolism (*see* Larsson-Cohn, 1975, for review). This may lead to a reduction in the level of 5-hydroxytryptamine in the brain. The precise role of this mecha-nism in the aetiology of a case of depression is debatable. The use of a combined oral contraceptive can relieve depression if a major cause is fear of pregnancy, so it is reasonable to try using the pill under strict supervision in cases of mild depression. Pyridoxine supplements (100 mg/day by mouth) may be effective in patients in whom oral contraceptives appear to cause depression.

We must also consider the feckless, for want of a better term. These include socially irresponsible women of low intelligence and drug addicts. Whilst they can readily agree to the undesirability of pregnancy these patients may not have the motivation or self-discipline to use either oral contraceptive or barrier methods properly and they may either themselves remove, or have removed, an intra-uterine device. They are at particular risk from the complications of intra-uterine devices in that they cannot be relied upon to report adverse symptoms promptly. Three monthly injections of a progestagen, either medroxyproges-terone acetate or norethisterone oenanthate, is often the method of choice for these patients. Domiciliary calls by visiting nurses can be used to check on any adverse effects and give the injections regularly.

Gynaecological Disorders

Patients presenting with a history of irregular periods or intermenstrual bleeding should rely on the use of condoms until the cause of the irregular bleeding has been elucidated. Patients with active or quiescent pelvic inflammatory disease should not have an intra-uterine device fitted because of the risk of exacerbation of their pelvic infection, with resulting tubal damage, and because of the small chance of developing peritonitis, septic emboli and septicaemia. Patients with intramural or submucous fibroids should not use an intra-uterine device. Risks of perforation at insertion and expulsion are increased, menorrhagia is a hazard, and the device may be ineffective because of the enlarged and distorted uterine cavity. The combined pill is contra-indicated, in theory at least, because of possible enlargement and necrosis of the fibroids. A trial may be the only way of deciding whether or not a low-dose oestrogen combined pill or a low-dose progestagen will produce unacceptable adverse effects. Low-lying fibroids may prevent effective fitting of a diaphragm and the only answer may be the use of condoms. For patients with anovulatory cycle bleeding or metropathia haemorrhagica, the pill is both good treatment and a contraceptive.

Patients with endometriosis usually benefit from taking a combined oral contraceptive cyclically (Potts *et al.*, 1975). By suppressing ovulation the pill can relieve mid cycle pain (mittelschmerz) and also primary spasmodic dysmenorrhoea. If these conditions are not improved by an oral contraceptive there is reason to suspect organic pathology. The progestagen supplements in the pill sometimes relieve premenstrual tension. Oral contraceptives are appropriate for patients who suffer from irregular menstruation or menorrhagia that is dysfunctional, organic causes having been excluded. Symptomatic improvement is usual with the pill, whilst an intra-uterine device will probably make things worse.

Patients who have had a hydatidiform mole evacuated are usually advised to avoid pregnancy for two years, so that assays of urinary HCG can be employed to ascertain that there is no persisting mole or trophoblastic tumour. In the past it has been common for these patients to be prescribed a combined oral contraceptive. It is now known that this not only delays the fall in HCG excretion but also increases the number of patients who will need chemotherapy for trophoblastic tumour (Stone *et al.*, 1976). Many gynaecologists would be unwilling on general grounds to disturb the uterine cavity with an intra-uterine device; these cases are probably best managed by advising rigid adherence to barrier precautions.

CONCLUSIONS

A few basic medical contra-indications should be observed in advising contraception for patients with major medical disorders. These usually are situations where oestrogen-containing oral contraceptives should be avoided. The list of conditions where it has been said that oestrogen-containing oral contraceptives can cause recurrence or exacerbation is now quite extensive, including, in addition to those already mentioned, a history of carcinoma of the breast, or of chloasma, herpes gestationis or cholestatic jaundice in pregnancy; hyperlipidaemia; acute intermittent, variegate and hereditary hepatic porphyria, Raynaud's disease, sickle cell disease; or a history of deep vein thrombosis or pulmonary embolism.

In many borderline situations it is reasonable to try the combined pill under strict supervision because of its low failure rate, and especially the 30 μg oestrogen preparations because of their potentially lower complication rate. There is some evidence that norgestrel causes fewer metabolic side-effects than other progestagens. It may tend to counteract the effects of oestrogen on the levels of plasma coagulation factors (Briggs, 1974), triglycerides, cholesterol, and on glucose tolerance (Wynn *et al.*, 1974). If this is the case, then a pill containing a low dose of oestrogen and norgestrel may be safer than the other combined preparations. More comparative biochemical and clinical evidence will be necessary before this claim can be substantiated.

The main problems with intra-uterine devices are linked with relative lack of long-term efficacy as a contraceptive, with local effects on the uterus and with creation of a portal of entry for infection. Their use may be acceptable in the presence of some medical conditions, for temporary postponement of pregnancy.

Of the other methods, the condom and the diaphragm, if used consistently and properly, have a much lower failure rate than is generally appreciated, and they can be an excellent method of spacing pregnancies. They may also be good methods in the long term, provided the patients have adequate motivation. They are totally free from medical side-effects, either immediate or accumulative. Low-dose progestagen pills are also useful for spacing pregnancies, but for long-term contraception they are only sufficiently effective if used in conjunction with a barrier method. They have the considerable benefit of being free from the metabolic side-effects of the combined pill, which are largely derived from the effects of oestrogen on liver cells.

The safe period, coitus interruptus, and spermicides are inadequate methods in this context. In the final analysis we return to the complex assessment of the relative risks to the patient of pregnancy and of the contraceptive method, and to her personal values.

REFERENCES

BARNES, C.G. (1974). *Medical Disorders' in Obstetric Practice, Fourth edition*, p. 11. Blackwell, Oxford

BRIGGS, M.(1974). Effect of oral progestogens on oestrogen induced changes in serum protein. *The Second International Norgestrel Symposium*, pp. 35—41. Excerpta Medica, Amsterdam

BRITISH MEDICAL JOURNAL (1969). Oral contraception and depression. *Br. med. J.*, iv, 380—381

GLASS, R., VESSEY, M. and WIGGINS, P. (1974). Use-effectiveness of the condom in a selected family planning clinic population in the United Kingdom. *Contraception*, 10, 591—598

GRANT, E.C.G. (1968). Relation between headaches from oral contraceptives and development of endometrial arterioles. *Br. med. J.*, iii, 402—405

JOHN, A.P.K. (1973). Contraception in general practice. *Jnl R. Coll. gen. Pract.*, 23, 664—675

LANE, M.E., ARICO, R. and SOBRERO, A.J. (1976). Successful use of the diaphragm and jelly by a young population: report of a clinical study. *Fam. Plann. Perspect.*, 8, 81—86

LARSSON-COHN, U. (1975). Oral contraceptives and vitamins: a review. *Am. J. Obstet. Gynec.*, 121, 84—90

MUMFORD, J.P.(1974). Drugs affecting oral contraceptives. *Br. med. J.*, ii, 333—334

POTTS, M., VAN DER VLUGT, T., PIOTROW, P.T., GAIL, L.J. and HUBER, S.C. (1975). *Population Reports*, series A, number 2, 30–51

STONE, M., DENT, J., KARDONA, A. and BAGSHAWE, K.D. (1976). Relationship of oral contraception to development of trophoblastic tumour after evacuation of a hydatidiform mole. *Br. J. Obstet. Gynaec.*, **83**, 913–916

VESSEY, M. and WIGGINS, P. (1974). Use-effectiveness of the diaphragm in a selected family planning clinic population in the United Kingdom. *Contraception*, **9**, 15–21

WYNN, V., ADAMS, P., OAKLEY, N. and SEED, M. (1974). Metabolic investigations in women taking 30 μg ethinyl oestradiol plus 150 μg d-norgestrel. *The Second International Norgestrel Symposium*, pp. 47–57. Excerpta Medica, Amsterdam

19 Clinical Trials

Physicians in family planning practice often wish to run or to participate in clinical trials. Fertility regulation is a specialty which lends itself readily to trials. Relatively large numbers of co-operative patients are available for the application of standardised clinical manoeuvres. Documentation is, in general, good and follow-up procedures are a routine part of good clinical practice. A well planned trial can enhance the efficiency with which services are provided to the patients. Further, there is a great need for cautious examination of new developments, and for large scale evaluation of established procedures.

On the other hand, trials of fertility regulating procedures require very considerable caution, lest any disadvantage, let alone any harm, befall a participant. The trial of a new antimitotic agent in terminal patients with malignant disease is a situation where the patient and his relatives will rightly consider that major risks, even of lethal unwanted effects, may be completely justified if there is a small chance of prolonging the patient's life. Trials of fertility regulating procedures are at the other extreme. In general, contraception and sterilisation are in the same class as cosmetic plastic surgery. They are elective contributions to well-being rather than medically necessary therapeutic procedures. In addition, established measures are always available which are very effective and carry very low rates of unwanted effects or failures, judged by the standards applied to most therapeutic agents. It follows that the greatest precautions must be taken in planning trials of new fertility regulating procedures to minimise any conceivable hazard to the participants.

In recent years a mystique has built up about clinical trials, generated primarily by an honest desire to improve the quality of the scientific information obtained, but clouded by the almost obsessional tendency of status-seeking individuals to introduce organisation, regimentation and administration into any developing field. The simplest trials, designed to test a single point, are often the most effective, and usually require nothing more than a combination of logic and common sense in their planning. Nonetheless, there is a virtue in those involved in planning and executing clinical trials becoming acquainted with some of the literature on this subject. Many mistakes have been made in apparently well-planned studies in the past, and acquaintance with standard procedures for avoiding recognised pitfalls can avoid much frustration and potential hazard to patients. Publications on the principles involved include the World Health Organization's (1968) report 'Principles for the Clinical Evaluation of Drugs' and the Medico-Pharmaceutical Forum's (1974) report on clinical trials. The

University of Exeter's (1974) report gives comprehensive recommendations for oral contraceptive trials and a detailed account of the statistical evaluation of contraceptive methods is presented by Tietze and Lewit (1974); some notes on the assessment of small studies of intra-uterine devices are included by Snowden *et al.* (1977).

GENERAL PRINCIPLES OF PLANNING CLINICAL TRIALS

Objective

Even the most general study is likely to produce meaningless results unless the question or questions being asked can be spelled out in simple terms at the start. To formulate these questions precisely is essential to the planning of the study.

Potential of the Field of Study

Innumerable clinical studies have been started without the investigator's appreciating that it is simply not possible, with the facilities and patients available, to obtain an answer to the question asked. This may be for statistical reasons, but it is often because the question, in the form put, is unanswerable!

Feasibility

Again, many investigations have failed because it has not been recognised that it is not possible to carry out the trial as planned for logistic reasons of personnel, time and facilities, or patient availability. Small pilot studies are sometimes of value in assessing this situation and perhaps reorganising the main trial appropriately.

Analysis

The data must be collected in a form suitable for answering the question posed. Where appropriate, the advice of a statistician must be obtained during the planning stage. The adequate analysis of data not infrequently takes longer than the trial itself and it is important that provision is made for expert help where necessary.

Interpretation

As many as possible of the difficulties that may arise in interpreting the results should be defined during the planning stage. Amendments to design can often obviate these difficulties.

Consultation

The advice of an individual experienced in clinical trials of the type envisaged is often invaluable. The pre-judgement of someone preoccupied with a given procedure – 'it doesn't qualify these days unless it's double-blind' – is of course useless. What is needed is an intelligent evaluation of the protocol for the trial in relation to the stated objective, and a sharp eye for any potential hazards to patients.

Publication

Although they may give satisfaction to the investigator, trials are of limited value unless the results can be communicated to the medical community. In general, unless the results will be of sufficient interest either to publish at least a short letter in a medical journal without 'diluting the literature' or to give a brief talk at a medical meeting then the justification for the labour involved should be. reviewed. There are exceptions to this principle, for example where definite information is required to assist changes or development of services in a clinic or a specific community.

Classification of Trials

It is currently convenient to classify some clinical trials of new procedures according to the recommendations of the United States Food and Drug Administration (see Medico-Pharmaceutical Forum, 1974).

Phase I trials cover the initial introduction of a drug to man. It is difficult to envisage this occurring in a fertility regulating context. Drugs should always have received full evaluation in humans before they are considered as fertility regulating agents.

Phase II is usually applied to early controlled clinical trials designed to demonstrate efficacy and relative safety in a limited, closely monitored sample of patients. Such trials often incorporate 100–200 patients.

Phase III means a large scale and less rigidly controlled trial of an agent whose efficacy and relative safety have been established. It is intended to assess efficacy under practical working conditions, and to establish the incidence of any low-incidence adverse effects.

Phase IV is a term for long-term surveillance of drugs whose usefulness is sufficiently well established that they are freely available for prescription by the medical community.

EFFECTS OF CLINICAL TRIALS ON FAMILY PLANNING BEHAVIOUR

Incorporation of patients in a well-conducted clinical trial can have a beneficial effect on their fertility regulating behaviour. This is mediated partly by the increased interest and support of the doctors conducting the trial and partly by the patient's sense of involvement, not only in her own family planning problems but also in those of others.

When a patient is admitted to a trial an extensive history is taken and full details specially recorded. Similar careful records are made of follow-up visits. In practice, this often means that patients in trials not only see the doctor — usually the same at each visit — but also are interviewed by ancillary staff whose function is documentation. This may be done with the patient fully dressed and perhaps accompanied by her children, in a private room separated from examination cubicles and waiting areas. Although the questions asked are routine, there is scope for the patients to ask questions about contraception, say how they feel about it and express any uncertainties they may have about birth control. Follow-up visits are of primary importance for clinical trials and special procedures are usually employed to contact defaulters. This alone can align the patient's attention to her contraceptive method and make her feel that her doctor has a special interest in her family planning performance. A good trial procedure can give strong reinforcement to the patient's motivation to undertake effective family planning.

In our own studies of the relationship between marital role relationships and fertility regulating behaviour (*see* Chapter 16, pp. 378–379) we examined some aspects of the behaviour of comparable groups of patients, some of whom were selected at random and incorporated in clinical assessments of intra-uterine contraceptive device effectiveness (Whitlock, Z.L. and Hawkins, D.F., unpublished observations). Our principal finding was that a proportion of women in whom poor attendance at the family planning clinic was associated with 'segregated' domestic role behaviour became good attenders as a result of participating in trials. The increased attention they received at the clinic appeared to compensate to a degree for the lack of emotional support from their husbands in the domestic situation. On the other hand, the trials did not affect the behaviour of women whose poor attendance was primarily associated with segregated — as distinct from 'joint' — marital behaviour with respect to the couple's sexual relationships. It seems that reinforcement given by the provider of the family planning service supports good attendance behaviour in the same way as 'jointness' in domestic behaviour, but cannot compensate for the influence of lack of 'jointness' in marital sexual behaviour.

ETHICAL CONSIDERATIONS IN CLINICAL TRIALS OF FERTILITY REGULATING AGENTS

The final arbiter in any ethical problem in relation to a clinical trial is the integrity of the physician with clinical responsibility for the patients involved. His deciding criterion must always be that the welfare of the individual patient, physical, mental or economic, takes precedence over scientific need, whatever may be the potential benefit to the human race. In the conduct of a trial, delegation of authority relating to any factor which may affect the patient to non-medical personnel or to physicians without direct clinical responsibility, is unacceptable. If such delegation occurs priority may be given to scientific, economic or even political needs, which could be to the detriment of an individual patient.

No set of rules covers every ethical situation which can arise in the planning, execution, analysis and reporting of a clinical trial. The principles conveyed by the World Medical Association's (1965) Declaration of Helsinki, the Medical

Research Council (1964) in Great Britain and the United States Department of Health, Education and Welfare (1973), supplemented by the opinions of local research committees (*see* World Health Organization, 1968) provide guidance which is of the greatest value in planning clinical trials. These codes of conduct have the virtue of giving a degree of legal protection in the event of accidental ill-consequences for the investigator who complies with their policies. By implication, they codify the problems which have been met in the past and indicate procedures which can protect both patients and investigators from repetition of mishaps from which others have suffered.

The functions that such codes cannot fulfil are:

(1) to provide such close restrictions that unethical consequences can never befall the patient;
(2) to define exactly the extent to which patients must be informed of the nature of an individual trial without having a deleterious effect on themselves, the trial or both;
(3) to cope with every possible type of trial, where circumstances can be such that an apparent transgression of the rules actually benefits the patient;
(4) to give judgements on the innumerable minor day to day problems, requiring decisions with an ethical connotation, which arise during the execution of a trial.

These are the circumstances where the investigating physician must act on behalf of the patient 'in good faith'.

GENERAL PRINCIPLES

The notes on consent, safety, rewards and other payments and compensation for injury given by the World Health Organization (1968) provide basic guidance, but there are certain characteristics that differentiate trials of procedures for controlling fertility from clinical trials in general.

Physical Consequences

In developed countries obstetric services are such that the morbidity of pregnancy is low and the mortality extremely low. Prevention of pregnancy seldom affects the physical health of a patient on a continuing basis and very rarely saves a life. It follows that for a fertility regulating procedure to convey actual physical benefit to a patient it must be singularly free from side-effects and physical sequelae, compared with agents used in the treatment of disease. This gives rise to strict limitations in the selection of agents which can reasonably be given clinical trials.

Psychological Consequences

The potential psychological benefits of effective contraceptive procedures may be greatly out of proportion to any potential physical effects. Most physicians would accept that physical ill-effects, even if minor in nature and rare in occurrence, should be given greater weight than psychological consequences. This conflict often leads the physician to make a major value judgement to justify a trial. It also introduces an ethical judgement into the selection of subjects, exclusion of individuals being to some extent dependent on the expressed values of the patient.

Management of Failures

When studying an agent or procedure intended to prevent conception consideration must be given to the management of failures, when the patient becomes pregnant. It is unethical to promise abortion to such patients in many countries, where, even if legal abortion is available, decisions cannot be made *ante hoc*. In many communities contraceptive failure *per se* is not considered adequate justification for therapeutic abortion. In these circumstances the implication that trial subjects will readily be granted abortion if they became pregnant should be scrupulously avoided. Only in an environment where abortion on demand is medically, legally and culturally acceptable as a primary procedure for family planning, equivalent to contraception, can the physician guarantee to terminate the unwanted pregnancy. Even then, the patient may not wish to have an abortion. Patients admitted to a trial should, in common with all those receiving family planning advice, be informed of prevailing circumstances when they are given an estimate of the chances of failure.

Risk of Teratogenesis

It follows that the trial of any contraceptive procedure is unethical where there is reason to believe that the chance of an abnormal fetus resulting from failure is greater than the chance of fetal abnormality arising from unprotected conception. The only exception to this is in environments where therapeutic abortion is available without restriction and the patients agree to this should they conceive. It may be a sad reflection that humanity has reverted to the primitive viewpoint that the generation of an infant with a disability is a greater calamity than the destruction of a fetus, but it is a fact that must be accepted. In Great Britain the physician is open to legal action for damages on behalf of an abnormal child whose defect may be attributed to medical management before conception, under the Congenital Disabilities (Civil Liability) Act of 1976. There is case law in many of the United States of America and in Canada and Australia, suggesting that the unborn child has a cause for action in these circumstances (Law Commission, 1973). In Great Britain, a medical practitioner is not answerable to the child if the parents know the risk of their child being born disabled. It is therefore important that the current state of knowledge about teratogenic potential of any fertility regulating procedure be conveyed accurately to the patients, however minute the risk. Actions in accordance with current professional opinion are also excluded from liability. This emphasises the importance of consultation with leading authorities.

The onus is on the physician to take reasonable steps to ascertain that no teratogenic risk is known. This includes making a search of the relevant medical literature. It is well known that tests for teratogenesis conducted in laboratory animals may be fallible. Negative tests do not exclude potential for causing an abnormal fetus in the human and positive results may be found in animals for a procedure which conveys no risk in humans. Nevertheless, the experimenter should ascertain that whatever standard of testing is acceptable in his community has been conducted with satisfactory results. If the animal tests show a teratogenic potential, exceptionally strong evidence should be available that the effect does not occur in humans before a clinical trial in patients is contemplated.

Future Fertility

Any therapeutic measure is associated with the possibility of long-term sequelae. Fertility control measures are applied to a population where specific assessment of possible effects on future reproductive capacity should be made as part of the appraisal of potential complications.

Physician—patient Confidentiality

Some women requesting contraceptive advice, abortion or sterilisation do not wish their consort to know. Others, attending clinics, do not wish their family practitioners to be informed. Views on the correctness of incorporating such patients in a clinical trial vary. The attitude of the physician should be clarified in the protocol of a trial to avoid conflict with the routine trial procedures. The physician who undertakes to refrain from advising the patient's general practitioner of any procedure is ethically responsible for providing full-time medical services to cover any possible consequences of his advice or therapy.

Confidentiality of Records

Whilst the doctor—patient relationship should ensure confidentiality in all clinical trials, a leak of information can always occur in work involving paramedical and technical personnel. Such inadvertent disclosures are particularly likely to have emotional, social and medico-legal consequences in studies involving reproductive behaviour. Reference to the statement on responsibility in the use of medical information for research by the Medical Research Council (1973) will be found useful in planning trials.

Patient Motivation

Contraception is a procedure in which patient motivation has basic importance. The investigator has a particular duty to ensure that highly motivated individuals are not exploited and poorly motivated subjects neglected, for the purposes of a trial.

Public Relations

Information on contraceptive measures dealing with either potential benefits or potential disasters, in common with other clinical manoeuvres associated with reproduction, is liable to rouse a profound emotional reaction, not only in trial subjects but also in the community at large. In addition to ensuring ethical validity by the usual standards, the investigator's duty to the community may require him to publicise his activities in advance in a way that will forestall extravagant reactions. It may also require him to abandon a valid trial to allay unjustified anxiety.

Community Mores

Although his primary duties are to the patient and to the health of the community, in that order, the physician also has a responsibility to respect the religious, social and legal mores of his community. Although there have been examples where clinical trials have been the means of introduction of enlightened attitudes in unfavourable environments, the investigator should appraise his position with great care before embarking on such a venture. He would do well to secure written support for his project from liberal but highly respected individuals who are prominent in the community.

Racial and Political Factors

A well designed trial takes account of the race of the subjects, either by controlling the variable and restricting the trial to patients of one racial group or by defining the racial distribution of the population studied. It is of importance that a trial in a mixed community be examined from the point of view of race relations. If it is to be restricted to a particular race, the scientific justification should be explicit, and there should be no evidence to support an allegation that a particular racial or political segment of the community are being used as 'guinea-pigs'. When testing fertility control agents a trial may easily be interpreted as threatening the future of a race.

Physician Attitudes

Emotional attitudes to fertility control are not the sole prerogative of patients. Investigators embued with enthusiasm for solving the present and future population problems of their community and the world sometimes lack perspective in their ethical judgements. It is often advantageous for trial projects to be reviewed by independent experts with a healthy scepticism for the predictions of economists and demographers and with a wide knowledge of human behaviour.

Technical Advance

Similar considerations apply to enthusiasm for technical advance in the field of fertility control. Consultation with physicians who have the experience to appraise the potential of a new approach against the dubious advantages of many past technical 'developments' will often call for a review of ethical decisions.

CONDUCT OF TRIALS

The nature of fertility regulating procedures, with particular reference to the preceding points, lays certain restrictions on actual trial procedure which do not necessarily apply to therapeutic trials in general.

Types of Trial

Initial studies in humans of a completely new drug for conception control can in general only be undertaken with volunteers in environments where abortion is an accepted primary fertility control procedure. Unless abortion can be guaranteed in the event of a pregnancy, and the trial subjects accept this, there is at least a remote risk of teratogenesis. A possible way of circumventing the difficulty is to solicit volunteers from patients shortly to undergo elective hysterectomy – the presence of a very early pregnancy makes little difference to the operation. Certain procedures, such as mechanical methods for preventing access of spermatozoa to the cervix, may be considered completely free from teratogenic potential and a trial in volunteers who are prepared to accept the risk of pregnancy is reasonable. It should be noted that devices or drugs which interfere with the tubal transport of ova do not fall into this class, since there is evidence that delay in transport conveys an increased risk of ectopic gestation and fetal abnormality.

In formal therapeutic trials of agents known to have some effect in regulating fertility, particular care should be taken to give the patient the best available prognosis and an account of the expected advantages and disadvantages of the new method, in comparison with established alternatives. Patients usually find comparative studies with random allocation to groups understandable and acceptable, provided that no clear advantage is known in advance to appertain to a particular group. Placebo-controlled trials are only applicable to the assessment of side-effects in volunteers who have been provided with alternative contraceptive protection.

Recruitment

However informed the consent of the patients, the physician must take some responsibility for conducting the trial in an appropriate population. A group of postpartum primiparae who merely desire to postpone their next pregnancy for a few months may be expected to accept a new procedure with a probable failure rate of a few per cent, if some compensating advantage is envisaged. To approach women who need to prevent pregnancy for years, or those who have already had a therapeutic abortion, with such a proposition may be unreasonable.

A study of a drug known to cause a proportion of women to develop menorrhagia or amenorrhoea in a community where these side-effects generate cultural sanctions would be unreasonable. To examine a procedure designed to reduce these side-effects of an accepted method in such a community would be very justified.

Women with unconventional sexual proclivities are unsuitable for trials of methods which convey no protection against venereal disease. If this is rife in the population then it is best that consent to the trials should include a statement that the method does not prevent acquisition of such a disease.

Consent

From an ethical point of view a physician's primary duty is to his patient, who is thereby entitled to give, on his or her own behalf, informed consent to participation in a trial. To obtain personally the consort's informed consent to participation by a subject in every case can sometimes cause considerable inconvenience to the patients and may result in unjustified selection. In trials of reversible anti-conception procedures, a reasonable compromise from both ethical and legal viewpoints is to obtain the subject's signed statement that the consort has been informed and agrees to the conditions of the trial. There are developed countries where a wife's consent to a fertility control procedure against her husband's wishes might provide grounds for divorce, and if this applies the patients should be so informed. In countries where culturally and legally a wife is the property of her husband, the physician should secure the husband's consent to participation in a trial.

It is generally accepted that minors — the age limit in a given community is usually defined — are not competent to consent to participation in an experimental trial and that their parents or guardians cannot give consent on their behalf. Similar considerations apply to the mentally incompetent and to individuals in underdeveloped countries who are incapable, by reason of lack of education or understanding, of giving informed consent. On the other hand knowledge about the best fertility control procedures for such groups is deficient. Provided the individuals concerned are capable of giving consent to temporary contraceptive measures, there is no reason why the physician should not attempt to determine in a comparative trial which of two apparently suitable procedures is the more appropriate.

Follow-up Procedures

The success of trials of fertility regulating procedures is heavily dependent on adequacy of follow-up. The ethical problems involved in tracing and questioning trial patients who default from follow-up attendance are best avoided by securing their agreement to appropriate follow-up procedures at the time of admission to the trial. Otherwise, it is ethically reasonable to ask the patient's family practitioner to request information about a subject who has ceased to attend the physician conducting the trial. If nurses or social workers attached to the study approach the patient to request an interview, then the purpose, confidentiality and voluntary nature of compliance must be made plain. Such manoeuvres as the employment of detectives to trace patients, whilst not illegal, could be considered as an invasion of privacy.

Low-incidence Major Complications

It is bitter experience that reporting of the most serious complications of a fertility control procedure is often unduly delayed. This is sometimes due to their low incidence rendering correlation of cause and effect difficult in small-scale trials, sometimes to a very long latent period before sequelae such as carcinogenesis become apparent, and sometimes due to conscious or sub-conscious reluctance of physicians to attribute consequences to a procedure in which they have faith. It is incumbent on those conducting small-scale trials to report any adverse reactions in the patients, however remote may be the chance of their being due to the trial procedure, and on those conducting large-scale trials to institute adequate long-term monitoring for low-incidence ill-effects.

Reporting of Results

It has become apparent that the major source of variation in results of trials of fertility control agents is 'between centre'. A valid report does not pool results from different centres of investigation but indicates how much of the variation can be attributed to this factor.

ETHICAL PROBLEMS ASSOCIATED WITH SPECIFIC FERTILITY REGULATION PROCEDURES

Whether or not a prospective patient is to be presented with data assessing the risk to life, however small, of a fertility regulation procedure, is a matter for the judgement of the physician. This should take into account the potential mistrust and anxiety which such information can create in susceptible patients, as well as the need for honesty in detailing the risks of a trial procedure. On the other hand, data must always be available for the patient who makes a positive request. The estimate of mortality must be constructed *de novo*, using the best infor-mation available. The consequences of failure of the method, derived using a maternal mortality figure from current statistics in the environment concerned should be added to any mortality arising from the method itself — an example of the calculation is given by Elder (1974). The mortality estimate should be significantly lower than that for the consequences of unprotected intercourse or the procedure cannot be considered for trial in the first place. To create further perspective, it is quite reasonable to make comparisons with risks of other features of everyday life such as driving an automobile or smoking.

Trials of certain types of fertility regulation procedure present special ethical problems.

Barrier Methods

Provided manufacturing, quality control and storage procedures are sound, failures with condoms, diaphragms and similar devices are nearly all due to 'patient failure'. Pregnancy results from misuse or non-use of the method at the mid cycle and can usually be linked with deficient motivation linked with overt or deep-seated desire for pregnancy. It is essential to convey these facts to the patients on admission to the trial and to inform them that alternative contraceptive procedures are available where the onus on the patient to determine her own destiny is less.

Intra-uterine Devices

Specific written consent for the actual procedure of insertion of the device should be obtained in the same way as for any minor surgery, in addition to the informed consent for participation in the trial.

The general properties of intra-uterine devices are now well established, and it is reasonable to expect a new device to share these properties, with the additional potential benefits or hazards of any new features. It follows that it is reasonable merely to inform a patient already acquainted with the use of the devices about the new feature, rather than presenting the matter as an entirely new contraceptive technique.

It is now generally accepted that 'closed ring' devices convey the additional hazard of bowel strangulation in the rare event of their perforating the uterus. It would be unethical to conduct a trial of such a device without informing the patients of this fact.

Should pregnancy occur with a device *in situ* abortion occurs spontaneously in a proportion of cases; in about half, the pregnancy will proceed normally with no ill-effects on the fetus. Although with some devices, removal in early pregnancy may increase the overall chance of the pregnancy continuing, removal can be followed by abortion. Removal of a new device might be construed as an attempt to procure abortion, if no valid medical reason for removal has previously been established.

Trials of devices containing chemical additives should be subject to the same precautions as trials of new drugs for regulating fertility and the risk of teratogenesis borne in mind.

Oral and Injectable Chemical Contraceptives

The tortuous history of the legal, medical, political and public relations implications in the United States of America of delayed recognition of the risk of thrombosis and embolism with oral contraceptives, during the decade after the association was first reported in 1961, is detailed by Katz (1972). This situation provides a model which applies by analogy to trials of any new drug preparation for controlling fertility. The far-reaching consequences of failure to exert full ethical control at all stages over the introduction of a new procedure, however beneficial on a world-wide basis, are well recorded by Katz.

When supplies of a drug are issued to patients they should be labelled with their composition. If by the nature of the trial, which may be a blind comparison, this is not possible, then the label should indicate a source where information on the contents can be obtained day and night. If a new drug, whose properties are not widely known, is incorporated, a similar precaution is desirable and the patient's family medical practitioner should be given full details of the trial and its implications.

Spermicides

Before considering a spermicidal preparation for clinical trial it is necessary that its efficacy *in vitro* shall have been established by standard tests, such as those recommended by the International Planned Parenthood Federation (1965). In addition it is particularly important that the possibility that the spermicide might be absorbed from the vagina has been examined experimentally and any potential systemic toxicity or teratogenicity studied. There should be adequate evidence, obtained *in vivo*, that the spermicide does not have an inflammatory or carcinogenic effect on the vaginal skin or cervix. Subjects with a history of skin allergy should be eliminated from the trial. Finally, not only should the effect of the spermicide on *Neisseria gonorrhoeae* and *Treponema pallidum* be known, but also its potential for masking the lesions caused by these organisms and for interfering with diagnosis.

No spermicide which is safe to use has yet been found to be really effective in preventing pregnancy when used alone. It is felt in some quarters (Drug and Therapeutics Bulletin, 1974) that the preparations presently available should be recommended only as adjuncts to other contraceptive procedures. The presumption must therefore be made when testing a new spermicide, however effective *in vitro*, that there will be a significant pregnancy rate, and patients in a trial must accept this possibility. The other way of testing spermicides is to use them in conjunction with a barrier method. It is reasonable to conduct a pilot or comparative trial of an apparently effective spermicide with patients who normally employ a diaphragm with a spermicidal preparation for contraception.

Postcoital Contraceptives

Spermatozoa can be present in the human fallopian tube as soon as five minutes after deposition in the vagina (Settlage *et al.*, 1973) and drugs administered postcoitally to prevent pregnancy must be assumed to be acting by preventing implantation of the fertilised ovum. Whether or not this can be considered as a process of abortion has not been and is unlikely to be tested in the courts. There are some environments where religious feeling against abortion is so strong that it would be unwise to attempt a trial of postcoital contraception.

It is surprising that trials of the use of diethylstilboestrol as a postcoital contraceptive have been undertaken in circumstances where therapeutic abortion is not available on demand, since this drug is a known teratogen. In addition to the ethical obligation not to test a procedure which might be teratogenic, the physician should bear in mind the possibility that a teenage girl whose birth resulted from a 'failure' and who developed a lesion such as an adenocarcinoma of the vagina might be in a position to undertake a civil action for damages. It would seem wise to restrict trials of hormonal agents as postcoital contraceptives to compounds whose lack of teratogenicity has been demonstrated by hundreds of women, who have become pregnant over the years whilst taking the drug as an ordinary oral contraceptive, unless therapeutic abortion is freely available.

The long-term ethical consequences of freely-available postcoital contraception are worth consideration by the physician who engages in trials of this procedure. It is a distressing but characteristic feature of human behaviour that to be widely accepted, a moral code is usually associated with a penalty for immorality. There are innumerable examples of this principle illustrated by circumstances where withdrawal of the penalty eventually results in the code being abandoned. Conversely, actions initially dictated by expediency tend to become community mores as the years pass. The penalty for unpremeditated sexual promiscuity has always been the risk of unwanted pregnancy, resulting in either undesirable social consequences or the unpleasantness of therapeutic abortion. The availability of postcoital contraception removes the penalty. Of all contraceptive procedures it is the one most likely to encourage sexual indulgence by a segment of the population whose behaviour was previously governed by unwillingness to premeditate the need for contraception and fear of pregnancy when the opportunity for coitus presented. Complete removal of the latter risk may eventually result in the abandoning by society of the taboos against completely free and permissive sexual behaviour.

Postconceptional Procedures

The argument as to whether or not the use of pharmacological or mechanical agents to ensure that the uterine cavity is emptied of its contents at the time of expected menstruation is contraception or abortion is specious semantics. There is no doubt that the intent is to remove a recently implanted conceptus should one be present. The point is even clearer if such methods are only employed when menstruation is delayed. The legal position varies with the environment. In countries such as Great Britain where it is illegal to operate with the *intent* to procure abortion then 'menstrual regulation' is illegal. In countries where knowledge of the existence of a pregnancy is required to establish criminality the physician should at present escape prosecution. The recent development of radioimmunoassays for the β sub-unit of human chorionic gonadotrophin in plasma which can detect a pregnancy reliably 12 days after conception (Braunstein *et al.*, 1973) will help to solve the problem. When these tests become available there will be no difficulty in deciding if abortion is being performed (Chez *et al.*, 1974).

If trials of menstrual regulating procedures are conducted within the law, it is important that the patients are informed that repeating intra-uterine instrumentation or incomplete evacuation of the uterine contents conveys a risk of infection. This could take the form of acute local or systemic illness or chronic pelvic inflammatory disease with its risk of subsequent infertility and of ectopic gestation.

Therapeutic Abortion

In the current climate of world opinion with respect to therapeutic abortion the absence of information in the medical and lay press on its long-term effects is quite striking. This is due to the wish of those patients undergoing the procedure to pass the responsibility for the moral and physical implications of the procedure on to their physicians, and a reluctance of those performing the abortions to recognise the consequences of actions which most of them sincerely believe are in the best interests of their patients. These attitudes do not relieve the ethical physician from the responsibility of informing his patients of the possible sequelae of abortion. Sufficient information is available to suggest that the main long-term hazards are chronic pelvic inflammatory disease and incompetence of the cervix, although the magnitude of these risks is far from clear.

It follows that the ethics of a trial of any procedure for the termination of pregnancy involving repeated or prolonged intra-uterine manipulation, in which there is a high risk of the retention of products of conception or in which the cervix is forcibly or rapidly dilated should be carefully considered. Comparisons with the potential long-term morbidity of established procedures are essential.

Only a very few of the traditional oral 'abortifacient' drugs are in fact capable of causing abortion and their ecbolic action is in general a consequence of severe toxic effects in the mother. Two groups of drugs, quinine and folic acid antagonists such as methotrexate, combine the risk of toxicity to the patient with a risk of fetal abnormality if, as is often the case, the pregnancy continues. It follows that, as has been so with the prostaglandins, an exceptionally wide knowledge of the experimental and clinical pharmacology of a proposed abortifacient must be required before it can be considered for clinical trial.

Agents Acting in the Male

The development of such agents has also proceeded with commendable caution. The reasons are:

(1) groups of drugs known to affect male fertility usually have general toxicity;
(2) the possible genetic and teratogenic consequences of drugs affecting spermatogenesis are largely unknown;
(3) complete reversibility of the effect cannot be guaranteed;
(4) potential fertility in the male persists to a much greater age than in the female, requiring a correspondingly greater degree of foresight;
(5) fear of impotence in the subjects.

Sterilisation

Most of the ethical and legal implications of irreversible procedures for male and female sterilisation are well established; it is necessary to ensure that local standards are satisfied by any clinical trial. The main difficulty is to provide the patients with a fair assessment of the failure rate of a new procedure, since accurate information will not be available until it has been employed in thousands of subjects over a period of years. It is reasonable that a new procedure for trial should possess significant advantages over conventional operations to compensate patients for the inability to predict the chances of failure which they must accept.

The old concept that sterilisation should always be treated as an irreversible procedure does not really conflict with recent developments of potentially reversible sterilisation operations. The difficulty is simply semantic. Reversible sterilisation is a long-term contraceptive manoeuvre, and in trials it is merely necessary to pay additional consideration to assess the likelihood that reversal may fail.

CONCLUSION

Development in the field of fertility regulation has now reached a point where reasonably effective and reasonably safe procedures can be made available to all. The advantages to be gained by further methodological advances are therefore marginal. It follows that the strictest ethical criteria should be applied to clinical trials of all fertility regulation procedures.

REFERENCES

BRAUNSTEIN, G.D., GRODIN, J.M., VAITUKAITIS, J. and ROSS, G.T. (1973). Secretory rates of human chorionic gonadotropin by normal trophoblast. *Am. J. Obstet. Gynec.*, **115**, 447–450

CHEZ, R.A., CALLARI, E. and BRANCH, B.N. (1974). Menstrual regulation/vacuum abortion: a valid distinction? *Contraception*, **9**, 643–649

CONGENITAL DISABILITIES (CIVIL LIABILITY) ACT (1976). Her Majesty's Stationery Office, London

DRUG AND THERAPEUTICS BULLETIN (1974). Spermicides: advertising and instructions for use. **12**, 96

ELDER, M.G. (1974). Contraception. In *Obstetric Therapeutics*, p. 574. Ed. Hawkins, D.F. Bailliére Tindall, London

INTERNATIONAL PLANNED PARENTHOOD FEDERATION (1965). *IPPF Medical Handbook*, 2nd edn, p. 71. Ed. Kleinman, R.L. IPPF, London

KATZ, J.H. (1972). *Experimentation with Human Beings*, Chapter 11, section B, pp. 736–793. Russel Sage Foundation, New York

LAW COMMISSION, THE (1973). *Injuries to unborn children. Working Paper No. 47*, Appendix, pp. i–viii. Law Commission, London

MEDICAL RESEARCH COUNCIL (1964). Responsibility in investigations on human subjects. *Br. med. J.*, **ii**, 178–180

MEDICAL RESEARCH COUNCIL (1973). Responsibility in the use of medical information for research. *Br. med. J.*, **i**, 213–216

MEDICO-PHARMACEUTICAL FORUM (1974). *A Report by the Forum's Working Party on Clinical Trials*. Royal Society of Medicine, London

SETTLAGE, D.S.F., MOTOSHIMA, M. and TREDWAY, D.R. (1973). Sperm transport from the external cervical os to the fallopian tubes in women: a time and quantitation study. *Fert. Steril.*, **24**, 655–661

SNOWDEN, R., WILLIAMS, M. and HAWKINS, D. (1977). *The IUD. A Practical Guide*, pp. 10–12 and 107–109. Croom Helm, London

TIETZE, C. and LEWIT, S. (1974). Statistical evaluation of contraceptive methods. *Clin. Obstet. Gynec.*, **17**, 121–138

UNITED STATES DEPARTMENT OF HEALTH, EDUCATION AND WELFARE (1973). Protection of human subjects. Policies and procedures. *Federal Register*, **38**, number 221, part II, 31738–31749

UNITED STATES FOOD AND DRUG ADMINISTRATION. Cited by Medico-Pharmaceutical Forum (1974), q.v.

UNIVERSITY OF EXETER, FAMILY PLANNING RESEARCH UNIT (1974). *The Control of Oral Contraceptive Clinical Trials. A Working Party Report*, p. 70. University of Exeter

WORLD HEALTH ORGANIZATION (1968). Principles for the clinical evaluation
  of drugs. *Wld Hlth Org. techn. Rep. Ser.*, number 403
WORLD MEDICAL ASSOCIATION (1965). Declaration of Helsinki. Recommendations guiding doctors in clinical research. *W.H.O. Chronicle*, **19**, 31–32

Part VII
The Future

20 Developments in Fertility Control Methods

In the course of reviewing the literature of the last ten years we have noted little in the way of major advances in techniques of fertility control. The main technical developments – oral contraceptives, plastic intra-uterine devices, suction and intra-amniotic injection techniques for abortion and perhaps laparoscopy for sterilisation – had already been made. As a result, the last decade has been one of modification, application and evaluation. The 'advances' that have occurred have mostly been either 'nine day wonders', whose deficiencies have become apparent within a year or two of their introduction, or procedures which have settled down to limited use in the small segment of the population in which they are advantageous. We have mixed feelings about the value of the return for the increase in world expenditure on reproductive research from $31 million in 1965 to $119 million in 1974 and some doubts about the justification for the projected need (Harkavy *et al.*, 1976) of $498 million *per annum* for research by 1980.

Development of oral contraceptives has been hamstrung by the complete lack of comparative trials of different preparations. This has made it impossible to make valid comparisons of the merits and side-effects of different formulations and to assess adequately the effects of reduction in dose of synthetic hormones. Nonetheless, considerable decreases in the hormone content have been achieved. It was predictable from the start what the outcome with depot injections of hormones would be. It is not possible to provide the relatively stable blood levels that can be achieved by daily oral administration. In order to achieve maintenance levels and compensate for erratic release there must be an overdose initially. This conveys unwanted effects which are in general unacceptable, and the use of depot injections will remain limited to individuals in whom for some reason their advantages outweigh their risks and side-effects. The outlook has been improved somewhat by the use of Silastic implants and more recently of organic polymer implants with progestagens in the matrix. These slowly disintegrate and do not require surgical removal. The main outcome with hormone-loaded intra-uterine devices was predictable – that they would add the problems of progestagen-only contraceptives to those of intra-uterine devices. The most important development in intra-uterine devices has been the recognition that 'between centre' variation in event rates far exceeds the variation between different devices. When this is taken into account there is little to choose between the devices that are available. It will be many years before the consequences of copper-containing devices are known, and many practitioners are

429

reverting to the use of the simplest plastic devices whose performance characteristics have been well documented over many years.

Legal abortion is an emotional topic, and objective data on its possible long-term sequelae is hard to come by. To accumulate valid statistics on such low incidence consequences as mortality, for which accurate figures should be available, is a long, slow process and this has delayed the evaluation of developments. It has taken ten years to determine that laparoscopic sterilisation has a higher failure rate than the orthodox operative sterilisation procedures, and comprehensive data on the complications of laparoscopy are only just becoming available. Fortunately the ill-consequences of most of the newer procedures for sterilisation have become apparent within two or three years of their introduction.

It seems likely that basic studies on fundamental mechanisms are more likely to result in the development of new techniques for fertility control than further modification of existing concepts.

FEMALE CONTRACEPTION

Controlled Interference with Hypothalamic Function

Since the hypothalamic gonadotrophin-releasing factors were identified as decapeptides the possibility has been raised of producing agents which interfere with their synthesis, immunological agents which would inactivate the releasing factors and competitive antagonists which would prevent stimulation of gonadotrophin release. To be generally acceptable the effects of such agents would have to be sufficiently controllable that they would prevent ovulation without otherwise interfering with the menstrual cycle. In addition they would have to be reversible. The end effect required would be similar to that of the combined oral contraceptives, but without the unwanted metabolic effects and without interference with the normal peripheral functions of the sex steroids.

Many agents which deplete amines in the brain, such as reserpine and a number of psychotropic drugs, are already known. Their use sometimes leads to loss of gonadotrophic function and interference with ovulation and menstruation as a side-effect. What is needed is an agent whose specific action is on the synthesis of the releasing factors. Attempts have already been made at immunological inactivation of LH releasing factor (Fraser, 1975). Analogues of LH releasing factor have been found which act as competitive antagonists in animals (Coy *et al.*, 1974; Vilchez-Martinez *et al.*, 1976). It may be possible to develop these agents to a point where they become useful clinically (Baird, 1976).

Preliminary tests have been made using the gonadotrophic secretion inhibitor danazol (Danol) as an oral contraceptive in women. The drug delays or blunts the pre-ovulatory surge of LH (Wentz *et al.*, 1976; Colle and Greenblatt, 1976). Doses of 50 or 100 mg/day are not very effective as a contraceptive; 200 mg/day inhibits ovulation but unwanted side-effects are common (Lauerson and Wilson, 1977). It seems possible that more specific agents of this type will be developed in the course of time.

The next logical step in this field would seem to be the development either of immunological agents which would inactivate LH or FSH, or of competitive antagonists of these gonadotrophins. At this level in the chain of events leading to ovulation, specificity of action would be possible and dose regimens might be found which would prevent ovulation without interfering with sex steroid synthesis to a degree that would affect systemic functions.

Interference with Steroid Hormone Activity

The term 'anti-oestrogen' has been applied to agents which interfere with oestrogen synthesis and release, agents which are competitive antagonists of oestrogens and androgens which exhibit physiological antagonism to oestrogen effects. In fact, the most specific use of such compounds as contraceptives is giving the combined oral contraceptive pill to prevent the pre-ovulatory surge of oestrogen secretion from the ovary. This is probably the main mechanism by which these agents prevent pregnancy. Less subtle use of anti-oestrogens is likely to lead merely to interference with required functions of the oestrogens or to exhibition of unwanted effects of the anti-oestrogen agents.

A great deal of animal work has been devoted to luteolytic drugs which interfere with the production of progesterone by the corpus luteum in the second half of the menstrual cycle. No drug that is sufficiently specific and effective for use to prevent implantation in humans has yet been produced, though the prostaglandins may yet be of interest in this respect. Little attention seems yet to have been paid to the possibility of developing specific progesterone antagonists or to immunological inactivation of this steroid. Recent information about progesterone receptors in the endometrium promises a possible approach to blocking the effects of this steroid.

Prostaglandins and the Ovary

The levels of prostaglandin $F_{2\alpha}$ increase markedly in ovarian follicles of rabbits and mice before ovulation (LeMaire *et al.*, 1973; Yang *et al.*, 1973; Saksena *et al.*, 1974). This rise may be stimulated by LH (Marsh *et al.*, 1974). Prostaglandin synthetase inhibitors such as indomethacin have been shown to prevent gonado-trophin-induced ovulation in rabbits (Armstrong *et al.*, 1974) and rats (Behrman *et al.*, 1972) as well as in rhesus (Wallach *et al.*, 1975) and marmoset monkeys (Maia, H., Jr., Barbosa, I., Lopes, T., Elder, M.G. and Coutinho, E.M., unpublished observations). In all these species the ova are retained within a normal luteinised follicle. Despite indomethacin treatment the pre-ovulatory LH surge occurs normally, indicating that interference with ovulation is at the ovarian level (Sato *et al.*, 1974). These facts suggest that prostaglandins produced by the ovary may play some part in the release of the ovum.

The ovaries of several mammalian species have been shown to contain smooth muscle cells in the stroma and in the follicle walls (Okamura *et al.*, 1972). These may be responsible for the inherent motility of the ovary *in vivo*, which varies throughout the human menstrual cycle, and for the altered ovarian motility and tone seen after administration of intravenous gonadotrophins (Coutinho and Maia, 1972) and prostaglandin $F_{2\alpha}$ (Virutamasen *et al.*, 1972; Coutinho and Maia, 1971). These observations suggest that increased ovarian motility, perhaps induced by locally released $F_{2\alpha}$, may cause rupture of the ripe Graafian follicle, allowing ovulation to take place.

Recent work (Elder, M.G. and Coutinho, E.M., unpublished observations) has shown that ovarian motility induced by intra-ovarian injection of prostaglandin

$F_{2\alpha}$ can be inhibited by oral flufenamic acid, which is a prostaglandin antagonist as well as a synthetase inhibitor. The development of a prostaglandin synthetase inhibitor acting primarily on the ovary may provide a non-steroidal oral contraceptive for the future.

Menstrual Induction with Prostaglandins

Oral or vaginal prostaglandins, taken monthly, have been suggested as a possible means of controlling fertility by causing very early abortion.

Experimental evidence in animals suggests that prostaglandin $F_{2\alpha}$ causes venous constriction, raising the venous pressure in the ovarian vessels and so affecting the vascular drainage of the corpus luteum. The ability of prostaglandin $F_{2\alpha}$ to cause luteolysis has been shown in rats, rabbits, hamsters, the rhesus monkey and the horse, and this may be related to its mode of action in the human. The dose of prostaglandin E_2 or $F_{2\alpha}$ necessary to stimulate the uterus to contract sufficiently to expel the implanting blastocyst causes side-effects such as nausea, vomiting and diarrhoea. These are more prevalent with oral and intravenous administration; vaginal and intra-uterine administration reduces the problem.

Prostaglandins E_2 and $F_{2\alpha}$ were administered vaginally by Karim (1971) to eight women who had a positive pregnancy test and four others who also had delayed menstrual periods. Vaginal administration into the posterior fornix of either 40 mg of prostaglandin E_2 or 100 mg of $F_{2\alpha}$ in two divided doses was advised at four hourly intervals. Two women were given a third dose on the second day because of the absence of uterine bleeding on the first day. A marked increase in uterine activity started within ten minutes of the insertion of prostaglandin and reached a peak after 60–90 minutes. The increased activity lasted for about four hours. In 10 out of the 12 women uterine bleeding began within 1–6 hours.

Csapo (1974) further developed the use of intra-uterine prostaglandins to induce menstruation, with the idea of altering the balance between endogenous prostaglandins and progesterone. The technique, which he calls 'prostaglandin impact' is based on the following hypothesis.

(1) The uterus synthesises its own intrinsic stimulant, in the form of prostaglandins, the rate of synthesis being controlled by the extent to which the uterine wall is stretched.
(2) Progesterone sustains a high myometrial threshold for excitation and so prevents activation of the pregnant uterus by endogenous prostaglandins.
(3) Withdrawal of progesterone decreases the threshold of uterine excitability, increasing the reactivity of the myometrium to stimuli, including endogenous prostaglandins. This effect can be blocked by substitution therapy with progesterone.
(4) The functioning of the corpus luteum is dependent on luteotrophic support from the conceptus. Compromising the conceptus may provoke luteolysis, and a reduction in progesterone output. This would allow the uterus to respond to prostaglandins.
(5) The increase in myometrial tone may compromise the blood supply to the conceptus and diminish its endocrine function. Progesterone production

may then be reduced by withdrawal of luteal and placental progesterone. The reduction in progesterone would increase the excitability of the myometrium, the uterus becoming highly sensitive to stimuli, and abortion or the onset of delayed menstruation would occur.

The doses used by Csapo (1974) were 5 mg of $F_{2\alpha}$ or 1 mg of E_2, instilled directly into the uterus. They caused painful contractions requiring analgesia; the more prolonged use of lower doses was unreliable. In 22 women whose menstrual period was an average of 12 days overdue and who had positive pregnancy tests bleeding began within a few hours and continued for an average of 8 days. The pregnancy tests became negative in 20 patients; the uterus was curetted in the other two. The fall in progesterone and oestradiol levels in these cases are shown in *Table 20.1*.

Table 20.1 PROGESTERONE AND OESTRADIOL-17β LEVELS BEFORE AND AFTER THE INTRA-UTERINE INJECTION OF 5 mg OF PROSTAGLANDIN $F_{2\alpha}$ IN 22 PATIENTS WHO WERE 6 MONTHS PREGNANT (CSAPO, 1974)

	Plasma progesterone (ng/ml)				*Plasma oestradiol-17β* (ng/ml)			
Hours	*0*	*3*	*6*	*24*	*0*	*3*	*6*	*24*
Mean	19.2	16.1	13.2	10.7	0.47	0.32	0.28	0.27
s.e.	± 2.2	± 2.4	± 2.1	± 1.9	±0.66	±0.04	±0.03	±0.03

All values are means ± s.e.m. Only 2 out of 22 patients had the uterus curetted, probably unnecessarily. There was a 44% reduction in plasma progesterone (P<0.05).

In larger studies, on 100 patients, similar results were obtained using either 5 mg prostaglandin $F_{2\alpha}$ or 1 mg prostaglandin E_2 (Csapo *et al.,* 1973; Mocsary and Csapo, 1973; Csapo, 1974).

Subsequent work has led to the development of a prostaglandin pellet of 5 mg of prostaglandin $F_{2\alpha}$ and an applicator so that it could be inserted into the uterus like an intra-uterine device. The pellet was found to be as effective as the solution. Halving the dose to 2.5 mg proved to be as efficient. The applicator is narrow and simple to use. Its use by the individual or by paramedical personnel may be feasible.

It seems unlikely that 'prostaglandin impact' in its present form will become a successful method of fertility control. Many women – and their doctors – do not like the idea of early abortion for birth control. The procedure is painful. It involves both intra-uterine manipulation and the likelihood of retained products of conception – a combination of circumstances which predisposes to chronic pelvic inflammatory disease.

On the other hand it is possible that prostaglandins may be the key to a method of fertility control. When their exact roles in human reproduction are better understood it may well be possible to pinpoint some mechanism which can either be blocked or exaggerated to a point where conception is prevented.

Prevention of Implantation of the Blastocyst

The possibility of active isoimmunisation with placental tissue as a method of fertility control was investigated in rats several years ago. Control of fertility was transient and reversible; autoimmune renal damage occurred in some cases. The next step in these studies was to focus on the human placenta and in particular human chorionic gonadotrophin. This hormone is secreted by the fertilised ovum before implantation, and is essential for the maintenance of pregnancy. If it could be neutralised by antibodies in the blood stream, while it was passing from the trophoblast to the corpus luteum, implantation would cease, and 'abortion' would take place. Hearn (1976) has reviewed much of the recent animal work on this topic.

The criteria necessary for a successful approach to immunological control of fertility are that the immunogenic stimulus should lead to the formation of antibodies capable of reacting with the β fraction of the HCG molecule, and neutralising its biological activity, and that the antibodies should not cross-react with other hormones, particularly LH. In addition the immunity should be of reasonable duration — at least six months; it should be reversible; and there should not be any toxicity or side-effects.

Initial experiments with varying proportions of dinitrophenyl groups tagged covalently to the β-subunit of HCG showed that they were immunogenic in the rhesus monkey and that the antibody response lasted for more than 14 months (Dubey *et al.*, 1976). The β-subunit is selected because this is the part of the HCG molecule which characterises its effects and distinguishes it from LH, FSH and thyroid stimulating hormones, all of which have an immunologically similar α-subunit to that of HCG. Further work resulted in the processing of the β-subunit to minimise the cross-reactivity with LH, and the use of tetanus toxoid as the conjugate. This combined vaccine induced antibody formation to both the HCG and the tetanus toxoid. The number of injections required varied according to the adjuvant used, one injection being adequate with Freund's complete adjuvant, but two or three injections being required with alum precipitate or sesame oil (Talwar *et al.*, 1976). Antibody titres reached a plateau at between 9 and 20 weeks after injection, began to decline after 6 months, and had virtually disappeared after 11 months. The antibodies raised to HCG-tetanus toxoid in goats and monkeys have been shown to inhibit the biological action of HCG. These antisera abolished the HCG-induced rise in ventral prostate weight of immature male rats and of uterine weight in prepubertal mice. The antisera were also effective in preventing the binding of radioactive-labelled HCG to receptors in rat testes and goat corpora lutea, and prevented *in vitro* progesterone production from slices of corpus luteum (Das *et al.*, 1976). Up to 64 times the human dose of the vaccine did not cause any increase in mortality in experimental animals (Dubey *et al.*, 1976) and there were no significant changes in liver function tests or many other biochemical and haematological tests (Sharma *et al.*, 1976). Post mortem studies on animals immunised for between 6 and 20 months showed no evidence of immunological or toxic damage (Nath *et al.*, 1976).

These encouraging results led to a trial of the vaccine in women.

Four subjects were immunised with the β-HCG-tetanus toxoid vaccine. All of them responded to active isoimmunisation by producing antibodies to both antigens. Thorough investigations of hepatic and renal function, and metabolic, endocrine and haematological studies for one year, have failed to show any abnormality (Kumar *et al.*, 1976). Anti-HCG antibodies were detectable in these women after 6 to 8 weeks, and they reached a maximum at 5 months. The titres then declined but were still high after 11 months in 3 of the 4 subjects. In one woman the titre had reached almost zero by 16 months, suggesting that the method may be reversible. The antibodies formed reacted immunologically with HCG and neutralised its biological activity. Three women continued to have normal menstrual periods and lactation was unimpaired in the fourth, who was puerperal, the antibodies not being secreted in the breast milk. The anti-tetanus immune response is of longer duration than, and is independent of, the anti-HCG response.

These results suggest that there is a future for immunisation against pregnancy as a method of fertility control. Much more work needs to be done but the results to date suggest that the combined vaccine is safe, and probably effective yet reversible with time. What is not known so far is the effectiveness of the method and how long it takes for the anti-HCG antibody titre to fall in a large number of women. Another unanswered question is whether or not a subsequent pregnancy, occurring in a woman whose antibody titre had fallen, will restimulate antibody production. The possibility of cross-reaction with LH must also be borne in mind, for whilst these initial experimental results suggest that there is minimal cross-reaction longer studies will be necessary before definite conclusions can be drawn. Significant cross-reaction with LH could lead to irreversible failure of ovulation and amenorrhoea.

The possibility of passive immunisation by the injection of antisera to HCG has also been raised (Hearn, 1976). This may be an advantageous approach since the onset of effectiveness might be expected to be more rapid, and reversibility more likely.

The potential advantages of an immunisation against pregnancy, especially if it can be made to be effective for two years and yet reversible, would be control of fertility and family spacing in the underdeveloped countries, provided the distribution and administration problems could be solved. These seem significantly less than with other contraceptive methods. The possibility of significantly fewer unwanted symptoms with immunisation also seems encouraging.

MALE CONTRACEPTION

The possible male methods of fertility control that may be used are hormonal, reversible vasectomy and retention within the vas deferens of some form of spermicidal agent such as filaments of copper or zinc.

Numerous hormonal methods have been tried in experimental animals and some in man (Fotherby, 1977). The methods which currently seem to be feasible can be summarised as follows.

(1) *Subdermal implant of an androgen.* This allows the release of an androgen from a silicone rubber implant over a period of months in a dose sufficient to suppress gonadotrophin secretion and inhibit spermatogenesis. Long-term treatment may have undesirable effects on erythropoeisis, lipid metabolism and the liver.

(2) *Injection of an androgen.* Testosterone oenanthate, acting for three to six months, has the same effect as a subdermal implant, spermatogenesis being suppressed.

(3) *Subdermal implant of a progestagen.* This allows the continuous release of low doses of progestagen, usually medroxyprogesterone acetate, which will

not suppress the production of gonadotrophins, but which will prevent the maturation of spermatozoa within the epididymis. Larger doses of either 17α-acetoxy- or 19-nor-progestagens do suppress gonadotrophin secretion. Loss of libido and gynaecomastia can result.

(4) *Androgen–progestagen oral preparations* act by depressing gonadotrophin levels, and so diminishing spermatogenesis, and by preventing maturation of sperm in the epididymis. The androgen counteracts the tendency of the progestagen to reduce libido and potency by gonadotrophin depression leading to reduced testosterone synthesis.

(5) *Oestrogens* are potent inhibitors of gonadotrophin release in the male, inhibiting spermatogenesis and reducing testosterone secretion. Used alone they tend to reduce libido and induce gynaecomastia.

(6) *Oestrogen–androgen oral preparations.* Twenty milligrams of ethinyl-oestradiol and 10 mg of methyltestosterone has been given twice daily to five volunteers. There was no loss of libido and no hepatotoxicity. Numbers of spermatozoa and motility were significantly diminished after 12 weeks. Spermatozoa did not reappear until 15 weeks after treatment was discontinued. Normal motility and normal numbers of spermatozoa returned after 35–40 weeks (Briggs and Briggs, 1974).

(7) *Danazol* (Danol) inhibits gonadotrophin release in men, but oral doses of 600 mg/day only produce a small reduction of spermatogenesis. In combination with an androgen, severe oligospermia or azoospermia can be produced in a few weeks (Skoglund and Paulsen, 1973; Paulsen and Leonard, 1976).

(8) *Anti-androgens.* Cyproterone acetate (Androcur) has been shown to produce reversible inhibition of spermatogenesis and a reduction in plasma testosterone (Petry *et al.*, 1972; Morse *et al.*, 1973). Cyproterone acetate blocks androgen receptors centrally and peripherally. In the hypothalamus it prevents endogenous androgens from inhibiting LH secretion, but increase in LH secretion does not occur since by virtue of its progestagenic properties cyproterone exerts a negative feedback on the hypothalamus (Brotherton and Harcus, 1973).

Other workers have suggested that cyproterone acts directly causing an inhibition of testosterone secretion (Morse *et al.*, 1973) and these authors observed a reduction in count of spermatozoa, libido and potency, after the administration of 200 mg/day. Doses used have varied from 50 to 200 mg/day.

Unwanted effects are serious disadvantages to the use of cyproterone in male fertility control, but the drug has been useful in the control of aggressive hypersexual behaviour in males. With a dose of 30 mg/day Petry *et al.* (1972) found that it took 7–15 weeks to obtain a significant reduction in spermatogenesis, and 4–5 months to regain a normal sperm count after cessation of therapy. Smaller doses (5–20 mg) can bring about rather slowly developing decreases in spermatozoa count without affecting libido or potency (Koch *et al.*, 1976; Roy *et al.*, 1976).

Other Experimental Procedures in Males

Immunisation with purified gonadotrophin could result in a gonadotrophin insufficiency and so diminish spermatogenesis. Reversibility will be a major problem.

Attempts are also being made to find a polypeptide that is an antagonist to gonadotrophin-release factors. In the male this would have the effect of diminishing spermatogenesis.

Another of the experimental methods currently being examined in animals is immunisation with testicular tissue or spermatozoa. Spermatozoal auto-antibodies may be the cause of diminished fertility following re-anastomosis after vasectomy. A similar state, induced by the administration of purified antigens, is being sought in animal experiments. With this procedure also, reversibility remains a major problem at the present time.

A certain amount of work, mainly in animals, has been done on drugs which act directly on the testis, interfering with production and maturation of spermatozoa (*see* de Kretser, 1976). Progress in this field is likely to be understandably slow — it is overshadowed by the risk, however small, of producing permanent testicular damage and interference with sexual potency.

Reversible Occlusion of the Vas Deferens

The use of liquid silicone rubber that vulcanises into a pliable plug at body temperature has been tried in animals. Removal of this leaves the vas undamaged.

The inclusion of a two-way gold tap fixed in the vas has also been tried, but the expense and possible irreversible fibrosis induced by its presence mean that this cannot be a very practical method.

Reversible Vasectomy

Re-anastomosis of the divided *vas* is not easy and can only be done if there has been a small segment of *vas* excised. Despite this, mobilisation may be difficult because of adhesions and fibrosis. If adequate union of the cut ends is achieved, the problem of diminished fertility due to auto-antibodies still remains. Vasectomy should not be thought of as a reversible procedure.

MOTIVATION

Most doctors who continue to be actively engaged in fertility control practice come to realise that the real problem which remains to be solved is neither that of technical advance nor that of provision of services. Again and again, detailed examination of the cause of failures reveals deep-seated or superficial reasons for acquiring a pregnancy or lack of any profound motivation for preventing one. Techniques already available are adequate for all ordinary purposes. In developed countries increasing availability of services is unnecessary for individuals who are already motivated to seek the means of controlling their family size and it will not help those who are not so motivated. Even in underdeveloped countries, where vast increases in education and provision of services are needed, consideration of motivational factors is important (Sai, 1976). As Potts (1976) puts it, to be effective, programmes must be consumer orientated.

In order to make progress in fertility control it will be necessary to achieve a far better understanding of the environmental and personal factors which contribute to contraceptive failure. The instinct to procreate is linked to the ego in the human, and the human female is physiologically ill-adapted to spend the greater part of her reproductive life in the non-pregnant state (Short, 1976). Only appreciation by individuals that many of the natural constraints to population increase have been removed and that they must assume responsibility for controlling their personal contributions to population is likely to solve the problem. In the next decade much more attention must be paid to the mechanisms involved in achieving this understanding.

REFERENCES

ARMSTRONG, D.T., GRINWICH, D.L., MOON, Y.S. and ZAMECNIK, J. (1974). Inhibition of ovulation in rabbits by intrafollicular injection of indomethacin and prostaglandin F antiserum. *Life Sci.*, **14**, 129–140

BAIRD, D.T. (1976). Manipulation of the menstrual cycle. *Proc. R. Soc. B.*, **195**, 137–148

BEHRMAN, H.R., ORCZYK, G.P. and GREEP, R.O. (1972). Effect of synthetic Gn–Rh on ovulation blockade by aspirin and indomethacin. *Prostaglandins*, **1**, 245–258

BRIGGS, M. and BRIGGS, M. (1974). Oral contraceptive for men. *Nature, Lond.*, **252**, 585–586

BROTHERTON, J. and HARCUS, A.W. (1973). Effect of oral cyproterone acetate on urinary FSH and LH levels in adult males being treated for hypersexuality. *J. Reprod. Fertil.*, **33**, 356–357

COLLE, M.L. and GREENBLATT, R.B. (1976). Contraceptive properties of danazol. *J. reprod. Med.*, **17**, 98–102

COUTINHO, E.M. and MAIA, H.S. (1971). The contractile response of the human uterus, fallopian tubes and ovary to prostaglandins *in vivo*. *Fert. Steril.*, **22**, 539–543

COUTINHO, E.M. and MAIA, H.S. (1972). Effects of gonadotrophins on motility of human ovary. *Nature: New Biology*, **235**, 94–96

COY, D.H., COY, E.J., SCHALLY, A.V., VILCHEZ-MARTINEZ, J., HIROTSU, Y. and ARIMURA, A. (1974). Synthesis and biological properties of (D-ARA-6, des-Gly-Na$_2$-10)-LHRH ethylamide, a peptide with greatly enhanced LH and FSH releasing activity. *Biochem. Biophys. Res. Commun.*, **57**, 335–340

CSAPO, A.I. (1974). 'Prostaglandin impact' for menstrual induction. *Population Reports*, series G, number 4, 33–40

CSAPO, A.I., MOCSARY, P., NAGY, T. and KAIHOLA, H.L. (1973). The efficacy and acceptability of the 'prostaglandin impact' in inducing complete abortion during the second week after the missed menstrual period. *Prostaglandins*, **3**, 125–139

DAS, C., SALAHUDDIN, M. and TALWAR, G.P. (1976). Investigations on the ability of antisera produced by Pr-β-HCG-TT to neutralize the biological activity of HCG. *Contraception*, **13**, 171–181

DE KRETSER, D.M. (1976). Towards a pill for men. *Proc. R. Soc. B.*, **195**, 161–174

DUBEY, S.K., SHARMA, N.C. and TALWAR, G.P. (1976). Survival of animals injected with Pr-β-HCG-TT. *Contraception*, **13**, 195–200

FOTHERBY, K. (1977). Androgen and progesterone compounds in male fertility control. *Br. J. Fam. Plann.*, **3**, 41 and 50–52

FRASER, H.M. (1975). Physiological effects of antibody to luteinising hormone releasing hormone. In *Physiological Effects of Immunity against Reproductive Hormones*, pp. 137–154. Ed. Edwards, R.G. and Johnson, M.A. Cambridge University Press

HARKAVY, O., JAFFE, F.S., KOBLINSKY, M.A. and SEGAL, S.J. (1976). Funding of contraceptive research. *Proc. R. Soc. B.*, **195**, 37–55

HEARN, J.P. (1976). Immunisation against pregnancy. *Proc. R. Soc. B.*, **195**, 149–160

KARIM, S.M.M. (1971). Once a month vaginal administration of prostaglandin E_2 and $F_{2\alpha}$ for fertility control. *Contraception*, **3**, 173–183

KOCH, U.J., LORENZ, F., DANEK, K., ERICSSON, R., HASON, S.H., KEYSERLINGK, D.v., LÜBKE, K., MEHRING, M., RÖMMLER, A., SCHWARTZ, U. and HAMMER-STEIN, J. (1976). Continuous oral low-dose cyproterone acetate for fertility regulation in the male? – A trend analysis in 15 volunteers. *Contraception*, **14**, 117–135

KUMAR, S., SHARMA, N.C., BAJAJ, J.S., TALWAR, G.P. and HINGORANI, V. (1976). Clinical profile and toxicology studies on four women immunized with Pr-β-HCG-TT. *Contraception*, **13**, 253–268

LAUERSON, N.H. and WILSON, K.H. (1977). Evaluation of danazol as an oral contraceptive. *Obstet. Gynec., N.Y.*, **50**, 91–96

Le MAIRE, W.J., YANG, N.S.T., BEHRMAN, H.H. and MARSH, J.M. (1973). Pre-ovulatory changes in the concentration of prostaglandins in rabbit Graafian follicles. *Prostaglandins*, **3**, 367–376

MARSH, J.M., YANG, N.S.T. and Le MAIRE, W.J. (1974). Prostaglandin synthesis in rabbit Graafian follicles *in vitro*. Effect of luteinizing hormone and cyclic AMP. *Prostaglandins*, **7**, 269–283

MOCSARY, P. and CSAPO, A.I. (1973). Delayed menstruation induced by prosta-glandin in pregnant patients. *Lancet*, **ii**, 683

MORSE, H.C., LEACH, D.R., ROWLEY, M.J. and HELLER, C.G. (1973). Effects of cyproterone acetate on sperm concentration, seminal fluid volume, testicular cytology, and levels of plasma and urinary ICSH, FSH, and testosterone in normal men. *J. Reprod. Fertil.*, **32**, 365–378

NATH, I., GUPTA, P.D., BHUYAN, U.N. and TALWAR, G.P. (1976). Autopsy report on Rhesus monkeys immunized with Pr-β-HCG-TT vaccine. *Contraception*, **13**, 213–219

OKAMURA, H., VIRUTAMASEN, P., WRIGHT, K.H. and WALLACH, E.E. (1972). Ovarian smooth muscle in the human being, rabbit and cat. *Am. J. Obstet. Gynec.*, **112**, 183–191

PAULSEN, C.A. and LEONARD, J.M. (1976). Clinical trials in reversible male contraception. I. Combination of Danazol plus testosterone. In *Regulatory Mechanisms of Male Reproductive Physiology*, pp. 197–211. Ed. Spilman, C.H., Lobl, T.J. and Kirton, K.T. Excerpta Medica, Amsterdam

PETRY, R., MAUSS, J., RAUSCH-STROOMAN, J.-G. and VERMEULEN, A. (1972). Reversible inhibition of spermatogenesis in men. *Hormone Metab. Res.*, **4**, 386–388

POTTS, D.M. (1976). The implementation of family planning programmes. *Proc. R. Soc. B.*, **195**, 213–224

ROY, S., CHATTERJEE, S., PRASAD, M.R.N., PODDAR, A.K. and PANDEY, D.C.

(1976). Effects of cyproterone acetate on reproductive functions in normal human males. *Contraception,* **14**, 403–420

SAI, F.T. (1976). The needs of the developing world. *Proc. R. Soc. B.,* **195**, 57–68

SAKSENA, S.K., LAU, I.F. and SHAIKH, A.A. (1974). Cyclic changes in the uterine tissue content of F-prostaglandins and the role of prostaglandins in ovulation in mice. *Fert. Steril.,* **25**, 636–643

SATO, E., TAYA, K., JYUJO, T. and IGARASHI, M. (1974). O.ulation block by indomethacin, an inhibitor of prostaglandin synthesis: a study of its site of action in rats. *J. Reprod. Fert.,* **39**, 33–40

SHARMA, N.C., GOEL, B.K., BAJAJ, J.S. and TALWAR, G.P. (1976). Metabolic endocrine and organ functions in monkeys immunized with Pr-β-HCG-TT vaccine. *Contraception,* **13**, 201–212

SHORT, R.V. (1976). The evolution of human reproduction. *Proc. R. Soc. B.,* **195**, 3–24

SKOGLUND, R.D. and PAULSEN, C.A. (1973). Danazol-testosterone combination: a potentially effective means for reversible male contraception. A preliminary report. *Contraception,* **7**, 357–365

TALWAR, G.P., DUBEY, S.K., SALAHUDDIN, M. and SHASTRI, N. (1976). Kinetics of antibody response in animals injected with processed beta-HCG conjugated to tetanus toxoid (Pr-β-HCG-TT). *Contraception,* **13**, 153–161

VILCHEZ-MARTINEZ, J.A., COY, D.H., COY, E.J., ARIMURA, A. and SCHALLY, A.V. (1976). Prolonged anti-luteinizing hormone/follicle-stimulating hormone-releasing activities of some synthetic antagonists of luteinizing hormone releasing hormone. *Fert. Steril.,* **27**, 628–635

VIRUTAMASEN, P., WRIGHT, K.H. and WALLACH, E.E. (1972). Effects of prostaglandins E_2 and $F_{2\alpha}$ on ovarian contractility in the rabbit. *Fert. Steril.,* **23**, 675–682

WALLACH, E.E., DE LA CRUZ, A., HUNT, J., WRIGHT, K.H. and STEVENS, V.C. (1975). The effect of indomethacin on HMG-HCG induced ovulation in the rhesus monkey. *Prostaglandins,* **9**, 645–658

WENTZ, A.C., JONES, G.S. and SAPP, K.C. (1976). Investigation of danazol as a contraceptive agent. *Contraception,* **13**, 619–630

YANG, N.S.T., MARSH, J.M. and LeMAIRE, W.J. (1973). Prostaglandin changes induced by ovulatory stimuli in rabbit Graafian follicles. The effect of indomethacin. *Prostaglandins,* **4**, 395–404

Epilogue

21 Doctors and Demography

'Every human society is faced with not one population problem but with two: how to beget and rear enough children and how not to beget and rear too many.' (Mead, 1949a).

This quotation puts the issue in a nutshell. Mead states mankind's perennial problem – how to keep births and deaths in balance with each other, and with the environment – and underlines the immediate problem – how to control the colossal explosion of numbers triggered off and continuously refuelled by the practitioners of medical science. This task presents not only great, possibly insuperable, practical problems but also important ethical questions. If people in general are held responsible for the foreseeable consequences of their actions, then all members of the health professions must take their individual share of the responsibility for this threatening outcome and ask themselves some fundamental questions; possibly those suggested at the end of the chapter.

THE BASIC FACTS. IS THERE A POPULATION PROBLEM?

Public opinion has moved so far in the last five years that there is now a very wide consensus that there is a problem of imbalance between population and resources although many would argue that there is no such thing as a 'pure' population problem. Ailments of the body politic have their demographic as well as their social, psychological, economic, political, religious and ethical aspects. The population problem should not be analysed or treated in isolation from its environmental and social matrix. Nevertheless it is true that there is a 'population problem' in that the numbers of mankind have doubled in the last 45 years, are expected to double once more in the next 35 to 45 years, and may even double again in the two or three generations after A.D. 2015, so that all of the net wealth mankind has created so far would have to be multiplied by four simply to maintain existing levels of poverty. Making an appreciable dent in world poverty would require at least one more doubling of wealth, increasing the requisite production multiplier to eight in not much more than one modern lifespan.

The demographic element in this equation sticks out like the proverbial sore thumb but as soon as we begin to ask why and how things happened as they did we are thrust into an almost intolerably complicated maze of social, cultural, psychological, ethical and economic interrelationships. If a society depends on a population for its existence, so the dynamics of a population depend on the character and behaviour of the related society *vis-à-vis* its own numbers and the environment. Fertility, mortality and migration, the three basic demographic variables, are all largely under social control, although this control is not always wielded consciously or purposefully, let alone intelligently.

The Three Population Explosions

On the world scale there have been three population explosions. The first was about a million years ago, the second some 10 000 years back, and the third, the one normally referred to, started just over three centuries ago. All of these were based upon waves of new technology; more precisely, upon technology directed outwards — from man towards his environment. The result has been that the carrying capacity of the environment has enormously increased, at least in the short term. This may be at the expense of the long-term carrying capacity of the environment because of technological man's profligate use of the earth's resources. Mumford (1934) analysed the later evolution of society along the scientific and technological continuum in his *Technics and Civilisation*. He calls the earlier phase the *eotechnic*, the middle the *paleotechnic*, and the third (and current) stage, the *neotechnic*. The 'modern' forms of birth-control, the pessary and the sheath, introduced into Western Europe from the Arab world by Fallopius (1523–1562), were '... the neotechnic answer to that vast, irresponsible spawning of Western mankind that took place during the paleotechnic phase, partly in response . . . to the introduction of new staple foods and the extension of new food areas, stimulated and abetted by the fact that copulation was the one art and the one form of recreation which could not be denied to the factory population, however it or they might be brutalised!' (Mumford, 1934).

A potent new factor entered the situation something over a century ago, gave the third population explosion a new impetus, and put an almost insupportable pressure upon our greatly enhanced support system. This was technology turned inwards — turned by man upon himself in order to understand the workings of his own body and to repair and improve upon natural processes so that life-expectancy at birth has more than doubled in the 'overdeveloped' countries, to use Ehrlich's (1970) phrase, and will soon have trebled in an even shorter period in the underdeveloped countries. I hope that Ehrlich's term for the latter, the 'never-to-be-developed' countries, is unduly pessimistic.

This increase in life-expectancy, not an increase in birth rates, is the 'cause' of the current explosion in numbers. People, once born, now tend to stay alive, increasing population size directly, and then to enter the reproductive phase, thereby swelling numbers still further.

The Bare Facts

The World

The United Nations mid year estimate for the world population in mid 1978 is just over 4200 millions. The crude annual birth and death rates are about 29 and

12 per 1000, respectively, giving a rate of growth of 1.7% per annum, a yearly natural increase of 72 millions, and a doubling-time of 41 years. The decrease in the doubling-time is a good indicator of the acceleration in the rate of increase of human numbers. Before the agricultural revolution around 8000 B.C. the doubling-time was some 75 000 years and as this time has decreased by a factor of about 2000 the *size* of each doubling has of course increased enormously, probably by a factor of 1600 as the estimated world population was only five millions in 8000 B.C.

What will happen in the future is unclear except for the one stark certainty that the world cannot possibly support population growth at these rates for much longer.

United Kingdom Population

It is important to be sure which territories are being referred to here as there is often confusion between the statistics for England, England and Wales (for which combined figures are published), Great Britain (England, Scotland and Wales) and the United Kingdom (which includes Northern Ireland in addition). Considering the territories that now comprise the United Kingdom as a single and historically continuous entity, our population was about 20 000 at the end of the New Stone Age, perhaps 400 000 at the time of the Roman Conquest, possibly increasing to two millions by the time the Romans left. Numbers decreased thereafter and were probably under one and a half millions at the time of the Domesday Survey.

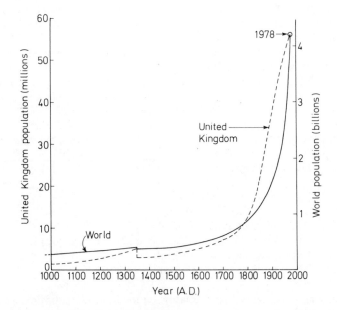

Figure 21.1 The World and the United Kingdom: population growth compared A.D. 1000 to 1978. (Adapted from Parsons, 1971b).

From A.D. 1286 they rose again to some five millions before, and three and a half millions after the Black Death. By A.D. 1600, two and a half centuries later, numbers had caught up again and from that point they rose rapidly, our population explosion proper dating from about A.D. 1700. The ten million mark was passed somewhat before 1800, 20 millions by 1847, 30 by 1882, 40 by 1911, and 50 millions by 1951.

The mid 1978 figure was nearly 56 millions and the outlook for the future is as unsettled on the demographic front as it is on the economic, social and political fronts.

Figure 21.1 shows that the United Kingdom has had a population explosion comparable to that of the world as a whole. In fact the United Kingdom led the way for well over a century but its population growth rate was already exceeded by that of the world as a whole by a factor of five or six even before the combined energy and economic crisis occurred in 1973 and the United Kingdom birth rate fell further.

UNDERSTANDING THE FACTS: THE ESSENTIALS OF DEMOGRAPHY

The history of population proper differs from the history of population studies. The former goes back at least one million years and possibly as much as four million, depending on where we draw the line regarding man's ancestors. The latter also has an ancient lineage as evidenced by the two tap roots of demography, analytically separate, if closely intertwined in real life. These are the 'problem' approach and the 'statistical-mathematical' approach (Hawley, 1968). The former studies population in terms of manpower, military might, prestige, poverty, prosperity, and so on, the socio-economic correlates of demographic variables, whilst the second relates to the numerical quantification and theoretical manipulation of the demographic variables themselves. Others have distinguished these as 'population studies' and 'formal demography' (Ford and de Jong, 1970). The first is prescriptive as well as descriptive, whilst the second is almost wholly descriptive.

Though demography proper is a newcomer compared with medicine or mathematics there is a case for regarding the problem approach to population — along with political science, well established by the time of Aristotle — as the most venerable of the social sciences. One of the oldest literary documents extant, impressed in cuneiform upon a clay tablet in Babylon between 1900 and 1500 B.C., is not only concerned with population problems, but calls for population control (Lambert and Millard, 1969):

> '... the people multipled ...
> Enlil heard their ... uproar
> And addressed the great gods,
> "The noise of mankind has become too intense for me.
> Cut off supplies for the peoples, ...
> There must be no rejoicing among them." '

Virtually all of the great commentators on the human condition have taken it for granted that a proper balance should be maintained between numbers and resources, and that these questions constitute proper matters for concern and appropriate action on the part of governments.

In the light of this ancient awareness there seems little point in listing the droves of scholars and men of affairs who later commented on population problems before Malthus capped them all with his great work in 1798.

Studies of past and contemporary so-called 'primitive societies', lacking both numeracy and literacy and analogous to civilised man's earlier stages of evolution, show that in the main they also had and often still have concern for population problems, coupled with appropriate mores and effective customs for the purpose of balancing numbers against resources in the light of their desired quality of life.

The statistical approach relates to two quite different types of activity, 'enumeration' and 'registration' (sometimes called 'vital' registration). Enumeration is the intermittent counting of heads whilst registration means keeping a continuous check on demographic change, individual marriages, births and deaths being recorded as they occur. Registration is equivalent to 'dead-reckoning' whilst the census checks the demographic position from time-to-time with a 'pinpoint' or 'fix'.

Enumeration had its earliest beginnings some 5000 years ago when the Sumerians started taking censuses as a basis for taxation (Pollard, 1973). Censuses are mentioned in the Bible and the ancient Romans also counted themselves to provide a basis for military conscription. In Britain there were many *ad hoc* counts, starting with the Domesday Survey, but the earliest example of an approximation to the modern periodic census, so far as I am aware, is provided by the Canadian French in 1665.

Ecclesiastical registration started in England in 1538 when Thomas Cromwell issued an injunction requiring all parish ministers to keep records of every marriage, christening and burial and these were further improved in 1558 under the orders of Elizabeth I. An attempt was made to institute civil registration as early as the 13th century, under Edward II, but it did not take root until 1837 when the appropriate civil departments were set up.

It was not until Malthus (1798) came along that demography's two strands were thoroughly fused. He was strongly problem-orientated but at the same time systematic, basing his deductions on a sound statistical basis, and he developed a coherent mathematical and theoretical framework. Of course he made some important mistakes but the central Malthusian point, as I understand it, is incontestable. This is, not that population *ought* to be controlled but that it is, always has been, and always must be controlled, for the simple reason that fecundity in all living things is invariably vastly greater than viable fertility. Keynes (1933) argued: 'If only Malthus, instead of Ricardo, had been the parent stem from which 19th century economics proceeded what a much wiser and richer place the world would be today. We have laboriously to discover and force through the obscuring envelopes of our misguided education what should never have ceased to be obvious!'

On the other side of the world the Chinese Malthus, Hung Liang Chi (1746–1809), put forward an almost identical thesis some five years earlier than Malthus himself (*see* Ping-Ti Ho, 1959), and from about this time population theories proliferated almost as rapidly as the human race. Great strides were also made in the mathematical handling of demographic data, one of the pioneers being Adolphe Quetelet (1796–1874), the Belgian astronomer, mathematician and meteorologist, who by 1830 was deeply immersed in population and social statistics. The word 'demography' itself was invented by Achille Guillard in 1855, some 50 years after the discipline of statistics was recognised and after 'sociology' was invented by Comte in 1838 (*see* Martineau, 1896), but a little before Haeckel (1834–1919) introduced the term 'ecology' in 1866 (Kormondy, 1969). The numerical branch has developed rapidly in complexity and sophistication from there into the computer age.

Despite all these great advantages it may not be out of place to offer a disclaimer on behalf of demographers who are all too often misunderstood and indeed maligned for their 'failure' to understand and forecast demographic trends some distance into the future. Demographers are not soothsayers and therefore cannot be expected to foretell the future any better than anyone else. Their techniques are for analysing past and present population dynamics, which are complicated enough in all conscience, and all they can tell us about the future is to say that on the assumption that present trends continue then population will be so-and-so at such-and-such a time, or, if the trends change in this way or that then the consequences will be different in this way or that. Demographers have no magic formula for determining whether present trends will continue or what new trends might replace them if they do not. Bagehot wrote, in 1876, 'The causes which regulate the increase in mankind are little short of all the causes, outward and inward, which determine human action.'

We do not expect political scientists to tell us which party will be in power in A.D. 2010, or even whether democracy will survive until then, so why should demographers be hounded for failing to prove an analogous public service in their field? The only way in which we can expect them to make reasonably firm projections is on the basis of structural properties. For example, they could say with virtual certitude in 1946 that, barring calamities, our post-war bulge would hit the junior schools in 1951 and the universities in 1964. They could also have added that it would hit the housing market around 1969 and help to force prices up still further, as the Population Stabilisation Group (1973) has subsequently pointed out. Demographers can project death rates and life-expectancies with considerable reliability, again barring calamities. They can also show that as around 37% of the world's population is under 15 years of age births will be greatly boosted when this generation starts to reproduce. Apart from these structure-determined probabilities, the great uncertainty is fertility, and this will remain so until we stop abusing our demographers and plan our population as we already try to plan all the other basic economic variables.

Balance of Births and Deaths: the Three Possibilities

There are only three possible relationships between births and deaths; births outnumber deaths, deaths outnumber births, or the two are equal. These three cases, together with their effects on population, are shown in *Figure 21.2*. Ignoring migration, when births outnumber deaths a population must increase, and *vice versa*, whilst in the special case, when the two are equal, it must remain stationary. This technical term is not equivalent to 'stable', a popular misnomer. A stable population is one in which, even though it may be growing or declining,

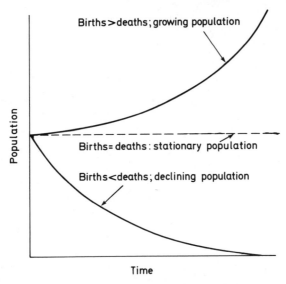

Figure 21.2 Balance of births and deaths. The three possibilities.

the vital rates are constant. From these simple and obvious relationships stems the inescapable fact that other than in the short run births must equal deaths.

If there is migration then births plus immigration must equal deaths plus emigration for a local population to remain stationary, and so on, *mutatis mutandis*, for the two other possibilities. Net migration must of course be zero for the world population. If there is fluctuation, regular or irregular, then the three curves shown in *Figure 21.2* could oscillate in an infinite variety of ways but the rules above would apply to their average relationship.

Life-expectancy and the Birth Rate

The birth rate required for a stationary population depends on the prevailing death rate, which is related to life-expectancy. If long life is valued (in many cultures it has not been) and death control is established, then either the birth rate must come down to match the new death rate, or population must rise. As population cannot rise indefinitely the birth rate must come down anyway – it is a question of when, rather than whether – or else deaths must rise again and life-expectancy decline.

Figure 21.3 shows the relationship between life-expectancy and birth and the crude death rate. The latter (in a stable population – an important proviso) is obtained by dividing 1000 by the life-expectancy at birth. The expectancy of 20 years, which appears to have characterised the Stone Age, would give a death rate of 50 per 1000 per year. This in turn would necessitate 50 births per 1000 per year – about four times the present level in Great Britain – simply to prevent a decline in numbers.

The average (male and female) life-expectancy at birth in Great Britain in 1978, about 72.5 years, would give a crude death rate of 13.8 per 1000 population per year in a stable population and requires, of course, a crude birth rate

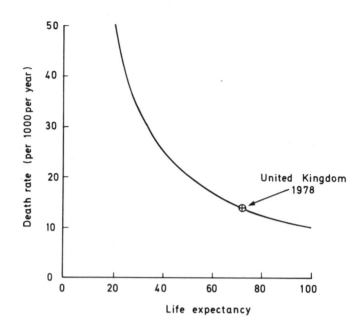

Figure 21.3 Relation between life-expectancy at birth (years) and crude death rate.

of the same figure to give a stationary population. The latter figure is the maximum we should aim for at present, and we should further reduce it if life-expectancy continues to increase. A few straws in the wind indicate that it may even decrease.

The Economics of Population

From time to time doctors concern themselves with the economic aspects of population problems, mostly without doing the necessary homework on these very complex matters. Despite this complexity, there are some straightforward cause and effect relationships and doctors can hardly be blamed for getting these wrong because nearly everyone else does, including many economists who egg us on with their fantasies of ever increasing wealth for an ever increasing number of consumers (Parsons, 1975, 1977b). In brief the main arguments are as follows:

Population Growth is Necessary to Stimulate Economic Growth

This belief sometimes takes the form that population growth is required, not merely to stimulate economic growth, but simply to keep the economy ticking over. With a stationary population we would find ourselves living in a society which is 'stagnant', a word with rather unpleasant connotations.

This argument grossly over-simplifies reality, ignoring all the other factors related to economic development and well-being; natural resources, terrain, climate, cultural variables, education, social behaviour, political factors, communications, technology – especially relating to inanimate energy – and so on. Arguing that all economic development is caused by population pressure is a very crude form of reductionism.

Population Growth is Necessary to Enable us to Bear the Burden of Aged Dependency

A number of doctors have been so concerned about this 'problem' that they have written to both medical journals and press arguing that the nation is approaching a crisis. They say we should put a stop to all talk of over-population, pollution, and scarce resources and concentrate on campaigning for more children.

Among these ardent pro-natalists are, for example, Dr. Iain Mackenzie, the Medical Officer of Health for Hereford, who created a furore in 1969 by urging people to increase the average family size in his area from two to four, backing this up with an appeal to the authorities to bring in 20 000 coloured workers to boost both numbers and fertility (Daily Mail, 1969; Daily Sketch, 1969).

Campbell (1973) has put the case in a more technical way. He argued recently '. . . there will be a gross unbalance in the structure of that enlarged population: there will be a deficiency of children and young adults who will have to bear the burden of dependency . . .'

These arguments are irrational and ignore virtually all the facts. The burden of dependency has two components: that of the old, obviously, and that of the young (under school-leaving age). The latter is at all times much greater than the former. It was nearly 14 times as great in 1821, six and a half times in 1906 and three times as great in 1931. Between 1941 and 1975 it has been around twice as great, and will remain at that level. The burden of the aged (over 65) group has indeed increased, from 3% of the population in 1821 to 13% in 1971 – that is by a factor of 4 – but the combined burden of dependency has declined over the whole of that period, from 44% in 1821 to 38% in 1971. The post-war increase in the burden of aged dependents has been from 11% in 1951 to 13.1% in 1970. The projected change from 1971 onwards is up to a peak of 14.3% in 1980 (up by 1.2%). By 1991 it will have gone down by 0.2%. By 2001 it will be 12.9% and by 2011, 12.6%. The 2011 figure is not only substantially less than the 1981 peak; it is less than the 1971 figure.

The combined burden of dependency will remain far less than it was in 1821 whilst, despite our economic tribulations, our productive power and surplus wealth for sustaining the so-called 'burden' of both young and old are vastly greater.

Far from creating insuperable social and economic problems, reduced birth rates bring marked benefits, as the Royal Commission on Population pointed out in 1949: 'The reduction in the number of children under 15 years from 12.6 million in 1911 to 10.4 million in 1947 has helped in raising standards in education and other services for children'. They also bring a substantial reduction in the demographic investment. This is the investment required with a rising population in order to maintain the level of investment *per capita*, a factor almost universally ignored by our economists and politicians.

The basic weakness of this argument is its parochialism: even if a stationary population did give rise to an uncomfortably large burden of dependency we would have to endure it because continued population growth is a physical impossibility.

Population Growth is Needed to Secure Economies of Scale

Another argument, this time with a modicum of truth in it, is also frequently trotted out: as enterprises become larger they can go in for ever greater specialisation, which in turn produces ever decreasing unit costs of production. Any decent elementary textbook in economics shows that 'returns to scale' can be both positive and negative. Up to the optimum size the returns are positive, whilst beyond it they are negative; unit production costs go up because of over-centralisation, bureaucracy, breakdown of communications, increasing transport costs and so forth.

Some of the smallest nations in the world are among those enjoying the highest material standards; Iceland, Luxembourg, Switzerland, Denmark, Norway and Sweden, for instance, whilst the largest are among the poorest, as we see in the cases of China, India and Indonesia.

Surely no argument, economic or otherwise, should rest upon a physically impossible basis — an ever increasing population.

Limits to Growth of World Population

Figure 21.4 shows some growth-curves giving hypothetical limits to the growth of world population, based on calculations made by Isaac Asimov (1971). It has

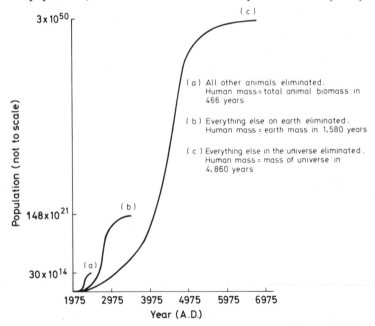

Figure 21.4 Three 'possible' limits to growth. All are impossible in real life.

been necessary to more or less ignore the correct proportions on the vertical axis as the numbers are so huge; a logarithmic scale would distort the shape of the 'S' curve. However, the time scale along the horizontal axis is a true linear representation, and the upper asymptotes are correct.

It would be absurd to contemplate any of these limits being approached, let alone reached. Asimov's point is that the present growth rate cannot possibly be sustained for more than a brief instant of historical time.

Automatic Versus Purposeful Control of Numbers

In addition to external checks to population — predation and food shortage, for example — all lower animals seem to have built-in population controls operating through such mechanisms as the instinct for territory. Indeed, the leading authority in this field, Wynne-Edwards (1962, 1964), has argued that the need to control numbers was the evolutionary imperative which led to communication and social behaviour. He thinks that *homo sapiens* may be the only living creature without a built-in population regulator, so that when man controls his numbers — as he mostly has done in the past — it must be through socially evolved values and institutions rather than biologically evolved instincts.

HUMAN POPULATION CONTROLS

These can be classified by their mode of operation under two broad headings, restriction of births and causation of deaths, with several important sub-headings.

Group 1. Some Typical Birth Prevention Measures

Keeping Potential Procreators Apart

The most efficient method of controlling numbers is simply to prevent potential procreators from coming together, and many measures have been used to attain this end. All known societies have imposed more or less onerous controls upon sexual activity, the most immediate and obvious of these being the incest taboo. Exogamy and endogamy put further obstacles in the way of finding a sexual partner, as do the minor variants of racial, class and religious endogamy.

The field of choice is narrowed by celibate religions, the dowry system, and many others. Two striking examples of the latter are provided by the Naga, whose girls used to mock any suitor who had not taken at least one human head, and the Galla of Ethiopia with whom the dowry had to include a spare pair of human testicles. Both of these provide double-acting population controls! Other drastic ways of keeping couples apart are to steer the sexually active towards a partner of the same sex, or towards members of other species, as in bestiality, and to make intercourse painful, difficult or impossible by means of female circumcision, infibulation, chastity belts and the like.

A milder custom adopted by cultures as far apart as post-famine Ireland and contemporary People's China is late marriage, which shortens the time available for procreation.

Prevention of Intercourse Between Established Couples

When couples have surmounted the hurdles keeping them physically apart, they often run into others keeping them sexually apart. One of these prevents intercourse with women with a child at the breast, often for quite inordinate periods by Western standards. Among the Arapesh, for example, the taboo is three years (Mead, 1939). This ensures widely spaced pregnancies, increases the offspring's life chances, and reduces the economic burden on both family and group.

Another way of preventing intercourse, still beloved of the Roman Catholic hierarchy, is to place a high value upon abstinence, as in the rhythm method of contraception.

Prevention of Conception During Intercourse

After these double barricades have been crossed and intercourse can take place, in many cultures further controls take over to prevent conception, sometimes by means of magical incantations and rituals, often with the aid of primitive birth control technology. As Draper (1965a) points out, cannibal societies tended to have more rational birth controls and population policies because of their gruesome but superior knowledge of human anatomy. Perhaps the logical beginning for an examination of these practices is with those permitting or even requiring 'aberrant' forms of heterosexual intercourse from which conception could not possibly follow, such as oral, anal and intercrural congress. Three other methods involve restriction during the sexual act proper, *coitus reservatus, coitus obstructus* (*coitus saxonicus*) and *coitus interruptus*.

Others again, requiring some knowledge of physiology, plus a simple technology, involve chemical, mechanical or combined barriers between sperm and ovum. Ancient papyri show that crocodile dung pessaries were used by ladies of the 12th Dynasty in Egypt, nearly 4000 years ago, and other societies have used a wide range of comparable techniques (Draper, 1965b).

Even more drastic methods requiring modification of bodily function by surgery have also been used. Among these are castration and sub-incision for males, and ovariotomy for females (Draper, 1965d).

Prevention of Birth After Conception

Most societies have been prepared to sanction abortion; many have actually required it in some circumstances, and it is still one of the most effective population controls ever evolved. Abortion has been procured in a wide variety of ways and the most picturesque which has so far come to my notice is that of the Kikuyu, who, it is said, to lighten their burden before a trek, used to lay their pregnant women on the ground and jump on their bellies until they aborted.

Group II. Causing Deaths

These controls may be grouped according to the point in the life-span at which they operate. No doubt some readers would want to include abortion under this heading.

Almost universal recourse has been had to infanticide, again by a very wide variety of methods. It is hard even to conceive of a practice more barbarous than the Madagascan habit of drowning unwanted babies in boiling water or burying them in ant-hills (Draper, 1965c).

Many cultures have applied general population controls at this stage, aimed at eliminating all members of a particular category rather than individual surplus infants. These have included infants born feet first, or on unlucky days, one or both of all twins, girls when boys were preferred, or *vice versa*, infants of mixed racial parentage and so forth. Australian aboriginals used to eat every tenth baby as a check on numbers (Whitmarsh, 1898; Sumner, 1906). The Todas used to lay nearly all their female infants in the mud for the buffaloes to trample to death, thereby creating such a shortage of wives that polyandry was necessary (Mead, 1949b).

Other controls have involved the reduction of numbers at later points in the life-span, long after the individuals concerned have become viable and accepted members of the group but before old age. These include dangerous exercises, rituals and trials of strength, compulsory emigration, which was the reason for much of the Viking predation in Europe (Parsons, 1971c), human sacrifice, cannibalism and institutionalised warfare. For a very interesting example of the last, coupled with other controls mediated through the size of a pig-herd, see the case of the Tsembaga in the highlands of New Guinea (Rappaport, 1968; Shantzis and Behrens, 1973).

The final category embraces methods used for killing, expelling or abandoning the old and the sick who were no longer able to look after themselves. Again the methods were sometimes very cruel but often a kindness was intended, and the deed had to be performed by the eldest son as an act of filial piety.

'MANIFEST' VERSUS 'LATENT' POPULATION CONTROLS

It will be clear by now that some of the measures described, such as abortion and infanticide, were designed to control numbers, whereas others, such as the Hindu rite of *suttee*, had the effect of controlling numbers although they were ostensibly designed for other ends. In sociological terms, this is the distinction between the 'latent' and 'manifest' functions of social mechanisms, defined as follows: 'Manifest functions are intended and recognised whilst latent functions are neither intended nor recognised' (Merton, 1967). A latent population control of particular relevance here was used by the Azande, who believed that all sickness and cures were caused by magic. They practised therapeutic techniques of such purblind inefficacy that a large proportion of the patients were killed so that society's medical agents were able to reduce population pressure whilst at the same time, by virtue of the mode of execution employed, furthering the value of solicitude for human life (Davis, 1956).

Possibility of Automatic Population Control in Man

I implied earlier that the Wynne-Edwards' (1962, 1964) thesis, that man is the only animal without built-in population control mechanisms, is generally accepted. There is in fact evidence that such mechanisms may exist in our species. Stott (1969) has argued: 'It may seem implausible to suggest that the appearance of lethal disabilities could have survival value . . . . but . . . for human beings we . . . reach the paradoxical conclusion that in times of . . . pressure . . . on food resources, any process which tended to lower the mental capacity, physical dexterity or perceptual acuity of a certain number of individuals might mean the saving of the race . . . Similarly, an increase in efficiency by natural selection may endanger the whole population if it reaches the point where the source of food is wiped out . . .'

Whilst admitting that population controls in man are mainly behavioural, he argues it is likely that, in addition, '. . . there is *regular genetic provision* for the production of malformation, or poor viability, in the offspring in times of stress.' Two of his examples are anencephaly and spina bifida. Other mechanisms described are periodic infertility, the '. . . self-banishing reaction . . .' in victims of parental rejection, and a lowering of intelligence in offspring (Stott, 1969).

Stott thinks the chief implication of his findings is that the catastrophe of a starving world is unlikely because these mechanisms will supervene and prevent the population explosion continuing up to that point. However this may be, the implications for medical people must surely be profound. On the one hand they have created the population explosion, and on the other hand they are doing their level best to negate, by ever more sophisticated means, the natural mechanisms which, if Stott is right, are operating as a countervailing force.

The Arithmetic of Procreation Control

Leaving aside those trusting souls who believe that population can grow for ever, people who agree that growth must stop sometime but who argue that it is unnecessary or wrong to control procreation, or both, surely must accept the responsibility of showing how a *laisser-aller* policy will produce the requisite end, a stationary population. Let us examine the procreative process from an arithmetical point of view.

Ignoring migration, the size of the United Kingdom population is determined by the procreative behaviour of around 11 million potential couples. Counting these as single decision-making units with the niggardly ration of one and three-quarters procreative decisions per week we have the round figure of 1000 million decisions each year, which, in 1977–78 gave us about 730 000 live births. Call this a round million to allow for miscarriages, stillbirths and induced abortions, and we have 1000 'nays' for every effective 'yea'. A 0.1% shift would either double our birth-rate or wipe us out. Asserting that population control will not be necessary must rest on the belief that our 1000 million procreative decisions each year will always sum to the social optimum, the births required for a stationary population.

Allowing for the hundreds of thousands of procreative accidents each year, and, according to apologists such as Campbell (1973), for the fact that couples are now making seriously sub-optimal decisions in failing (by some 11%) to replace themselves, we see that without social control the probability of a permanently optimal outcome is rather low.

Most medical people will know the old story of the woman who went to her doctor complaining of morning sickness and all the other symptoms of early pregnancy, whilst denying that they could be anything to do with having a baby because she was unmarried, until, eventually, under the doctor's creeping barrage of questions, she coyly admitted that she might possibly be 'just a tiny bit pregnant'. Most doctors (not to mention most demographers and social scientists) seem to think in an analogous way about the birth rate. If it is 'only a tiny bit' above the replacement level it does not count. *Figure 21.5* illustrates the 'tiny bit' syndrome with respect to a population of the smallest viable size

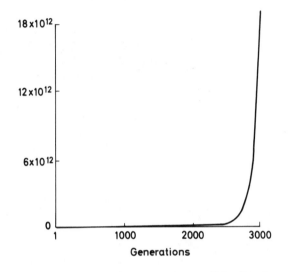

Figure 21.5 Growth of world population with very small families (Parsons, 1971a).

slightly overdoing the replacement function by producing one-hundredth of a child per person extra, giving an average of 2.02 children per couple. For 2000 generations there is no visible growth (This is an artefact, of course. Growth is exponential from the beginning but a scale chosen to show the earlier growth would not do for the later growth.) Around 2700 generations the growth curve leaps into a near-vertical exponential and in only 300–400 generations total numbers increase from somewhere near zero up to 18 thousand billions, increasing at that instant, by 180 billions per generation. It follows inexorably that, other than in the very short run, if man does not arrange for births to balance deaths, natural mechanisms will do it for him.

The Population Flywheel

Biosocial systems are such that even after innovations destined to produce great change they may appear to go on for some time behaving exactly as they did before. In engineering terminology there is a 'lag' in the control mechanism. This is equally true of demographic change and produces what has been called the population 'flywheel' effect. *Figure 21.6* shows the outcome of achieving replacement level fertility at four different dates, A.D. 1980, 2000, 2020, and 2040, with population levelling out at about 6.25, 8, 11.25, and 15.75 billions

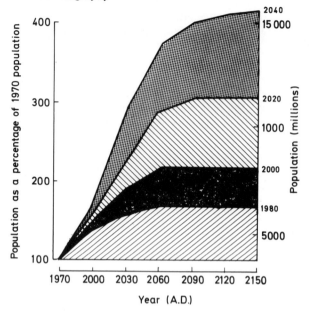

Figure 21.6 Alternative paths of approaching a stationary world population. Two-child family average achieved by A.D. *1980, 2000, 2020 and 2040 (Population Council, 1971).*

respectively, after various time lags. This shows that, barring calamities, it is virtually impossible for world population growth to be halted before at least one more doubling has taken place.

Completed Family Sizes and Future United Kingdom Populations

What follows is not a prediction. The only prediction I want to make is that population size, composition and distribution are virtually certain to come out wrong unless we plan them. It is possible to make various reasonable assumptions and show what would be the outcome if they turned out to be correct. An interesting set of projections was produced by Beral (1973) in a series of computer runs. These data (*Figure 21.7*) are for England and Wales but they are relevant to the whole country, and they show that if procreative motivations and practices remained steady at their 1973 levels our population would continue to grow so as to give us three or four millions more by A.D. 2000. Even at the long-term replacement level (2.1 children) it takes the better part of a life span for numbers to stabilise.

The curves related to the three below-replacement family sizes should comfort those who fear a population crash. At two children per family it is 60 or 70 years before the decline becomes visible. At 1.8 the population is more or less stationary for about 50 years before beginning to show a significant drop, and even at 1.6 children per family, appreciably below the present level, it would be 40–50 years before numbers started to decline sharply. Great Britain is unable to feed herself, and in the present state of the world is grossly overpopulated. We probably could feed ourselves if we tightened our belts, gave up most of our meat, and generally behaved unselfishly and rationally but there is little chance of any of these things happening except through Hobson's choice. My view is that we are over-populated by a factor of at least three, preferably four, a ratio implying an optimum population one-quarter of the present size. At this level we could not only live well on our own resources but enjoy a comfortable safety margin *vis-à-vis* such factors as unfavourable climatic change (Parsons, 1971d). We can only welcome a below-replacement fertility, provided it does not decline to and remain at unheard of levels.

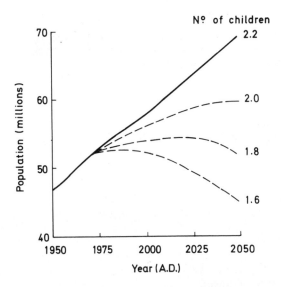

Figure 21.7 Population predictions by family size, in England and Wales (Beral, 1973).

We seem to be very irrational about the birth-population equation and there may be deep forces at work inside us to prevent our particular tribe from diminishing in size and power, as measured by some primitive index such as the number of arms to wield hoes and spears. We may have a fear amounting almost to dread of the demographic stationary state in which, of course, births match deaths exactly. In psychological terms it is rather like floating on one's back. If the base of the nostrils is exactly at water level we breathe in air and do not drown, the stationary state. It feels a whole lot safer, however, if the nostrils are at least a few millimetres above the waterline. If we do have an instinctive fear of a decline in numbers then a birth rate well above the replacement level must be very comforting. We have to get over this hurdle and though it may now appear to be a high one it ought to present little difficulty, even in the medium short term, because man has evolved in, and is therefore well adapted to, an economic and demographic steady state (Parsons, 1975).

The Fertility Reservoir

One way of mitigating these atavistic fears, and indeed of curing the problem if it should ever arise, is to ponder over the reservoir of fertility reflected in the abortion figures. Legal abortions for residents of England and Wales alone are running at about 120 000 a year, equivalent to about 2.2 per 1000 population per year. If the crude birth rate should fall as low as 2.0 below the replacement level of 13.8 per 1000 per year, with our current life-expectancy, it would still be unnecessary to revert to a pro-natalist policy. What we ought to do — bearing in mind that a controlled decline in numbers is desirable — is to introduce a policy of selective avoidance of abortion, which would meet several important needs:

(1) Population size could be controlled exactly, within the limits imposed by the number of those seeking abortions, by the simple expedient of measuring the birth deficit in any year and then saving the appropriate number of abortion candidates next year.
(2) The onerous medical task of destroying potentially viable fetuses, would be reduced to a minimum.
(3) A eugenic policy could be pursued, if desired, through the choice of candidates with the best genetic inheritance.
(4) The backlog of adoptions might be filled.

The policy should obviously be voluntary: would-be abortees being urged to bear their child in the national interest and given sufficient support to go through with the pregnancy. Some of the babies would turn out to be wanted after all, and would be reared in the ordinary way, whilst the others would be adopted, brought up by foster parents, or reared like orphans at the present time.

The great thing is to avoid panic and a pro-natalist backlash. There is no need whatever to worry about fertility at anything like the present levels, indeed it is a blessing — not even in disguise — and members of the health professions should ignore or quietly sit on the pro-natalist fanatics in their midst.

If it is dogmatic to insist that population will never level out without a deliberate policy of control — an allegation sometimes thrust into the teeth of us neo-Malthusians — it is doubly dogmatic to insist that it will spontaneously enter the stationary state without such a policy and remain there indefinitely into the future. This is to supplant Adam Smith's (1776) 'invisible hand' with the 'invisible condom' of the population apologist, an equally improbable device.

Even if the double dogma happened to encapsulate a demographic truth, which cannot be ruled out, it seems very unlikely indeed that the population would be not only stabilised but optimised.

DEMOGRAPHY AND THE HEALTH PROFESSIONS

Surely the implications of these facts for the medical profession cannot be other than profound. Livingstone (1951) has defined a technician as a person '. . . . who understands everything about his job except its ultimate purpose and its place in the order of the universe' and — in complete contrast to the wide-ranging humanitarian and environmental philosophy of the founding fathers of the medical arts and sciences — doctors have become technicians in just the sense described. There is virtually no concern about the relation between medical practice and the ecosystem, the evolutionary process, or man's spiritual needs. Even at the nuts and bolts level there is no sort of balance in the apportionment of scarce resources between curative and preventive medicine on the one hand, or between death control and birth control on the other. The health professions confine themselves almost solely to short-term goals, exemplified in the profligate use of the new antibiotics, making resistant strains an increasingly serious hazard, and ignore the probable consequences of their actions.

Hill (1952, 1969) has drawn attention to the ethical dilemma which is rarely faced in this context: 'If ethical principles deny our right to do evil in order that good may come, are we justified in doing good when the foreseeable consequence is evil?'

We are moral agents and must be held responsible for the natural consequences of our acts and failures to act, and the medical practitioner, who every day intervenes in the balance of nature and the evolutionary process, cannot be excused from this universal principle because he likes to believe that his intentions are good. He has spear-headed the attack on the earlier balance of nature which has created the current population explosion. His reluctance to face this fact, let alone initiate reasonable corrective action, lays him open to the charge of *hubris* partly in the pursuit of the self-interested goals of money, prestige and power.

The traditional ethic of Western Medicine rests on the teaching of Hippocrates, who, according to Dubos (1968), developed the code and practice of the lay Asclepiads who in turn borrowed and adapted to Greek life the even earlier medical sciences of Egypt and Mesopotamia. The lay Asclepiads practised under the aegis of the two goddesses, Hygeia, the goddess of health and preventive medicine, and Panacea who symbolised man's power over injury and disease through knowledge. These two complementary strands are found in the medical sub-cultures of all the great civilisations. In the Greek instance, Hygeia was a manifestation of Pallas Athena, the great divinity of wisdom, according to whom men will be healthy and contented if they live wisely and without excess.

Hippocratic medicine seems to be inspired much more by the teachings of Hygeia than of Panacea, and the avoidance of over-population would naturally come under her rubric. The collection of authors loosely called 'Hippocrates' advocate the practice of a medicine based on the natural sciences and pre-eminent among those, if only the name had been invented, would surely have been ecology a word which is derived, as is 'economics', from the Greek root *oikos* meaning household or dwelling place.

The essence of the practical side of Hippocratic medicine is summarised by Dubos (1968) under five headings, no less than four of which stress ecological balance. '1. The well-being of man is influenced by all environmental factors: . . . air, water and food; the winds . . . and topography . . . Understanding their effects . . . on man is thus the fundamental basis of the physician's art. 2. Health is the expression of harmony among the environment, the ways of life, and the various components of man's nature . . . 3. Whatever happens in the mind influences the body and the body has a like influence on the mind . . . (Health) can be achieved only by governing all activities of life in accordance with natural laws so as to create an equilibrium between . . . the organism and . . . the environment. 4. Whenever equilibrium is disturbed, rational therapeutic procedures should be used to restore it . . .'.

The need for a balanced approach and an understanding of man's place in nature are the very things which have become etiolated almost to vanishing point in modern medicine. The proliferation of specialisms, drugs, techniques and jargon has meant that practitioners no longer see the trees, let alone the wood.

The first law of ecology is that everything affects everything else, an over-statement in most everyday contexts, but a useful starting point for both science and for an examination of the effects stemming from a purposely intro-duced change in an ecosystem. Leach (1967) has coined the term 'biological backlash', the unforeseen and undesirable consequences of a change introduced to attain some good end. This concept has special relevance for the medical profession, as we see in the related process of iatrogenesis, the introduction of disease by the physician. The classic case of this, as Semmelweis showed, was that of the high mortality from puerperal fever in 19th century Austrian lying-in houses. A later and more insidious variant on this theme is the introduction of completely new and increasingly intractable problems. John Maynard Smith (1967), dean of the School of Biological Sciences, University of Sussex, has remarked '. . . it's getting to the stage when it's actually dangerous to go into hospital . . .' because of the proliferation of drug-resistant strains of bacteria.

If modern medicine has developed over the last two and a half centuries then this development has taken place during a great change in the situation regarding births, life-expectancy and death, which the French writer Fourastié has described in dramatic terms. 'At the end of the 17th century, the average man . . . living until 52 . . . will have seen about nine people die in his immediate family (not counting uncles, nephews and cousins) among whom would have been one grandparent (the three others being dead before his birth), both his parents and three of his children . . . Nowadays . . . the only deaths the average man of 50 . . . has seen have been those of his four grandparents.' He concludes that in future the average man will be between 55 and 60 when his father dies (Fourastié, 1959).

There is a strong tendency for cultural change to lag behind material change and we must question whether the Western medical value-system is in tune with the contemporary situation. If it is not, in what ways ought it to be modified?

WHAT SHOULD MEMBERS OF THE HEALTH PROFESSIONS DO?

All citizens are responsible to some degree for the state of our society and for the problems we have created and failed to tackle. The more intelligent and informed we are then the greater is our share of this responsibility. It follows from what has gone before, that the health professions must bear an extra burden of moral responsibility in this field as they are in the front line — they are the agents employed by society to tamper with the biological balance of nature and after all this discussion and criticism it would be remiss not to put forward some concrete proposals. These are grouped under two headings, general principles and particular instances.

General Principles

Members of the health professions should:

(1) Give themselves a reasonable grounding in basic ecological and demographic facts so that they can begin to understand the population—resources problem.

(2) Likewise with respect to the basic elements of economics, sociology, psychology and politics so that they have some insight into their social and cultural aspects.

(3) Reinterpret medical theory, values and practice in the light of the teachings of the earliest pioneers who aimed for a sound mind in a sound body in a health-giving environment.

(4) Re-examine their attitudes towards individual patients so that they are seen as members of a biosocial system, not, of course, to the extent of ignoring or riding rough-shod over their individual needs and value, but in such a way that the social dimension is present as well as the individual. The medical ethic should be more socio-centric and less ego-centric.

In essence doctors should ask themselves two basic questions:

(1) Taking the long view, are my activities doing more good than harm, or *vice versa*?

(2) What actions ought I personally to pursue, and urge my colleagues to pursue, in order to ameliorate the harm which has been done already and to ensure that in the future, as far as is humanly possible, the good outweighs the harm?

The answer must surely entail a switch from a simple, uncritical, short-term numerical philosophy, pro-natalism and life-prolongation regardless of the consequences; not to anti-natalism, but to a critical, flexible, self-aware and long-term philosophy of what one might call *equi-natalism*, a balancing of births against deaths, informed by a deeper concern for the quality of life rather than the quantity of life.

To those doctors who ask with feeling and more than a little justice, where in their 70 hour working week they are going to find time for all this study and concern, I would answer that they might consider the particular points listed below, or, at the very least, refrain from expressing hasty judgements or ill-considered opinions concerning these vital questions.

Particular Instances

Ethical Pro-natalism

The health professions must now ask themselves whether or not the original commitment to the preservation of existing human life, through the Hippocratic Oath, has evolved into a dedication to the production and preservation of an ever-increasing quantity of human life.

Economic Pro-natalism

Do the health professions have a vested interest in pro-natalism? More babies mean more hard cash for the legion of obstetricians, midwives, paediatricians and others. The passionate tone of much of the argumentation against family planning and induced abortion indicates that this vested interest does exist. It is difficult to account on other grounds for the irrationality of the argument that induced abortion uses resources needed in the maternity wards and elsewhere. The typical abortion uses far less resources than the birth which would otherwise take place, apart from saving a lifetime of medicine for the resulting person.

Allocation of Scarce Resources

By what arguments can doctors justify the gigantic effort in pro-natalist and life-prolonging research and practice, in comparison with the minuscule allocation of funds for the discovery and improvement of safe, cheap, effective, and aesthetically pleasing birth-control appliances and techniques?

Population Optimisation

The health professions are very well placed to help solve the thorny problem of the optimum population. Traditionally this has been defined in economic terms (Carr-Saunders, 1964), more specifically in terms of *per capita* income (when this is maximised population is optimised) but the concept has been rejected for all practical and most theoretical purposes. This is short-sighted: the fact that we cannot give a precise, universally agreed, and permanently valid definition to the notion of an optimum population does not make it useless. Not one of our major policies is precisely defined, unanimously accepted, or permanently relevant, so why should not a population policy with numerical goals be adopted and pursued on a temporary, rule of thumb basis in precisely the same way?

To optimise our numbers we must maximise our quality of life and the health professions could help in various ways, for instance, by working out some ground rules about how much space and what sort of amenities we need for a full and healthy life. In particular they can determine by epidemiological criteria the optimum numbers, distribution and mobility of the population in order to minimise the spread of disease in the light of the evolution of the new immune strains of dangerous pathogens.

Ill-effects of Large Families

Are doctors aware, and do they inform their patients, how unsatisfactory an environment is provided for a growing child by a large family? (Parsons, 1977a). By virtually every measurable criterion the child in the large family is appreciably worse off than his opposite number in a small family. He is shorter, lighter, less healthy, less emotionally developed, less able to cope with schoolwork and less likely to stay on the right side of the law. The only two positive things I have found in favour of children in the large family are reductions in the incidence of obesity and of pyloric stenosis.

Doctors should surely study these facts and — without pressuring their patients — advise them accordingly.

Relaxation of Closed Shop

Are you, for the purpose of making the most effective use of our scarce resources, prepared to reconsider and possibly to relax the near monopolistic hold of the medical profession on the dispensation of drugs and medicaments and, in particular, of contraceptives of proven safety? (Speiden *et al.*, 1973).

'. . . It would be a responsible and constructive step forward in medical practice to widen the range of those empowered to dispense oral contraceptives to include state registered nurses, midwives, and health visitors who have had some additional training in contraceptive practice.' (Smith *et al.*, 1974).

The pill is already off prescription in Bangladesh, Pakistan, the Philippines, Thailand and a number of other countries. Of course the situation is not the same here as in the poor countries and there could be snags but on the other hand we have a much larger reserve of moderately well educated manpower and if paramedical staff could be more widely used then both doctors and patients — not to mention taxpayers — would be better off.

Two-way Population Control

Most people think that population control refers only to activities intended to reduce births but this is one-sided. All population policies are designed to attain certain social, economic, or political goals, and there is no moral distinction between policies for raising numbers and for reducing them. Doctors must ask themselves what their response would be if our birth rate fell some way below the long-term replacement level and the government of the day, backed by public opinion, asked them to encourage people to have more babies and fewer abortions in the national interest. Only those doctors who can declare, hand on heart, that they would have nothing to do with it are entitled to ethical objections to a policy of stabilising or reducing numbers.

CONCLUSION

This chapter is called 'Doctors and Demography' but in my heart I feel that perhaps it really ought to be called 'Doctors and the Balance of Nature' because much more than demography or population in general or fertility control in particular is involved. Mankind is rapidly approaching a great turning point in what Lapp (1973) has called the 'Logarithmic Century' perhaps a re-turning point would be a more apposite description. The population explosion will be controlled, by one means or another, massive and general economic growth will stop, severe resource and pollution constraints will make themselves felt in no uncertain way, and we shall re-enter some new approximation to our normal demographic, social and economic steady state.

Medical practitioners have been one of the main agents in triggering off the explosion and I hope they will play an equally important part in shepherding mankind back into a saner, quieter, more neighbourly and more permanently viable world.

The requisite moral and philosophical resources are not only there to be re-discovered in the thought and work of the founding fathers of medicine but cast a luminous glow over the centuries. I hope that the medical profession will pause, observe, reflect and react in accordance with the current moral and ecological imperatives.

REFERENCES

ASIMOV, I. (1971). The end. *Penthouse,* 5, No. 10, January, pp. 22–24 and 52.

BAGEHOT, W. (1876). The preliminaries of political economy. In *Economic Studies* (1888) p. 86. Ed. Hutton, R.H. Longmans, Green, London and New York

BERAL, V. (1973). Cited by Allaby, M., Blythe, C., Hines, C. and Wardle, C. (1975). 'Losing Ground'. *Family Planning,* 24, Number 1, April, 3–13

CAMPBELL, H. (1973). Letter to the editor. *The Times,* 26th March

CARR-SAUNDERS, Sir A. (1964). *World Population. Past Growth and Present Trends*, 2nd impression, pp. 330–331. Frank Cass, London

DAILY MAIL (1969). Please have more babies, country told! 8th December.

DAILY SKETCH (1969). Poser over the size of families. 10th December

DAVIS, K. (1956). *Human Society*, chapter 20. Macmillan, New York

DRAPER, E. (1965a, b, c and d). *Birth Control in the Modern World,* pp. 59, 88, 102 and 117 respectively. Penguin Books, London

DUBOS, R. (1968). *Man, Medicine and Environment*, pp. 76–83. Penguin Books, London

EHRLICH, P. (1970). *Population, Resources, Environment.* W.H. Freeman, San Francisco

FORD, T.R. and DE JONG, G.F. (1970). Editors, *Social Demography*, Preface. Prentice Hall, New Jersey

FOURASTIÉ, J. (1959). De la vie traditionelle à la vie tertiaire. *Population,* July–September. Cited by Pressat, R. (1973). *Population,* pp. 51–52. Pelican Books, London

GUILLARD, A. (1855). *Éléments de Statistique Humaine ou Demographie Comparée.* Guillaumin, Paris

HAECKEL, E. (1866). *Generelle Morphologie der Organismen,* p. 286. George Reiner, Berlin. See also Kormondy, E.J. (1969)

HAWLEY, A.H. (1968). *Roderick D. McKenzie on Human Ecology,* p. 36. University of Chicago Press, Chicago and London

HILL, A.V. (1952). The ethical dilemma of science. *Nature, Lond.,* 170, 388–393

HILL, A.V. (1969). Cited by Hardin, G. (1969). *Population, Evolution and Birth Control,* p. 77. Freeman, San Francisco

HOLY BIBLE. II Samuel, 24, 2–8

KEYNES, J.M. (1933). *Essays in Biography.* p. 121. Norton, London

KORMONDY, E.J. (1969). *Concepts of Ecology,* p. viii. Prentice Hall, New Jersey

LAMBERT, W.G. and MILLARD, A.R. (1969). *The Babylonian Story of the Flood.* Cited by Adler-Karlsson, (1974) in *Harrying and Carrying Capacity*, p. 69. Swedish Royal Ministry for Foreign Affairs, Stockholm

LAPP, R. (1973). *The Logarithmic Century.* Prentice Hall, New Jersey

LEACH, G. (1967). In *Biological Backlash.* A series of four programmes broadcast in March, 1967, in the British Broadcasting Corporation Third Programme

LIVINGSTONE, Sir R. Cited in Vogt, W. (1951), *The Road to Survival,* p. 272. Gollancz, London

MALTHUS, T.R. (1798). *Essay on the Principle of Population*, 2 volumes, pp. 692, 693. Everyman's Library (1967) London. *See also* Flew (1970), editor, *Malthus, An Essay on the Principle of Population.* Penguin Books, London

MARTINEAU, H. (1896). *Comte's Positive Philosophy,* volume 2, p. 201. George Bell, London

MEAD, M. (1939). *Sex and Temperament in Three Primitive Societies.* Mentor Books, New York and London

MEAD, M. (1949a, b). *Male and Female*, pp. 210 and 223, respectively. Penguin Books, London

MERTON, R.K. (1967). *Social Theory and Social Structure,* chapter 1. Free Press, New York: Collier Macmillan, London

MUMFORD, L. (1934). *Technics and Civilisation,* pp. 260–261. Routledge, London

PARSONS, J. (1971a, b, c and d). *Population versus Liberty,* pp. 21, 41, 116 and 208–211 respectively. Pemberton, London

PARSONS, J. (1975). *The Economic Transition.* Conservation Trust, Chertsey, Surrey

PARSONS, J. (1977a, b). *Population Fallacies,* chapters 7 and 14, respectively, pp. 74–96. Elek/Pemberton, London

PING-TI HO (1959). *Studies on the Population of China 1368–1953.* Harvard University Press, Cambridge, Massachusetts

POLLARD, J.H. (1973). *Mathematical Models for the Growth of Human Population.* Cambridge University Press, London

POPULATION COUNCIL (1971). *Annual Report,* p. 38. New York

POPULATION STABILISATION GROUP (1973). *Overpopulation . . . It's Costing us the Earth.* London

RAPPAPORT, R.A. (1968). *Pigs for the Ancestors.* Yale University Press, Newhaven

ROYAL COMMISSION ON POPULATION (1949). Paragraph 462. Her Majesty's Stationery Office, London

SHANTZIS, S.B. and BEHRENS, W.W. (1973). Population control mechanisms in a primitive agricultural society. *Toward Global Equilibrium*, pp. 257–288. Ed. Meadows, D.L. and Meadows, D.H. Wright-Allen, Cambridge, Massachusetts

SMITH, ADAM (1776). *The Wealth of Nations.* Everyman's edition, (1950), volume 1, p. 400. Dent, London; Dutton, New York

SMITH, J.M. (1967). In *Biological Backlash.* A series of four programmes broadcast in March 1967, in the British Broadcasting Corporation Third Programme

SMITH, M. *et al.* (1974). Distribution and supervision of oral contraceptives. *Br. med. J.,* iii, 161, Also in Smith, M. and Kane, P. (1975). *The Pill off Prescription,* p. 16. Birth Control Trust, London

SPEIDEN, L., RAVENHOLT, R.T. and TERRY, M.I. (1973). Non-clinical distribution of oral contraceptives. *Advances in Planned Parenthood,* 8, 28–29

STOTT, D.H. (1969). Cultural and natural checks on population growth. In *Environment and Cultural Behaviour,* pp. 90–120. Ed. Vayda, A.P. Natural History Press, New York

SUMNER, W.G. (1906). *Folkways.* (1959 edition). Dover Publications, New York

WHITMARSH, M.P. (1898). *The World's Rough Hand,* p. 178. Century, New York

WYNNE-EDWARDS, V.C. (1962). *Animal Dispersion in Relation to Social Behaviour.* Oliver and Boyd, London

WYNNE-EDWARDS, V.C. (1964). Population control in animals. *Scientific American,* **211**, August, number 2, 68–74

Index

Abortifacient drugs, 297
Abortion Act 1967, 57, 117, 237, 239, 245, 265
Abortion, legal, 237–313
  abdominal hysterotomy, 300
  abortifacient drugs, 297
  alcohol injection, 293
  bougie, 296
  clinical trials, 422
  complications, 267
  contraception after, 393
  counselling, 237–262
    aftermath of abortion, 246
    circumstance of conception, 243
    consequences of pregnancy, 244
    contraception after abortion, 247
    depression, 245
    environmental pressures, 245
    equivocation, 245
    examination, 246
    late abortions, 249
    married women, 248
    mentally incompetent patients, 249
    objectives of interview, 243
    rejection of request, 247
    sterilisation after abortion, 247
    teen-age girls, 247
    type of operation, 246
  cytotoxic agents, 297
  dilatation and curettage, 271
    mid-trimester, 299
  dextrose injection, 293
  ethacridine lactate, extra-amniotic, 294
  fructose injection, 294
  grounds for, 238–243
    contraceptive failure, 189
    injury to children's health, 242
    injury to mental health, 241
    injury to physical health, 240
    preservation of life, 243
    risk of handicapped child, 242
    risk to life, 239
  hormone withdrawal for, 298
  hypertonic saline, extra-amniotic, 295
  hypertonic saline, intra-amniotic, 284–293

Abortion, legal,
  hypertonic saline, intra-amniotic (*cont.*)
    cervical damage, 293
    complications, 290
    contra-indications, 288
    haemorrhage, 292
    hypernatraemia, 291
    infection, 292
    injection difficulties, 290
    management, 290
    procedures, 288
    systemic effects, 287
    vaginal approach, 289
    water and electrolytes, 291
  hysterotomy, 300
    complications, 301
    vaginal, 302
  intrauterine device insertion at, 202
  Karman catheter, 264
  legal background, 238
  mannitol injection, 294
  married women, 248
  menstrual regulation, 265
  mentally incompetent patients, 249
  metreurynter, 296
  mortality, 246, 251
  older women, 389
  operative
    first trimester, 264
    mid-trimester, 298
  oxytocin, 296
  prostaglandins, 272–284
    extra-amniotic, 280
    intra-amniotic, 274
    intramuscular, 274
    intravaginal, 281
    intravenous, 272
    intravenous with oxytocin, 273
  rejection of request, 247
  rhesus isoimmunisation and, 263
  sequelae, 246, 252
    cervical incompetence, 255, 271
    depression, 259
    ectopic gestation, 253, 270
    infertility, 246, 252, 253, 263, 270
    hysterotomy scars, 258

Abortion, legal
  sequelae (*cont.*)
    pelvic inflammatory disease, 253,
        263, 270
    perinatal mortality, 258
    premature labour, 256
    psychiatric, 246, 258
    spontaneous abortion, 255
  soft soaps, 295
  special cases, 247–249
  sterilisation with, 247, 355
  techniques, 263–313
  teen-age girls, for, 247
  type of operation, 246
  urea injection, 293
  use of products for research, 249
    placenta, 251
  vacuum curettage, 266
  vaginal hysterotomy, 302
Abortion, septic, associated with intra-
    uterine devices, 229
Abortion, spontaneous
  after legal abortion, 255
  incidence, 58
  intra-uterine devices and, 215
Abruptio placentae, after legal abortion,
    259
Abstinence,
  periodic, 153
    advantages, 156
    disadvantages, 157
    infertile periods, 154
    use-effectiveness, 155
  psychological stress and, 157
  total, 158
17-Acetoxyprogesterone derivatives, 94,
    96, 97
Acid phosphatase activity, intra-uterine
    devices and, 169, 171
Acne and combined pill, 64
Actinomycosis, intra-uterine devices and,
    223
Aerosol spermicides, 145
Age, combined pill and, 73, 76
Aged dependency, 451
Albumin, oestrogen and, 21
Alcohol injections for abortion, 293
Aldosterone, 27, 63
Alkaline phosphatase, oestrogen and, 22
Allergy, condoms, causing, 137
Amenorrhoea,
  post-pill, 56, 57, 67–68
  sterilisation, after, 322
American tips, 134
Amino acids,
  oestrogen action on, 21
  progestagen action on, 37
Aminocaproic acid, reducing intermenstrual
    bleeding, 220
Aminotransferase, oestrogen and, 22

Androgens,
  lipoproteins, action on, 20
  subdermal implants of, 435
Androgen-progestagen preparations,
  male use, 36
Androstenedione, structure, 8
Anti-androgens, 436
Antigon device, 183
  expulsion of, 217
Antiplasmin, quinestrol and, 94
Antithrombin III, oestrogen action on, 16
Ascorbic acid, oestrogen action on, 22
Atherosclerosis, and combined pill, 20
Autoimmunity, vasectomy and, 362, 363

Bacterial endocarditis, and intra-uterine
    devices, 187
Bactericidal agents, as spermicides, 146
Barbiturates, combined pill and, 66
Birnberg bow, 164, 181
  expulsion of, 217
  pregnancy and, 213, 215
Birth defects, and progestagen pill, 105
Birth rate,
  balance with death rate, 448
  life-expectancy and, 449
Blastocyst, prevention of implantation of,
    433
Blood coagulation,
  cascade mechanism, 14
  disorders of, sterilisation in, 328
  oestrogen action on, 14–18
  prostaglandins affecting, 278
Blood coagulation factors,
  combined pill and, 69
  oestrogen action on, 15
  progestagen action on, 35
  stilboestrol affecting, 16
Blood dyscrasias, intra-uterine devices and,
    188
Blood groups, thrombo-embolism and, 72
Blood platelets,
  adhesiveness, and combined pill, 15
  chlormadinone acetate action on, 15
  oestrogen action on, 15
Blood pressure,
  combined pill and, 62, 80
  continuous low dose progestagens and,
      104
  oestrogen action on, 13
  progestagen action on, 35
Body weight, progestagens affecting, 38
Bowbent diaphragm, 139
Breakthrough bleeding,
  combined pill and, 56, 61, 66
  intra-uterine devices and, 168
Breast cancer,
  implanted hormones, from, 5
  oestrogens and, 81

Breast tenderness,
depot progestagens causing, 108
Bronchiectasis, sterilisation and, 329
Bronchospasm, prostaglandins and, 276,
278

C-films, 147
Caesarean section,
intra-uterine devices after, 186
repeated, sterilisation and, 331
Candida infection, and intra-uterine device,
221
Caps, *see under* Diaphragms, Cervical caps,
Vault caps, etc.
Carbohydrate metabolism,
combined pill and, 53, 75, 129
depot progestagens and, 109
oestrogen action on, 18, 76
progestagen action on, 36, 76
sequential pill and, 92
Carcinogenesis, combined pill and, 80
Cardiovascular disorders, contraception
and, 401
Cardiovascular system,
oestrogen action on, 13
progestagen action on, 35
Carpal tunnel syndrome, combined pill
and, 62
Censuses, 447
Cerebral thrombosis, 403
age and, 73
combined pill and, 69, 72, 74
Cerebral vascular abnormalities,
sterilisation and, 329
Cervical caps, 133, 142–143
Cervical cytology, annual check, 55
Cervical erosion, intra-uterine devices and,
221
Cervical incompetence,
post abortion, 255
vacuum curettage, following, 271
Cervical mucus,
combined pill affecting, 52
continuous low dose progestagens,
effects of, 97
intra-uterine devices affecting, 166
observation of in rhythm method, 155,
156
oestrogen affecting, 10, 13
progesterone affecting, 27, 35
Cervical shock, insertion of intra-uterine
device causing, 206
Cervicitis,
contra-indicating IUD, 185
intra-uterine devices, insertion and, 203
Cervix,
carcinoma,
aetiology, 136
depot progestagens and, 109

Cervix
carcinoma (*cont.*)
intra-uterine devices and, 186, 228
oral contraceptives and, 81
damage to,
hypertonic saline abortion, in, 293
prostaglandins causing, 279
vacuum curettage causing, 267, 269
virus infections of, 136, 185
Chlormadinone, 3, 29
action on,
blood pressure, 35
carbohydrate metabolism, 36
cervical mucus, 35
liver function, 37
ovulation, 32
platelet behaviour, 15
sperm transport, 34
continuous use, 95
side effects, 103
structure, 29
vaginal ring containing, 113
Cholecystitis, combined pill and, 79
Cholestatic jaundice,
combined pill and, 78
oestrogen causing, 22
sequential pill and, 92
Cholesterol, 25
oestrogen action on, 20
Chromosomal abnormalities, ageing of
sperm and, 157
Clinical trials of contraceptives, 409–425
agents acting in males, 423
analysis of, 410
barrier methods, 419
classification of, 411
community mores and, 416
conduct of, 417
confidentiality of records, 415
consultation, 411
ethical considerations, 412
specific procedures, 419–423
family planning behaviour, effects on,
411
feasibility, 410
field of study, 410
follow-up procedures, 418
future fertility, 415
general principles, 413–417
interpretation, 410
intra-uterine devices, 420
low-incidence major complications and,
419
management of failures, 414
oral contraceptives, 420
patient motivation, 415
patient's consent, 418
physical benefits of, 413
physician attitudes, 416
physician–patient confidentiality, 415

Clinical trials of contraceptives (*cont.*)
  planning, 410
  postcoital contraceptives, 421
  postconceptional procedures, 422
  psychological consequences, 413
  publication, 411
  public relations, 416
  racial and political factors, 416
  recruitment for, 417
  reporting of results, 419
  risk of teratogenesis, 414
  spermicides, 421
  sterilisation, 423
  technical advances, 416
  types of, 417
Clogestone, 98, 117
  fallopian tube, effect on, 34
Clostridium Welchii, 294
Coarctation of the aorta, 326
Coeliac disease, 402
Coital timing, sex of child and, 156
Coitus interruptus, 151–153
  advantages and disadvantages, 152
  effectiveness, 153
  incidence of use, 135, 152
  reasons for failure, 153
Combined Multiload CU-250, 183
Combined pill, 3, 49–90
  abortion after, 394
  action on, 52; *see also* side-effects
    carbohydrate metabolism, 19, 75, 129
    cervical mucus, 52
    endometrium, 52, 55
    hypothalamus, 129
    liver function, 21
    ovulation, 52
    plasma proteins, 21
    renin-angiotensin system, 62, 63
  age factors, 126
  benign tumours of liver and, 79
  breakthrough bleeding and, 56, 61
  carcinogenesis and, 80
  carpal tunnel syndrome and, 62
  cerebral thrombosis and, 69, 72, 74
  changing, 55
  clinical management, 53
  clinical trials, 420
  composition of preparations, 49
  congenital abnormalities and, 58, 129
  contra-indications to, 69
    age factors, 73, 76, 128
    Hodgkin's disease, 82
    hypertension, 62, 80, 402
    malignant melanoma, 82
    obesity, 75, 77
    plasma coagulation factors, 69
    psychological, 80
    risk of diabetes mellitus, 75
    risk of liver damage, 78
    thrombo-embolism, 69

Combined pill
  contra-indications to (*cont.*)
    varicose veins, 73
  coronary thrombosis and, 128
  depression and, 56, 80, 404
  drug interaction, 66
  effectiveness of, 127
  failure of, 56
    outcome of pregnancy, 56
  failure to take, 66
  fibroids and, 405
  gynaecological disease and, 405
  heart disease and, 401
  initial preparation prescribed, 54
  initial prescription, 53
  management of patients on, 55
  menopause and, 59
  migraine and, 404
  mode of action of, 52
  neonatal jaundice and, 58
  oestrogen content of, 49
  older woman, for, 59, 388
  post-partum, 390
  post-pill amenorrhoea following, 56, 67
  pre-eclamptic toxaemia and, 63
  pregnancy following cessation of, 57
  progestagen content of, 49
  psychological effects of, 64
  replacement therapy, as, 60
  side effects of, 54, 60–68
    age factors, 59
    change of pill, 55
    depression, 65
    headache, 61
    hypertension, 62
    irregular bleeding, 61
    lactation, on, 61
    leg aches and cramps, 63
    loss of libido, 56, 65
    nausea, 65
    psychological, 64
    skin lesions, 64
    urinary tract infections, 23, 63
    weight gain, 55
  stopping, 57
  surgery and, 58
  teenagers, for, 384
  thrombo-embolism and, 127, 128
    age affecting, 73
  tuberculosis and, 402
Communication, marital, 376
Condoms, 133–139
  advantages and disadvantages, 136
  allergy from, 137
  failure rate, 137, 401
  gynaecological disease and, 404
  older couples, for, 388
  plastic, 134
  post-partum use, 392
  quality control, 133
  teenagers, for, 385

Condoms (*cont.*)
    use of, 134
    venereal disease and, 134, 136
Congenital abnormalities, combined pill
    and, 56, 58, 129
Congenital Disabilities (Civil Liability)
    Act, 1976, 57, 414
    postcoital pill and, 118
Congenital heart disease,
    indicating sterilisation, 325, 400
Congenital limb reduction, 58
Contact lenses, combined pill and, 64
Contraceptive pill, combined, *see* Combined
    pill
    postcoital, *see* Postcoital pill
Cooperative Statistical Program for the
    Evaluation of Intra-Uterine Devices,
    176
Copper,
    endometrial effects of, 171
    intra-uterine devices containing, 170
        perforation by, 226
        postcoital use, 211
        pregnancy rates, 214
        replacement, 208
        vaginal discharge from, 221
Copper Omega, 183
Copper T device, 183
Coronary thrombosis,
    combined pill and, 60, 69, 74, 128
Corpus luteum,
    continuous low dose progestagens,
        effects of, 96
Cortisone metabolism, oestrogens affecting,
    23
Creams, spermicidal, 145, 146
Crohn's disease, 402
Cyproterone acetate, 436
Cytotoxic agents inducing abortion, 297

Dalkon shield, 182
    additional precautions with, 207
    expulsion of, 217
    expulsion rates, 201
    insertion of, 205
    perforations by, 182, 224
    pregnancy and, 215
    pregnancy rate, 164, 173
    removal during pregnancy, 215
Danazol, 430, 436
Dehydroepiandrosterone, structure, 8
Demography, 443–467, *see also* Population
    balance of births and deaths, 448
    essentials of, 446
    health professions and, 460
        action required, 462
Depot hormonal contraception, 105–114
    combined oestrogen-progestagen
        injections, 110
    intramuscular progestagen, 106

Depot hormonal contraception (*cont.*)
    mode of action, 106, 110, 112
    post-partum, 393
    subcutaneous implants, 113
    vaginal rings, 111
Depression,
    abortion, grounds for, 245
    combined oestrogen-progestagen
        injections causing, 111
    combined pill and, 55, 56, 65, 80, 404
    post abortion, 259
Developments in fertility control, 429–440
Diabetes mellitus,
    combined pill and, 75, 78
    contraception and, 403
    latent, 77, 78, 99
    oestrogens and, 18
    progestagens and, 36
    sterilisation and, 330
Diaphragms, 133, 139–142
    advantages and disadvantages, 141
    failure rates, 141, 401
    fitting, 139
    older woman, for, 388
    post-partum use, 393
    side-effects, 142
    spermicides applied to, 140
    teenagers, for, 385
    use, 140
Diarrhoea, prostaglandins causing, 278, 281
p-Diisobutylphenoxypolyethoxyethanol,
    146
Dilatation and curettage, 271
    mid-trimester pregnancy, in, 299
Dutch cap, *see* Diaphragm
Dysmenorrhoea,
    intra-uterine devices and, 221
    following sterilisation, 335

Ebstein's anomaly, 326
Eclampsia, sterilisation and, 331
Economic pro-natalism, 463
Ectopic gestation,
    continuous low-dose progestagens and,
        101
    incidence, 227
    intra-uterine devices and, 176, 221, 226
    legal abortion, after, 253, 270
    postcoital pill, 116
    progestasert and, 172
    progestagens and, 392
    rhythm method and, 157
Eisenmenger's syndrome, 326, 400
Endocrine disorders, sterilisation and, 330
Endocrine system,
    oestrogen action on, 23
    progestagen action on, 38
Endometriosis, hysterotomy, following, 301
Endometritis,
    chronic, 169, 170
    virus origin of, 172

Endometrium,
  carcinoma of, 82
    sequential pill and, 91
  combined pill and, 52, 55
  copper, and, 171
  intra-uterine devices and, 168
  long-acting oral contraceptives and, 93
  oestrogen action on, 13
  progestagen action on, 33
  progesterone action on, 28
Epilepsy, 64
  contraception and, 404
  sterilisation and, 330
Ethacridine lactate inducing abortion, 294
Ethical pro-natalism, 463
Ethinyloestradiol, 3, 10, 116
  actions of,
    blood coagulation, 14–18
    plasma coagulation factors, 15, 69
    plasma proteins, 21
    thyroid gland, 24
  combined pill, 4, 49, 50
  thrombo-embolism and, 73
Ethynodiol, 4
  action on protein metabolism, 37
  low dose pills, 102
  potency, 32
  structure, 29
Evaluation of contraceptive practices,
  definitions, 178
  intra-uterine devices, 173–179
  Pearl's index, 177

Fallopian tube,
  continuous low-dose progestagens,
    and, 97
  intra-uterine devices and, 165
  progestagen action on, 34
Fallot's tetralogy, 326
Fat embolism, 295
'Female pills', 298
Fertility,
  combined pill, after, 57
  decline in, 151–152
  following removal of intra-uterine
    device, 210
  post abortion, 246, 252, 253, 263, 270
  proof of, 374
Fertility reservoir, 459
Fetal abnormality risk, abortion and, 242
Fetus, viable,
  abortion and, 250
  definition of, 249, 250
Fibrinogen,
  combined pill affecting, 16, 69
  hypertonic saline and, 287
  oestrogen and, 16, 17
Fibrinolysis,
  intra-uterine devices and, 219
  oestrogen action on, 15, 17
  triglycerides affecting, 20

Fibroids, 405
  intra-uterine devices and, 186
Fimbriectomy, 353
Foam aerosols, 145, 147
Foam tablets, 145
Follicle stimulating hormone, 10, 430
  combined pill and, 52
  oestradiol secretion and, 10
  oestrogen action and, 53
  oestrogen production and, 10
  progestagen action on, 32
  progesterone affecting, 27
  releasing factor, 12
  sequential pill and, 91
Free fatty acids, oestrogen action on, 19
Fructose, abortion induced with, 294

Galactorrhoea, oral contraceptives and, 67
Gall bladder disease, oral contraceptives
  and, 79, 403
Gallstones, 79
Gastro-intestinal disorders, sterilisation and,
  330
Genetic problems, sterilisation and, 331
Glucose, abortion induced by, 293
Glucose tolerance,
  combined pill and, 76
  oestrogens affecting 18
  progestagens affecting, 36
Gonadotrophins,
  in post-pill amenorrhoea, 68
  production of, 11
Gonorrhoea, 222, 223
  C-films and, 148
Grafenberg hooks, use of, 210
Grafenberg ring, 163, 188
  complications, 175
  composition, 170
  pregnancy and, 213, 215
  pregnancy rates, 164
  use, 179
Gravigard, 183
  insertion, 204
  pregnancy rates, 164
Grecian tips, 134
Gynaecological disorders, contraception
  and, 404

Haematological disease,
  contraception and, 402
  sterilisation and, 328
Haemorrhage,
  hypertonic saline abortion causing, 292
  hysterotomy, following, 301
  insertion of intra-uterine device, after,
    206, 218
  laparoscopic sterilisation, 351
  vacuum curettage, with, 267
Hall rings, 179

Headache, combined pill causing, 61
Heart disease,
    intra-uterine devices and, 187
    pregnancy and, 239, 241, 401
    sterilisation and, 325, 400
Hepatitis, infective, 79, 403
Herpesvirus hominis,
    cervical carcinoma and, 136
    cervical infection with, 185
    copper containing devices and, 222
Hexoestrol, action on coagulation factors,
    16
Hodgkin's disease, combined pill and, 82
Homosexuality and abstinence, 158
Hormonal contraception, effectiveness and
    risks of, 127–130
Hormones, injectable, 5, 105–111
Human chorionic gonadotrophin, 434
Hydatidiform mole, 405
Hydronephrosis, 400
17α-Hydroxypregnenolone, structure, 8
17α-Hydroxyprogesterone, structure, 8
Hydroxyprogesterone derivatives,
    combined pill, in, 52
    metabolism, 30
    structure, 28, 29
Hypernatraemia following hypertonic saline
    for abortion, 291
Hypertension,
    combined pill causing, 62
    contraception in, 80, 402
    sterilisation and, 329
Hypertonic saline in abortion, 284–293
    complications, 290
        cervical damage, 293
        haemorrhage, 292
        hypernatraemia, 291
        infection, 292
        injection difficulties, 290
        water and electrolytes, 291
    contra-indications, 288
    extra-amniotic, 295
    management of, 290
    mode of action, 285
    procedures, 288
    systemic effects of, 287
    vaginal approach, 289
Hypothalamic function, controlled
    interference with, 430
Hypothalamus,
    combined pill and, 52, 129
    oestrogen acting on, 11
    progestagen action on, 32
    progesterone action on, 26
Hysterectomy,
    mortality rate, 356
    psychological sequelae, 353, 357
    sterilisation by, 346, 353, 356
    termination, 356
    uterine perforation, for, 269
Hysteroscopy for sterilisation, 352

Hysterotomy, 299, 300
    abdominal, 300
    complications, 301
    scars, sequelae of, 258
    uterine perforation, for, 268
    uterine rupture following, 301
    vaginal, 302

Immunological control of fertility, 433
    male aspects of, 436
Implanted hormones, 5, 113
Indomethacin, 168
Infanticide, 455
Infection,
    hypertonic saline abortion, after, 292
    hysterotomy, following, 301
    intra-uterine devices and, 163, 182,
        221–223
    vacuum curettage, after, 267, 270
Infective hepatitis, 79, 403
Infertile period, pre- and post ovulatory,
    154
Insulin levels,
    progestagens affecting, 36
Insulin, oestrogen and, effect on,
    triglyceride synthesis, 20
Insulin resistance, oestrogen and, 19
Intra-uterine devices, 163–233, *see also*
    under specific names
    abortion, inserted after, 394
    acid phosphatase activity and, 169
    additional precautions with, 207
    cancer and, 228
    clinical trials, 420
    clinic attendance, motivation and, 378
    complications, 175, 179, 213–233
        age and parity factors, 184
        bleeding, 218
        discomfort to husband, 228
        ectopic gestation, 226
        pelvic inflammatory disease, 222,
            225
        pelvic pain, 220
        pregnancy, 213
        vaginal discharge, 221
    containing copper, 170, 183
        pregnancy rates, 214
        replacement of, 208
    containing progesterone, 172
    contra-indications, 185
    endometrium affected by, 168
    ethical and legal considerations, 189
    evaluation of, 173
        definitions, 178
        sources of data, 176
    expulsion, 175, 201, 216
        abortion and, 184
        disappearance of transcervical
            appendage, 216
        management, 217

Intra-uterine devices
    expulsion (*cont.*)
        pregnancy and, 214
        unnoticed, 191
    failures, 174, 401, *see also* Intra-
            uterine devices, Pregnancy rates
    heart disease and, 401
    history of, 163
    infection with, 163, 182, 221–223
        insertion and, 201, 202, 222
        postpartum insertion and, 201
        severe and unusual, 223
    inflammatory changes with, 166, 170
    insertion, 201
        advice after, 207
        after legal abortion, 202
        difficulties, 205
        examination of uterus, 204
        facilities, 202
        follow-up visits, 208, 209
        haemorrhage following, 206, 218
        infection, 201, 202, 222
        inserters, 204
        pain following, 206, 220
        perforation following, 207
        postpartum, 201, 393
        preparation of devices, 202
        procedure, 203
        timing, 201
    intermenstrual bleeding and, 220
    intra-uterine environment and, 166
    leucocyte proliferation and, 169
    menopause and, 209
    menorrhagia and, 218
    metallic, 170
    mode of action, 165
        cervical mucus, 166
        mechanical, 167
        myometrial activity, 167
        tubal factors, 165
    mortality associated with, 228
    motivation and, 174, 175, 186, 188,
            205, 377–379
    older women for, 389
    perforation by, 163, 191, 214, 224,
            229
        diagnosis, 225
        incidence, 224
        management, 226
        postpartum insertion and, 201
        predisposing factors, 225
    perforation rate, 182
    postcoital use, 211
    post-partum use, 393, 201
    pregnancy and, 213
        management, 215
    pregnancy rates, 164, 173, 213, 214
        surface area and, 166
    procedures for, 201–213
    progesterone containing, 172
    prostaglandins and, 165, 168, 171

Intra-uterine devices (*cont.*)
    psychiatric problems and, 188
    removal, 209
        complications, for, 175
        during pregnancy, 191, 215
        fertility following, 210
        procedure, 210
        uterine damage during, 183
    replacement, 209
    selection of patients, 184
        age and parity, 184
        environmental factors, 185
        ethical and legal considerations, 189
        medical complications, 187
        social and personal factors, 188
    silicone rubber device, 172
    teenagers, for, 385
    tubal transport of ova and, 165
    types, 179
    use, 135
    use-effectiveness, 177
    uterine damage on removal, 183
    vaginal cytology and, 167, 209
Irving procedure, 345
Isoimmunisation with placental tissue, 433

Jaundice,
    combined pill and, 78
    oestrogens causing, 22
Jellies, spermicidal, 145

Karman catheter for abortion, 264

Labour, premature, after abortion, 256
Lactation, combined pill affecting, 61, 390
Lactate dehydrogenase, 171
Leg aches and cramps, combined pill and, 63
Leucocyte proliferation, intra-uterine
        devices and, 169
Leukaemia, sterilisation and, 328
Levonorgestrel, 97; *see also* Norgestrel
    action, 34
    fallopian tube, effect on, 34
    postcoital pill, in, 117
Libido, loss of,
    combined pill and, 56, 65
    continuous low dose progestagens
            causing, 104
    sterilisation and, 322, 324, 336, 358
Life-expectancy and birth rate, 449
Lippes loops, 164, 180
    causing discomfort to husband, 228
    expulsion of, 217
    expulsion rates, 168, 201
    intra-uterine environment and, 166
    intra-uterine pressure and, 167
    mechanical mode of action, 167
    perforation by, 224

Lippes loops (*cont.*)
  pregnancy and, 215
  pregnancy rates, 164, 173, 213
    size and, 168
  removal during pregnancy, 216
  replacement, 209
  spontaneous abortion and, 215
  structure, 180
Liver, benign tumours of, combined pill
    and, 79
Liver damage, risk from combined pill, 78
Liver disorders, contraception and, 403
Liver function,
  oestrogen action on, 21
  progestagens affecting, 36
  sequential pill and, 92
Lipid metabolism,
  oestrogen action on, 19
  progestagens affecting, 36
Lipoproteins,
  androgen action on, 20
  oestrogen action on, 20
Lipoprotein lipase, 20
Long-acting oral contraception, 92
  mode of action, 92
  side-effects, 94
  use-effectiveness, 93
Lung disease, sterilisation and, 329
Luteinising hormone,
  combined pill affecting, 52
  low dose progestagens and, 96
  plasma levels, oestrogen and, 11
  progestagen action and, 32
  progesterone affecting, 27
  surge of production, 10, 53
Luteinising hormone releasing factor, 430
Luteolytic drugs, 431
Lynoestrenol,
  low dose pills, 102
  metabolism, 30
  potency, 32

M-213 intra-uterine device, 170
  spermicides used with, 207
M device, 181
  perforation by, 224
  removal of, 183, 210
Madlener operation, 343
  results, 345
Majzlin spring, 181
  inflammatory changes from, 170
  removal, 183, 210
Malabsorption syndromes, 98, 100, 402
Male contraception,
  clinical trials, 423
  future developments, 435
Malignant disease, sterilisation and, 331
Malignant hypertension, 62
Malignant melanoma, combined pill and, 82

Malthus, Thomas R., 447
Mannitol in abortion, 294
Margulies spiral, 164, 181
Mastalgia from combined pill, 54
Matrisalus diaphragm, 139
Medical disorders, contraception and,
    75–82, 187, 399–407
Medroxyprogesterone,
  action on,
    cervical mucus, 35
    carbohydrate metabolism, 36
    endocrine system, 38
    plasma proteins, 21
    protein metabolism, 37
  continuous use, 95
  depot contraception, in, 105, 107
  duration of action, 106
  injected in puerperium, 393
  structure, 29
  vaginal rings containing, 112
Megestrol, 100, 103
  action of on cervical mucus, 35
  subcutaneous implant of, 113
Melanoma, malignant, 82
Menopause,
  combined pill and, 59
  intra-uterine devices and, 209
Menorrhagia,
  intra-uterine devices and, 218
  sterilisation, following, 333, 335
Menstrual cycle,
  irregular,
    combined pill and, 61
    combined oestrogen-progestagen
        injections and, 110
    continuous low-dose progestagens
        and, 103
    intramuscular progestagen depots
        causing, 108
    vaginal rings, with, 112
  intra-uterine devices and, 175
  sterilisation, following, 333
Menstrual regulation, 155, 265, 281, 422
  prostaglandins in, 281
Menstruation,
  following combined pill, 57
  induction with prostaglandins, 432
  intra-uterine devices and, 218
  long-acting oral contraceptives and, 93
  sterilisation, after, 322
Mestranol, 3, 10
  action on,
    ascorbic acid levels, 22
    protein metabolism, 21
  combined pill, in, 4, 49, 50
  cortisol, and, 23
  metabolism, 11
  thrombo-embolism and, 73
p-Methanylphenylpolyoxyethylene ether,
    146
Methoxypolyoxyethylene glycol, 146

Methyl-prostaglandin $F_{2\alpha}$, 274, 279
     abortion, for, 274, 279, 281, 283, 284
Migraine, 62, 404
Mittelschmerz, 154
Mood changes, progesterone and, 27
Motivation for contraception, 373–381,
     437
     attributes of fertility regulating methods
          and, 376
     barrier methods and, 133, 400
     clinic attendance, 378
     decision making, 375
     domestic roles and, 378
     intra-uterine devices and, 205, 377, 378
     marital communication and, 376
     sexual relationship and, 379
     rewards for childbearing versus contra-
          ception and, 374
     unwanted pregnancies and, 373
Multiple sclerosis, 330
Myometrial activity, intra-uterine devices
     and, 167

National Health Service (Family Planning)
     Amendment Act, 1972, 319
Nausea and vomiting,
     combined pill causing, 55, 65
     continuous low dose progestagens and,
          104
     depot progestagens causing, 108
     long-acting oral contraceptives causing, 94
     prostaglandins causing, 278, 281
Neonatal jaundice, combined pill and, 58
Neurological disease, 403
     sterilisation and, 330
Nonylphenoxypolyethoxyethanol, 146
Norethisterone, 3, 100
     action on
          blood coagulation, 35
          blood pressure, 35
          carbohydrate metabolism, 36
          endometrium, 32
          lipid metabolism, 36
          liver function, 37
          ovulation, 32
          plasma coagulation factors, 36, 69
          plasma proteins, 21
     continuous use, 95
     duration of action of injections, 106
     low dose pills, 4, 95, 102
     metabolism, 11, 30
     potency, 32
     structure, 29
     subcutaneous implant of, 113
Norethisterone oenanthate, 107, 108
Norethynodrel, 3
     structure, 28, 29
Norgestrel,
     action on
          blood pressure, 35

Norgestrel
     action on (*cont.*)
          cervical mucus, 35
          endometrium, 34
          ovary, 33
          ovulation, 32
     continuous use, 95
     low dose pills, in, 4, 95, 102
     metabolism, 30
     potency, 32
     structure, 29
     subcutaneous implant of, 113
19-Nortestosterone derivatives,
     action, 30, 32
     metabolism, 30
     structure, 28, 29

Obesity, combined pill and, 75, 77
Oestradiol,
     incorporation into tissue, 9
     structure, 7, 8
Oestradiol benzoate, post-coital, 116
Oestrane, structure, 7
Oestriol, structure, 7
Oestrogens, 7–24
     action on
          amino-acid levels, 21
          anterior pituitary, 11
          ascorbic acid levels, 22
          blood platelets, 15
          carbohydrate metabolism, 18, 76
          cardiovascular system, 13
          cervical mucus, 10, 13
          coagulation system, 14–18
          endocrine system, 23
          endometrium, 13
          fibrinolytic activity, 15, 17
          FSH levels, 12, 53
          free fatty acid levels, 19
          glucose tolerance, 18
          hypothalamus, 11
          lipid metabolism, 19
          liver function, 21
          ovary, 12
          pancreas, 24
          phospholipids, lipoproteins and
               cholesterol, 20
          plasma proteins, 21
          skin arterioles, 13
          thyroid gland, 23
          triglycerides, 19
          urinary system, 23
          water and electrolytes, 22
     breast cancer and, 81
     carpal tunnel syndrome and, 62
     causing insulin resistance, 19
     cholestatic jaundice, 22
     clinical pharmacology, 7–24
     content of combined pill, 3, 49
     contra-indications, 73

Oestrogens (*cont.*)
  coronary thrombosis and, 74
  depot preparation, in, 106
  diabetes mellitus and, 18, 403
  endometrial cancer and, 82
  epilepsy and, 404
  headache, 61
  levels in pregnancy, 10, 13
  liver disorders and, 403
  metabolism, 9
  ovarian biogenesis, 8
  pharmacological actions, 11
  physiological role, 9
  postcoital pill, in, 115
  sequential pill, in, 91
  structure, 7
  synthetic, 10
  systemic effects, 13
  thrombo-embolism and, 18, 23, 73
Oestrogen-progestagen combinations,
    postcoital pill, in, 117
Oestrogen-progestagen injections, 110–112
Oestrone,
  metabolism, 9
  structure, 7, 8
Oil of Juniper, 298
Oral contraceptives, *see also under specific
    names and compounds*
  clinical trials, 420
  combined pill, *see* Combined pill
  long-acting, 4, 92
  sequential pill, *see* Sequential pill
  types, 3
  use, 135
Ota rings, 179, 209
Ova,
  fertilisation of, age factors, 157
  tubal transport of, intra-uterine devices
    and, 165
Ovarian function, breast cancer and, 81
Ovary,
  long-acting oral contraceptives affecting,
    92
  oestrogen action on, 12
  progestagens action on, 33
  prostaglandins and, 431
Ovulation,
  continuous low dose progestagens and,
    95
  inhibition of, 33
    combined pill, by, 52
    progestagens, by, 32
    intramuscular depots and, 106
    sequential pill, by, 91
Oxytocin, abortion induced by, 296

Pain following insertion of intra-uterine
    device, 206, 220
Pancreas, oestrogen action on, 24
Pancreatitis, acute, 24

Pastes, spermicidal, 146
Patent ductus arteriosus, 326
Pathfinder Fund, 176
Pearl's index, 177
Pelvic congestion syndrome, 152
Pelvic inflammatory disease,
  abortion, following, 253, 263, 270
  contraception and, 405
  intra-uterine devices and, 186, 222
  sterilisation, following, 336
  vacuum curettage, following, 270
Perinatal mortality, abortion and, 258
Peritonitis,
  associated with intra-uterine devices,
    226, 229
  foreign body granuloma with, 137
Pessaries,
  spermicidal, 145, 146
  stem and wishbone, 163
Petal devices, 183
  postpartum insertion, 201
Phospholipids, oestrogen action on, 20
Pituitary gland,
  continuous low dose progestagens,
    effects of, 96
  oestrogen action on, 11
  progestagen action on, 32
  tumours, 68
Placenta, use for research, 251
Placental tissue, isoimmunisation with, 433
Placenta praevia, 157, 259
Plasma proteins,
  oestrogen action on, 21
Plasminogen, quinestrol and, 94
Pomeroy operation, 343, 349, 355
  failure rates, 345, 355
Population,
  balance of births and deaths, 448
  censuses, 447
  control of, 453
    arithmetic of, 456
    automatic, 455
    birth prevention measures, 453
    causing deaths, by, 454
    manifest versus latent, 455
    two-way, 465
  economics, 450
  fertility reservoir, 459
  flywheel, 457
  Great Britain, 445
    future growth, 458
  growth and aged dependency, 451
  ill effect of large families, 464
  life-expectancy and birth rate, 449
  limits to growth, 452
  optimisation, 464
  predictions, 458, 459
  world, 444
    limits to growth, 452
Population explosions, 443
Population flywheel, 457

Population problem, 443
  facts of, 444
Porphyria, 64
Postcoital contraception, 114–118
  clinical trials, 421
  ethical and legal considerations, 117
  intra-uterine devices for, 211
  oestrogen-progestagen combinations
    in, 117
  teenagers, for, 386
Postcoital pill, 5, 114–118
  oestrogens in, 115
  progestagens in, 116
Post ovulatory infertile period, 154
Post-partum oral contraception, 390
Pre-eclampsia,
  combined pill and, 63
  sterilisation and, 331
Pregnancy,
  carbohydrate metabolism, effects on, 18
  following combined pill, 57
  heart disease and, 239, 241, 326
  immunisation against, 435
  intra-uterine devices and, 213
    management, 215
  oestrogen levels in, 10, 13
  outcome following failure of combined
    pill, 56
  progesterone role in, 27
  pruritis, 78, 79
  recurrent jaundice of, 78
  renal disease and, 239, 329
  risks of, 128, 399
  sterilisation in relation to, 354
  teenagers, 383
  unwanted,
    motive for contraception, 373
    wilful exposure to, 374
Pregnancy, uterine perforation in, 224
Pregnancy rates, difficulty of establishing,
  173
Pregnenolone, structure of, 8
Pre-menstrual tension, 104
  progesterone levels and, 27
Pre-ovulatory infertile period, 154
Progestagens,
  action on, 28–38
    amino acid metabolism, 37
    anterior pituitary gland, 32
    blood pressure, 35
    body weight, 38
    carbohydrate metabolism, 36, 76
    cardiovascular system, 35
    cervical mucus, 35
    coagulation factors, 35
    endocrine system, 38
    endometrium, 33
    hypothalamus, 32
    lipid metabolism, 36
    liver function, 36
    ovary, 33

Progestagens,
  action on (*cont.*)
    ovulation, 32
    protein metabolism, 37
  clinical pharmacology, 32–38
  combined pill, in, 3, 49
  combined with intra-uterine devices,
    207
  combined with oestrogen, injections of,
    110–111
  continuous low-dose, 94–105
    clinical use, 98
    ectopic gestation and, 101
    failure rates, 99, 101
    mode of action, 95
    post-partum, 391
    side-effects, 103
    therapeutic ratio, 95
  continuous oral contraception with,
    94–105
  depot preparations, in, 106
  depression caused by, 80
  groups, 4
  haematological disorders and, 402
  hypertension and, 402
  indices of potency, 30, 31
  intramuscular depots, 106
    metabolic complications, 109
    mode of action, 106
    side-effects, 108
    use effectiveness, 107
  low-dose, 4, 94–105
    side-effects, 129
    post-partum, 391
  metabolism, 30
  postcoital pill, in, 116
  sequential pills, in, 91
  structure of, 28
  subdermal implants of, 435
  systemic actions, 35
  thrombo-embolism and, 36
  vaginal rings, in, 111
Progestasert, 172
Progesterone, 3
  actions, 24–28
    catabolic, 26
    cervical mucus, on, 27
    systemic, 26
    thermogenic, 26
    water and electrolytes, on, 27
  hypnotic effect, 26
  intra-uterine devices containing, 172
  metabolism, 25
  physiological role, 26
  production, by corpus luteum, 154
  rôle in pregnancy, 27
  structure, 8, 24
Prolactin, action, 11
Pro-natalism, 463
Prostaglandins,
  abortion in, 272–284

Prostaglandins,
  abortion in (*cont.*)
    contra-indications, 275
    extra-amniotic, 280
    first trimester, 272, 280, 281
    intramuscular administration, 274
    intra-uterine, 274
    intravaginal, 281
    intravenous administration, 272
    middle trimester, 272, 280, 283
    with oxytocin, 273
  future developments, 431
  intra-uterine devices and, 165, 168, 171
  menstrual induction with, 432
  side effects, 276, 280, 281
  uteroplacental ischaemia, causing, 275
Prostaglandin E_2
  abortion, in, 272, 273, 277–278
    283
  menstrual inductions with, 432
Prostaglandin $F_{2\alpha}$,
  abortion, in. 272, 273, 277–278
  future developments, 431
  menstrual induction with, 432
  methyl derivatives, 274, 279, 281,
    283, 284
  side-effects, 278, 281
Prostatic hypertrophy, benign, 153
Protein metabolism, progestagens affecting,
  37
Protein synthesis, oestrogens and, 23
Pruritis of pregnancy, 78, 79
Puerperal psychosis, 327
Pulmonary embolism,
  age and, 73
  combined pill and, 60, 69

Quinestrol, 92, 94
  long-acting contraceptives, in, 93
Quingestanol acetate,
  low dose pills, 102
  ovulation, effect on, 32
  postcoital pill, 116
Quinine, 146, 298

Radiotherapy, fetal injury from, 242
Raynaud's disease, 64
Renal dialysis, 400
Renal disease,
  pregnancy and, 239
  sterilisation in, 326, 329
Renal failure, contraception and, 403
Renin-angiotensin system, combined pill
  and, 62, 63
Respiratory disease, contraception and, 402
Rhesus isoimmunisation,
  abortion and, 263
  sterilisation and, 331

Rheumatic heart disease,
  contraception in, 401
  indicating sterilisation, 326
Rheumatoid arthritis, 64
Rhythm method, 153–158
  advantages, 156
  disadvantages, 157
  use-effectiveness, 155
  use, 135
Rifampicin, oral contraceptive and, 66, 402
'Risk taking', 138

Safe period, 153–158
  advantages, 156
  disadvantages, 157
  use-effectiveness, 155
Saf-T-Coil, 181
  causing discomfort to husband, 228
  expulsion rates, 201
  perforation by, 224
  spontaneous abortion rates and, 215
Salpingectomy, 352
Salt retention, oestrogens causing, 22
Sequential pill, 4, 91–92
  contents of, 12
  diabetics, in, 18
Sex of offspring, control of, 156
Sickle cell anaemia, 326
Silver nitrate, sterilisation by, 346
Skeletal disorders, sterilisation and, 330
Skin arterioles, oestrogen action on, 13
Skin lesions, combined pill causing, 64
Smoking, combined pill and, 70, 71, 128,
  388
Soft soaps for inducing abortion, 295
Sperm, ageing of, 157
  transport,
    chlormadinone acetate affecting, 34
Spermicides, 133, 145–150
  action of, 145
  advantages and disadvantages, 148
  aerosols, 145, 147
  applied to diaphragms, 140
  applied to vault and cervical caps, 142,
    143
  bactericidal agents as, 146
  clinical trials, 421
  creams and pastes, 145, 146
  C-films, 147
  foam tablets, 145
  irritation from, 142
  jellies and pastes, 145
  used with intra-uterine devices, 207
  use-effectiveness, 146, 148
Status epilepticus, 240
Stem pessaries, 163
Sterilisation, 317–369
  by vaginal route, 346
  chemical, 346
  clinical trials, 423

Sterilisation (*cont.*)
  cornual resection, 352
  counselling, 317–341
    detection of equivocation, 323
    failure rate, 322
    in practice, 320
    irreversibility, 321
    loss of children, 322
    marital breakdown, 322
    mentally incompetent, 325
    minors, 324
    nature of operation, 321
    preservation of menstrual and sexual
      function, 321
    reason for request, 321
    sequelae, 322
    single women, 324
    special cases, 323
    vasectomy as alternative, 323
    young women, 323
  failure rate, 322
  fimbriectomy, 353
  hysterectomy, 346, 353, 356
  hysteroscopy, 352
  incidence, 317
  indications, 325–333, 400
    cardiovascular disorders, 329
    congenital heart disease, 325, 400
    endocrine disorders, 330
    gastro-intestinal disorders, 330
    genetic problems, 331
    haematological disorders, 328
    malignant disease, 331
    neurological disease, 330
    obstetric, 331
    psychiatric illness, 327
    pulmonary disease, 329
    relative, 327
    renal disease, 326, 329
    rheumatic heart disease, 326
    skeletal disorders, 330
    systemic lupus erythematosus, 326,
      329
  laparoscopic, 347
    advantages and disadvantages, 350
    application of silicone rubber bands,
      348, 349
    clips, 348, 349
    failure rates, 349
    problems of, 351
    puerperium, in, 356
    tubal coagulation and division, 348
  legal abortion, following, 247, 355
  legal aspects, 318
  male, 318, *see also* Vasectomy
  medical indications for, 317, 325–333
  methods, 343–369
  older women, in, 398
  relation to pregnancy, in, 354
  relative irreversibility, 321

Sterilisation (*cont.*)
  reversal of, 357, 358
    requests for, 336
  reversible, 357
  salpingectomy, 352
  sequelae, 333
    gynaecological, 333
    pelvic inflammatory disease, 336
    physical, 322, 333–336
    psychological, 321, 322, 333
  tubal, 343–352
    failure rate, 345
    mortality rates, 337
    requests for reversal, 336
    reversal of, 358
    techniques, 344
    with or without partial salpingec-
      tomy, 343
Steroid diabetes, 75
Steroid hormone activity, interference with,
  431
Stilboestrol, 10
  plasma factor IX affected by, 16
  postcoital pill, in, 116, 117
Streptococcal infection, 223
Subcutaneous implants, 113
Suicide, threatened, 240
Suppositories, spermicidal, 145
Surgery, combined pill and, 58
Systemic lupus erythematosus, sterilisation
  and, 326, 329

Teenagers,
  contraception for, 383
    counselling, 386
    legal position, 384
    postcoital, 386
  diaphragms for, 385
  intra-uterine devices for, 190, 385
  legal abortion for, 247
  oral contraception for, 384
  pregnancy among, 383
  use of condoms, 385
Temperature, rhythm methods and, 154
Testosterone, 11
  structure, 8, 29
Thrombo-embolism, 3, 53, 99, 105, 401
  age factors, 59
  combined pill and, 69–75, 127, 128,
    390
    epidemiological studies, 70
  incidence, 70, 72, 75
  menopause and, 60
  oestrogens and, 14–18, 23, 73
  progestagens and, 36
  sequential pill and, 92
  sterilisation and, 328
  surgery, following, 58
Thrombosis, *see also* Thrombo-embolism
  intravascular, 22

Thyroid gland, oestrogens and, 23
Triglycerides,
    atherosclerosis and, 20
    insulin and, 20
    oestrogen action on, 19
Triiodothyronine, oestrogens and, 23
Tri-isopropylphenoxypolyethoxyethanol,
    146
Tubal pregnancies, *see* Ectopic gestation
Tuberculosis, 329, 402

Uchida procedure, 345
Ulcerative colitis, 402
Urea injections for abortion, 293
Ureters, dilatation of, 23
Urinary system, oestrogen action on, 23
Urinary tract infections,
    combined pill and, 63
    oestrogens and, 23
Uterine environment, intra-uterine devices
    and, 166
Uterine pressure, intra-uterine devices and,
    167
Uteroplacental ischaemia, prostaglandins
    causing, 275
Uterotubal implantation, 359
Uterotubal junction, coagulation of, 352
Uterus,
    examination of, before intra-uterine
        device insertion, 204
    perforation of, 163, 191, 207, 214, 224
        following hysterotomy, 301
        post-partum, 393
        vacuum curettage, during, 267, 268

Vacuum aspiration in abortion, 264
Vacuum curettage, 266–271
    cervical incompetence following, 271
    cervical laceration during, 269
    complications, 267
    haemorrhage, 267
    mortality rates, 271
    retained products of conception causing
        haemorrhage, 269
    technique, 266
    uterine perforation during, 268
    vaginal haematoma caused by, 269

Vagina,
    carcinoma, stilboestrol causing, 116
    cytology, intra-uterine devices and, 167,
        209
    haematoma, vacuum curettage, during,
        267, 269
Vaginal discharge, intra-uterine devices and,
    221
Vaginal epithelium, progesterone affecting,
    27
Vaginal rings, 111
Varicose veins, 73, 105
Vas deferens, reversible occlusion of, 437
Vasectomy, 319, 337–338, 359–363
    advantages and disadvantages, 360
    complications, 362
    failures, 361
    indications for, 337
    legal aspects, 339
    operative procedure, 359
    psychological sequelae, 338
    reversal of, 362, 437
    type of patient, 338
Vault caps, 142–143
Vault haematoma, vacuum curettage, after,
    267, 269
Venereal disease,
    condoms protecting against, 134, 136,
        386
    intra-uterine devices and, 191
Venous thrombosis, combined pill and, *see*
        Thrombo-embolism
    oestrogens and, 14–18
Vimules, 142
Virus infections, combined pill and, 64

Water and electrolytes,
    hypertonic saline affecting, 291
    oestrogen action on, 22
    progesterone affecting, 27
Weight gain, combined pill and, 54, 55
    depot progestagens, and, 108
'Whore syndrome', 385
Wilson's disease, 188
Wishbone pessaries, 163
Withdrawal, *see* Coitus interruptus

Yusei rings, endometrial reaction, 209